CONCEPTS AND ISSUES
IN NURSING PRACTICE

SECOND EDITION

Dedicated to my mother, Joan Koernig who has always been there, and to my many RN-BSN students in their quest for excellence.

KB

Project Editor: Wendy Earl
Executive Editor: Patricia L. Cleary
Production Editor: Gail Carrigan
Interior Designer: Victoria Ann Philp
Cover Designer: Yvo Riezebos
Editoral Assistant: Bradley Burch
Compositor: Graphic Typesetting Services, Inc.

Library of Congress Cataloging-in-Publication Data

Kozier, Barbara.
   Concepts and issues in nursing practice / Barbara Kozier, Glenora Erb, Kathleen Blais. — 2nd ed.
      p.   cm.
   Includes bibliographical references and index,
   ISBN 0-8053-3520-X
   1. Nursing—Philosophy.   I. Erb. Glenora
Lea, 1937– .
II. Blais, Kathleen.   III. Title.
   [DNLM: 1. Nursing Process.   2. Nursing
   Theory.   WY 100 K88c]
RT84.5.K69   1992
610.73—dc20
DNLM/DLC
for Library of Congress   91-44371
                                                 CPI

ISBN 0-8053-3520-X
   4 5 6 7 8 9 10-DO-95 94

Addison-Wesley Nursing
A Division of the Benjamin/Cummings
Publishing Company, Inc.
390 Bridge Parkway, Redwood City, CA 94065

CONCEPTS AND ISSUES IN NURSING PRACTICE

SECOND EDITION

BARBARA KOZIER
RN, MN

GLENORA ERB
BSN, RN

KATHLEEN BLAIS
RN, EdD

Addison-Wesley Nursing
A Division of The Benjamin/Cummings Publishing Company, Inc.
Redwood City, California · Menlo Park, California
Reading, Massachusetts · New York · Don Mills, Ontario
Wokingham, U.K. · Amsterdam · Bonn · Sydney · Tokyo · Madrid · San Juan

BRIEF CONTENTS

DETAILED CONTENTS

PREFACE

". . . nursing has a great destiny but one that cannot be fulfilled until nurses–you and I and all of us–change what we are. For us to change what we are, we must change the way we think, the way we feel, and the way we act."

Margretta M. Styles*

Concepts and Issues in Nursing Practice was written for nursing students, with particular reference to nurses in transition or in bridge courses of BSN programs. This edition, adapted from the fourth edition of *Fundamentals of Nursing,* may be useful in basic nursing programs that present concepts and psychomotor skills as separate courses. If a skill text is needed, *Techniques in Clinical Nursing,* may provide an effective complement to this book.

NEW FEATURES

Five New Chapters

- Historical and Societal Influences on Nursing
- Advocacy and Change
- Contemporary Health Care Delivery System
- Managing and Directing
- Healthy Aging

* Styles, M. M. 1982. *On nursing toward a new endowment.* St. Louis: C.V. Mosby Co.

Increased Application of the Nursing Process

- Assessment interview boxes in question format, to help students obtain nursing history data and conduct interviews.
- Expanded lists of nursing diagnoses with contributing factors and tables showing assessment data clusters and related nursing diagnoses. Rather than providing detailed information about each diagnosis, which is readily available from other sources, the focus is on applying nursing diagnoses.
- Expanded lists of outcome criteria in the planning sections.

Increased Emphasis on Wellness

- See Chapter 13; Health, Wellness, Illness, and Disease, and Chapter 15; Health Promotion. Wellness diagnoses are included in Chapter 15.

Increased Application of Nursing Research

- In each chapter, a box summarizes a related research study and explains its clinical application. Each chapter concludes with a list of related research.

Learning Activities

- Each chapter provides two or more learning activities to expand the learner's understanding of the content and to encourage critical thinking about nursing issues.

Appendices

- Significant Events in Nursing History
- American Nurses Association publication on Nursing's Agenda for Health Care Reform

Organization

This edition is organized in seven units. Units and chapters are organized so that they can be used independently or in a sequence. The steps of the nursing process are a major organizational element in many chapters.

Unit 1, Professionalism in Nursing focuses on concepts of professionalism, definitions and descriptions of nursing, historical and societal influences on nursing, and professional socialization.

Unit 2, Theoretical Foundations for Professional Nursing Practice presents theories and conceptual frameworks for nursing, including theories about caring and other theories that affect nursing practice. A chapter on the research process emphasizes the investigative roles of all nurses and describes how to find researchable problems in clinical practice and how to become an intelligent research consumer.

Unit 3, The Nursing Process highlights essential information about each of the five nursing process components: assessing, diagnosing, planning, implementing, and evaluating. This unit lays the groundwork for application of the nursing process in subsequent chapters.

Unit 4, Professional Accountability and Advocacy includes information about essential ethical and legal aspects of nursing practice and introduces topics such as the acquisition of personal and professional values, nursing codes of ethics, and ethical issues and dilemmas. Also included are descriptions of the many facets of the law affecting nursing. A new chapter combines the concepts of advocacy, the process of change, and power and professional influence.

Unit 5, Health Perceptions and Health Promotion focuses on concepts of health, health beliefs, wellness, well-being, illness, and disease. Chapters in the unit discuss current health trends, health care systems, and health care problems, and address future challenges and implications for nursing. Chapters on health promotion, family health, and community health emphasize the role of the nurse in promoting and maintaining the health of individuals, families, and communities.

Unit 6, Interactive Processes focuses on the skills needed to establish and maintain a helping relationship and to implement a teaching plan. It includes a section on types of health care groups and features of effective groups. A new chapter on managing and directing client care includes sections on management practices, nursing management systems, use of computers in nursing, mentors and preceptors, networking, and work related social support groups.

Unit 7, Contemporary Concepts of Well-Being discusses both psychosocial and biophysical concepts that help the learner gain an understanding of human differences and responses. Specific chapters address self-concept and role relationships; stress tolerance and coping; ethnic and cultural values; sexuality; spirituality and religion; and loss, grieving, and death. Because of the increasing elderly population, we include a new chapter entitled *Healthy Aging*.

As the health care revolution continues, nursing will redefine itself in response to the world it serves. So, too, will books needs to change. Thus we welcome comments and suggestions from students and faculty using this text; they are essential to increasing the book's effectiveness.

ACKNOWLEDGMENTS

We would like to extend our warmest appreciation and sincere thanks to the many people who participated in the development of this book.

- Patti Cleary, sponsoring editor, whose commitment to professionalism and sensitivity to the needs of this book was greatly appreciated.

- Wendy Earl, whose expertise as project editor was invaluable to the authors. Her management of the editorial process greatly facilitated completion of this book.

- Gail Carrigan, the production editor whose meticulous attention to detail has been greatly appreciated.

- Bradley Burch, editorial assistant, for his gracious help whenever it was needed.

- The nurse educators who supported and confirmed the need for this book.

- The nurse experts who contributed chapters to this book: Holly Skodol Wilson, RN, PhD: Chapter 5; The Research Process. Janice Denehy, RN, PhD: Chapter 16; Family Health.

- Our typist, Mary Tobin, who was so accommodating in preparing manuscript.

- Our family and friends, whose patience and support sustained us through the writing schedule.

PROFESSIONALISM IN NURSING

A Growing Profession

CONTENTS

AN EMERGING DEFINITION OF NURSING

Nursing today is far different from nursing as it was practiced 50 years ago, and it takes a vivid imagination to envision how the nursing profession will change in the next 50 years in an ever-changing world. To comprehend present-day nursing and at the same time prepare for nursing in tomorrow's world, one must understand not only past events but also contemporary nursing practice and the sociologic factors affecting it.

Florence Nightingale defined nursing over 100 years ago as "the act of utilizing the environment of the patient to assist him in his recovery" (Nightingale 1860). Nightingale considered a clean, well-ventilated, and quiet environment essential for recovery. Often considered the first nurse theorist, Nightingale raised the status of nursing through education. Nurses were no longer untrained housekeepers but people trained in the care of the sick.

Virginia Henderson was one of the first modern nurses to define nursing. In 1960, she wrote, "The unique function of the nurse is to assist the individual, sick or well, in the performance of those activities contributing to health or its recovery (or to peaceful death) that he would perform unaided if he had the necessary strength, will, or knowledge, and to do this in such a way as to help him gain independence as rapidly as possible" (Henderson 1966, p. 3). Like Nightingale, Henderson described nursing in relation to the client and the client's environment. Unlike Nightingale, Henderson saw the nurse as concerned with both well and ill individuals, acknowledged that nurses interact with clients even when recovery may not be feasible, and mentioned the teaching and advocacy roles of the nurse.

In the latter half of the twentieth century, a number of nurse theorists developed their own views of nursing. Certain themes are common to many of these definitions: that nursing is caring, adaptive, individualized, holistic, family- and community-interrelated; that it involves teaching and direct/indirect services; and that it is a science as well as an art concerned with health promotion, health maintenance, health restoration, and the care of the dying. See Table 1–1 for definitions of nursing by selected nurse theorists.

Professional nursing associations have also examined nursing and developed their definitions of nursing. The American Nurses' Association (ANA) describes nursing practice as "direct, goal oriented, and adaptable to the

TABLE 1–1 *Definitions and Descriptions of Nursing**

Nursing Theorist and Theory	Definition/Description
Hildegard Peplau (1952): Psychodynamic nursing	A therapeutic, interpersonal process. It functions cooperatively with other human processes that make health possible for people in communities. An educative instrument, a maturing force that aims to promote forward movement of the personality in the direction of creative, constructive, productive, personal, and community living.
Faye Abdellah (1960): Twenty-one nursing problems	Service to individuals and families; therefore, to society. An art and science that molds the attitudes, intellectual competencies, and technical skills of the individual nurse into the desire and ability to help people, sick or well, cope with their health needs. May be carried out under general or specific medical direction.
Virginia Henderson (1960): Fourteen basic needs	The unique function of the nurse: to assist clients, sick or well, in the performance of those activities contributing to health, its recovery, or peaceful death that clients would perform unaided if they had the necessary strength, will, or knowledge. Also, to do so in such a way as to help clients gain independence as rapidly as possible.
Martha Rogers (1970): Unitary human beings, an energy field	A humanistic science dedicated to compassionate concern with maintaining and promoting health, preventing illness, and caring for and rehabilitating the sick and disabled. Nursing seeks to promote symphonic interaction between the environment and the person, to strengthen the coherence and integrity of the human beings, and to direct and redirect patterns of interaction between the person and the environment for the realization of maximum health potential.
Imogene King (1971, 1981): Goal attainment theory	A helping profession that assists individuals and groups in society to attain, maintain, and restore health. If this is not possible, nurses help individuals die with dignity. Nursing is perceiving, thinking, relating, judging, and acting vis-a-vis the behavior of individuals who come to a nursing situation. A nursing situation is the immediate environment, spatial and temporal reality, in which nurse and client establish a relationship to cope with health states and adjust to changes in activities of daily living if the situation demands adjustment. It is an interpersonal process of action, reaction, interaction, and transaction whereby nurse and client share information about their perceptions in the nursing situation.
Dorothea Orem (1971, 1980, 1985): Self-care theory	A helping or assisting service to persons who are wholly or partly dependent—infants, children, and adults—when they, their parents, guardians, or other adults responsible for their care are no longer able to give or supervise their care. A creative effort of one human being to help another human being. Nursing is deliberate action, a function of the practical intelligence of nurses, and action to bring about humanely desirable conditions in persons and their environments. It is distinguished from other human services and other forms of care by its focus on human beings.

▶

*The definitions are listed in chronological order.

needs of the individual, the family, and community during health and illness" (ANA 1973, p. 2). In 1980, the ANA published this definition of nursing: "Nursing is the diagnosis and treatment of human responses to actual or potential health problems" (ANA 1980, p. 9). In its 1987 House of Delegates, the ANA adopted a statement on the scope of nursing practice: "There is one scope of clinical nursing practice. The core, or essence, of that practice is the nursing diagnosis and treatment of human responses to health and to illness" (ANA 1987a, p. 76). The new statement further describes the differences between professional and technical nurses: The "depth and breadth to which the individual nurse engages in the total scope of the clinical practice of nursing are defined

TABLE 1–1 *continued*

Nursing Theorist and Theory	Definition/Description
Myra Levine (1973): Four conservation principles	A human interaction; a discipline rooted in the organic dependency of the individual on relationships with other human beings. A subculture reflecting ideas and values unique to nurses, even though the values mirror the social template that created them.
Sister Callista Roy (1976, 1984): Adaptation theory	A theoretical system of knowledge that prescribes a process of analysis and action related to the care of the ill or potentially ill person. As a science, nursing is a developing system of knowledge about persons used to observe, classify, and relate the processes by which persons positively affect their health status. As a practice discipline, nursing's scientific body of knowledge is used to provide an essential service to people, that is, to promote ability to affect health positively.
Jean Watson (1979, 1985): Science of caring	Nursing is concerned with promoting and restoring health and preventing illness. *Caring* is a nursing term representing all the factors the nurse uses to deliver health care to the client. In contrast, *curing* is a medical term that refers to the elimination of disease. See also Theories of Caring in Chapter 4.
Dorothy E. Johnson (1980): Behavioral system theory	An external regulatory force that acts to preserve the organization and integration of the client's behavior at an optimal level under those conditions in which the behavior constitutes a threat to physical or social health or in which illness is found.
Rosemarie Rizzo Parse (1981): Man-Living-Health	Nursing is a human science that focuses on Man as a living unity and Man's qualitative participation with health experiences. The responsibility to society relative to nursing practice is guiding the choosing of possibilities in the changing health process. Nursing practice is directed toward illuminating and mobilizing family interrelationships in light of the meaning assigned to health and its possibilities as languaged in the co-created patterns of relating.
Bette Neuman (1982): Systems theory	A unique profession in that it is concerned with all of the variables affecting an individual's response to stressors, which are intra-, inter-, and extrapersonal in nature. The concern of nursing is to prevent stress invasion, or, following stress invasion, to protect the client's basic structure and obtain or maintain a maximum level of wellness. The nurse helps the client, through primary, secondary, and tertiary prevention modes, to adjust to environmental stressors and maintain client system stability.
Madeleine Leininger (1984): Transcultural care theory	A learned humanistic art and science that focuses on personalized (individual and group) care behaviors, functions, and processes directed toward promoting and maintaining health behaviors or recovery from illness. Behaviors have physical, psychocultural, and social significance or meaning for those being assisted generally by a professional nurse or one with similar role competencies.

by the knowledge base of the nurse, the role of the nurse, and the nature of the client population within a practice environment" (ANA 1987a, p. 76). The Canadian Nurses' Association (CNA) published a definition in 1984 that serves as the professional standard for nurses in Canada.

"Nursing" or "the practice of nursing" means the identification and treatment of human responses to actual or potential health problems and includes the practice of and supervision of functions and services that, directly or indirectly, in collaboration with a client or providers of health care other than nurses, have as their objectives the promotion of health, prevention of illness, alleviation of suffering, restoration of health and optimum development of health potential and includes all aspects of the nursing process. (CNA Connection 1984, p. 8)

GROWTH OF PROFESSIONALISM

The profession of nursing has evolved over centuries. The traditional nursing role was one of humanistic caring, nurturing, comforting, and supporting. To these must be added specific characteristics of true professionalism, including education, a code of ethics, mastery of a craft, an informed membership involved in the organized profession, and accountability for actions (Flaherty 1979, p. 61).

There are a number of ways to differentiate a profession from an occupation. A *profession* is a calling that requires special knowledge, skill, and preparation. Medicine and law have consistently been recognized as learned professions. The terms *vocation* and *occupation* are often used synonymously. A vocation is the work that a person regularly performs or the work that especially suits him or her. An occupation is an activity in which one engages, e.g., a business. Thus, an occupation does not necessarily hold a special interest for the person and may be temporary, whereas a vocation often denotes employment in an area of interest on a regular basis. In this chapter, the more commonly used term *occupation* will be used to denote nonprofessions.

A profession is generally distinguished from other kinds of occupations by (a) its requirement of prolonged, specialized training to acquire a body of knowledge pertinent to the role to be performed and (b) an orientation of the individual toward service, either to a community or to an organization. The standards of edu-

cation and practice for the profession are determined by the members of the profession, rather than by outsiders. The education of the professional involves a complete socialization process, more far-reaching in its social and attitudinal aspects and its technical features than is usually required in other kinds of occupations. In 1915, Abraham Flexner stated that professions are organized primarily for the achievement of social ends and secondarily for the assertion of rights and the protection of special interests (Flexner 1915, p. 901).

Styles (1983) writes that nursing organizations must perform the following five functions for the preservation and development of the profession:

1. Professional definition and regulation through the setting and enforcing of standards of education and practice for the generalist and the specialist. Regulation is largely achieved in the United States and Canada through licensure of individual nurses, certification, and accreditation. See the section on credentialing of nurses in Chapter 10. Regulation is also achieved through the adoption of codes of ethics and norms of conduct (Styles 1983, p. 570).

2. Development of the knowledge base for practice in its broadest and narrowest components. Major contributions to the development of nursing knowledge have been made by various theorists. The primary purpose of nursing theories is to generate nursing knowledge. The challenge for nurses in the future is to generate questions and formulate hypotheses from these published theories and then test the hypotheses through nursing research. Since only research can determine the usefulness of a theory, research makes a major contribution to the development of nursing knowledge. Another significant contribution to nursing knowledge is the work of the North American Diagnosis Association (NANDA) (see Chapter 7). This group is generating and expanding a taxonomy of nursing diagnoses. Research is required to determine the validity and reliability of these diagnoses.

3. Transmission of values, norms, knowledge, and skill to neophytes and members of the profession for application in practice. This function is largely performed through the education of nurses and the socialization processes. Socialization is the development in the individual of those qualities (skills, beliefs, habits, requirements) necessary to belong to and function in a group. See Chapter 3.

4. Communication and advocacy of the values and contributions of the field to several publics and constituencies. This function requires that nursing organiza-

tions speak for nurses from a position of broad agreement. It is essential for nurses to participate actively in the formulation of health legislation and policy.

5. Attendance to the social and general welfare of their members. This function is carried out by the professional nursing organizations of the country. Professional associations give their members social and moral support to perform their roles as professionals and to cope with their professional problems. See the inside front cover for a list of selected nursing organizations. Association journals, for example, disseminate updated knowledge, new ideas, and professional concerns. By participating in the collective bargaining process, nurses can improve their economic and working conditions.

In 1970, Moore and Rosenblum identified six elements of a profession. A profession should (a) have a systematic theory, (b) exert authority, (c) command prestige, (d) have a code of ethics, (e) have a professional culture, and (f) be the major source of income by those who practice it (Moore and Rosenblum 1970).

Kramer (1974) identified the following characteristics of a profession:

- Specialized competence having an intellectual component
- Extensive autonomy in exercising this special competence
- Strong commitment to a career based on special competence
- Influence and responsibility in the use of special competence
- Development of training facilities that are controlled by the professional group
- Decision-making governed by internalized standards

More recently Miller (1985) stated that the critical attributes of professionalism in nursing are the following:

- Gaining a body of knowledge in a university setting and a science orientation at the graduate level in nursing
- Attaining competencies derived from the theoretical base wherein the "diagnosis and the treatment of human responses to actual or potential health problems" (ANA 1980) can be accomplished
- Delineating and specifying the skills and competencies that are the boundaries of expertise (Miller 1985, p. 25)

In summary, the growth of professionalism in nursing can be viewed in relation to specialized education, knowledge base, ethics, and autonomy.

PROFESSIONAL BEHAVIORS OF NURSES

Miller states that the degree to which a nurse behaves as a professional is reflected in the following five behaviors. The professional:

1. Assesses, plans, implements, and evaluates theory, research, and practice in nursing. These behaviors are reflected in the entire nursing process. See also Chapters 6 through 9.

2. Accepts, promotes, and maintains the interdependence of theory, research, and practice. These three elements make nursing a profession and not a task-centered activity (Miller 1985, p. 26).

3. Communicates and disseminates theoretical knowledge, practical knowledge, and research findings to the nursing community. Professionalism must be demonstrated by supporting, counseling, and assisting other nurses (Miller 1985, p. 26).

4. Upholds the service orientation of nursing in the eyes of the public. This orientation differentiates nursing from an occupation pursued primarily for profit. Many consider altruism the hallmark of a profession. Nursing has a tradition of service to others. This service, however, must be guided by certain rules, policies, or a code of ethics (Miller 1985, p. 26). The nursing code of ethics is formulated by national nursing associations. In addition, society is protected by licensure and certification of nurses. These self-regulatory provisions give nurses the autonomy to function in the public's best interests rather than in the best interests of an institution or other profession.

5. Preserves and promotes the professional organization as the major referent. Operation under the umbrella of professional organization differentiates a profession from an occupation (Miller 1985, p. 26). In nursing, the American Nurses' Association in the United States and the Canadian Nurses' Association in Canada perform the self-regulatory functions.

See also Critical Values of Professional Nursing and Roles of the Professional Nurse in Chapter 3.

SPECIALIZED EDUCATION

The nurse's function today is so complex that a nursing student requires knowledge in the biologic, physical, and social sciences, in addition to nursing theory and practice. It is not possible for nurses to acquire a safe level of skill through empiric (experience and observation) means alone. They require specific knowledge and skills that can be gained only through an organized nursing curriculum.

The traditional focus of nursing education has been on teaching the skills required in hospitals. However, considerable evidence shows that the need for community and home services is increasing and that using these services overcomes some of the negative aspects of hospitalization, such as separation from family. As a result, nursing curricula now focus more broadly on health as well as illness and community as well as hospital, in addition to appropriate knowledge from the biologic, social, and physical sciences.

ANA Position Paper

The ANA (1965) published "Educational Preparation for Nurse Practitioners and Assistants to Nurses: A Position Paper," which concluded the following:

> The education for all of those who are licensed to practice nursing should take place in institutions of higher education; minimum preparation for beginning professional nursing practice should be a baccalaureate degree; minimum preparation for beginning technical nursing practice should be an associate degree in nursing; education for assistants in health service occupations should be short, intensive preservice programs in vocational education rather than on-the-job training. (American Nurses' Association)

The thrust to make the baccalaureate degree the minimum entry level for professional nursing practice has significantly increased the need for post-RN baccalaureate programs. Providing programs to meet these needs and demands is a challenge for universities, especially since the profile of returning nursing students indicates that most are married women in their 30s and 40s who have dependent children and hold either full-time or part-time jobs (Dugas 1985, p. 18). Universities must be flexible in planning and providing such programs for these adult learners. Some universities now offer courses in off-campus sites for post-RN baccalaureate and MSN students and use distance delivery techniques such as teleconferencing and shipments of basic reference materials to remote areas (Kerr 1985, p. 30).

Although baccalaureate nursing education programs were established in universities in both the United States and Canada in the early 1900s, it was not until the 1960s that the number of students enrolled in these programs increased markedly. The 1965 ANA position paper provided considerable impetus to move nursing education out of hospitals and into the general education system.

Another impetus toward baccalaureate education for all nurses was a resolution of the ANA, passed in 1978, stating that the minimum educational preparation for entry into professional nursing practice by 1985 be a baccalaureate degree (BSN). The 1978 delegates also endorsed a resolution that diploma and associate degree graduates who are licensed to practice before 1985 not be affected. In 1984, the ANA House of Delegates adopted a different time frame for this change. The goal was to implement the requirement of a BSN for entry into professional nursing practice in 5% of states by 1986, 15% by 1988, 50% by 1992, and 100% by 1995 (Hood 1985, p. 592).

Technical and Professional Levels of Practice

In 1985, the ANA House of Delegates proposed that two levels of nurses be delineated: technical and professional. The technical nurse is to be prepared in an associate degree program, and the professional nurse is to be prepared in a baccalaureate degree program. This proposal, if implemented by the state nursing associations, has many implications. One implication concerns "grandfathering" to protect those nurses already licensed to practice. Because at present both technical and professional nurses are licensed as registered nurses, there is substantial agreement about grandfathering those already licensed. However, even with a grandfather clause in place, many nurses fear that they will not be protected from discrimination when they compete with recent graduates for jobs.

In its 1985 proposal, the ANA endorsed that the professional nurse with a baccalaureate degree be licensed under the legal title *registered nurse* (RN) and that the technical nurse with an associate degree be licensed under the legal title *associate nurse* (AN). As a professional organization, however, the ANA cannot legislate these changes. It is the responsibility of each state to define the legal boundaries of nursing practice and to designate the titles to be used by those practitioners who meet the individual state's criteria for licensure. Thus, if this proposal is to be accepted nationally, each state will need to implement its own changes. Such changes have major implications for diploma nurses and LPNs, because their status is not discussed in the proposal. In addition, this proposal means that new standardized examinations must be developed to test the two levels of competence.

Timelines for Transition

The National Commission on Nursing Implementation Project (NCNIP 1987) recommended in its *Timeline for Transition into the Future System for Two Categories of Nurses* a time frame for systematic transition of the present system of nursing education into a future system of education of technical and professional nursing. See Figure 1–1. According to the paper's recommendations, the educational preparation of the professional and technical nurse will differ from the current preparation. Professional nurses will be prepared in liberal arts and nursing education. They will have baccalaureate or higher degrees with majors in nursing. Technical nurses will be prepared in general education courses and natural and behavioral sciences as well as nursing. They will be graduates of associate degree programs in nursing.

In Canada in 1982, the Board of Directors of the CNA endorsed the recommendations of the Committee on Entry to Practice that the baccalaureate degree be the minimum entry level for professional nursing practice by the year 2000. Although many nurses recognize the move toward a baccalaureate degree as a requirement for entry into professional nursing practice, the issue of titling and licensure has yet to be resolved by individual state or provincial legislation. In addition, there are nurses who believe that the appropriate entry level for nursing should be at the master's or doctoral level.

Economic Constraints

Stevens (1985, p. 124) states that "what is best for nursing may not coincide with what is best for society at large," and that "one can no longer assume that the *best* for society—at any price—is a feasible goal." Recognizing that no discipline has ever achieved professional status outside of the traditional academic institutions, Stevens (1985, pp. 125–26) points out that 4-year baccalaureate programs are more costly than 2-year programs, BSN graduates require higher salaries, and the financial resources of the health care industry are shrinking. For these reasons, the nursing profession must substantiate to the general public the claim that the BSN nurse can

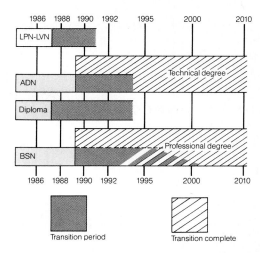

Figure 1–1 Timeline for transition into the future: nursing education system for two categories of nurse. ***Source:*** National Commission on Nursing Implementation Project. (Milwaukee: NCNIP, 1987) Reprinted with permission.

deliver qualitatively different care from that provided by the ADN nurse. The 2-year associate degree program, however, can potentially effect cost savings that can offset the high cost of educating and hiring the BSN nurse. How the two roles can be redesigned to best complement each other is a question that needs to be answered. The 1987 ANA statement on the scope of practice (see page 5) begins to answer this question and calls for further differentiation between the professional and technical practice of nursing (ANA 1987, pp. 76–79).

Specialization

Basic nursing education programs are designed to develop nurses as generalists, not specialists in any aspect of nursing. Traditionally, educators and employers have perpetuated the idea that nurses should be generalists who can rotate among services and shifts with minimal preparation. Yet, with the technological advances affecting nursing practice over the past 10 years, the market demand for nurses with specialized knowledge and skills has grown significantly.

There is a bewildering array of educational programs to prepare specialists. Aims, length, and content of the programs differ. Once prepared, the specialists are employed in a wide number of capacities and have a variety of job titles. There is a need for the national association to establish priorities for specialty development, program standards, credentialing mechanisms, and an accompanying need for employers to provide appropriate economic rewards for the performance of specialty services.

Graduate Programs

Education at the graduate level requires critical thinking. Most graduate programs are conducted by departments within the graduate school of a university, and the applicant must first meet requirements established by the graduate school. Although all graduate schools have somewhat different requirements, common requirements for admission to graduate programs in nursing include the following (DeYoung 1985, p. 120):

- The applicant must be a registered nurse.
- The applicant must hold a baccalaureate degree in nursing from an approved college or university and have had an acceptable upper division major in nursing at the baccalaureate level.
- The applicant must give evidence of scholastic ability (usually a minimum grade point average of 2.7 to 3.0 on a 4.0 scale).
- The applicant must demonstrate satisfactory achievement on a qualifying examination.
- Additionally, graduate nursing programs may also require introductory courses in statistics and computers, and demonstrated proficiency in physical assessment.

Master's programs generally take from $1\frac{1}{2}$ to 2 years to complete. Degrees granted are the Master of Arts (MA), Master in Nursing (MN), Master of Science in Nursing (MSN), and Master of Science (MS).

Master's degree programs may focus on an area of advanced clinical practice, e.g., psychiatric mental health nursing, or on functional areas such as administration or nursing education.

The number of nurses obtaining master's degrees has increased. In 1988, 20,182 students were pursuing master's study, as compared to 5085 who obtained master's degrees in 1983 (Poteet and Hodges 1990, p. 145; ANA 1985, p. 155).

Doctoral programs in nursing, which award the degrees of doctor of philosophy (PhD), doctor of nursing science (DNS or DNSc), or nursing doctorate (ND), began in the 1960s in the United States. These programs further prepare the nurse for advanced clinical practice, administration, education, and research. Before 1960, nurses acquired doctoral degrees in such related fields as psychology, sociology, physiology, and education.

The number of doctoral programs in nursing has greatly increased in the past decade. Between 1977 and 1987, the number of doctoral programs increased 156% from 18 to 46 (Lenz 1990, p. 114).

Content and approach vary among doctoral programs. One may focus on usual clinical areas, such as medical-surgical nursing, while others emphasize such nontraditional areas as transcultural nursing. Some programs emphasize theory development, but all emphasize research (DeYoung 1985, p. 119). In 1988, 2077 nurses were pursuing doctoral degrees (Poteet and Hodges 1990, p. 145).

BODY OF KNOWLEDGE

As a profession, nursing is establishing a well-defined body of knowledge and expertise. A number of nursing conceptual frameworks (discussed in Chapter 4) contribute to the knowledge base of nursing and give direction to nursing research and nursing education.

Increasing research in nursing is contributing to this body of knowledge. In the 1940s, nursing research was at a very early stage of development. In the 1950s, increased federal funding and professional support helped to establish centers for nursing research. In 1952, *Nursing Research,* the first journal to report findings of nursing studies, was founded. Since that time, more nurses with doctorates are carrying out nursing research.

Early research focused on the needs and resources of nursing and nursing education. In the 1960s, studies were often related to the nature and veracity of the knowledge base underlying nursing practice (Gortner 1980, p. 205). During the 1970s and 1980s, research was largely practice-related, and nursing's involvement in research continues to grow. See Chapter 5 for additional information about research.

ETHICS

Nurses have traditionally placed a high value on the worth and dignity of others. The nursing profession requires integrity of its members; that is, a member is expected to do what is considered right regardless of the personal cost. Nurses must respect the professional judgment of others and must develop nursing standards and establish mechanisms for identifying and dealing with unethical behavior.

Ethical codes change as the needs and values of society change. Nursing has developed its own codes of ethics and in most instances has set up means to monitor the professional behavior of its members. See Chapter 11 for additional information on ethics.

AUTONOMY

A profession is autonomous if it regulates itself and sets standards for its members. Providing autonomy is one of the purposes of a professional association. If nursing is to have professional status, it must function autonomously in the formation of policy and in the control of its activity. To be autonomous, a professional group must (a) be granted legal authority to define the scope of its practice; (b) describe its particular functions and roles; and (c) determine its goals and responsibilities in delivery of its services. The amount of autonomy a professional group possesses depends on its effectiveness at governance. *Governance* is the establishment and maintenance of social, political, and economic arrangements by which practitioners control their practice, their self-discipline, their working conditions, and their professional affairs. Nurses, therefore, must work within their professional organizations.

To practitioners of nursing, autonomy means independence at work, responsibility, and accountability for one's actions.

The ANA statement on the scope of practice describes the accountability of professional and technical nurses:

> Professional nurses develop nursing policies, procedures, and protocols and set standards for nursing care for all client populations in all practice settings. . . . Technical nurses use policies, procedures, and protocols developed by professional nurses in implementing an individual's plan of care. Technical nurses are accountable for practicing within these guidelines. (ANA 1987b, p. 77)

Scope of Nursing Practice

Nursing involves an interrelationship of many people concerned with a client's responses to potential or actual health problems. Because people are seen as biopsychosocial beings, nursing practice involves a complex of knowledge and skills applied to the whole client. Nurses are also involved with support persons and the community as a whole. For this reason, nurses must be aware of how the support persons and community affect the client's well-being and consider the well-being of these support persons and the community.

Nursing practice involves four areas related to health (health is discussed in Chapter 13):

1. *Health promotion*. Health promotion means helping people develop resources to maintain or enhance their well-being. The goal of health promotion is to move people toward their own optimum level of health and well-being or wellness (Black and McDowell 1984, p. 19). An example of a nursing action that promotes health is explaining the benefits of an exercise program to a client. Health promotion is discussed in more detail in Chapter 15.

2. *Health maintenance*. Health maintenance nursing activities are those actions that help clients to maintain their health status. An elderly person in a long-term care facility can be taught and encouraged to exercise to maintain muscle strength and mobility.

3. *Health restoration*. Health restoration means helping people to improve health following health problems or illness. Examples of activities that help restore health are teaching a client to protect an incision and to change a surgical dressing or assisting handicapped individuals to attain the highest level of physical strength and independence of which they are capable.

4. *Care of the dying*. This area of nursing practice involves comforting and caring for people of all ages while they are dying. Nurses carrying out these activities work in homes, hospitals, and extended care facilities. Some agencies, called hospices, are specifically designed for this purpose.

Standards of Nursing Practice

Establishing and implementing standards of practice are also major functions of a professional organization. Nursing practice standards provide exact criteria against which clients, nurses, and employers can evaluate care for effectiveness and excellence.

In the ANA publication *Standards of Nursing Practice,* the association comments on this responsibility of the nursing profession to society:

> Nursing's concern for the quality of its services constitutes the heart of its responsibility to the public. The more expertise required to perform the service, the greater society's dependence upon those who carry it out. Nursing must control its practice in order to guarantee the quality of its service to the public.

TABLE 1–2 *American Nurses' Association Standards of Nursing Practice*

Standard	Rationale	Standard	Rationale
1. The collection of data about the health status of the client/patient is systematic and continuous. The data are accessible, communicated, and recorded.	Comprehensive care requires complete and ongoing collection of data about the client/patient to determine the nursing care needs of the client/patient. All health status data about the client/patient must be available for all members of the health care team.	5. Nursing actions provide for client/patient participation in health promotion, maintenance, and restoration.	The client/patient and family are continually involved in nursing care.
2. Nursing diagnoses are derived from health status data.	The health status of the client/patient is the basis for determining the nursing care needs. The data are analyzed and compared to norms when possible.	6. Nursing actions assist the client/patient to maximize his health capabilities.	Nursing actions are designed to promote, maintain, and restore health.
3. The plan of nursing care includes goals derived from the nursing diagnoses.	The determination of the results to be achieved is an essential part of planning care.	7. The client/patient's progress or lack of progress toward goal achievement is determined by the client/patient and the nurse.	The quality of nursing care depends upon comprehensive and intelligent determination of nursing's impact upon the health status of the client/patient. The client/patient is an essential part of this determination.
4. The plan of nursing care includes priorities and the prescribed nursing approaches or measures to achieve the goals derived from the nursing diagnoses.	Nursing actions are planned to promote, maintain, and restore the client/patient's well-being.	8. The client/patient's progress or lack of progress toward goal achievement directs reassessment, reordering of priorities, new goal setting, and revision of the plan of nursing care.	The nursing process remains the same, but the input of new information may dictate new or revised approaches.

Source: From Standards of Nursing Practice, 1973, American Nurses' Association, Kansas City, Mo. Reprinted with permission.

Behind that guarantee are the standards of the profession, which are directed toward assurance that service of a good quality will be provided. This is essential both for the protection of the public and for the profession itself. A profession which does not maintain the confidence of the public will soon cease to be a social force. (ANA 1973, p. 1)

The profession's responsibilities inherent in establishing and implementing standards of practice include (a) to establish, maintain, and improve standards, (b) to hold members accountable for using standards, (c) to educate the public to appreciate the standards, (d) to protect the public from individuals who have not attained the standards or willfully do not follow them, and (e) to protect individual members of the profession from each other (Phaneuf and Lang 1985, p. 2).

TABLE 1–3 *Canadian Nurses' Association Standards for Nursing Practice*

I.	Nursing practice requires that a conceptual model(s) for nursing be the basis for that practice.
II.	Nursing practice requires the effective use of the nursing process.
III.	Nursing practice requires that the helping relationship be the nature of the client-nurse interaction.
IV.	Nursing practice requires nurses to fulfill professional responsibilities.

Source: Canadian Nurses' Association, February 1987. A definition of nursing practice: Standards for nursing practice. Ottawa, Ontario: CNA. Pub. #ISBN 0-919 108-51-2. Reprinted with permission.

Nursing standards clearly reflect the specific functions and activities that nurses provide, as opposed to the functions of other health workers. The ANA's Standards of Nursing Practice are set forth in Table 1–2, and those of the CNA are summarized in Table 1–3. These standards apply to the practice of all registered nurses.

When standards of professional practice are implemented, they serve as yardsticks for the measurements used in licensure, certification, accreditation, quality assurance, peer review, and public policy (Phaneuf and Lang 1985, p. 7). Licensure, certification, and accreditation are discussed in Chapter 10. Quality assurance and peer review are discussed in Chapter 9.

CHAPTER HIGHLIGHTS

▸ Florence Nightingale may be thought of as nursing's first nurse theorist, since she emphasized such independent nursing functions as preventive health care, humanistic care, comfort, and support of the client.

▸ There are many definitions and descriptions of nursing, but the essence of nursing is caring for and caring about people as holistic beings in matters related to health promotion, health maintenance, health restoration, and dying.

▸ A desired goal of nursing is professionalism, which necessitates a unique body of knowledge including specific skills and competencies, autonomous regulation, and formulation of a code of ethics.

▸ Although the majority of nurses today are employed in hospital settings, more nurses are working in other areas, such as home health care and community clinics.

▸ Standards of nursing practice provide criteria against which the effectiveness of nursing care can be evaluated.

▸ Educational programs for nurses must reflect the health care demands and needs of a changing society, accommodate changes in the health care delivery system, and adhere to professional standards yet be responsible to concerns about rising costs of health care.

▸ Flexibility in nursing curricula and innovation in implementing curricula are needed to upgrade the educational achievement of nursing graduates from programs below the baccalaureate degree level.

▸ Participation in the activities of nursing associations enhances the growth of involved individuals and helps nurses collectively influence policies affecting nursing practice.

LEARNING ACTIVITIES

■ Utilizing the characteristics of a profession as identified by Kramer (1975) and Miller (1985), review your beliefs and knowledge about nursing. Does nursing meet each of the identified criteria? In what ways are each criteria met? If a criterion is not met, how will you participate in the fulfillment of the criteria?

■ Compare the roles filled by Registered Nurses with different educational backgrounds: Diploma graduates, associate degree graduates, and baccalaureate degree graduates. Are there differences in role expectations? Performance? Compensation? What is your expectation of role change as you make the transition through an RN-BSN program?

READINGS AND REFERENCES

SUGGESTED READINGS

Cahill, C. A., and Palmer, M. H. 1989. Individual professionalism: Part of the solution to the nursing shortage crisis. *Nursing Forum* 24:27–31.

The authors point out that nursing is currently faced with a number of problems, including who is to control nursing practice and its scope. The authors quote Styles: "If nursing is to become a profession, each nurse must be required to exhibit the characteristics of 'professionhood'" (1982,

p. 119). The article further states that nurses must attain an understanding and mastery of their role.

Diers, D. January 1990. Learning the art and craft of Nursing. *American Journal of Nursing* 90:65–66.

Diers writes about the *art* of nursing, which is described in part as self-discipline. The tool of the nurse in this context is the intellect. Diers describes the discipline of nursing as the constant attention to difference and unpredictability.

Orlando, I. J., and Dugan, A. B. February 1989. Independent and dependent paths: The fundamental issue for the nursing profession. *Nursing and Health Care* 10:76–80.

Orlando and Dugan address the dilemma of dependent versus independent nursing function. They write that the distinct function of nursing must be stated. In addition, the product of professional nursing practice must be identified.

Zwolski, K. Winter 1989. Professional nursing in a technical system. *Image: Journal of Nursing Scholarship* 21:238–42.

Zwolski discusses four principles that describe a technical system: (a) technique is distinguishable from technology; (b) a technique cannot produce the philosophy that directs it; (c) technology at its incomplete and imperfect stages creates new problems; and (d) technology produces fragmentation. The author points out that the more technical the health care system becomes, the greater the need for professionally prepared nurses.

RELATED RESEARCH

Baer, E. D. January/February 1987. "A cooperative venture" in pursuit of professional status: A research journal for nursing. *Nursing Research* 36:18–25.

Fenton, M. V. March/April 1987. Development of a scale of humanistic nursing behaviors. *Nursing Research* 36:82–87.

Keefe, M. R.; Pepper, G.; and Stoner, M. November 1988. Toward research-based nursing practice: The Denver Collaborative Research Network. *Applied Nursing Research* 1:109–15.

Moody, L. E.; Wilson, M. E.; and Smyth, K. November/December 1988. Analysis of a decade of nursing practice research 1977–1986. *Nursing Research* 37:374–79.

Reverby, S. January/February 1987. A caring dilemma: Womanhood and nursing in historical perspective. *Nursing Research* 36:5–11.

Schank, M. J., and Weis, D. January/February 1989. A study of values of baccalaureate nursing students and graduate nurses from a secular and a nonsecular program. *Journal of Professional Nursing* 5:17–22.

SELECTED REFERENCES

American Journal of Nursing. February 1985. ANA gears up new drive for entry-level change: Despite opposition, some SNAs see success soon. *American Journal of Nursing* 85:194, 200–201.

American Nurses' Association. December 1965. American Nurses' Association first position on education for nursing. *American Journal of Nursing* 65:106–11.

———. 1973. *Standards of nursing practice.* Kansas City, Mo.: ANA.

———. 1980. *Nursing: A social policy statement.* Kansas City, Mo.: ANA.

———. 1987a. *Facts about nursing 86–87.* Kansas City, Mo.: ANA.

———. 1987b. *Proceedings of the 1987 House of Delegates.* Kansas City, Mo.: ANA.

Balasco, E. M. January/February 1990. The nurse in relationship. *Journal of Professional Nursing* 6:4.

Barritt, E. R. 1973. Florence Nightingale's values and modern nursing education. *Nursing Forum* 12:6–47.

Baumgart, A. J., and Larsen, J. 1988. *Canadian nursing faces the future.* St. Louis: C. V. Mosby Co.

Black, A., and McDowell, I. April 1984. Healthstyles: Moving beyond disease prevention. *Canadian Nurse* 80:18–20.

Canadian Nurses' Association. February 1981. *CNA Position Statements.* Ottawa: CNA.

———. 1987. *A definition of nursing practice: Standards for nursing practice.* Ottawa CNA.

Chaska, N. J., editor. 1990. *The nursing profession: Turning points.* St. Louis: C. V. Mosby Co.

CNA Connection. April 1984. Canada health act. CNA appears before commons committee. *Canadian Nurse* 80:8–9.

DeBack V. 1990. Debate: Entry into practice: Will the 1985 proposal ever happen? In McCloskey, J. C., Grace, H. K., editors. *Current Issues in Nursing.* 3d ed. St. Louis: C. V. Mosby Co.

DeCrosta, T. May/June 1985. Megatrends in nursing: Ten new directions that are changing your profession. *Nursing Life* 5:17–21.

Diers, D. 1979. *Research in nursing practice.* Philadelphia: J. B. Lippincott Co.

Dugas, B. W. May 1985. Baccalaureate for entry to practice: A challenge that universities must meet. *Canadian Nurse* 81:17–19.

Ellis, J. R., and Hartley, C. L. 1988. *Nursing in today's world: Challenges, issues and trends.* 3d ed. Philadelphia: J. B. Lippincott Co.

Flaherty, M. J. 1979. The characteristics and scope of professional nursing. *Journal for Nursing Leadership and Management* 1:61, 63, 69.

Flexner, A. 1915. Is social work a profession? *School Society* 1:901.

Gortner, S. R. July/August 1980. Nursing research: Out of the past and into the future. *Nursing research* 29:204–207.

Hall, L. November 1963. A center for nursing. *Nursing Outlook* 11:805–806.

Henderson, V. 1966. *The nature of nursing: A definition and its implications for practice, research, and education.* New York: Macmillan Co.

———. April 1990. Excellence in nursing. *American Journal of Nursing* 90:76–7.

Hood, G. May 1985. At issue: Titling and licensure. *American Journal of Nursing* 85:592, 594.

Huxley, E. 1975. *Florence Nightingale.* New York: G. P. Putnam's Sons.

Inglehart, J. K. September 1987. Problems facing the nursing profession. *New England Journal of Medicine* 317:646–51.

Kerr, J. May 1985. Taking the campus to the student. *Canadian Nurse* 81:30–31.

King, I. M. 1971. *Toward a theory for nursing: General concepts of human behavior.* New York: John Wiley and Sons.

———. 1981. *A theory for nursing: Systems, concepts, process.* New York: John Wiley and Sons.

Kinney, C. D. May/June 1985. A reexamination of nursing role conceptions. *Nursing Research* 34:170–76.

Kramer, M. 1974. *Reality shock.* St. Louis: C. V. Mosby.

Leddy, S., and Pepper, J. M. 1989. *Conceptual bases of professional nursing.* 2d ed. Philadelphia: J. B. Lippincott Co.

Leininger, M. 1989. *Care: The essence of nursing and health.* 2d ed. Thorofare, N.J.: Charles B. Slack.

Lenz, E. R. 1990. Doctoral education: Present views, future trends. In Chaska, N. L., editor. *The nursing profession: Turning points.* St. Louis: C. V. Mosby Co.

Levesque, V. D. June 1985. Specialization and certification: A review of CNA's activities. *Canadian Nurse* 81:26–28.

Lewis, E. P. September/October 1983. News outlook: The issue that won't go away. A report on the 1983 NLN convention. *Nursing Outlook* 31:246–47.

———. September/October 1985. Taking care of business: The ANA House of Delegates. *Nursing Outlook* 33:239–43.

Merton, R. K. January 1958. The function of the professional organization. *American Journal of Nursing* 58:50–54.

Miller, B. K. April 1985. Just what is a profession? *Nursing Success Today* 2:21–27.

Montag, M. L. April 1980. Looking back: Associate degree education in perspective. *Nursing Outlook* 28:248–50.

Moore, W. E., and Rosenblum, G. W. 1970. *The professions: Roles and rules.* New York: The Russell Sage Foundation.

National Commission on Nursing: Summary report and recommendations. July 1983. American Hospital Association. Chicago: The Hospital Research and Educational Trust, and American Hospital Supply Corporation.

National Commission on Nursing Implementation Project. 1987. Timeline for transition into the future: Nursing education system for two categories of nurse. Milwaukee: National Commission on Nursing Implementation Project.

National League for Nursing. March/April 1975. 1974 Annual Report. *NLN News* 23:3.

———. 1978. *Characteristics of graduate education in nursing leading to the master's degree.* New York: NLN.

———. 1979. *Characteristics of baccalaureate education in Nursing.* New York: NLN

Neuman, B. 1982. *The Neuman systems model: Application to nursing education and practice.* New York: Appleton-Century-Crofts.

Nightingale, F. 1860. *Notes on nursing: What it is, and what it is not.* London: Harrison. Reprinted in Bishop, F. L. A., and Goldie, S. 1962. *A bio-bibliography of Florence Nightingale.* London: Dawsons of Pall Mall.

Nyberg, J. May 1990. The effects of care and economics on nursing practice. *Journal of Nursing Administration* 20:13–18.

Orem, D. E. 1985. *Nursing: Concepts of practice.* 3d ed. New York: McGraw-Hill.

Palmer, I. S. June 1981. Florence Nightingale and international origins of modern nursing. *Image: Journal of Nursing Scholarship* 8:28–31.

Parse, R. R. 1981. *Man-living-health: A theory of nursing.* New York: John Wiley and Sons.

Perlich, L. J. M. March 1986. Catalyzing educational change . . . Issues of health care economics. *Journal of Nursing Administration* 16:6.

Phaneuf, M. C., and Lang, M. 1985. *Issues in professional nursing practice 7: Standards of nursing practice.* Kansas City, Mo.: American Nurses' Association.

Poteet G. W., and Hodges, L. E. 1990. How to choose a graduate program. In McClosky, J. C., and Grace, H. K. *Current issues in nursing.* 3d ed. St. Louis: C. V. Mosby Co.

Poulin, M. A. 1985. *Issues in professional nursing practice 5, Configurations of nursing practice.* Kansas City, Mo.: American Nurses' Association.

Primm, P. L. May/June 1986. Entry into practice: Competency statements for BSNs and ADNs. *Nursing Outlook* 34:135–37.

Riehl, J. P., and Roy, C. 1980. *Conceptual models for nursing practice.* 2d ed. New York: Appleton-Century-Crofts.

Rogers, M. E. 1970. *An introduction to the theoretical basis of nursing.* Philadelphia: F. A. Davis Co.

———. 1980. Nursing: A science of unitary man. In Riehl, J. P., and Roy, C. *Conceptual models for nursing practice.* 2d ed. New York: Appleton-Century-Crofts.

Roy, C. 1984. *Introduction to nursing: An adaptation model.* 2d ed. Englewood Cliffs, N.J.: Prentice-Hall.

Segal, E. T. June 1985. Is nursing a profession? Yes no. *Nursing 85* 15:40–43.

Snyder, M. E., and LaBar, C. 1984. *Issues in professional nursing practice 1. Nursing: Legal authority to practice.* Kansas City, Mo.: American Nurses' Association.

Stevens, K. R. May/June 1985. Does the 1985 education proposal make economic sense? *Nursing Outlook* 33:124–27.

Stull, M. K., May/June 1986. Entry skills for BSNs. *Nursing Outlook* 34:138, 153.

Styles, M. M. January 1978. Dialogue across the decades. *Nursing Outlook* 26:28–32.

———. 1982. *On nursing: Toward a new endowment.* St. Louis: C. V. Mosby Co.

———. November 1983. The anatomy of a profession. *Heart and Lung* 12:570–75.

Watson, J. 1979. *Nursing: The philosophy and science of caring.* Boston: Little-Brown.

———. 1985. *Nursing: Human science and health care.* Norwalk, Conn.: Appleton-Century-Crofts.

Young, W. B. 1987. *Introduction to nursing concepts.* Norwalk, Conn.: Appleton & Lange.

Historical and Societal Influences on Nursing

CONTENTS

THE DEVELOPMENT OF EARLY NURSING

One of the irrefutable laws of nature is dynamism, or change. Individual and group elements of society respond and adapt to historical events that may alter the behaviors, values, laws, beliefs, and even the daily living habits of society. Influential events may be related to natural disasters, such as floods, earthquakes, famine, or epidemic disease, or they may be invented by people, such as the discovery of fire, the wheel, the printing press, the microscope, and penicillin. War, political upheaval, religious intolerance, and economic instability are systemic events that can alter individuals' lives and group progress.

As a subgroup of society, nursing must also respond and adapt to the influences of society. Nursing has been a continuous thread linking the past with the present—from the tribal groups of early societies to modern societies linked by jet-powered transportation and instant telecommunications. And just as human history has shown tremendous progress over the centuries, so has nursing evolved from the art of comforting, caring for, and nurturing the sick to a synthesis of this art with the science and technology of contemporary thinking.

Nursing in Primitive Societies

It is impossible to describe nursing practice or the role of the nurse prior to recorded history. It is also difficult to differentiate between the role of the physician and that of the nurse, or even to determine if there were two distinctly different roles. It is probable that any differentiation that existed was based on male-female role proscriptions, such as medicine man or herb woman. It may be postulated that individuals provided care or cure based on experience and oral transmission of available knowledge about health and disease. Traditional female roles of wife, mother, daughter, and sister always included the care and nurturing of other family members. The term *nurse* derives from the care mothers gave to their helpless infant children. Dolan, Fitzpatrick, and Hermann (1983) suggest that the very survival of the human species is evidence of the existence of nursing throughout history—"the art of nurturing has been essential to the preservation of life." Further, they postulate "that the nurse figure in the community was a very capable, concerned, and compassionate woman who assumed the nurse role as a societal assignment."

Nursing in Ancient Civilizations

In the early recordings of ancient civilizations, there is little information about those who cared for the sick. It is known that midwives provided care for the mother and infant during birthing, and that wet nurses often suckled and cared for infant children of wealthy families. Often these roles were filled by female slaves. This fact contributes to the lack of recorded information about nursing, because slaves had no status and as such their work was not worthy of documentation. The slave-nurse was dependent upon the master, healer, or priest for instruction or direction in the care of her charge. Often the care provided for the sick was related to physical maintenance and comfort.

During this time, beliefs about the cause of disease were imbedded in superstition and magic and thus treatment often required magical cures. The priest or witch doctor enjoyed great status in ancient societies. But as these societies evolved, practical theories of medical care emerged as non-magical causes of disease were observed. The earliest recording of healing practices is a 4000-year-old clay tablet attributed to the Sumerian civilization. It contains healing prescriptions but, unfortunately, neglects to describe the illnesses for which they were prescribed.

The earliest documentation of law governing the practice of medicine is the Code of Hammurabi, attributed to the Babylonians and dating to 1900 BC. The Code recorded regulations related to sanitation and public health, the practice of surgery, the differentiation between the practice of human and veterinary medicine, a table of fees for operations, and penalties for violators of the code. There is no specific record of nursing in the Babylonian civilization, however, there are references to tasks and practices traditionally provided by nurses. Medical illustration from that period often includes a nurse-like figure providing patient support or comfort.

Important historic findings related to the Egyptian culture include the Ebers papyrus and the practice of mummification. The Ebers papyrus, which dates to approximately 1550 BC, is believed the oldest medical text in the world. It describes many diseases known today and it identifies specific symptomatology. It also lists over 700 substances that were used as drugs and describes their preparation and medicinal use. Mummification, or embalming, derived from the belief in life after death. The development of effective solutions to preserve the body from decay and the subsequent ability of modern day anthropologists to examine the mummified body indicate a high level of knowledge of human anatomy, physiology, and pathophysiology.

The ancient Hebrew culture contributed the Mosaic Health Code to the history of health care. This code is considered the first sanitary legislation and contains the first record of public health requirements. The Code, which covered every aspect of individual, family, and community health, differentiated between "clean" and "unclean." Principles of personal health related to rest, sleep, and cleanliness were also provided. There were rules for women related to menstruation and childbearing. Dietary laws were a significant part of the Mosaic Code and provided for the "kosher" slaughter of animals, as well as preparation and preservation of animal and plant foods.

The use of quarantine as a prevention against the transmission of communicable diseases, such as leprosy and diphtheria, is recorded in the Bible. Nurses are mentioned occasionally in the Old Testament as women who provided care for infants and children, for the sick and dying, and as midwives who assisted during pregnancy and at delivery.

In ancient African cultures, the nurturing functions of the nurse included roles as midwives, herbalists, wet nurses, and carers for children and the elderly (Dolan, Fitzpatrick, and Hermann 1983, p. 19). In ancient India, early hospitals were staffed by male nurses who were required to meet four qualifications: (1) "knowledge of the manner in which drugs should be prepared for administration, (2) cleverness, (3) devotedness to the patient, and (4) purity of mind and body" (Donahue 1985, p. 61). Indian women served as midwives and nursed ill family members. There is no mention of the nurse role in ancient China; however, the contribution of ancient China to health care knowledge includes the effects of some 365 herbal remedies in the Pen Tsao (c. 2700 BC), the use of acupuncture as a treatment method, and the publication of the Nei Ching (Canon of Medicine), which detailed the four steps of examination—look, listen, ask, and feel.

In the histories of ancient Greece and Rome, care of the sick and injured was advanced in mythology *and* reality. The Greek mythic God Asklepios was the chief healer; his wife, Epigone, was the soother. Hygeia, the daughter of Asklepios, was the goddess of health and was revered by some as the embodiment of the nurse. Temples built to honor Asklepios became centers for healing, and the priests of Asklepios provided healing through natural and supernatural remedies (Donahue 1985, p. 68). The ancient Greek physician, Hippocrates, is honored today as the "Father of Medicine." He believed that disease had a natural cause, in contrast to the magical and mystical causes pronounced by the priest healers of the temples.

After they conquered Greece in 200 BC, the Romans borrowed gods from the Greeks, including Aesculapius (Asklepios) and Hygeia. Greek physician-slaves brought medical practices to the Roman empire. The Romans' contribution to health care was in public sanitation, the draining of marshes, and the building of aqueducts, public and private baths, drainage systems, and central heating.

THE ROLE OF RELIGION IN THE DEVELOPMENT OF NURSING

Many of the world's religions encourage benevolence, but it was the Christian value of "love thy neighbor as thyself" that impacted significantly on the development of Western nursing. The principle of caring was established with Christ's parable of the Good Samaritan providing care for a tired and injured stranger. Christianity converts during the third and fourth centuries included several wealthy women of the Roman Empire. See the accompanying box.

Women were not the sole providers of nursing services; in the third century in Rome there was an organization of men called the Parabolani brotherhood. This group of men provided care to the sick and dying during the great plague in Alexandria. During the Crusades, Knighthood orders—such as the Knights Hospitalers of St. John of Jerusalem, the Teutonic Knights, and the Knights of Lazarus—were often composed of brothers in arms who provided nursing care to their sick and injured comrades. These orders were responsible for building great hospitals, the organization and management of which set a standard for the administration of hospitals throughout Europe at that time.

As the Christian church grew, more hospitals were built, as were specialized institutions providing care for orphans, widows, the elderly, the poor, and the sick. It is unfortunate that the religious beliefs of the Church were in conflict with scientific thought and education during this period. The Church encouraged care and comfort of the sick and poor but did not allow for the

---

Dedicated Women of the Roman Empire

- *Marcella* converted her palace into a monastery, and encouraged other Roman matrons to join her in caring for the sick poor. She is considered by some to be the first nurse educator, as she taught her followers how to care for the sick. She was also literate in Latin, Greek, and Hebrew and encouraged the education of women.

- *Fabiola,* a follower of Marcella, also contributed her great wealth to the care of the poor and sick. She is credited with establishing the first public hospital in Rome in 390 AD. She is said to have personally nursed patients whose wounds and sores were ugly and repugnant. She was considered the patron saint of nursing (Donahue 1985, p. 110).

- *Paula* was a wealthy and learned friend of Fabiola. Upon the death of her husband, she converted to Christianity. She, too, studied with Marcella. In 385 AD she moved with her daughter to Palestine, where she built hospitals for the sick and hospices for the pilgrims who followed the road to Bethlehem. She also provided direct care to the sick.

advancement of knowledge in preventing illness or curing disease. This attitude pervaded the period known as the Dark Ages, which endured for approximately 500 years.

During the Middle Ages (500–1500 AD), male and female religious, military, and secular orders with the primary purpose of caring for the sick were formed. Conspicuous among them were the Knights Hospitalers of St. John; The Alexian Brotherhood (organized in 1431); and the Augustinian sisters, which was the first purely nursing order.

In 1633 the Sisters of Charity were founded by St. Vincent de Paul in France. It was the first of many such orders organized under various Roman Catholic church auspices and largely devoted to caring for the sick.

The deaconess groups, which had their origins in the Roman Empire of the third and fourth centuries under Marcella, Fabiola, and Paula, were suppressed during the Middle Ages by the Western churches. However, these groups of nursing providers reoccurred occasionally throughout the centuries, most notably in 1836 when Theodor Fliedner reinstituted the Order of Deaconesses and opened a small hospital and training school in Kaiserswerth, Germany. Florence Nightingale received her "training" in nursing at the Kaiserswerth School.

THE DEVELOPMENT OF MODERN NURSING

In the eighteenth and nineteenth centuries, the world underwent a renaissance. The discoveries of Copernicus, Galileo, Newton, Kepler, Briggs, and Descartes precipitated an intellectual revolution. Vesalius, Harvey, Hooke, and van Leeuwenhoek contributed to the scientific revolution in medicine. With the discovery and exploration of new continents, an economic revolution evolved, after which nations became more interdependent through trade and mercantilism. The Industrial Revolution displaced workers from cottage craftsmen to factory laborers. With these changes came stressors to health. New illnesses, transmitted in the holds of ships by seamen and stowaway rodents, jumped national boundaries and continents. The closeness of factory work, the long hours, and the unhealthy working conditions led to the rapid transmission of communicable diseases such as cholera and plague. Lack of prenatal care, inadequate nutrition, and poor delivery techniques resulted in a high rate of maternal and infant mortality. Orphaned children died in workhouses of neglect or cruelty. These conditions have been effectively portrayed in the writings of Dickens, including *Oliver Twist* and *David Copperfield*.

A "proper" woman's role in life was to maintain a gracious and elegant home for her family. The common women worked as servants in private homes or were dependent on their husband's wage. The provision of care for the sick in hospitals or private homes fell to the uncommon women—often prisoners or prostitutes who had little or no training in nursing and even less enthusiasm for the job. Because of this, nursing had little acceptance and no prestige. The only acceptable nursing role was within a religious order wherein services were provided to the hospital for little or no cost.

The development of the Deaconess Institute at Kaiserswerth, Germany changed all this. Associated with a religious organization, the Order of Deaconesses ignited recognition of the need for the services of women in the care of the sick, the poor, children, and female prisoners. The training school for nurses at Kaiserswerth included care of the sick in hospitals, instruction in visiting nursing, instruction in religious doctrine and ethics, and pharmacy. The deaconess movement eventually spread to four continents, including North America, North Africa, Asia, and Australia.

Florence Nightingale, the most famous Kaiserswerth pupil, was born to a wealthy and intellectual family. Her education included the mastery of several ancient and modern languages, literature, philosophy, history, science, mathematics, religion, art, and music. It was expected that she would follow the usual path of a wealthy and intelligent woman of the day: marry, bear children, and maintain an elegant home. She was determined, however, to become a nurse in order to "lift the load of suffering from the helpless and miserable." As a well-traveled young woman of the day in 1847 she opportuned to visit Kaiserswerth, where she received three months training in nursing. In 1853 she studied in Paris with the Sisters of Charity, after which she returned to England to assume the position of superintendent of a charity hospital for ill governesses.

During the Crimean War, there was public outcry about the inadequacy of care for the soldiers. The death rate, estimated at 42–60%, was attributed to wounds, infection, cholera, inadequate nutrition, lack of drugs, and lack of care. Florence Nightingale was asked by Sir Sidney Herbert of the War Department to recruit a contingent of female nurses to provide care to the sick and injured in the Crimea. In spite of opposition from the Army medical officers, she and her nurses transformed the environment by setting up diet kitchens, a laundry, recreation centers, and reading rooms, and organizing classes. She trained the orderlies to scrub the wards and empty wastes. In the course of six months, the mortality rate decreased to less than 2%.

When she returned to England, Nightingale was given an honorarium of 4500 pounds by a grateful English public. This was later used to develop the Nightingale Training School for Nurses, which opened in 1860. The school served as a model for other training schools. Its graduates traveled to other countries to manage hospitals and institute nurse training programs. The efforts of Florence Nightingale and her nurses changed the status of nursing to a respectable occupation for women.

THE DEVELOPMENT OF NURSING IN THE AMERICAS

Between the American Revolution and the Civil War nursing in America probably paralleled nursing in Europe (Kelly 1985, p. 38). In 1639, the Augustinian sisters migrated to Canada and eventually established the first hospital, the Hotel Dieu, in Quebec City. In 1644 in the United States, Mother Elizabeth Seton established the first American order of the Sisters of Charity of St. Joseph in Maryland. Also in 1644, Jeanne Mance, known as the Florence Nightingale of Canada, founded the Hotel Dieu in Montreal.

See Appendix A for a complete listing of significant events in nursing history, from 1 AD through 1990.

THE IMPACT OF WAR ON NURSING

War has influenced and enhanced the development of organized nursing. Throughout history, individuals have responded to the need to care for soldiers wounded on the battlefield. During the Roman conquest of the known world, the wives of soldiers, women camp followers, or comrades in arms provided comfort and care. The value of nurses escalated as they provided care to the heroes who risked their lives in defense of their nation's values or territory.

The Knighthood orders of the Middle Ages combined religion, chivalry, militarism, and charity. Their original purpose was to carry the wounded from the battlefield to the hospitals and to provide care. During the period of the Crusades, the organization and management of their battlefield hospitals became the standard for the development of hospitals throughout Europe. Other branches of the Knights defended the wounded from the enemy and defended pilgrims under attack.

The development of the Nightingale Training School was a direct result of the Crimean War, as the public, grateful for the care Florence Nightingale and her nurses provided the soldiers, gave the funds necessary to start the school.

During the Civil War, Dorothea Dix was appointed superintendent of the first nurse corps of the United States Army. She recruited only women that were over 30 and plain-looking. Miss Dix was able to recruit 2000 women to care for the armed forces. These nurses dressed wounds, gave medicines, and attended to diets. In addition to war wounds, the soldiers suffered from dysentery and smallpox, and many nurses died as a result of disease contracted in the line of duty.

An additional group that provided service was The Women's Central Association for Relief. This group pleaded with the government to establish a commission to investigate the sanitary conditions of the Army hospitals. In response, the United States Sanitary Commission was established in 1861. The Women's Central Association became a branch of the U.S. Sanitary Commission and assumed the responsibility of recruiting and training nurses for the war effort.

As with Nightingale in the Crimea, the nurses in the Civil War met with much opposition from the male physicians. Hospital ships were used to transport the wounded to hospitals, and nurses provided the care along with medical orderlies. Many assertive women, who are known not only for their ability to nurse but also for their influence in other arenas, provided nursing service during the Civil War. Some of the most influential were Jane Stuart Woolsey, one of many nurses from the Woolsey family; Louisa May Alcott, who eventually became an important literary figure; Harriet Tubman, who as a nurse and abolitionist provided care and comfort to her fellow blacks on the Underground Railroad; Sojourner Truth, another black nurse who provided care for the wounded soldiers of the Union Army and was active in the early roots of the women's movement; and Margaret Breckinridge, granddaughter of a U.S. senator, who later became Attorney General of the United States. In 1901 the United States Army Nurse Corps was formally established by act of Congress, and in 1908 the United States Navy Nurse Corps was established.

During World War I, approximately 20,000 nurses were assigned to military service (Donahue 1985, p. 398). After the war, many of these nurses continued to provide care with relief programs in Europe and Asia. The need for trained nurses placed a strain on the supply of nurses, resulting in a fear of a decrease in the admission and graduation standards of nurse training. Rather than sacrifice the quality of nurses, a committee composed of M. Adelaide Nutting, Annie Goodrich, and Lillian Wald met to develop an alternative training program combining university and hospital training. The first such program was the "Vassar Training Camp" under the direction of Isabel Stewart. In 1918, in response to the need for trained nurses, the Secretary of War authorized the Army School of Nursing, with Annie Goodrich as its first dean.

World War II had a tremendous impact on nursing. Nurses served at the war front in field hospitals, on hospital ships, and in air ambulances. Again the need for nurses impacted on nursing education, resulting in the development of the United States Cadet Nurse Corps, a training program for nurses funded by federal funds under the Nurse Training act of 1942. This was a forerunner of federal funding programs aiding nursing education. Provisions of this act forbade discrimination on the basis of race and marital status, required minimum educational standards, and forced nursing schools to review and revise their curricula (Kelly 1985, p. 63). In 1947 female nurses were recognized by the military as comparable to other male officers and were granted full commissioned officer status. It is interesting to note, however, that male military nurses were not admitted to full officer rank until 1954.

As with previous wars, nurses demonstrated their bravery and heroism in the care of the wounded. Eleven Navy nurses were held as prisoners of war for 37 months, while continuing to provide nursing care to fellow POWs. Two hundred and one nurses died during World War II, 16 as a result of enemy action. During World War II, the military experimented with frontline resuscitation stations (the forerunner of the MASH units) to provide rapid care to war casualties. The success of these units resulted in the establishment of postanesthesia recovery rooms.

During the Korean Conflict, a new type of Army Medical Unit was tested. The Mobile Army Surgical Hospital (MASH) unit provided rapid and urgent care to the war wounded. Physicians, nurses, and corpsmen were located within 8 to 12 miles of the front, and a helicopter unit attached to each MASH unit provided rapid movement of incoming casualties from the battlefield and outgoing treated casualties to staging areas far behind the front lines. This unit effectively reduced the numbers of war dead in both the Korean and Vietnam Conflicts. The Korean Conflict also saw the emergence of the Air Force Nurse Corps, whose responsibility was to provide care during aeromedical evacuation of war wounded to definitive treatment centers in the United States. The success of these units impacted on nursing and health care in the United States with the advent of hospital-based mobile intensive care units.

During the Vietnam Conflict and the Persian Gulf War military nursing services were consolidated. Army physicians, nurses, and medics set up and maintained field hospitals close to the war front to provide immediate care to war wounded. Air Force nurses provided care during aeromedical evacuation to definitive treatment centers behind the lines and then during the long flight home. Navy nurses provided nursing care on board floating hospital ships near the war front.

Large influxes of wounded during the aforementioned wars and conflicts stressed the military medical complex, and increased the autonomy of the nurse in the care of the wounded. Nurses initiated care based on standard care algorithms, and they provided that caring touch so longed for by young soldiers far from home. In addition, nurses provided care to the civilian casualties of war.

FACTORS INFLUENCING CONTEMPORARY NURSING PRACTICE

To understand nursing as it is practiced today and as it will be practiced in the next century requires not only a historic perspective of nursing's evolution but also an understanding of some of the social forces currently influencing this progression. These forces usually affect the entire health care system, and nursing, as a major component of that system, cannot avoid the effects.

Economics

Greater financial support provided through public and private health insurance programs has increased the demand for nursing care. Health services such as emergency room care, mental health counseling, home health care, and preventive physical and diagnostic examinations are used increasingly by people who could not have afforded them in the past. Federal governments recognized this need and markedly increased their budgets for health care in the 1970s and early 1980s. Changes in health care legislation have enabled some providers of nursing services to obtain third party reimbursement from governmental and private insurance providers. This increase in expenditure is accompanied by increased employment opportunities for those who provide health services.

Costs of health care have also increased during this period. In response to these increasing costs, the Medicare payment system to hospitals was revised in 1982, establishing fees according to diagnostic related groups (DRGs). With the implementation of this legislation, clients in hospitals are more acutely ill than before, and clients once considered sufficiently ill to be hospitalized are now treated at home.

These changes present challenges to nurses. Currently, the health care industry is shifting its emphasis from inpatient care of acutely ill clients to outpatient services designed to promote and maintain healthy living behaviors and prevention of disease with preadmission testing, posthospitalization rehabilitation, home health care, health maintenance, and physical fitness (Powell 1984, p. 33). Nurses need to adapt their knowledge and skills to these settings. Since the 1950s an increasingly larger percentage of nurses are working in outpatient settings. Rogers (1985, p. 10) suggests that soon a large majority of nurses will not work in hospitals. This change in the nature of employment has implications for nursing education, nursing research, and nursing practice.

The Nursing Shortage

In the United States, 58% of hospitals report an acute shortage of registered nurses, particularly in areas such as intensive care, emergency, and operating rooms. A similar shortage exists in Canada. These shortages may be the result of many factors, e.g., a decline in student enrollment, and an increase in the number of nurses leaving the profession (Graham and Sheppard 1990, pp. 440–41). Another factor impacting on the perceived shortage of nurses is nurses' increased practice in community settings, both in traditional milieus such as public health services and school nursing, and in newly evolving settings such as hospice care, homeless shelters, prison health services, and entrepreneurial home health agencies.

The declining interest in nursing is a multifaceted problem. Students have wider career choices than in previous years. Inglehart (1987) points out that nurses' salaries and benefits do not reflect their levels of education, experience, or performance. In addition, weekend and shift work appear unattractive to many prospective students. Another factor considered to affect recruitment is nursing's public image. The public often has difficulty differentiating the "generic" nurse from other nursing personnel, e.g., nursing assistants and support personnel. This inability to identify and explain nursing's effect on society is also reflected in declining nursing school enrollment.

Nursing associations, government agencies, employers, and nursing educators have studied the problem. The major organizations of the Tri-Council for Nursing have plans to address the nursing shortage. The Ad Council has developed public service posters and radio and television spots to recruit candidates for nursing as well as to enhance the public image of nursing as a profession. The American Nurses' Association (ANA) has developed highly motivating videotapes to recruit potential nurses. The American Association of Critical Care Nurses (AACN) has developed the McMurphy Project to acquaint high school students with the career options in nursing.

Some hospitals are testing strategies to change the role of the hospital nurse and to improve the practice environment. In addition, some nursing schools, in order to attract more students to nursing, have designed new models for nursing education, flexible scheduling of courses, and alternative support for students, including work-study programs, child care, nurse mentors, and tuition assistance.

Nurses themselves need to take a more proactive role in the recruitment and retention of nurses. Negative statements need to be reconsidered before being spoken. Nurses should instead be supportive and provide accurate information about nursing to civic groups such as Girl Scouts, Boy Scouts, PTA groups, teen groups, and the general public.

Consumer Demands

Consumers of nursing services (the public) have become an increasingly effective force in changing nursing practice. People are better educated and have more knowledge about health and illness today, and consumers have become more aware of others' need for care. The ethical and moral issues raised by poverty and neglect have made people more vocal about the needs of minority groups, the poor, and the homeless.

The public's concepts of health and nursing have also changed. Most people now believe that health is a right of all people, not just a privilege of the rich. The media emphasize the message that individuals must assume responsibility for their own health by obtaining a physical examination regularly, checking for the seven danger signals of cancer, and maintaining their mental well-being by balancing work and recreation. Furthermore, many people now want more than freedom from disease—they want increased energy, vitality, and a feeling of wellness. Interest in health and nursing services is therefore greater than ever.

Increasingly, the consumer has become an active participant in making health and nursing care decisions. Planning committees concerned with providing community nursing services usually have active consumer membership. Recognizing the legitimacy of public input, many state and provincial nursing associations and regulatory agencies now have consumer representatives on their governing boards.

Changing Family Structures

The need for nursing services is being influenced by new family structures. An increasing number of people are living away from the extended family and the nuclear family, and the husband and father is no longer necessarily the family breadwinner. An extended family may consist of parents or step-parents, children or siblings, grandparents, and sometimes aunts and uncles. A nuclear family consists of one or more parents and their children.

Today many single women and men rear children, and in many two-parent families both parents work. It is also common for young parents to live far away from their own parents, and these young families need support services, such as day-care centers. Many young families do not have grandparents or other relatives readily available to help in times of illness or to offer advice about childbearing and child health. These new parents usually get this advice from physicians, nurses, or other health care professionals. Similarly, grandparents who live alone and far from other members of the family require homemaker and visiting nurse services when they are ill because the younger members of their family may be unable to provide this care.

Adolescent mothers need specialized nursing services. In addition to their needs as new mothers, these young people have the normal needs of teenagers as well. In 1960 13.9% of all births were to teenage mothers; this percentage has increased steadily despite the fact that an increasing number of women are choosing to delay motherhood. Many teenage mothers are raising their children alone with inadequate financial resources because of poor or no job skills. This type of single-parent family is especially vulnerable to health crises as motherhood compounds the difficulties of adolescence.

Science and Technology

Advances in science and technology affect nursing practice. For example, wide-spread immunization for poliomyelitis decreased the morbidity of that disease and the need for specialized nursing care. As medical and nursing knowledge bases expand, nurses acquire knowledge and skills as they adapt to meet the clients' new needs.

The space program has developed advanced technologies for space travel based on the need for long-distance monitoring of astronauts and space craft, lighter materials, and miniaturization of equipment. Health care has benefited as this new technology has been adapted in health care aides such as Viewstar (an aid for the visually impaired), the insulin infusion pump, the voice-controlled wheelchair, magnetic resonance imaging, laser surgery, filtering devices for intravenous fluid control devices, and intensive care monitoring systems (Haggerty 1989). In some settings, technologic advances have required that nurses become highly specialized; today's nurses often use sophisticated computerized equipment to monitor or treat clients. As technologies change, nursing education changes, and nurses require further education to provide effective, safe nursing practice.

Advances in technology are exemplified by the variety of machines used to help clients maintain life. With the knowledge explosion of the twentieth century has come the charge that medical services—and some health professionals—have become dehumanized. Yet an increasing understanding of the psychologic, emotional, and spiritual aspects of care has developed to balance the technology. It is the responsibility of all health professionals—and nurses in particular—to remember that clients are human beings requiring warmth, care, and acknowledgment of self-worth. Often equipment is frightening to clients and their support persons, and medical vocabulary appears mysterious and is frequently misunderstood. The nurse who interacts with clients daily is in an ideal situation to humanize technology by offering explanations, communicating support, and recognizing the clients' needs for understanding and support. This is the "high touch" aspect of a "high tech" environment.

Problems created by technologic change present new nursing challenges. For example, some industries are hazardous to employees because of dangerous equipment or harmful chemical residues. Trauma and disease are frequently the direct result of advanced technology; the classic example is automobile accidents, which are among the top five causes of death in North America. In addition, our life-styles frequently create high levels of stress, which has been associated with major physical illnesses such as heart disease, cancer, and gastrointestinal disturbances, as well as psychologic problems such as depression.

Legislation

Legislation about nursing practice and health matters affects the public and the nursing profession. Changes in legislation relating to health also affect nursing. For example, laws requiring the use of seat belts and slower speed limits have reduced the morbidity and mortality rates for automobile accidents. Currently, two areas of legislative and ethical controversy are related to abortion and the termination of life in the brain dead, or "vegetative," client. The decade of the 90s will see much discussion in state, provincial, and national legislatures and courts as these issues are resolved. Whatever the outcome, there will be significant impact on nursing practice.

Legislation regarding the Medicare payment system according to DRGs has had an enormous influence on nursing practice in hospitals and communities. Many clients leave hospitals earlier than they did in the past. As a result, more clients in hospitals are seriously ill, and more clients require complex home care. Although this trend has contributed to a shortage of nurses in acute care settings, it has opened new opportunities for nurses in home health care.

Legislation related to the funding of health care may affect nursing as the federal government considers the direct reimbursement of nurse practitioners for care provided to the elderly, infants, and pregnant women.

Demography

Demography is the study of population, including statistics about distribution by age and place of residence, mortality, and morbidity. Demographic data can be used to assess the need for nursing services. For example:

> The total population in North America has increased since 1900. The proportion of elderly people has also increased. It is anticipated that by the year 2000, 15% of the population of the United States will be 65 or older, resulting in an increased need for nursing services for this group.

> The population is shifting from rural to urban settings. This shift signals increased needs for nursing services related to problems caused by pollution and the changing environment.

> Mortality and morbidity studies reveal the presence of "risk factors," e.g. smoking, that are major causes of death and disease that can be prevented through life-style changes. Nurses now assume a major role in helping clients assess personal health risk factors and make appropriate life-style changes.

Nursing Associations

Professional nursing associations (see the inside front cover) have provided leadership that affects many areas of nursing. Voluntary accreditation of nursing education programs by the NLN and by mandatory accreditation licensing boards in each state have also influenced nursing. Over the years many programs have steadily improved to meet the standards for accreditation. As a result, graduate nurses are better prepared to meet the demands of society.

In 1979 the ANA published findings of a credentialing committee, which recommended the establishment of a center for credentialing in nursing (ANA 1979, p. 682). The credentialing of expanded nursing roles, such as that of the nurse practitioner, is carried out by the ANA and several nursing specialty organizations, including the American Association of Critical Care Nurses, the American Association of Operating Room Nurses, and the Emergency Nurses Association.

To influence health care policy-making, a group of professional nurses organized formally to take political action in the nursing and health care arenas. Nurses for Political Action (NPA) was formed in 1972 and became an arm of the ANA in 1974, when its name changed to Nurses Coalition for Action in Politics (N-CAP). In 1986 the name was changed to ANA-PAC. Through this group, nurses have lobbied actively for legislation affecting health care. A number of nursing leaders hold positions of authority in government. Maintenance of such positions is essential for nurses to continue to exert ongoing political influence.

The impetus for increased autonomy comes from the nursing profession itself. During the past 20 years, the increased autonomy is evident in nurses' function in specialty care units (e.g., intensive care) and in their expanded roles (e.g., nurse practitioner). Many states have rewritten their nurse practice acts to reflect such changes in nursing practice.

The Feminist Influence

The history of nursing is intertwined with the history of women. Throughout history nursing has been associated with women. The Knighthood orders of the Middle Ages, while committed to providing care and comfort to their wounded soldiers, were more strongly linked to their military traditions. Wherever women challenged society's notion of the "proper" role of women, the ancient roots of the women's movement emerged. Marcella, Fabiola, and Paula, all proper women of Rome, challenged the prescribed family role of women and chose to serve the poor, the sick, and the weak. Florence Nightingale, a proper young woman of Victorian England, contradicted the norms of society to become a nurse. She changed the world of health care. Black nurses Sojourner Truth and Harriet Tubman elected to risk their lives in the care of slaves and soldiers during the Civil War. Lavinia Dock, an early author of nursing texts and a major force in the American Nurses' Association and the International Council of Nurses, was also committed to the women's suffrage movement. She believed that women's subjugation to men was the cause of many of the problems affecting nursing.

The feminist movement has brought public attention to human rights in all areas, particularly in educational, political, economic, and social equality. Because the majority of nurses are women, this movement has altered nurses' economic and educational perspectives. As a result, nurses are increasingly asserting themselves as professional people who have a right to equality with men in health professions, and nurses are demanding more autonomy in client care. Sampselle (1990, p. 243) suggests that "incorporating feminist philosophy into practice can make it more likely for women to become full partners in sexual, social, and economic relationships and to be valued for a wide range of contributions to society." Nurses who integrate feminist philosophy into their practice may also view their female clients from a feminist perspective, challenging stereotypical characteristics of women in relation to ability, beauty, and health (Sampselle 1990). Recently the federal government has been challenged regarding funding for research in women's health problems. As a result, a new concern for women's issues has emerged.

Professions that were once almost inaccessible to women are now actively recruiting women. Nursing now competes with law, medicine, technology, science, and business for qualified applicants to nursing education programs. Gordon (1991, p. 48) suggests that women are now empowered to promote caring ideals in our society—"we need to value care not only to save the caregiving professions, but because we must protect, defend, and expand this human activity upon which society depends."

In summary, the feminist movement challenges nurses to integrate the characteristics of caring, nurturing, power and empowerment, assertiveness and advocacy, and independence and collaboration into a holistic approach to client care and personal care. To care for the client is to improve self, and to improve self is to care for the client.

CHAPTER HIGHLIGHTS

▶ Nursing as a subgroup of society has existed throughout the history of humankind.

▶ From primitive to contemporary societies, care of the sick has been influenced by many factors, such as superstition and magic, Greek and Roman mythology, religion, male-female role proscriptions, legislation, wars, and so on.

▶ Male-female role proscriptions traditionally attributed the care and nurturing functions to women, although in the third century in Rome the Parabolani brotherhood provided care to the sick and dying during the great plague in Alexandria, and early hospitals in India were staffed largely by male nurses.

▶ The first sanitary legislation, the Mosaic Health Code, was contributed by ancient Hebrew culture. This code differentiated "clean" and "unclean."

▶ The Christian value of "love thy neighbor as thyself" and the parable of the Good Samaritan impacted greatly on the development of Western nursing.

▶ During the Dark Ages, religious beliefs of the Church encouraged comfort of the sick and poor but little was done to prevent illness or cure disease.

▶ During the Middle Ages, male and female religious, military, and secular orders with the primary purpose of caring for the sick were established. Examples are the Knights Hospitalers of St. John, the Alexian Brotherhood, the Augustinian Sisters, and the Sisters of Charity founded by St. Vincent de Paul in France.

▶ In 1836 the Order of Deaconesses operated a small hospital and training school in Kaiserwerth, Germany, where Florence Nightingale "trained."

▶ The eighteenth and nineteenth centuries contributed a scientific revolution in medicine, the industrial revolution, and economic revolution, all of which impacted on nursing.

▶ The Nightingale Training School for nurses was opened in 1860 as a result of public funds and influenced nursing practices during the Crimean War.

CHAPTER HIGHLIGHTS *(continued)*

▸ The development of nursing in the Americas started with the Augustinian Sisters in Canada. Jeanne Mance founded the Hotel Dieu in Montreal in 1644 and Mother Elizabeth Seton established the first American order of the Sisters of Charity of St. Joseph in Maryland.

▸ Wars have influenced nursing practice substantially, the first result being the Nightingale Training School. In addition, nurse corps were developed for the armed forces. Army hospitals were established, and programs of nursing education were developed.

▸ Contemporary nursing practice is influenced by many factors, including economics, the nursing shortage, consumer demands, changing family structures, science and technology, legislation, demography, the women's movement, and the leadership of professional nursing associations.

LEARNING ACTIVITIES

■ Interview a nurse who has been practicing for several years to determine the changes that she or he has observed in nursing practice, nursing education, and nursing administration, then give possible reasons for the changes.

■ Review a current newspaper for local, regional, and national events that may impact nursing and health care. Events may be economic, political, legislative, scientific, environmental, and so on. How will these events affect nursing? Will they have a positive or negative impact? How can nurses and the nursing profession meet these challenges?

■ In your opinion, what impact has the feminist movement had on nurses and the nursing profession? What are the positive effects? Are there negative effects? How might the nurse incorporate the positive aspects of the feminist movement in the enhancement of professional nursing practice?

READINGS AND REFERENCES

SUGGESTED READINGS

Dolan, J. A., Fitzpatrick, M. L., and Hermann, E. K. 1983. *Nursing in society: A historical perspective.* 15 ed. Philadelphia: W. B. Saunders Co.

This text provides a concise, yet systematic history of nursing. Nursing is depicted against the societal setting and the cultural and scientific background of the history of humankind. This text links the history of nursing to social history.

Donahue, P. M. 1985. *Nursing: The finest art: An illustrated history.* St. Louis: C. V. Mosby.

This book, according to Donahue, is the "demonstration of the historical development of nursing from primitive times to the present through an integration of a variety of selected illustrations and written text."

REFERENCES

American Nurses' Association. April, 1979. Credentialing in nursing: A new approach. Report of the Committee for the Study of Credentials in Nursing. *American Journal of Nursing* 79:674–683.

Baer, E. D. February, 1991. Even her feminist friends see her as "only" a nurse. *International Herald Tribune.*

Baly, M. 1986. *Florence Nightingale and the nursing legacy.* London: Croom Helm Ltd.

Chaska, N. J., editor. 1990. *The Nursing profession: Turning points.* St. Louis: C. V. Mosby.

Davis, A. T. April, 1991. America's first school of nursing: The New England Hospital for Women and Children. *Journal of Nursing Education* 30:158–61.

De Crosto, T., May/June 1985. Mega trends in nursing: Ten new directions that are changing your profession. *Nursing Life* 5:17–21.

Dolan, J., Fitzpatrick, M. L., and Hermann, E. 1983. *Nursing in society: A historical perspective.* 15th ed., Philadelphia: W. B. Saunders.

Donahue, B., and English D., 1973. *Nursing: The finest art: An illustrated history.* St. Louis: C. V. Mosby.

Ehrenreich, B., and English, D. 1973. *Witches, midwives, and nurses: A history of women healers.* Old Westbury, N.Y. The Feminist Press.

Ellis, J. R., and Hartley, C. L. 1988. *Nursing in today's world:*

Challenges, issues and trends. 3d ed. Philadelphia: J. B. Lippincott.

Gordon, S. February, 1991. Fear of caring: The feminist paradox. *American Journal of Nursing* 91:44–48.

Graham, N. O., and Sheppard, C. 1990. Realities in retention and recruitment. In Chaska, N. L., editor. *The nursing profession: Turning points.* St. Louis: C. V. Mosby.

Haggerty, J. J. 1989. *Spinoff.* National Aeronautics and Space Administration. Washington, D.C.: U.S. Government Printing Office.

Inglehart, J. K. September, 1987. Problems facing the nursing profession. *New England Journal of Medicine* 317:646–51.

Kelly, L. Y. 1985. *Dimensions of professional nursing.* 5 ed. N.Y.: Macmillan.

Lindberg, J. B., Hunter, M. L., and Kurszewski, A. Z. 1990. *Introduction to nursing: Concepts, issues, and opportunities.* Philadelphia: J. B. Lippincott.

McCloskey, J. C., and Grace, H. K. 1990. *Current issues in nursing.* 3d ed. St. Louis: C. V. Mosby.

National Aeronautics and Space Administration. Aerospace spinoffs: *Twenty-five years of technology transfer.*

Nornhold, P. January, 1990. 90 predictions for the 90's. *Nursing* 90:34–41.

Powell, D. J. January/February 1984. Nurses–"high touch" entrepreneurs. *Nursing Economics* 2:33–36.

Rogers, M. E. 1985. High touch in a high-tech future. Paper presented at the National League for Nursing convention, San Antonio, Texas.

Sampselle, C. M. Winter, 1990. The influence of feminist philosophy on nursing practice. *Image* 22:243–47.

Smolan, R., Moffitt, P., and Naythons, M. 1990. *The power to heal: Ancient arts and modern medicine.* New York: Prentice-Hall.

Will, G. F. August, 1988. The dignity of nursing. *Nursing 88* 18:64.

Professional Socialization

CONTENTS

TYPES AND CHARACTERISTICS OF SOCIALIZATION

Socialization can be defined as the process by which people learn to become members of society (Berger and Berger 1975) or as the process by which people learn the social rules defining relationships into which they will enter (Tepperman and Richardson 1986). In short, socialization makes people skilled at following the rules for living. Although socialization goes on throughout life, the changes are most dramatic in childhood. By the time children begin school, they have learned to follow the rules given by people in authority (primarily adults),

to cooperate with others, especially peers, to accept certain responsibilities, and to carry out assigned tasks at home.

The rules and roles learned in socialization are compatible with the values learned in acculturation. *Acculturation* is the process by which members of a society learn its culture and norms (Tepperman and Richardson 1986). The learning of cultural values is largely an unstructured and unconscious process. For example, young children are unaware that they are learning to speak the society's language. Related to acculturation and socialization is *assimilation,* the process by which members of non-dominant cultural groups learn the values and behaviors of the dominant culture into which they have relocated.

Sociologists have categorized socialization into primary and secondary phases. *Primary socialization* is early socialization that occurs from birth to adolescence. It is the process during which "children learn language, symbols, mores, norms, and values and develop a diverse set of cognitive skills that enable them to cope with the wide range of interactions they will experience during their lifetime" (Shaffir and Turowetz, 1987, p. 136). Because children have less power than adults and are unaware of alternatives, early primary socialization is largely imposed. However, socialization can also be *reciprocal*. Mutual learning usually occurs between peers but may also occur between children and parents or between students and teachers. Children influence parents and teachers in many ways, especially in situations where there is mutual respect, when the adult's exercise of power is not excessive, and when affection is high. Children may, for example, influence parents in their involvement in sports, leisure, personal care, politics, and attitudes toward handicapped persons, drugs, sexuality, and minority groups. Socialization therefore is usually considered a two-way process.

Characteristics of Socialization

- It is a lifelong process by which a person learns the ways of a group or society in order to become a functioning participant.

- It is a reciprocal learning process brought about by interaction with other people.

- It involves all of a person's interactions with various agents of socialization—family, teachers, peers, media. Interactions may be conscious or unconscious, formal or informal.

- It is a universal process that varies according to a person's social class, ethnic origin, sex, and religion.

- It is a process that produces attitudes, values, knowledge, and skills required to participate effectively as an individual or a group member.

- It establishes boundaries of behavior.

- It develops a social self or awareness of others and their expectations.

- It is basic to group continuity and stability.

Secondary, or *adult, socialization* is the ongoing process of learning to adjust to new situations. Secondary socialization differs from primary socialization in that adults bring to new situations an accumulation of previous learning experiences and certain preconceptions about each new role. In secondary socialization, new values and appropriate behavior are developed for adult positions and group memberships. Every time a person enters a new group or assumes a new role (for example, becomes a nursing student, starts a new job, gets married, becomes a parent or grandparent), that person undergoes a period of formal or informal preparation or socialization for this new role. Even when an adult learns about a new set of beliefs through another person or exchanges ideas in a new social setting, the person is becoming socialized. Socialization is therefore an ongoing series of processes that continues throughout the life cycle. It is an adaptive process in which people learn about new and varied ways to look at the world. Characteristics of socialization are summarized in the accompanying box.

Anticipatory socialization is the process by which people prepare themselves for roles to which they aspire but which they do not yet occupy (Lundy and Warme 1986). In anticipatory socialization, there is some conscious motivation on the part of the person to acquire the skills and values of a given role. The person imagines what the new experience will be like.

Resocialization entails learning a different way of looking at the world and is the process of changing behavior in rather dramatic ways. This becomes necessary whenever a person starts a new job, joins a club, changes marital status, or immigrates to another country, for example. Resocialization may or may not be a matter of free choice. For example, families generally choose to relocate for school or work. In other cases, however, resocialization is brought about by social changes beyond a person's control, as when the nature of a job is completely altered by technology.

In some situations, resocialization can create conflict with earlier experiences. Thus, conflict may be experienced by a worker promoted to supervisor or a staff nurse promoted to charge nurse. As a worker or staff nurse, the person may have felt loyal to workers and opposed to management, but as a supervisor or charge nurse the nurse must feel loyal to management. The structure and rules associated with specific roles and relationships, i.e., worker/supervisor or staff nurse/charge nurse, create conflict. People usually resolve conflict through resocialization and accomplish the transition even though it may not always be smooth.

SOCIALIZATION FOR PROFESSIONAL NURSING PRACTICE

Professional (or occupational) socialization is a very important part of adult socialization. People's work identities can be one of the most important parts of their social identities, since they are often judged by the ways in which they do their jobs and by how successful they are at achieving their goals. Watson (1981, p. 19) defines *professional socialization* as "the process whereby the values and norms of the profession are internalized into one's own behavior and concept of self; it is the process whereby the knowledge, skills, and attitudes characteristic of a profession are acquired." Hinshaw (1986, p. 20) defines socialization as "the process of learning new roles and the adaptation to them, and as such, continual processes by which individuals become members of a social group." She points out that from the perspective of professional nursing, the adult socialization/resocialization process focuses on the provision of values and behaviors basic to the delivery of quality client care. Standards for this process are derived from the norms of service professions and guide the specific role of professional nurses. Styles (1978, p. 29) in her analysis of the socialization process referred to this phenomenon simply as "the development of a professional soul."

Obviously, each person enters a nursing education program with many personal values that reflect the person's culture. Some of these values influence the person's choice of nursing as a career and during ongoing professional development through life-long learning. The professional educational concept of the nurse is one who does the following (Hinshaw 1977, p. 5):

- Defines clients in terms of health and promoting and maintaining health
- Views the relationship between the nurse and clients as a therapeutic and analytic process
- Learns technical mastery of procedures and tools from the aspect of principles guiding their use
- Uses critical inquiry and creativity processes to manipulate knowledge in relation to the client's concerns
- Accepts responsibility and accountability for client care decisions

The socialization process therefore involves changes in knowledge, skills, attitudes, and values—changes that are often associated with strong emotional reactions and conflict.

Critical Values of Professional Nursing

It is within the nursing educational program that professional values are developed, clarified, and internalized. Specific professional nursing values are stated in nursing codes of ethics (see Chapter 11), in standards of nursing practice (see Chapter 1), and in the legal system itself (see Chapter 10). Watson (1981, pp. 20–21) outlines four values critical for the profession of nursing:

1. A strong commitment to the service that nursing provides for the public
2. Belief in the dignity and worth of each person
3. A commitment to education
4. Autonomy

The first value, a strong commitment to the service that nursing provides for the public, is considered essential. Nursing is a helping, humanistic service directed to the health needs of individuals, families, and communities. The nurse's role is therefore focused on *health* and *care*. Nurses, being responsible for assessing and promoting the health status of all humans, need to value their contribution to the health and well-being of people. Since "care and caring is the central core and essence of nursing" (Watson 1979), nurses also need to value the caring aspect of nursing.

The second value—the dignity and worth of each person—is based on Judeo-Christian philosophy of the sacredness of human life and the worth of the individual. Because nursing is a person-oriented profession, a basic value of the worth of each person regardless of nationality, race, creed, color, age, sex, politics, social class, and health status is basic to nursing. Applied to nursing practice this value means that the nurse always acts in the best interest of the client.

Commitment to education, the third value, reflects the lifelong value of learning in North American society. In terms of professional nursing, continuous education is needed for graduates to maintain and expand their level of competencies to meet professional criteria, to anticipate the role of the nurse in the future, and to expand the body of professional knowledge. Nurses need to question nursing knowledge and practice critically, to contribute to nursing's theoretical base, and to test theories in nursing practice.

The fourth value—autonomy, or the right of self-determination as a profession—is "the one where the greatest emphasis should be placed at this time" (Watson 1981, p. 21). Watson points out that "nurses must have freedom to use their knowledge and skills for human betterment and the authority and ability to see that nursing service is delivered safely and effectively." A future challenge for nurses is to become more assertive in promoting nursing care and to develop the ability for independent behavior.

Process of Socialization

Several models have been developed to explain the initial process of socialization into professional roles. The models described here include those of Simpson, Davis, Hinshaw, and Dreyfus. Each model outlines a sequential set of phases or "chain of events" beginning at the role of a lay person and ending at the role of a professional. Table 3–1 summarizes each model.

Ida Harper Simpson   Simpson (1967) outlines three distinct phases of professional socialization. In the first phase, the person concentrates on becoming proficient in specific work tasks. In the second phase, the person becomes attached to significant others in the work or reference group. In the third and final phase, the person internalizes the values of the professional group and adopts the prescribed behaviors.

Fred Davis   Davis (1966) describes a six-stage doctrinal conversion process among nursing students.

Stage 1: Initial innocence   When students enter a professional program, they have an image of what they expect to become and how they should act or behave.

Nursing students usually enter a nursing program with a service orientation and expect to look after sick people. However, educational experiences often differ from what the students expect. During this phase students may express disappointment and frustration at experiences provided and may question their value.

Stage 2: Labeled recognition of incongruity
In this phase students begin to identify, articulate, and share their concerns. They learn that they are not alone in their value incongruencies: peers share the same concerns.

Stages 3 and 4: "Psyching out" and role simulation   At this point, the basic cognitive framework for the internalization of professional nursing values begins to take shape. Students begin to identify the behaviors they are expected to demonstrate and through role modeling begin to practice the behaviors. In Davis's terms, this process becomes a matter of "psyching out" the faculty. The more effectively the role simulation is done, the more authentic the person believes the behavior to be, and it becomes part of the person. However, students may feel they are "playing a game" and are being "untrue to oneself," resulting in feelings of guilt and estrangement.

Stage 5: Provisional internalization   In stage five, students vacillate between commitment to their former image of nursing and performance of new behaviors attached to the professional image. Factors that increase the students' use of the new professional image

TABLE 3–1   *Models of Socialization into Professional Roles*

Simpson (1967) Model	Davis (1966) Doctrinal Conversion Model	Hinshaw (1986) Model	Dreyfus (1980) Model
Stage 1 Proficiency in specific work tasks	*Stage 1* Initial innocence	*Phase I* Transition of anticipatory role expectations to role expectations of societal group	*Stage 1* Novice
Stage 2 Attachment to significant others in the work environment	*Stage 2* Labeled recognition of incongruity		*Stage 2* Advanced beginner
Stage 3 Internalization of the values of the professional group and adoption of the behaviors it prescribes	*Stage 3* "Psyching out" and role simulation	*Phase II* Attachment to significant others/Labeling incongruencies	*Stage 3* Competent
	Stage 4 Increasing role simulation		*Stage 4* Proficient
	Stage 5 Provisional internalization	*Phase III* Internalization of role values/behaviors	*Stage 5* Expert
	Stage 6 Stable internalization		

are an increasing ability to use professional language and an increasing identification with professional role models, e.g., nursing faculty.

Stage 6: Stable internalization   During stage six, the student's behavior reflects the educationally and professionally approved model. However, preparation of the student for the work setting is only the initial process in socialization. New values and behaviors continue to be formed in the work setting.

Ada Sue Hinshaw   Hinshaw (1986) provides a three-phase general model of socialization that is an adaptation of Simpson's model.

Phase I: Transition of anticipatory role expectations to role expectations of societal group
During the first phase, individuals change their images of the role from anticipated concepts to the expectations of the persons who are setting the standards for them. Hinshaw states that (a) adults entering a profession have already learned a number of roles and values that help them to evaluate new roles and (b) these individuals are actively involved in the socialization process, having chosen to learn the new role expectations and enter the socialization process.

Phase II: Attachment to significant others/ Label incongruencies   This phase has two components: (a) learners attach themselves to significant others in the system, and at the same time (b) they label situations that are incongruent between their anticipated roles and those presented by the significant others. In the initial professional socialization, significant others are usually a group of faculty; in the work setting, they are selected colleagues or immediate supervisors. Hinshaw emphasizes the importance of appropriate role models in both educational programs and work settings. At this stage, individuals are able to verbalize the expected role behaviors are not what they anticipated. It is a stage that often involves strong emotional reactions to conflicting sets of expectations. Successful resolution of conflicts depends on the existence of role models who demonstrate appropriate behaviors and who show how conflicting systems of standards and values can be integrated.

Phase III: Internalization of role values/behaviors   In this final phase the student internalizes the values and standards of the new role. The degree to which values and standards are internalized and the extent to which incongruencies in role expectations are re-

solved is variable. Kelman (1961) defines three levels of value orientation. Individuals may demonstrate one or a blend of three levels:

1. *Compliance.* The person demonstrates the expected behavior to get positive reactions from others but has not internalized the values. Compliance behavior can be dismissed when it no longer elicits positive responses.
2. *Identification.* The person selectively adopts specific role behaviors that are acceptable to that person. The person may accept only expected behaviors rather than values. Identification behavior usually changes as role models change.
3. *Internalization.* The person believes in and accepts the standards of the new role. The standards are a part of the person's own value system.

Stuart and Hubert Dreyfus   The Dreyfus model of skill acquisition is based on a study of chess players and airline pilots (Dreyfus and Dreyfus 1980). Benner (1984) has applied this model to nursing and discusses implications for teaching and learning. Five levels of proficiency are described: novice, advanced beginner, competent, proficient, and expert.

Stage 1: Novice   A novice may be a nursing student or any nurse entering a clinical setting where that person has no experience. Behavior of the novice is extremely limited, inflexible, and governed by rules. Because novices have no experience for the situations they face, their performance must be guided by rules.

Stage 2: Advanced beginner   The advanced beginner can demonstrate marginally acceptable performance. The beginner has had experience with enough real situations to be aware of the meaningful "aspects" of a situation. "Aspects" require prior experience in real situations to be recognized.

Stage 3: Competent   Competence is manifested by the nurse who has been on the job in a similar situation for 2 or 3 years. It develops when the nurse consciously and deliberately plans nursing care and coordinates multiple complex care demands. The nurse at this stage demonstrates organizational ability but lacks the speed and flexibility of the proficient nurse. The competent nurse knows which aspects of care are to be considered most important and which ones can be delayed.

Stage 4: Proficient   The proficient nurse perceives situations as wholes rather than in terms of aspects. The nurse focuses on long-term goals and is oriented toward managing the nursing care of a client rather than performing specific tasks. This holistic understanding improves the decision making of the proficient nurse. Maxims are used as guides but can be applied only after a deep understanding of the situation is acquired. Maxims provide direction to what must be taken into consideration. To the competent or novice performer, maxims appear as unintelligible nuances of a situation; they can mean one thing at one time and another thing at a different time.

Stage 5: Expert The expert performer no longer relies on rules, guidelines, or maxims to connect an understanding of the situation to an appropriate action. The expert nurse intuitively grasps each situation and focuses on the accurate area of the problem without wasteful consideration of large ranges of unnecessary alternative diagnoses and solutions. The expert nurse may be inclined to say that a certain action was taken because "it felt right." Expert nurses have highly developed perceptual acuity or recognitional ability and their performance is fluid, flexible, and highly proficient. However, the nurse's highly skilled analytic ability is used in situations with which the nurse has had no previous experience.

Resocialization in the Employment Setting

When the new graduate enters the work setting, further socialization occurs. In the work setting, the nurse is faced with the need to put the values of the profession into operation in primarily bureaucratic settings that may not be supportive of professional career development (Leddy and Pepper 1989, p. 67). Various models of career stages have been developed. Two models by Dalton, Thompson, and Price (1977) and Kramer (1974) are summarized in Table 3–2.

ROLES OF THE PROFESSIONAL NURSE

The following nurse roles are ways of describing the nurse's activities in practice. Each role is described as a separate entity for the sake of clarity. However, the roles are not in actuality exclusive of one another. In practice, several roles often coincide. For example, the nurse may be acting as a client advocate while also caring, communicating, teaching or counseling, and acting as a change agent and a leader.

Carer

The caring/comforting role of the nurse has traditionally included those activities that preserve the dignity of the individual and those often referred to as the "mothering actions" in nursing. However, caring involves knowledge and sensitivity to what matters and what is important to clients. (See caring theories in Chapter 4.) The caring role is difficult to define specifically. It is the role of human relations. The chief goal of the nurse in this role is to convey understanding about what is important

TABLE 3–2 *Models of Career Development*

Dalton, Thompson, and Price Model	Kramer Model
Stage I Performs fairly routine duties under the direction of a mentor	*Stage I* Skill and routine mastery or development of technical expertise
Stage II Works independently as a competent colleague	*Stage II* Social integration; peer recognition of competence and acceptance into the group as the major concerns
Stage III Takes responsibility for influencing, guiding, directing, and developing others	*Stage III* Moral outrage at incongruities between conceptions of *bureaucratic* role associated with rules and regulations, *professional* role committed to continued learning, and *service* role concerned with the client as a person
Stage IV Influences the direction of the organization or a segment of it; has one of three roles: manager, internal entrepreneur, or idea innovator	*Stage IV* Conflict resolution by surrendering behaviors and/or values or by learning to use both the values and behaviors of the professional and bureaucratic system in a politically astute manner

Sources: G. W. Dalton, P. H. Thompson, and R. L. Price, The four stages of professional careers—A new look at performance by professionals, *Organ Dynamics,* Summer 1977 :19–42; and M. Kramer, *Reality shock: Why nurses leave nursing* (St. Louis: C. V. Mosby Co., 1974).

RESEARCH NOTE

How Similar Are the Nursing Role Identities of Students and Faculty Members?

In this study, the authors sought to determine the relationship between nursing role identities of students and faculty members in the baccalaureate nursing program at Fairleigh Dickinson University in Rutherford, N.J. The participants in the study included 309 students and 23 full-time faculty members. With the exception of the department chairperson, all of the faculty members had clinical responsibilities. Most of the faculty were members of professional organizations (83%), belonged to the nursing honor society (74%), and had recently participated in workshops (95%). To measure the congruence between the student nurses' perceptions and faculty members' opinions of the professional nursing role, Crocker and Brodie's 59-item Nurses Professional Orientation Scale (NPOS) was used.

Results indicated the following: (a) the further students had advanced in the program, the more closely their responses correlated with those of the faculty; (b) during the first year, when students begin taking nursing courses, students started to substitute a professional view of nursing for a traditional view; (c) the congruency of scores of students who had completed their sophomore year and who had taken their first clinical nursing course were significantly higher than those of entering freshmen; (d) there was a statistically significant higher relationship between students' congruency scores and the following variables: previous work experience as a nurses' aide, post–high school education before enrollment, high verbal scores on scholastic aptitude tests (SATs), high grade point averages, and high scores on the state board examination; and (e) the congruency scores of graduating seniors did not change between the time of the first survey and the time of the second, one year later, indicating that they had developed realistic role identities during the program.

Implications: Professional socialization is a complex process, and students need time to assimilate their professional identities. These authors suggest, therefore, that programs should offer both nursing courses and clinical experience under faculty guidance early on. To serve as effective role models, furthermore, faculty members should be expert clinicians as well as educators and have clinical responsibilities.

Source: B. J. Cohen and C. P. Jordet, Nursing schools: Students' beacon to professionalism? *Nursing and Health Care,* January 1988, 9:38–41.

and to provide support. The nurse supports the client by attitudes and actions that show concern for client welfare and acceptance of the client as a person, not merely a mechanical being.

Benner and Wrubel (1989, p. 4) state that "caring is central to effective nursing practice. . . . Nursing can never be reduced to mere technique and scientific knowledge because humor, anger, 'tough love,' administering medications, and even client teaching have different effects in a caring context than a noncaring one." Caring is central to most nursing interventions and an essential attribute of the expert nurse.

Communicator/Helper

Effective communication is an essential element of all helping professions, including nursing. Communication shapes relationships between nurses and clients, nurses and support persons, and nurses and colleagues. It plays a role in every action the nurse undertakes. The communication process, listening and responding skills, and ways to establish helping relationships are discussed in detail in Chapter 18.

Communication facilitates all nursing actions. The nurse communicates to other health care personnel the nursing interventions planned and implemented for each client. Planned nursing interventions are written on the client's care plan. Once the interventions are implemented, the nurse documents them on the client's record. Assessment findings, procedures implemented, and the client's responses are recorded. Pertinent information is communicated verbally by nurses at change of shift reports, when client's are transferred to another unit, at client rounds, and when clients are discharged to another health care agency. This type of communication needs to be concise, clear, and relevant.

Teacher

Teaching refers to activities by which the teacher helps the student to learn. It is an interactive process between a teacher and one or more learners in which specific learning objectives or desired behavior changes are achieved (Redman 1988, pp. 9 and 15). The focus of the behavior change is usually the acquiring of new knowledge or technical skills. The teaching process has four components—assessing, planning, implementing, and evaluating—which can be viewed as parallel to the parts of the nursing process. In the assessment phase, the nurse determines the client's learning needs and readiness to learn. During planning, specific learning goals and teaching strategies are set. During implementation, teaching strategies are enacted, and, during evaluation, learning is measured. See Chapter 19 for detailed information about the teaching/learning process.

Many factors have increased the need for health teaching by nurses. Today, there is a new emphasis on health promotion and health maintenance rather than on treatment alone; as a result, people desire and require more knowledge. Shortened hospital stays mean that the clients must be prepared to manage convalescence at home. The increase in long-term illnesses and disabilities often require that both the client and the family understand the illness and its treatment.

Counselor

Counseling is the process of helping a client to recognize and cope with stressful psychologic or social problems, to develop improved interpersonal relationships, and to promote personal growth. It involves providing emotional, intellectual, and psychologic support. In contrast to the psychotherapist, who counsels individuals with identified problems, the nurse counsels primarily healthy individuals with normal adjustment difficulties. The focus is on helping the person develop new attitudes, feelings, and behaviors rather than on promoting intellectual growth. The client is encouraged to look at alternative behaviors, recognize the choices, and develop a sense of control.

Counseling can be provided on a one-to-one basis or in groups. Often nurses lead group counseling sessions. For example, on the individual level, the nurse counsels clients who need to decrease activity levels, stop smoking, lose weight, accept changes in body image, or cope with impending death. At the group level, the nurse may be a leader, member, or resource person in any self-help group in which the nurse may assume the role of structuring activities and fostering a climate conducive to group interaction and productive work.

Obviously, counseling requires therapeutic communication skills. In addition, the nurse must be a skilled leader, able to analyze a situation, synthesize information and experiences, and evaluate the progress and productivity of the individual or group. The nurse must also be willing to model and teach desired behaviors, to be sincere when dealing with people, and to demonstrate interest and caring in the welfare of others. The nurse-leader needs an inventive mind, a flexible attitude, and a sense of humor to deal with the varied experiences of people. Essential to leadership abilities is self-awareness, self-assurance, and self-understanding.

Client Advocate and Change Agent

An *advocate* pleads the cause of another, or argues or pleads for a cause or proposal. Advocacy involves concern for and defined actions on behalf of another person or organization to effect change. A *client advocate* is an advocate of clients' rights. Kohnke (1982) describes the role of the advocate as "informing the client and then supporting him in whatever decision he makes." According to Disparti (1988), advocacy involves promoting what is best for the client, ensuring that the client's needs are met, and protecting the client's rights. Many clients need an advocate to protect their rights and to help them speak for themselves. Advocacy is discussed in greater detail in Chapter 12.

A *change agent* is a person or group who initiates changes or who assists others in making modifications in themselves or in the system (Kemp 1986). Brooten, Hayman, and Naylor (1978) describe a change agent as a professional who relies on a systematic body of knowledge about change to guide the change process. Types, theories, and the process of change are discussed in Chapter 12.

Nurses are obligated to advocate for their clients and their profession to ensure that the health needs of the client are met. Nurses are agents of change as they assist clients to modify health-destructive behaviors, and as they act to improve the quality of nursing and health care provided.

Leader

The leadership role can be applied at many different levels: individual, family, groups of clients, professional colleagues, or the larger society. At the client level, *nursing leadership* is defined as a process of interpersonal influence through which a client is assisted in the establishment and achievement of goals toward improved well-being (Leddy and Pepper 1989, p. 336). On a larger scale, leadership can be defined as translating innovative ideas into action or as influencing individuals or groups to take an active part in the process of achieving agreed-upon goals (Epstein 1982, p. 2).

Effective leadership is a learned process requiring an understanding of the needs and goals that motivate people, the knowledge to apply the leadership skills, and the interpersonal skills to influence others. The leadership role of the nurse will be discussed in Chapter 20.

Manager

There is often confusion between management and leadership, because in much of the literature, leadership is associated with group interaction within an organizational setting. *Management* is defined as "the use of delegated authority within the formal organization to organize, direct, or control responsible subordinates . . . so that all service contributions are coordinated to attain a goal" (Yura, Ozimek, and Walsh 1981, p. 5). Leadership, by contrast, may or may not require delegated authority within a formal organization.

The nurse manages the nursing care of individuals, families, and communities. The nurse-manager also delegates nursing activities to ancillary workers and other nurses, and supervises and evaluates their performance. Managing requires knowledge about organizational structure and dynamics, authority and accountability, leadership, change theory, advocacy, delegation, and supervision and evaluation. The role of the nurse as manager will be discussed in Chapter 20.

Researcher

The majority of researchers in nursing are prepared at the doctoral and postdoctoral level, although an increasing number of clinicians with master's degrees are beginning to participate in research activity as part of their nursing role. However, "if nursing is to emerge in society as a socially significant, credible, scientific, and learned profession with a commitment to high-quality patient care, then research (for all nurses) is a necessity" (Starzomski 1983). It may be unrealistic to expect each nurse to conduct a study in the clinical setting. Many constraints in clinical settings must be reckoned with before research can become a legitimate and comfortable activity. However, if nursing is to develop as a research-based practice, it is not unreasonable to expect the nurse in the clinical area to (a) have some awareness of the process and language of research, (b) be sensitive to issues related to protecting the rights of human subjects, (c) participate in the identification of significant researchable problems, and (d) be a discriminating consumer of research findings.

Nursing students learn these investigative functions early in their careers to establish the connection that "knowing how we know is fundamental to doing what we do" (Wilson 1985, p. viii). See Chapter 5 for more detailed information about the role of the researcher in nursing.

CHAPTER HIGHLIGHTS

▶ Socialization is a lifelong process by which people become functioning participants of a society or a group. It is a reciprocal learning process brought about by interaction with other people and establishes boundaries of behavior.

▶ Primary socialization occurs from birth to adolescence and is largely imposed by authority figures.

▶ Secondary socialization is the ongoing process of learning to adjust to new situations.

▶ Anticipatory socialization prepares people for the roles to which they aspire but do not yet occupy.

▶ Resocialization is the process of adapting to a very different social situation and may or may not be a matter of free choice. The most extreme form occurs in institutions that control every aspect of a person's existence.

▶ Professional socialization is the process whereby the values and norms of the profession are internalized into one's own behavior and concept of self. Knowledge, skills, and attitudes characteristic of the profession are acquired.

▶ Socialization for professional nursing requires the development of critical values, including a strong commitment to the service that nursing provides to the public, a belief in the dignity and worth of each person, a commitment to education, and autonomy.

▸ Various models of the socialization process have been developed. Such models may serve as guidelines to establish the phase and extent of an individual's socialization.

▸ In nursing practice, the nurse functions in a variety of roles that are not exclusive of one another; in reality, they often occur together. The roles serve to clarify the nurse's activities and include carer, communicator/helper, teacher, counselor, client advocate and change agent, leader, manager, and researcher.

LEARNING ACTIVITIES

■ In a small group, use Watson's four values of professional nursing (see page 31) as a framework and identify behaviors that represent these values.

READINGS AND REFERENCES

SUGGESTED READINGS

Benner, P. 1984. *From novice to expert: Excellence and power in clinical nursing practice.* Menlo Park, Calif.: Addison-Wesley Publishing Co.

This book is a major contribution to nursing. It provides a lucid description of nursing practice as it is rendered by expert nurses. It provides profound implications for nurses in administration, education, and practice.

Wierda, L. 1989. BSN students find a way to lessen the severity of reality shock. *Nursing Forum* 22:11–14.

Fear of "reality shock" influenced a group of BSN students to develop different variations in their clinical experience. The most successful and well-liked alternative was a module consisting of two students and three clients. Students said they felt more independent and liked having another person, other than the clinical instructor or staff nurses, with whom they could discuss their problems.

RELATED RESEARCH

Cohen, B. J., and Jordet, C. P. January 1988. Nursing schools: Students' beacon to professionalism? *Nursing and Health Care* 9:38–41.

Dobbs, K. K. April 1988. The senior preceptorship as a method for anticipatory socialization of baccalaureate nursing students. *Journal of Nursing Education* 27:167–71.

Langston, R. A. 1990. Comparative effects of baccalaureate and associate degree educational programs on the professional socialization of nursing students. In Chaska, N. L. *The nursing profession: Turning points.* pp. 53–58. St. Louis: C. V. Mosby Co.

SELECTED REFERENCES

Batra, C. January 1990. Socializing nurses for nursing entrepreneurship roles. *Nursing Health Care* 11:34–37.

Benner, P. 1984. *From novice to expert: Excellence and power in clinical nursing practice.* Menlo Park, Calif.: Addison-Wesley Publishing Co.

Benner, P., and Wrubel, J. 1989. *The primacy of caring: Stress and coping in health and illness.* Redwood City, Calif.: Addison-Wesley Nursing.

Berger, P., and Berger, B. 1975. *Sociology: A biographical approach.* 2d ed. New York: Basic Books.

Brooten, D. A.; Hayman, L.; and Naylor, M. 1978. *Leadership for change: A guide for the frustrated nurse.* Philadelphia: J. B. Lippincott, Co.

Cohen, B. J., and Jordet, C. P. January 1988. Nursing schools: Students' beacon to professionalism? *Nursing and Health Care* 9:38–41.

Dalton, G. W.; Thompson, P. H.; and Price, R. L. Summer 1977. The four stages of professional careers—A new look at performance by professionals. *Organ Dynamics* pp. 19–42.

Davis, F. September 1966. Professional socialization as subjective experience: The process of doctrinal conversion among student nurses. Sixth World Congress of Sociology Paper. Evian, France.

Disparti, J. 1988. Nutrition and self care. In Caliandro, G., and Judkins, B. L. *Primary nursing practice.* Glenview Ill.: Scott, Foresman & Co.

Dreyfus, S. E., and Dreyfus, H. L. February 1980. A five-stage model of the mental activities involved in directed skill acquisition. Unpublished report supported by the Air Force Office of Scientific Research (AFSC), USAF (Contract F49620–79–C–0063), University of California at Berkeley.

Hinshaw, A. S. November 1977. *Socialization and resocialization of nurses for professional nursing practice.* National League for Nursing Pub. no. 15–1659. New York: National League for Nursing.

———. 1986. Socialization and resocialization of nurses for professional nursing practice. In Hein, E. C., and Nicholson, M. J., editors. *Contemporary leadership behavior: Selected readings.* 2d ed. Boston: Little, Brown and Co.

Kelman, H. 1961. Process of opinion changes. *Public Opinion Quarterly* 25:57.

Kemp, V. H. 1986. An overview of change and leadership. In Hein, E. C., and Nicholson, M. J., editors. *Contemporary leadership behavior: Selected readings.* 2d ed. Boston: Little, Brown and Co.

Kohnke, M. F. November 1980. The nurse as advocate. *American Journal of Nursing* 80:2038–40.

Kohnke, M. F. 1982. *Advocacy: Risk and Reality.* St. Louis: C. V. Mosby Co.

Kozier, B., and Erb, G. 1988. *Concepts and issues in nursing practice.* Redwood City, Calif.: Addison-Wesley Nursing.

Kramer, M. 1974. *Reality shock: Why nurses leave nursing.* St. Louis: C. V. Mosby Co.

Leddy, S., and Pepper, J. M. 1989. *Conceptual bases of professional nursing.* 2d ed. Philadelphia: J. B. Lippincott Co.

Redman, B. K. 1988. *The process of patient education.* 6th ed. St. Louis: C. V. Mosby Co.

Shaffir, W. B., and Turowetz, A. 1987. Socialization and the self. In Rosenberg, M. M.; Shaffir, W. B.; Turowetz, A.; and Weinfeld, M., editors. *An introduction to sociology.* 2d ed. Toronto: Methuen Publications.

Simpson, I. H. Winter 1967. Patterns of socialization into professions: The case of student nurses. *Sociological Inquiry* 37:47–54.

Starzomski, R. September 1983. The place of research in nursing. *Canadian Nurse* 79:34–35.

Styles, M. M. June 1978. Why Publish? *Image: Journal of Nursing Scholarship* 10:28–32.

———. 1982. *On nursing: Toward a new endowment.* St. Louis: C. V. Mosby Co.

Tepperman, L., and Richardson, R. J., editors. 1986. *The social world: An introduction to sociology.* Toronto: McGraw-Hill Ryerson Ltd.

Watson, I. Summer 1981. Socialization of the nursing student in a professional nursing education programme. *Nursing Papers* 13:19–24.

Watson, J. 1979. *Nursing—The philosophy and science of caring.* Boston: Little, Brown and Co.

Wilson, H. S. 1985. *Research in Nursing.* Menlo Park, Calif.: Addison-Wesley Publishing Co.

———. 1989. *Research in Nursing.* Redwood City, Calif.: Addison-Wesley Nursing.

Yura, H.; Ozimek, D.; and Walsh, M. B. 1981. *Nursing leadership: Theory and process.* New York: Appleton-Century-Crofts.

Zusman, J. November/December 1982. Want some good advice? Think twice about being a patient advocate. *Nursing Life* 6:46–50.

THEORETIC FOUNDATIONS FOR PROFESSIONAL NURSING PRACTICE

Nursing Theories and Conceptual Frameworks

CONTENTS

NURSING THEORIES AND CONCEPTUAL FRAMEWORKS

Theory development is considered by many nurses to be one of the most crucial tasks facing the profession today. Historically, knowledge used by nurses has been derived from the physical and behavioral sciences. As an increasingly emerging profession, nursing is now deeply involved in identifying its own unique knowledge base—that is, the body of knowledge essential to nursing practice—or a so-called nursing science. Identification of this knowledge base requires the development and recognition of concepts and theories specific to nursing.

Theory development gained momentum in the 1960s and has progressed markedly since then through the work of several nurse theorists and the participation of nurses in theory conferences and in research to refine or validate the theories. Three approaches may be used to develop nursing theory:

1. Borrowing conceptual frameworks from other disciplines and applying them to nursing problems. The problem with this approach is that many theories are not easily applied to nursing practice.

2. Using an inductive approach; that is, looking at various aspects of nursing in nursing practice settings to discover theories and concepts that explain phenomena important to nurses.

3. Using a deductive approach; that is, looking for the compatibility or fit of a general theory of nursing with various aspects of nursing.

Nursing theories serve several essential purposes. Nursing theory (King 1978):

- Generates knowledge that facilitates improved practice
- Organizes information into logical systems
- Discovers knowledge gaps in the specific field of study
- Provides a rationale for collecting reliable and valid data about the health status of clients, which are essential for effective decision making and implementation
- Provides a measure to evaluate the effectiveness of nursing care
- Develops an organized way of studying nursing
- Guides nursing research to expand knowledge

Conceptual frameworks and models offer ways of looking at (conceptualizing) a discipline (e.g., nursing) in clear, explicit terms that can be communicated to others. Although most nurses have a clear idea of what nursing is, its uniqueness needs to be clearly stated to other health care workers and the public. Professionalism and a desire for collegial status with other health professionals have made the need for conceptual frameworks of nursing to be explicit. If nurses are to be considered health professionals, they must communicate exactly what makes their place in the interdisciplinary team unique and important.

Before conceptual frameworks are discussed, the terms *concept, model, framework, conceptual model* or *framework,* and *theory* must be clarified. A *concept* is an abstract idea or mental image of phenomena or reality. Many concepts apply to nursing: concepts about human beings, health, helping relationships, and communication. The concepts that influence nursing most significantly and determine its practice include: the *person* receiving nursing care, the *environment* in which the person exists, *health* at the time of interaction with the nurse, and *nursing actions*. Together these concepts form the *metaparadigm of nursing*. The metaparadigm is the most global perspective of any discipline, its encapsulating unit or framework. It singles out the phenomena with which the discipline deals in a unique manner. Most disciplines have a single metaparadigm, but several conceptual models provide different views of the metaparadigm concepts.

A *model is* a pattern of something to be made, an abstract outline or architectural sketch of a genuine article, or an approximation or simplification of reality. A model can also show the features of a discipline. Nursing models include only those concepts that the model builder considers relevant and that aid understanding by others.

A *framework* is a basic structure supporting anything. A *conceptual framework* is a set of concepts and statements that integrate the concepts into a meaningful configuration (Fawcett 1984, p. 2). Conceptual frameworks, however, are not made up only of concepts. They are also made up of *propositions,* statements that express the relationships between concepts. Each nurse theorist's conceptual framework proposes a different view of the metaparadigm concepts.

A conceptual model gives clear and explicit direction to the three areas of nursing: practice, education, and research. (Some nurses add a fourth field of nursing, administration; however, many consider administration a component of each of the three areas.) All conceptual models are frames of reference (conceptual and theoretical), but not all frames of reference are models in that some are not specific enough to give clear direction to practice, education, and research.

A *theory,* like a conceptual model, is made up of concepts and propositions; however, a theory accounts for phenomena with much greater specificity. The primary purpose of a theory, as opposed to a conceptual framework, is to generate knowledge in a field. A conceptual framework, by contrast, provides a guide for nursing practice, education, and research. Numerous definitions of theory exist in the literature. Most definitions include three elements:

1. A set of well-defined constructs or concepts. For example, the constructs in Imogene King's (1981) theory of goal attainment include perception, communication, interaction, transaction, self, role, growth and development, stress, time, and space.

2. A set of propositions that specify the relationships among the constructs. For example, here are a few examples of the eight propositions King developed to describe the relationship among the concepts in her theory of goal attainment (Austin and Champion 1983):

   a. If perceptual accuracy is present in nurse-client interactions, transactions (goal attainment) will occur.

   b. If role expectations and role performance as perceived by the nurse and client are congruent, transactions will occur.

c. If transactions are made in nurse-client interactions, growth and development will be enhanced.

3. Hypotheses that test the relationships between the constructs and propositions. Because theory is abstract, it cannot be applied to practice. Instead, hypotheses derived from the theory are tested. For example, here are some testable hypotheses derived from King's goal-attainment theory (King 1981):

    a. Perceptual accuracy in nurse-client interactions increases mutual goal setting.

    b. Communication increases mutual goal setting between nurses and clients and leads to satisfaction.

    c. Goal attainment decreases stress and anxiety in nursing situations.

In summary, the major distinction between a theory and a conceptual model is the level of abstraction. A conceptual model is an abstract system of related concepts. A theory is based on a conceptual model but is more limited in scope. It contains more concrete concepts with definitions and detailed explanations of the premises or hypotheses linking them together.

As there are varying opinions on the nature and structure of nursing, theories continue to be developed. Each theory bears the name of the person or group who developed it and reflects the beliefs of the developer. Some well-known theories are Virginia Henderson's (1966) complementary-supplementary model; Dorothy E. Johnson's (1980) behavioral systems model; Imogene King's (1971, 1978, 1981, 1987) systems interaction model; Madeleine Leininger's (1984) transcultural care theory; Myra Levine's (1973) conservation theory; Betty Neuman's (1982) health care systems model; Dorothea E. Orem's (1971, 1980, 1985) self-care model; Martha Roger's (1970, 1980) life process theory; and Sister Callista Roy's (1976, 1984) adaptation model. Each nursing education program is based on a conceptual framework selected or developed by the program's faculty to guide student learning and to provide a nursing model for graduates.

Components of Nursing Models

Conceptual models have three components: assumptions, a value system, and major units.

Assumptions   *Assumptions* are statements of facts (premises) or suppositions that people accept as the underlying theoretical foundation for conceptualizations about nursing. Assumptions are derived from scientific theory or practice or both, and either have been or can

be verified. Some nursing models draw assumptions from adaptation theories; others from general systems theories. Most models also draw assumptions from practice.

Assumptions differ greatly from model to model, since they are drawn from different premises. For example, assumptions about human beings (the client) vary considerably: Henderson views the client as a being with 14 fundamental needs; Roy, as a being with four modes of adaptation; Johnson, as a being with eight behavioral subsystems; and Orem, as an agent with six universal self-care requisites.

Value System   The beliefs underlying a profession are its value system. Generally, these beliefs are similar from model to model. Some of them are the following:

- Nurses have a unique function even though they share certain functions with other health professionals.

- Nursing is a service directed toward meeting the needs of well or ill persons or groups (families and communities) rather than directed toward specific aspects of disease or illness.

- Nursing uses a systematic process (see Chapter 6) to operationalize its conceptual model.

- Nursing involves a series of interpersonal relationships. The nurse-client relationship (helping relationship) is of major importance. See Chapter 18.

Margretta Styles believes that the nursing profession must have a common ideology, just as nations have their pledges of allegiance, societies their oaths, and religions their creeds. Styles proposes a series of beliefs about the nature and purpose of nursing, as outlined in the box on the following page.

Major Units   Seven major units of nursing models are constructed from the assumptions and values: (a) Goal of nursing, (b) client (patient), (c) role of the nurse, (d) source of difficulty of the client, (e) intervention focus, (f) modes of intervention, and (g) consequences of nursing activity. A summary of these units in the major conceptual models is given in Table 4–1 on page 48.

Goal of nursing   The goal is the end or aim of nursing, what nursing is trying to achieve. This goal has to agree with the goals common to all health professionals—to improve health, to maintain health, to prevent health problems, to restore health, etc. However, each health discipline has a goal distinct enough to justify the presence of that discipline on the health team. Specific nursing goals vary from model to model, depending on its assumptions about people. Goals need to be broad enough (a) to indicate what end the nursing profession is working toward, (b) to indicate what to teach future practitioners, and (c) to apply to nursing practice in all practice settings (community, hospital, home, health center, etc.). Before the 20th century, Florence Nightingale believed the goal of nursing was to make the patient as comfortable as possible and to put the patient in the best possible condition for nature to act and for the physician's treatment to take effect. For current goals of nursing, see Table 4–1.

Client   The client unit refers not only to the intended recipient(s) of nursing service but also to conceptions about that person or group. Most models indicate that the client is a biopsychosocial being, but they differ in exactly how the client is conceptualized as such. Henderson views the client as a whole, complete, independent being who has 14 fundamental needs, while John-son views the client as a behavioral system composed of eight subsystems. See Table 4–1 for further information.

Role of the nurse   The role of the nurse must be wanted, needed, and accepted by society just as the physician's curative role or the lawyer's defending role is wanted and accepted. Many nurses consider their role to be one of "caring"; however, caring is a vague concept that is difficult to operationalize. In Orem's self-care model, the role of the nurse is to provide assistance to influence the client's development in achieving an optimal level of self-care; in Roy's adaptation model, the nurse's role is to promote the client's adaptive behaviors by manipulating stimuli. See Table 4–1 for additional information.

Source of difficulty   The source of difficulty resides with the client, not the nurse. In other words, it is the probable origin or cause of any client problems amenable to nursing intervention. Clients in health care agencies have health problems that may be subcategorized as medical, psychologic, dietary, nursing, etc. The physician deals with medical problems, the psychologist or psychiatrist with psychologic problems, the dietitian with dietary problems, and the nurse with nursing problems. The source of difficulty is an explicit statement of the nursing problem. For example, in Henderson's model, the origin of the client's problem is lack of strength, will, or knowledge; in Johnson's model, it is functional or structural stress. Table 4–1 lists the sources of difficulty identified by other theorists.

Intervention focus   Another unit of each model is the target or focus of nursing intervention. The universally accepted intervention focus for the physician is the client's pathology. In Orem's self-care model, the intervention focus for nurses is a deficit in the client's ability to maintain self-care; in Roy's adaptation model, it is the stimuli the client is having difficulty adapting to. See Table 4–1 for additional information.

Modes of intervention   The modes of intervention unit clarifies the means at the nurse's disposal when intervening. It is closely allied to the intervention focus and spells out specific ways in which the nurse helps the client. For example, in Roy's adaptation model the intervention focus is stimuli and the mode of intervention is manipulation of the stimuli. In contrast, Florence Nightingale believed the mode of intervention was manipulation of the environment. This was done by providing warmth, fresh air, light, food, and sanitation. See Table 4–1 for other intervention modes.

Consequences   The last unit states the expected consequences of nursing actions. It reflects the nursing goal and the concept of the client. See Table 4–1 for the consequences identified by specific models.

One Model Versus Several Models

Many nurses believe that there are advantages to having a single, universal model for nursing for these reasons:

- It would further the development of nursing as a profession.
- It would give all nurses a common framework, enhancing communication and research.
- It would promote understanding about the nurse's role in nontraditional nursing settings, such as independent nurse practitioner practice, self-help clinics, and health maintenance organizations (HMOs), since

many people believe nurses provide care for only sick persons.

In contrast, advocates of several different conceptual models point out the following:

- Most disciplines have several conceptual models, which allow members to explore phenomena in different ways and from different viewpoints.
- Several models increase an understanding of the nature of nursing and its scope.
- Several models foster development of the full scope and potential of the discipline.

It is possible that in the 21st century many more models for nursing will be developed or that existing ones will be refined in accordance with societal needs and with their tested usefulness.

Relationship to the Nursing Process

Conceptual models for nursing are abstractions that are operationalized or made real by the use of the nursing process. See Chapters 6–9 for detailed information on the nursing process. This systematic process, similar to the scientific or problem-solving process, consists of five steps:

1. *Assessing.* The specific data collected about a client's health needs relate directly to the second unit of the conceptual model for nursing, the client. For example, if the client is seen as having 14 fundamental needs, data are collected about these 14 needs.
2. *Diagnosing.* In this step, the assessment data are analyzed to identify actual, potential, and possible nursing diagnoses. The client's actual or potential health problems are outlined or written as a nursing diagnostic statement in accordance with the nursing model used.
3. *Planning.* Planning also relates directly to the conceptual nursing model. Goals for resolution of client problems, nursing interventions aimed at achieving those goals, and outcome criteria by which the nurse can evaluate whether or not the goals are met are established in accordance with the modes of intervention outlined in the conceptual model.
4. *Implementing.* Implementing the planned interventions draws on scientific knowledge that is not part of the nursing model. The nursing model instructs the nurse what to do and directly influences what nursing interventions are planned, but it does not tell the nurse how to do it.

(continued on page 52)

TABLE 4-1 *Summary of Major Units from Selected Conceptual Models for Nursing* *

Theorist	Goal of Nursing	Client	Role of the Nurse
Virginia Henderson (1966): Complementary-supplementary model	Independence in the satisfaction of human beings' 14 fundamental needs	A whole, complete and independent being who has 14 fundamental needs to breathe, eat and drink, eliminate, move and maintain posture, sleep and rest, dress and undress, maintain body temperature, keep clean, avoid danger, communicate, worship, work, play, and learn	A complementary-supplementary role to maintain or restore independence in the satisfaction of clients' 14 fundamental needs
Martha Rogers (1970, 1980): Science of unitary human beings	Achievement of maximum health potential	A unified whole possessing integrity and manifesting characteristics that are more than and different from the sum of its parts; an organized patterned energy field that continually exchanges matter and energy with the environmental energy field, resulting in continuous repatterning. The human being has the capacity for abstraction and imagery, language and thought, and sensation and emotion	To help clients develop patterns of living that accommodate environmental changes rather than conflict with them
Imogene King (1971, 1978, 1981, 1987): Systems interaction model	Attainment, maintenance, or restoration of health to allow clients to achieve maximum potential for daily living and to function in social roles	Three interacting systems: individuals (personal systems), groups (interpersonal systems), and society, (social systems); the personal system is a unified, complex, whole self who perceives, thinks, desires, imagines, decides, identifies goals, and selects means to achieve them	An interaction process

*The models are listed in chronologic order.

TABLE 4-1 *(continued)*

Source of Client Difficulty	Intervention Focus	Modes of Intervention	Consequences of Nursing Activity
Lack of strength, will, or knowledge	The deficit that is the source of client difficulty	Actions to replace, complete, substitute, add, reinforce, or increase strength, will, or knowledge	1. Increased independence in satisfaction of the client's 14 fundamental needs, or 2. Peaceful death
Unharmonious person-environment interactions that are determined by social values	Coordinating environmental field and human field rhythmicities	Actions to promote harmonious interaction between the client and environment, to strengthen the integrity of the human field, and to direct and redirect patterning of the human and environmental fields	Maximum health potential, unity, and increasing complexity of organization
Stressors in the internal and external environment	Perception of client difficulty and goal setting through communication	Interaction process in which both client and nurse perceive and communicate, thus creating action; actions result in reactions, and, if there is no disturbance, goals may be set, means to achieve them explored and agreed upon, and transactions made	Goal attainment

Theorist	Goal of Nursing	Client	Role of the Nurse
Dorothea Orem (1971, 1980, 1985): Self-care model	Achievement of optimal client self-care so that clients can achieve and maintain an optimal health state	A unity who can be viewed as functioning biologically, symbolically, and socially and who initiates and performs self-care activities on own behalf in maintaining life, health, and well-being; self-care activities deal with air, water, food, elimination, activity and rest, solitude and social interaction, hazards to life and well-being, and being normal (the tendency to conform to the norm)	To provide assistance to influence clients' development in achieving an optimal level of self-care
Myra Levine (1973): Conservation model	Promotion of wholeness	Holistic being: an open system of systems that in its wholeness expresses the organization of all its parts; the person retains personal integrity through adaptive capability; the life process of the system is unceasing change that has direction, purpose, and meaning	Therapeutic, i.e., to influence adaptation favorably or move client toward renewed social well-being; or supportive, i.e., to maintain the status quo
Sister Callista Roy (1976, 1981, 1984): Adaptation model	Adaptation in each of the four adaptive modes in situations of health and illness	A biopsychosocial being who is in constant interaction with the environment and who has four modes of adaptation, based on: physiologic needs, self-concept (physical self, moral-ethical self, self-consistency, self-ideal and expectancy, and self-esteem), role function, and interdependence relations	To promote clients' adaptive behaviors by manipulating focal, contextual, and residual stimuli
Dorothy Johnson (1980): Behavioral systems model	Behavioral system equilibrium and dynamic stability	A behavioral system composed of seven subsystems: affiliative, achievement, dependence, aggressive, eliminative, ingestive, and sexual	A regulator and controller of behavioral system stability and equilibrium

TABLE 4-1 *(continued)*

Source of Client Difficulty	Intervention Focus	Modes of Intervention	Consequences of Nursing Activity
Any interference with self-care, by a person, object, condition, event, circumstance, or any combination of interferences	Inability to maintain self-care (a deficit in the self-care agency)	Five general ways of assisting: acting for or doing for, guiding, supporting, providing a developmental environment, and teaching	Achievement of the client's optimal level of self-care
Altered relationship with the internal and external environment	Enhancing patterns of adaptive response	Four conservation principles: actions to conserve energy, structural integrity, personal integrity, and social integrity	Adaptive responses that retain wholeness
Coping activity that is inadequate to maintain integrity in the face of a need deficit or excess	The focal, contextual, and residual stimuli	Manipulation of the stimuli by increasing, decreasing, and/or maintaining them	Adaptive responses to stimuli by the client
Functional or structural stress; inadequate development or stimulation of the system or its parts; breakdown in regulatory system; exposure to noxious influences; lack of environmental input	1. The mechanisms of control and regulation 2. The functional requirements	Imposing external regulatory control mechanisms; changing structural units; fulfilling functional requirements; helping to regulate subsystem balance	Efficient and effective client behavior

▶

Theorist	Goal of Nursing	Client	Role of the Nurse
Betty Neuman (1982): Health care systems model	Attainment and maintenance of client system equilibrium	Open system consisting of a basic structure or central core of survival factors surrounded by concentric rings that are bounded by lines of resistance, a normal line of defense, and a flexible line of defense. The total person is a composite of physiologic, psychologic, sociocultural, and developmental variables	To identify intrapersonal, interpersonal, and extrapersonal stressors and assist the individual to respond to stressors
Rosemarie Parse (1987): Human-living-health model	Transforming or changing health patterns	An open being, more than and different from the sum of its parts, in mutual simultaneous interchange with the environment, who chooses from options (value priorities) and bears responsibility for choices	Guided by three principles: meaning, rhythmicity, and cotranscendence; exploration of personal meanings of lived experiences (meaningful moments); helping clients to illuminate different rhythms; presenting energizing ways of becoming or reaching beyond what *is* toward the possible; helping clients to experience a shift in everyday rhythms.

5. *Evaluating.* Evaluating is a continuous nursing function. How is the client adjusting and reacting? What does the client see as needs? How does the client see these needs changing? Has the client achieved the desired consequences? The answers to these questions help the nurse evaluate the effectiveness of the total nursing process and the nursing model.

Relationship of Nursing Theory to Research

Because the primary purpose of nursing theory is to generate scientific knowledge, nursing theory and nursing research are closely related. Scientific knowledge is derived from testing hypotheses generated by theories for nursing. Research determines the utility of those hypotheses, and research findings may be developed into theories for nursing. In the research process, comparisons are made between the observed outcomes of research and the relationship predicted by the hypotheses.

Several approaches can be used to test or develop theory:

- *Inductive.* Research is first conducted, and the findings are used to develop a theory. In this inductive method, a theory is developed from multiple data. The following premise and conclusion illustrate the inductive method: If X (e.g., low self-esteem) is true of persons A1, A2, . . . , A100, and if the persons are all members of the same class (e.g., rape victims) then X is true of all members of that class.

- *Deductive.* A theory is devised, hypotheses generated, and then research is conducted. For example, in deductive research a premise (hypothesis) is first proposed, e.g., all rape victims have low self-esteem. Among many others, Mary, Joan, Ellen, and Judy are

TABLE 4-1 *(continued)*

Source of Client Difficulty	Intervention Focus	Modes of Intervention	Consequences of Nursing Activity
Intrapersonal, interpersonal, and extrapersonal stressors in the internal and external environments	Strengthening normal and flexible lines of defense and reducing stress factors	Primary intervention, i.e., strengthening the person's flexible line of defense; secondary prevention, i.e., strengthening internal lines of resistance; and tertiary prevention, i.e., maintaining the person's existing energy resources	Reconstitution, i.e., movement from a variance of wellness to the desired level of wellness and client system stability
Patterns of relating and values at a given moment	Provision of attentive listening (true presence) or empathetic sounding board for clients to express and therefore uncover the meaning of thoughts, feelings, values, and changing views	Illuminating meaning by explicating what is happening through language; synchronizing rhythms by *dwelling with* the flow of connecting-separating; mobilizing transcendence by moving toward possibles in transforming	Changed health patterns

rape victims, and their level of self-esteem is tested. Because it is low, it is concluded that the hypothesis is valid.

■ *Combined.* Both inductive and deductive methods are used.

SELECTED THEORETICAL VIEWS OF HUMAN BEINGS

The nurse's view of human beings influences the focus of nursing interventions. Although most nurses agree that humans are biopsychosocial beings, they differ in how they view human beings as recipients of nursing services. Nursing theorists have developed these viewpoints from systems, adaptation, and interactive theories. The conceptualizations of the client according to

selected nursing theorists are summarized in Table 4–1, above.

The Person as a System

The human being is an *open system* in constant interaction with a changing environment (Roy 1980, p. 180). Systems theory is discussed later in this chapter. In other words, the individual engages in a dynamic interchange with the environment, and this interchange is an essential factor of the system's viability, reproductive ability or continuity, and ability to change. Constant input (stimuli) into the system and feedback to it maintain the system in a state of dynamic equilibrium. This premise directs the nurse to look at environmental factors influencing the system and to provide nursing interventions that help the client maintain and achieve a state of dynamic equilibrium.

Human beings interact with the environment by adjusting themselves to it or adjusting it to themselves (Neuman 1980, p. 122). This premise directs the nurse to look at ways the client handles changing situations. Does the client withdraw from the environment, alter the environment, or alter self?

Humans are open systems with many interrelated subsystems. Because humans are biopsychosocial beings, their biologic, psychologic, social, and spiritual components can be regarded as systems with hierarchic subsystems. (See systems theory later in this chapter.)

The *biologic system* can be subdivided into the neurologic, musculoskeletal, respiratory, circulatory, gastrointestinal, and urinary subsystems, among others. Each subsystem can in turn be subdivided. For example, the urinary system consists of the kidneys, the ureters, and the bladder. The biologic system can also be subdivided into categories of needs or functional health patterns or activities of daily living, such as nutrition and hydration, sleep/rest, activity/exercise, elimination, etc.

The *psychologic and social systems* consist of subsystems that include thinking, feeling, and interaction patterns. Names of the psychologic and social subsystems vary considerably according to the individual nursing theorist and model. For example, Johnson (1980, p. 228), who describes the human system in terms of behaviors, lists the following psychologic subsystems: affiliative, dependency, aggressive/protective, and achievement. Orem (1980, p. 316) categorizes the psychologic and social systems as conditions of being alone or with people, situations that threaten the well-being of the individual, and the tendency to conform to the norm. (See Table 4–1.)

According to King (1976, p. 51) the primary concerns of nursing are human behavior, social interactions, and social movements. Therefore, she includes three dynamic interacting systems in her concept of person: individuals (*personal systems*), groups (*interpersonal systems*), and society (*social systems*). Each of these systems has a set of related concepts that King sees as relevant for understanding human beings.

The Person as an Adaptive System

Adaptation is a process of change allowing the individual to respond to environmental changes yet retain personal integrity or wholeness (Levine 1969, p. 95). In this sense, *environment* means all the conditions, circumstances, and influences surrounding and affecting the development of an organism or group of organisms. It refers to both the internal and external environments. Roy states that the person, as an adaptive system, func-

tions as a totality. *Adaptive behavior* is the behavior of the whole person. Roy identifies two major internal processor subsystems of the adaptive system: the regulator and the cognator (Roy and Roberts 1981, p. 43). The individual uses these subsystems to adapt to or cope with internal and external environmental stimuli. The regulator mechanism has neural, endocrine, and perception-psychomotor components. The cognator mechanism encompasses psychosocial pathways and apparatus for perceptual/information processing, learning, judgment, and emotion. These two mechanisms are linked by the process of perception.

Concept of Holism

Nurses are concerned with the individual as a whole, complete, or holistic person, not as an assembly of parts and processes. The terms *holistic* and *holism* are derived from the Greek word meaning "whole." The term holism itself was coined by Jan Smuts, a South African statesman, in his book *Holism and Evolution* (1926). In holistic theory, all living organisms are seen as interacting, unified wholes that are more than the mere sums of their parts. Viewed in this light, any disturbance in one part is a disturbance of the whole system; in other words, the disturbance affects the whole being.

When applied to humans and health, the concept of holism emphasizes the fact that "nurses must keep the self-identity of the 'whole' person in mind and must strive to understand simultaneously the relationship of the 'part' of the individual under concern to the totality of that individual's interactions and the relationship of the whole to its parts" (Krieger 1981, p. 4). Therefore, when studying one part of an individual, the nurse must consider how that part relates to all others. The nurse must also consider the interaction and relationship of the individual to the external environment and to others. For example, a nurse helps a man who is recuperating from a heart attack to consider his life-style and other contributing factors so that he can improve his health in the future. The nurse asks the client why he thinks the attack happened, what stresses he feels in his life, whether he smokes, what his eating habits are, and how much exercise he normally gets. Using the holistic approach, the nurse considers all contributing factors so that the client can prevent a recurrence.

Holistic health involves the total person: the whole of the person's being and the overall quality of life-style. It includes physical fitness, primary prevention of negative physical and emotional states, stress management, sensitivity to the environment, self-awareness, and spiritual insight (Smith 1984, p. 5). Many holistic health centers have been established across North America. They help clients to take responsibility for their health, to seek alternative, healthy, self-fulfilling behaviors, and to mobilize inner healing capacities.

Human Needs

Although each individual has unique characteristics, certain needs are common to all people. Nursing theorists define *need* in various ways. Orlando defines a need as "a requirement of the person which, if supplied, receives or diminishes his immediate distress or improves his immediate sense of adequacy or well-being." (Orlando 1961, p. 5). King defines need as "a state of energy exchange within and external to the organism which leads to behavioral responses to situations, events, and persons" (King 1971, p. 80). Roy defines a need as "a requirement within the individual which stimulates a response to maintain integrity" (Roy 1980, p. 184). For the purposes of this book, a need is something that is desirable, useful, or necessary.

The humanist Abraham Maslow developed his theory of human needs in the 1940s. To Maslow, needs motivate the behavior of the individual. His model of human needs includes both physiologic and psychologic needs, which he ranks according to how critical to survival they are. Maslow believes that the needs at one level must be met before the needs on the next level can be met. Thus,

the physiologic needs must be met before the safety needs are met. Maslow's five categories or levels of needs, in hierarchical order, are physiologic needs, safety and security needs, love and belonging needs, self-esteem needs, and the need for self-actualization (1970, p. 37). See Figure 4–1.

Throughout life, people strive to meet their needs at each level; however, the dominant needs *within one level* may vary at different times of life. Maslow sees humans as beings who continue to grow and develop from conception until death. Once a need is completely met, Maslow believes, the individual is no longer aware of it. Needs can be completely met, partially met, or not met at all. An individual usually persists in behavior to meet a need until it is met.

Maslow also states that an individual who apparently meets all needs still looks further to self-actualization. Maslow discusses two additional needs: the need to know and the need to understand. He believes that these needs are always present and permit people to meet the other needs more efficiently.

Maslow includes air, food, water, shelter, rest and sleep, activity, and temperature maintenance as the basic physiologic needs. A person who is starving or deprived of fluid for an extended time will center all activities around meeting that need. After the physiologic needs are met, the need to feel safe in one's environment emerges. This need for safety has both physical

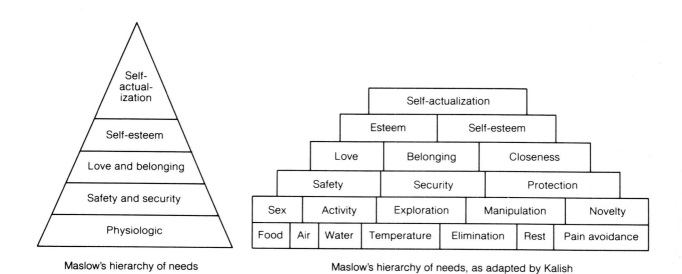

Maslow's hierarchy of needs

Maslow's hierarchy of needs, as adapted by Kalish

Figure 4–1 Maslow's needs. ***Source:*** From *The Psychology of Human Behavior,* 5th ed., by R. A. Kalish. Copyright © 1966, 1970, 1973, 1977, 1983 by Wadsworth, Inc. Reprinted by permission of Brooks/Cole Publishing Company, Monterey, Calif. 93940.

and psychologic aspects; the person needs to *be* safe and to *feel* safe, both in the physical environment and in relationships.

The third level of needs (for love, affection, and belonging) emerges after the needs for safety are met. According to Maslow, the need for love encompasses both giving and receiving. Belonging needs include attaining a place in a group, e.g., having a family and the feeling of belonging. The need for esteem is at the fourth level. The individual needs both *self-esteem* (i.e., feelings of independence, competence, and self-respect) and *esteem from others,* i.e., recognition, respect, and appreciation.

When the need for esteem is satisfied, the individual strives for *self-actualization.* Self-actualized persons have realized their full potential. Such a person has the ability to connect the past and the future to the present while living fully in the present, is inner-directed, and is autonomous in contrast to being other-directed.

To be inner-directed means that the individual is guided by a few basic values and principles, whatever the situation. To be autonomous is to be free from parental and social pressures and to apply these values or principles to behavior in a manner that appears appropriate to the individual. The other-directed individual is influenced by outside pressures, accepts guidance and direction from others, and adheres to this guidance to gain approval.

Not all people become fully self-actualized, and Maslow does not believe that intelligence is required for self-actualization. However, if all the "lower" needs are met, an individual may aspire to become self-fulfilled or self-actualized. Maslow sees self-actualization as a product of maturity that comes about through relating to people in autonomous and time-competent ways.

The fully self-actualized person may not always be happy, successful, or well adjusted. Maslow views many of the subjects he believes to be self-actualized as prideful, vain, and possessing doubts and fears. However, they are able to deal positively with their fears, doubts, and failures. See the accompanying box for the major characteristics of a self-actualized person.

In later research, Maslow identified the growth needs, in contrast to the deficiency needs. He calls the growth needs *Being values* (*metaneeds,* B-values). These "being values" resemble needs because, when metaneeds are not met, the person has a "sickness of the soul," or *metapathology* (Maslow 1971, p. 43). Maslow believes that for some people being values give meaning to life. There are 14 "being values:" truth, goodness, beauty, wholeness, aliveness, uniqueness, perfection, completion, justice, simplicity, richness, effortlessness, playfulness, and self-sufficiency. These needs are not ranked (Goble 1970, pp. 47–48).

Richard Kalish (1977, p. 32) has adapted Maslow's hierarchy and suggests an additional category of needs between the physiologic needs and the safety and security needs. This category includes sex, activity, exploration, manipulation, and novelty. See Figure 4–1. Kalish em-

---

Maslow's Characteristics of a Self-Actualized Person

- Is realistic, sees life clearly, and is objective about his or her observations
- Judges people correctly
- Has superior perception, is more decisive
- Has clear notion of right and wrong
- Is usually accurate in predicting future events
- Understands art, music, politics, and philosophy
- Possesses humility, listens to others carefully
- Is dedicated to some work, task, duty, or vocation
- Is highly creative, flexible, spontaneous, courageous, and willing to make mistakes
- Is open to new ideas
- Is self-confident and has self-respect
- Has low degree of self-conflict; personality is integrated
- Respects self, does not need fame, possesses a feeling of self-control
- Is highly independent, desires privacy
- Can appear remote and detached
- Is friendly, loving, and governed more by inner directives than by society
- Can make decisions contrary to popular opinion
- Is problem centered rather than self-centered
- Accepts the world for what it is

Source: Based on Chapter 3, "The Study of Self-Actualization," from *The Third Force. The Psychology of Abraham Maslow,* by Frank Goble. Copyright © 1970 by Thomas Jefferson Research Center. Reprinted by permission of Viking Penguin, a division of Penguin Books U.S.A., Inc.

phasizes that children need to explore and manipulate their environments to achieve optimal growth and development. He notes that adults, too, often seek novel adventures or stimulating experiences before considering their safety or security needs. Maslow, by contrast, includes the pursuit of knowledge and aesthetic needs in the category of self-actualization needs.

Halbert Dunn's (1958) model presents a series of needs that the individual must meet to achieve a state of maximum functioning or high-level wellness. Dunn's basic needs are survival, communication, fellowship, growth, imagination, love, balance, environment, communication with the universe, philosophy of living, dignity, freedom, and space. At any specific time, different needs assume a greater relative importance to the individual.

Jourard (1963) believes that people rank their needs according to their relative importance in their lives. He adds the needs for health (physical and mental), freedom, challenge, cognitive clarity, and varied experience to Maslow's list.

Characteristics of Basic Needs
All people have the same basic needs; however, each person's needs are modified by that person's culture. A person's perception of a need varies according to learning and the standards of the culture. For example, professional achievement may be important in one culture or subculture and unimportant in another.

- People meet their own needs relative to their own priorities. For example, during a drought, a mother might give up her share of water and die so that her child might have sufficient water to live.

- Although basic needs generally must be met, some needs can be deferred. An example is the need for independence, which an ill person can defer until well.

- Failure to meet needs results in one or more homeostatic imbalances, which can eventually result in illness.

- A need can make itself felt by either external or internal stimuli. An example is the need for food. A person may experience hunger as a result of thinking about food (internal stimulation) or as a result of seeing a beautiful cake (external stimulation).

- A person who perceives a need can respond in several ways to meet it. The choice of response is largely a result of learned experiences and the values of the culture. For example, the professional woman who comes home from work feeling tired may meet the need for relaxation by having a cocktail. This response reflects her experience and culture.

- Needs are interrelated. Some needs cannot be met unless related needs are also met. The need for hydration can be seriously altered if the need for elimination of urine is not also met. Likewise, the need for security can be markedly altered if the need for oxygen is threatened by a respiratory obstruction.

Needs can be satisfied in healthy and unhealthy ways. Individuals can succeed in their profession as a way of meeting the needs for belonging and self-esteem. Ways of meeting basic needs are considered healthy when they are not harmful to others or to self, conform to the individual's sociocultural values, and are within the law. Conversely, unhealthy behavior has one or more of the following characteristics: It may be harmful to others or to self, does not conform to the individual's sociocultural values, or is not within the law. Maslow found that people who satisfy their basic needs are healthier, happier, and more effective than those whose needs are frustrated (Goble 1970, p. 50).

Factors Affecting Needs Satisfaction
Gauging whether physiologic needs are met is largely an objective judgment by the nurse, although it may be subjective for the client. For example, the nurse can judge whether an individual's need for food has been met by weighing that person, using calipers to measure body fat, or reviewing the results of laboratory tests that analyze the metabolic processes of the body. Gauging whether psychologic needs have been met, however, is largely a subjective judgment. If a person believes a psychologic need (e.g., for love) is not satisfied, then for that person it is not met, regardless of external appearances. Several factors affect people's abilities to satisfy their needs. Four of these are illness, significant relationships, self-concept, and development stage.

Illness frequently interferes with people's abilities to meet their own needs. Nurses help ill clients to meet their physiologic needs on a number of levels. The man recovering from abdominal surgery probably requires oxygen, intravenous fluids, assistance in moving, and reassurance immediately after surgery. Enacting each of these interventions helps to meet a different need. As he recovers, his requirements for nursing help will decrease. As his physiologic needs are met, the client attends to needs at the next level (e.g., safety needs, according to Maslow) and so on. Ailing people often direct all their energies to meeting physiologic (survival) needs and may not identify needs at higher levels until later.

A second variable affecting needs satisfaction is *significant relationships.* Often these relationships are with family and support persons. Nurses also frequently establish significant relationships with clients because they are present at critical times in people's lives. Through these relationships, nurses can help clients become aware of their needs and establish healthy ways of meeting them.

A person's *self-concept* affects not only the ability to meet basic needs but also the awareness of whether or not these needs are satisfied. People who feel good about themselves are more likely to change, to recognize needs, and to establish healthy ways of meeting those needs. Those with a poor self-concept are less likely to meet these needs independently and may require more assistance from the nurse. Self-concept is discussed with greater depth in Chapter 22.

A fourth variable is an individual's *developmental stage.* According to Erikson's model of psychosocial human development, if an individual satisfactorily achieves the developmental task of learning to trust, then the basic needs of feeling safe and secure are readily resolved. The person who has already learned to trust others transfers those feelings to the health personnel caring for the person. As another example, if the developmental tasks of establishing identity and intimacy have been achieved, the individual has an increased sense of belonging and being loved at a time of illness.

Assigning Priorities to Needs
Although Maslow's needs are presented in a hierarchy, sometimes clients and nurses must adjust the priority of the needs. People are continually changing and growing; thus, their needs do not stay constant but also continually change. Depending upon the situation, the nurse may be able to help a client meet several needs at once, partially meet one need and then go on to another, or deal with one need at a time. Needs related to life-threatening situations, e.g., a suffocating client's need for air, always assume first priority.

In many situations, one need does not stand out as priority one. In these cases, the client and nurse consider several factors, such as the client's health, the client's and support persons' perceptions about health and areas of need, and the client's sociocultural background. A person may not perceive a specific need. If so, the nurse may allocate it a low priority, often deferring action until the person is ready. For example, a man who smokes heavily might not see the need to stop.

Socioeconomic and cultural backgrounds affect how people rank their needs. For example, a man may place his need to return to work ahead of his need to learn exercises. A woman may perceive that getting her husband's breakfast is more important than resting in bed. See Chapter 24 for more information about cultural influences.

Applications in Nursing
A knowledge of human needs helps nurses in several ways. First, it helps nurses understand themselves so that they can meet personal needs outside of the client situation. Second, by understanding human needs, nurses can understand people's behavior better. Recognizing the causes of certain behavior helps nurses be less judgmental and more objective. In addition, understanding the reason for behavior helps nurses respond therapeutically rather than emotionally. For example, by repeatedly turning on his signal light, a man may be reflecting a need for safety (he feels frightened), a need for belonging or affection, or a need for esteem. The nurse can discuss his feelings to determine what his need is and thus how to respond. If the client is turning on his light because he is frightened, the nurse can employ a variety of methods to reassure him, including explaining about the hospital, answering his call promptly, anticipating some of his needs, and telling him when the nurse will return and returning at that time.

Third, knowledge of basic needs can provide a framework for, and be applied in, the nursing process at the individual and family levels. Human needs can serve as a framework for assessing, assigning priorities to problems, and planning nursing interventions. A client's unmet need for blood can be of high priority and calls for immediate nursing action, whereas the same client's self-esteem needs are of lower priority during that emergency.

Fourth, nurses can apply their knowledge of human needs to relieve distress. To meet or help a client meet unmet needs and thereby alleviate distress, the nurse requires a knowledge not only of needs but also of the situations that bring about these unmet needs and the manner in which the client conveys the need.

Fifth, the nurse can use a knowledge of human needs to help people develop and grow. Sometimes people are unaware or only partially aware of their own needs. Nurses can often help clients move toward self-actualization by helping them to find meaning in their illness experience. To encourage the client's growth toward self-actualization nurses can help them to (a) understand what is happening to them, (b) maintain some control over events affecting them, (c) maintain their identities and self-respect, (d) accept inevitable outcomes, and (e) feel good about themselves.

THEORIES ABOUT CARING

Humanistic Theory

<u>Humanism is a concern for human attributes</u>, for those characteristics that are considered human. Some of these attributes are universal, that is, they occur in all cultures. Examples of humanistic behaviors are empathy, compassion, sympathy toward other people, and respect for life.

Humanism has received increased attention in nursing in response to the technologic advances that have affected nursing practice. <u>Humanism in nursing refers to an attitude and an approach to the client and support persons recognizing them as human beings with human needs,</u> rather than as "the appendectomy in Room 192" or "the catheterization in bed 6A."

North American societies are multiethnic (i.e., they comprise diverse ethnic groups). They are person-centered in their humanism and embody human rights concepts. This means that individuals are seen as autonomous and have certain rights and freedoms; in fact, each person has the right to be treated as an individual. By contrast, in certain societies, the tribe or the family, not the person, is the primary unit endowed with values and rights. Other characteristics of American humanism—though not necessarily unique to it—are belief in helping the poor and the suffering and respect for the ways and values of others, even if these differ from one's own.

The nurse who takes a humanistic approach to nursing practice takes into account all that is known about a client—thoughts, feelings, values, experiences, likes, desires, behavior, and body (La Monica 1985, p. 2). This humanistic approach, <u>the traditional "caring" aspect of nursing, is characterized by understanding and action</u>. Understanding requires the ability to listen to another and perceive that person's feelings. Action requires the ability to respond to another with genuineness and warmth to promote optimal well being (Slevin and Harter 1987, p. 24). The caring aspect of nursing is a core construct upon which the nurse builds the knowledge and skill of professional practice.

Caring Constructs

The terms *nursing care* and *caring* have been used by nurses for more than a century. Leininger (1984, p. 3) states: "Care is the essence and the central, unifying, and dominant domain to characterize nursing: it is an essential human need for the full development, health maintenance, and survival of human beings in all world cultures . . . yet care has not received the same degree of attention by professionals and the public as cure." In an address to the 75th Annual Registered Nurses' Association of Nova Scotia, Benner (1984, p. 3) made this statement: "Caring is often frankly curative because it facilitates healing." Leininger (1984, p. 6) says that there can be <u>no curing without caring, but there may be caring without curing</u>.

Definitions and a clear understanding of the terms *care* and *caring* have been lacking. Systematic research is needed to describe caring behaviors, values, and practices in nursing so that this knowledge can be incorporated into nursing education and practice areas. Some definitions of care and caring are provided in Table 4–2.

In her <u>transcultural care theory,</u> Leininger (1984, pp. 5–6) <u>points out that human caring, although a universal phenomenon, varies among cultures in its expressions, processes, and patterns;</u> it is largely culturally derived. These differences in caring values and behaviors lead to differences in the expectations of those seeking care. For example, cultures that perceive illness primarily as a personal and internal body experience—caused by physical, genetic, and intrabody stresses—tend to use more medications and physical techniques than cultures that view illness as an extrapersonal experience.

Leininger identifies many caring and nursing care constructs. Examples are comfort, compassion, concern, coping behaviors, empathy, enabling, involvement, health acts (consultative, instructive, maintenance), love, nurturance, presence, sharing, tenderness, touching, and trust. Each of these constructs has many subdescriptions. Leininger believes the goal of health care personnel should be to work toward an understanding of care and the health of different cultures so that each culture's care, values, beliefs, and life-styles will be the basis for providing culture-specific care.

Watson (1979, pp. 10–208; 1988, p. 75) identifies ten caring factors in nursing:

1. Forming a <u>humanistic-altruistic system of values.</u> This factor relates to <u>satisfaction through giving and extending the sense of self</u>. Although the values are <u>learned early in life, t</u>hey can be greatly influenced by educators.

2. <u>Instilling faith and hope.</u> Feelings of faith and hope promote wellness by helping the client to adopt health-seeking behaviors. By developing an effective nurse-client relationship, the nurse facilitates feelings of optimism, hope, and trust.

3. <u>Cultivating sensitivity to one's self and others.</u> Nurses who are able to recognize and express their feelings are better able to allow others to express theirs.

TABLE 4-2 *Definitions and Descriptions of Care and Caring*

Delores Gaut	There is no clear-cut rule for the use of *caring* in common language, but the family of meanings is related to the notion of caring in three senses: (a) attention to or concern about; (b) responsibility for or providing for; and (c) regard or fondness for.
	The term *caring* in both lay and scholarly literature is found in discussions of: (a) certain feelings or dispositions within a person; (b) the doing of certain activities that seem to identify that person as a caring individual; or (c) a combination of both attitudes and actions in which caring about the other disposes the one to carry out activities for the other.
	Caring is intentional activity.*
Madeleine Leininger	*Care* in a generic sense refers to those assistive, supportive, or facilitative acts toward or for another individual or group with evident or anticipated needs to ameliorate or improve a human condition or lifeway.
	Caring refers to the direct (or indirect) nurturant and skillful activities, processes, and decisions related to assisting people in such a manner that reflects behavioral attributes that are empathetic, supportive, compassionate, protective, succorant, educational, dependent upon the needs, problems, values, and goals of the individual or group being assisted.
	Professional caring embodies the cognitive and deliberate goals, processes, and acts of professional persons or groups providing assistance to others, and expressing attitudes and actions of concern for them, in order to support their well-being, alleviate undue discomforts, and meet obvious or anticipated needs.
	Scientific caring refers to those judgments and acts of helping others based on tested or verified knowledge.
	Humanistic caring refers to the creative, intuitive, or cognitive helping process for individuals or groups based upon philosophic, phenomenologic, and objective and subjective experiential feelings and acts of assisting others.†
M. Mayeroff	We sometimes speak as if caring did not require knowledge, as if caring for someone, for example, were simply a matter of good intentions or warm regard. . . . To care for someone, I must know many things. I must know, for example, who the other is, what his powers and limitations are, what his needs are, and what is conducive to his growth; I must know how to respond to his needs and what my own powers and limitations are.
	Caring is an important means for self-growth. To help another person grow is at least to help him to care for something or someone apart from himself, and it involves encouraging and assisting him to find and create of his own in which he is able to care. Also, it is to help that other person to come to care for himself, and by becoming responsive to his own needs, to care and to become responsible for his own life.‡
Jean Watson	Human caring in nursing is not just an emotion, concern, attitude, or benevolent desire. Caring connotes a personal response. Human caring involves values, a will and a commitment to care, knowledge, caring actions, and consequences. All of human caring is related to intersubjective human responses to health-illness conditions; a knowledge of health-illness; environmental-personal interactions; a knowledge of the nurse caring process; self-knowledge; [and] knowledge of one's power and transaction limitations.
	The ideal and value of caring is a starting point, a stance, an attitude, which has to become a will, an intention, a commitment, and a conscious judgment that manifests itself in concrete acts. The most abstract characteristic of a caring person is that he or she is somehow responsive to a person as a unique individual, perceives the other's feelings, and sets apart one person from another from the ordinary. The uncaring person is by contrast insensitive to another person as a unique individual, [not] perceptive of the other's feelings, and does not necessarily distinguish one person from another in any significant way.§

Sources:
*D. Gaut, A theoretic description of caring as action, in M. Leininger, *Care: The essence of nursing and health* (Thorofare, N. J.: Charles B. Slack, 1984), pp. 27–28.
†M. Leininger, *Care: The essence of nursing and health* (Thorofare, N. J.: Charles B. Slack, 1984), pp. 4, 46.
‡M. Mayeroff, *On caring* (New York: Harper and Row, 1971), P. 13.
§J. Watson, *Nursing: Human science and human care—A theory of nursing* (National League for Nursing, 1988), pp. 29, 31, 32, 34.

4. Developing a helping-trust (human care) relationship. This kind of relationship involves effective communication, empathy, and nonpossessive warmth. It promotes and accepts the expression of positive and negative feelings.

5. Expressing positive and negative feelings. Sharing feelings of sorrow, love, and pain is a risk-taking experience. The nurse must be prepared for negative feelings.

6. Using a creative problem-solving caring process. Caring linked to the nursing process contributes to a creative problem-solving approach to nursing care.

7. Promoting interpersonal teaching-learning. This factor separates caring from curing and shifts responsibility for wellness to the client.

8. Providing a supportive, protective, or corrective mental, physical, sociocultural, and spiritual environment. Because the client can experience change in any aspect of the internal and external environments, the nurse must assess and facilitate the client's abilities to cope with mental, emotional, and physical changes.

9. Assisting with gratification of human needs. Caring is conveyed by recognizing and attending to the physical, emotional, social, and spiritual needs of the client.

10. Being sensitive to existential-phenomenologic-spiritual forces. Phenomenology describes data of the immediate situation that help people understand the phenomena in question. The *phenomenal field* is the individual's frame of reference; this field can be known only to the person. Existential psychology is a science of human existence that employs the method of phenomenologic analysis. Persons possess three spheres of being: mind, body, and soul (Watson 1988, p. 54). Allowing for expression of these forces leads to a better understanding of self and others.

Benner and Wrubel examine the relationship among caring, stress and coping, and health and claim that caring is primary. To Benner and Wrubel, caring means that persons, events, projects, and things matter to people (1989, p. 1). They state that caring is *primary* for any health care practice and view it as central to human expertise, to curing, and to healing. Caring is primary in three ways:

1. "Since caring sets up what matters to a person, it also sets up what counts as stressful, and what options are available for coping."

2. It is an enabling condition of connection and concern. When there is caring and concern, people find ways to cope. "Coping based on caring may not abolish loss and pain but it allows for the possibility of joy and the satisfactions of attachment."

3. "It sets up the possibility of giving and receiving help. A caring relationship sets up the conditions of trust that enable the one cared for to accept the help offered and to *feel* cared for" (Benner and Wrubel 1989, pp. 1–4).

The Power of Caring

Benner (1984, pp. 209–15) identifies six different qualities of power associated with caring:

1. *Transformative power.* With this power, the nurse can help clients to regain a sense of control and to participate actively in situations they thought were beyond their control. For example, clients often need help to realize that they have a choice and can abandon whatever role they wish.

2. *Integrative caring.* Caring can also reintegrate individuals into their own social world. For example, when prolonged or permanent disability is inevitable, the nurse can help clients to continue with meaningful life activities despite their limitations.

3. *Advocacy power.* Clients and families frequently need the nurse to act on their behalf. They may be confused by medical jargon, or their understanding may be hampered by anxiety or fear. The nurse can interpret necessary information to the client and to the physician. Advocacy removes obstacles; it is a standing alongside and enabling of the client.

4. *Healing power.* To establish a healing relationship and climate, the nurse (a) mobilizes hope within the self, the staff, and the client; (b) finds an interpretation or understanding of the situation (e.g., illness, pain, fear, or other stressful emotion) that is acceptable and clarifying to the client; and (c) helps the client find social, emotional, and spiritual support. A healing relationship helps the client to mobilize internal and external resources by bringing hope, confidence, and trust.

5. *Participative/affirmative power.* By participating, a nurse finds meanings in specific events. The nurse may experience pain but may also experience strength and affirmation. A detached, avoiding approach usually offers only frail protection and develops no positive inner resources.

6. _Problem solving._ Caring is the prerequisite for creative problem solving. The most difficult problems require perceptual ability as well as conceptual reasoning, and perception requires involvement and attentiveness. Caring provides a sensitivity to cues that allows persons to search for solutions and even makes it possible to recognize solutions when they are not directly sought.

OTHER THEORIES THAT AFFECT NURSING PRACTICE

Many other theories have a potential impact on nursing practice. These include theories about health and wellness in Chapter 13, change theory in Chapter 12, stress and adaptation theory in Chapter 23, and growth and development theories. This section includes the following theories: general systems theory, problem-solving and decision-making theory, and perception theory.

General Systems Theory

General systems theory explains the breaking of whole things into parts and the working together of those parts in systems. The theory explains the relationship between wholes and parts, a description of concepts about them, and predictions about how the parts will behave

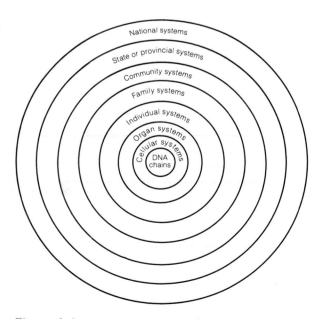

Figure 4-2 A common system hierarchy.

and react. This theory is relevant in the nursing process as it is applied to the individual, family, and community.

The basic concepts of systems theory were proposed in the 1950s. One of its major proponents, Ludwig von Bertalanffy (1969) introduced systems theory as a universal theory that could be applied to many fields of study. Systems theory is being used increasingly by nurses as a way of understanding not only biologic systems but also systems in families, communities, and nursing and health care. General systems theory provides a way of examining interrelationships and deriving principles.

A *system* is a set of interacting identifiable parts or components. A system can be an individual, a family, or a community. The fundamental components of a system are matter, energy, and communication. Without any one of these, a system does not exist. The individual or the human system has matter (the body), energy (chemical or thermal), and communication (e.g., the nervous system). The *boundary* of a system, such as the skin in the human system, is a real or imaginary line that differentiates one system from another system or a system from its environment.

Systems may be complex and therefore are often studied as *subsystems*. Each subsystem belongs to a higher system. In the individual or human system, the subsystems (or lower level systems) are the organ systems, such as the respiratory system and the digestive system; the *suprasystems* are the family systems. See Figure 4–2 for a hierarchy of the human system.

Because all the parts of a system are interrelated, the whole system responds to changes in one of its parts. This interrelatedness is the basis for nursing's holistic view of the client. For example, a tumor of the liver affects the whole individual, that is, the person may be nauseated, tired, anxious, and so on. A psychologic problem such as stress or anxiety may also manifest itself by physiologic symptoms such as sleeplessness, nausea, or changes in cardiac function.

There are two general types of systems: closed and open. A *closed system* does not exchange energy, matter, or information with its environment; it receives no input from the environment and gives no output to the environment. An example of a closed system is a chemical reaction that takes place in a test tube. In reality, no closed systems exist. In an *open system,* energy, matter, and information move into and out of the system through the system boundary. All living systems, such as plants, animals, people, families, and communities, are open systems, since their survival depends on a continuous exchange of energy. They are, therefore, in a constant state of change.

For its functioning, an open system depends on the quality and quantity of its input, output, and feedback. *Input* consists of information, material, or energy that enters the system. After the input is absorbed by the system, it is processed in a way useful to the system. This process of transformation is called *throughput*. For example, in the digestive system, food is input; it is digested (throughput) so that it can be used by the body. *Output* from a system is energy, matter, or information given out by the system as a result of its processes. Output from the digestive system is feces and caloric energy.

Feedback is a process that enables a system to regulate itself by redirecting the output of a system to determine the input of the same system, thus forming a feedback loop. Numerous examples of this feedback mechanism are found within individual, family, and community systems. In the individual, for example, the autonomic nervous system relies on a feedback system to balance the effects of the sympathetic and parasympathetic centers, which regulate, among other processes, heart and respiratory rates. In the family system, parents provide feedback to children to regulate behavior. In the community, laws, rules, and regulations regulate the behavior of citizens.

To survive, open systems must maintain a special balance often referred to as *dynamic equilibrium, homeostasis,* or *homeodynamics.* In the human being, examples of this balance include maintenance of normal body temperature, regardless of variations in environmental temperature from freezing to 85 F, and regulation of heart and respiratory rate within normal limits, in spite of varying degrees of physical exertion from watching television to running a marathon.

The nursing process has some of the characteristics of an open system: it is open, flexible, and dynamic; it is planned and goal directed; it interacts with the environment; and it emphasizes feedback. The nursing process can be viewed as a system with input, throughput, output, and feedback. Input (data) from the client and nurse is then transformed by the processes of analyzing, planning, and implementing, all of which are throughput. The output (client's response) is then evaluated.

Problem-Solving and Decision-Making Theory

Problem solving and decision making are used in applying the nursing process. Although these two terms are often used interchangeably, they are separate processes that are related in some situations. Solving a problem may require making a number of decisions, and making a decision may involve solving a number of problems. In addition, not all decisions involve problem solving. In many nursing situations, however, decision making is an aspect of problem solving.

Problem-Solving Methods There are various approaches to problem solving. Four of the most commonly used are trial and error, intuition, experimentation, and the scientific method.

Trial-and-error problem solving One way to solve problems is to try a number of approaches until a solution is found. However, the reason one solution works is not known when alternatives are not considered systematically. Trial-and-error methods in nursing care can be dangerous because the client might suffer harm if an approach is inappropriate.

Intuitive problem solving Intuition as a problem-solving method has not been considered either sound or legitimate. Rather, it has been viewed as a form of guessing and, as such, an inappropriate basis for nursing decisions. However, according to recent investigations, intuition appears to be an essential and legitimate aspect of clinical judgment acquired through knowledge and experience (Benner and Tanner 1987). *Intuitive judgment* in nursing is developed through clinical experience with similar types of situations. In other words, expertise in a specialty area, such as cardiovascular nursing, is developed by continuous and meaningful exposure to clients who have experienced cardiovascular problems.

Intuition is based on experience and knowledge. The nurse must first have the knowledge base necessary to practice in the clinical area, then use that knowledge in clinical practice. Clinical experience allows the nurse to recognize cues and patterns and begin to make correct decisions.

Experimentation Experimentation is more controlled than trial and error. It is based on knowledge and research, and it is therefore a more valid method than trial-and-error or intuitive problem solving. Examples of experimentation are pilot projects or limited trials in an effort to solve a problem. For example, a nurse caring for a client with intractable pain may try one specific nursing intervention for 3 days to reduce the pain. If the pain is not reduced, the nurse may then implement a second plan for another 3 days. Many research projects designed and implemented by nurse researchers are done to determine the most effective nursing interventions and ultimately improve nursing care.

RESEARCH NOTE

Is Intuition Used In Nursing?

Intuition is the ability to recognize and understand something immediately without using analysis. People say, "I had a feeling that this was the appropriate choice." This statement describes intuition. In this study, the researchers wanted to determine if nurses use intuition while providing nursing care. They discovered that nurses do use intuition very effectively. They also found that nurses (a) recognized that the clients' signs and symptoms were falling into a particular pattern; (b) were able to draw on their experience to recognize how a particular client's symptoms were similar to those of other clients that they had cared for; (c) were able to identify quickly the most important pieces of information about the client to consider; and (d) anticipated that certain events would occur.

Implications: The researchers of this project suggest that although experience plays a very important role in improving this skill, some of these techniques can be taught. This teaching is most effective when students are given a complete description of all the factors surrounding the client's situation. In addition, experienced nurses should work with students and let them know whether their intuitions were correct or incorrect.

Source: P. Benner and C. Tanner. Clinical judgment: How expert nurses use intuition, *American Journal of Nursing,* January 1987, 87:23–31.

Scientific method   The *scientific method* is a logical, systematic approach to solving problems. The classic scientific method is most useful in a laboratory where the scientist is working in a controlled situation. The steps of the scientific method are outlined in Table 4–3.

Although the scientific method has certain applications in nursing, there are differences between the scientist's laboratory setting and the nurse's practice setting. Three of these differences are as follows:

1. The nurse's time frame is often shorter than the scientist's. The scientist may take months or even years to carry out a study, whereas a nurse, for example, must give immediate help to a client in pain.
2. The nurse's environment makes complete scientific control impossible, whereas the scientist strives to establish precise scientific controls in experiments. For

example, a home care nurse striving to help regulate a client's diabetes through diet and insulin injections can outline a regimen and teach the client to administer insulin but has no control over whether the client will follow instructions later.

3. The nurse deals with multiple, complex problems, especially since most clients have more than one problem when they are ill. The scientist often isolates and studies a single aspect of a problem.

The scientific method, therefore, must be adapted for nursing practice. The nurse requires a problem-solving system that is scientific, systematic, yet flexible enough to deal with the complex situations in the health care system.

Modified scientific method (problem-solving process)   Health professionals require a modified approach of the scientific method for solving problems. This modified scientific problem-solving method is used in the nursing process as well as the medical process. Like the scientific process, it has seven steps. See Table 4–3 for a comparison of the problem-solving process, the nursing process, and the scientific method.

Decision-Making Process   *Decision making* is a process of choosing a particular and best action to meet a desired goal. Three conditions must prevail: freedom, rationality, and voluntary (Schaefer 1974, p. 1852). Freedom means that the individual makes the decision without pressure from others and has the authority to make the decision. Rationality, in the context of decision making, means that the best or optimal decision is made and that it is consistent with the decision maker's values and preferences. Rationality involves both deliberation and judgment. Voluntary is making a choice voluntarily.

Decision making involves two types of reasoning: inductive and deductive. In *inductive reasoning,* generalizations are formed from a set of facts or observations. When viewed together, certain bits of information suggest a particular interpretation. For example, the nurse who observes that a client has dry skin, poor turgor, sunken eyes, and dark amber urine may make the generalization that the client is dehydrated. *Deductive reasoning,* by contrast, is reasoning from the general to the specific. The nurse starts with a conceptual framework—for example, a self-care framework—and makes descriptive interpretations of the client's condition in relation to that framework. For example, the nurse who uses a self-care framework might categorize data and define the client's problems in relation to the client's

TABLE 4–3 *Comparison of Steps in the Problem-Solving Process, the Nursing Process, and the Scientific Method*

Problem-Solving Process	Nursing Process	Scientific Method
1. Encounter the problem	1. Assessing	1. Recognize and define the problem
2. Collect data		2. Collect data from observation and experimentation
3. Analyze information and identify exact nature of the problem	2. Diagnosing	3. Formulate hypothesis (an assumption made to test the logic of a proposition)
4. Determine a plan of action	3. Planning	4. Select plan to test the hypothesis
5. Carry out the plan	4. Implementing	5. Test the hypothesis
6. Evaluate the plan and its outcomes	5. Evaluating	6. Interpret test results (evaluate whether the hypothesis is correct)
7. Terminate or modify the plan		7. Conclude or modify hypothesis

abilities to perform self-care activities involving food, elimination, activity, and rest.

Several authors have described the decision-making process. For the purposes of this text, a three-phase decision-making process is chosen: deliberation, judgment, and discrimination (choice).

Deliberation During this initial phase, the nurse considers all the available data. The data are categorized and any gaps, inconsistencies, or conflicts are identified. At this time, solutions are considered, including all alternative actions and their consequences.

Judgment During the judgment phase of the decision-making process, each course of action is analyzed in terms of (a) effectiveness related to the goal of the action and (b) efficiency of the action. Included in the analysis are the risk factors involved.

Discrimination (choice) The third phase in the decision-making process is choosing one alternative action and the consequences. Insufficient deliberation and judgment can lead to poor choices, and inadequate consideration of the consequences can also lead to poor choices. However, thorough deliberation and judgment can lead to an effective choice of action.

Decision-making, like the nursing process, is cyclical. Assessing, the gathering of data about a client, is similar to the deliberation phase of the decision-making process (see Table 4–4). The analyzing stage of the nursing process is parallel to the judgment phase of decision-making. Planning, in the nursing process, is like the discrimination (choice) phase. Intervention involves continuous collection of data, analyses of the data, and nursing judgments regarding the effectiveness of the intervention. Any change in data may change the plan and the intervention. All three phases of decision-making apply to this stage of the nursing process. During evaluation, the nurse continues to gather data, reassess the effectiveness of the intervention, and make decisions about it. In effect, the nurse also evaluates the effectiveness of the decision-making process itself.

Perception Theory

Perception is a major means by which people gain information about themselves, their needs, and the environment. *Perception* is the process of selecting, organizing,

TABLE 4–4 *A Comparison of the Steps of the Nursing Process and Decision Making*

Nursing Process Steps	Decision-Making Phases
1. Assessing	Deliberation
2. Diagnosing	Judgment, discrimination
3. Planning	Discrimination
4. Implementing	Deliberation, judgment, discrimination
5. Evaluating	Deliberation, judgment, discrimination

and interpreting sensory stimuli into a meaningful and coherent picture of the world. When looking around, a person sees a whole range of different objects, forms, and colors. People also see depth; all objects appear three-dimensional. Why does the world look the way it does to a person? A superficial answer is that things look the way they do because that is the way they are; they mirror reality.

Perception, however, is more complex than a response to sensory stimuli. It is also the interpretation of the sensation in the light of previous learning. Perception is a person's conscious awareness of reality and is based on an individual's knowledge and past experiences.

People tend to see what they want to see. What people anticipate as a result of past experience can become so firmly embedded into their thinking that people can be "blinded" to reality. Differences in people's perceptual fields are evident when, for example, witnesses to an accident give different reports of the same event. Often, there are as many different reports as witnesses. Observers are prone to make inferences from fragments of information, and the inferences are influenced by what the observer expects to perceive.

Three main factors influence people's perceptual fields: (a) the persons' needs, (b) their values or beliefs, and (c) their self-concept. People who have a low self-concept, i.e., think of themselves as weak, will selectively ignore stimuli that refute it.

An understanding of perceptual theory is essential for the nurse who wishes to communicate with clients and acquire and interpret data about them. Analysis of data is an inductive process. To share information accurately with a client, the nurse must perceive what the client intends to be perceived.

To enhance the ability to collect data and the accuracy of inferences made about the client, nurses must continually strive to increase their observational or perceptual field. This can be achieved by the following:

1. Using all senses—sight, smell hearing, touch, and taste—when collecting data.

2. Not focusing attention on only particular events or aspects of a stimulus.

3. Resisting the expectation that certain types of stimulation or responses will occur.

4. Asking for feedback about the client's perceptions, sharing and comparing perceptions, and reaching a common understanding. When eliciting feedback, the nurse can say, "I don't understand" or nonverbally indicate a question with a raised eyebrow or other gesture.

5. Being aware of their own values, beliefs, and biases, which may affect how nurses interpret what they see and hear. Nurses need to overcome the tendency to attend only to a person's positive attributes (that is, those that are similar to the nurse's own values) or to attend overly to negative attributes (that is, those in conflict with the nurse's values).

CHAPTER HIGHLIGHTS

▶ Three directions have been used to develop nursing theories: borrowing from conceptual frameworks in other disciplines, using an inductive approach, and using a deductive approach.

▶ A conceptual framework is a way of looking at a discipline in clear, explicit terms that can be communicated to others.

▶ Concepts that influence nursing most significantly include the person, the environment, health, and nursing actions. Together these concepts form the metaparadigm of nursing.

▶ A conceptual model gives clear and explicit directions to the three areas of nursing: practice, education, and research.

▶ A theory is made up of concepts, propositions, and hypotheses. Whereas a conceptual framework provides guidelines, a theory serves to generate knowledge in a field.

▶ A number of models have been developed by nurse theorists, including Henderson, Johnson, King, Levine, Neuman, Orem, Parse, Rogers, and Roy.

▶

CHAPTER HIGHLIGHTS *(continued)*

▶ The three basic components of nursing models are assumptions, a value system, and major units. The seven major units of nursing models (constructed from the assumptions and values) are goal of nursing, client, role of the nurse, source of difficulty of the client, intervention focus, modes of intervention, and consequences of nursing activity.

▶ Conceptual models for nursing are operationalized by the nursing process. This process consists of five steps: assessing, diagnosing, planning, implementing, and evaluating.

▶ Much research must be conducted before the usefulness of a conceptual model for nursing can be realized.

▶ Nursing involves viewing the individual holistically.

▶ How nurses view human beings influences how they assess and intervene.

▶ Humans can be viewed as open systems with many interrelated subsystems.

▶ Maslow defined a hierarchy of human needs, from physiologic (survival) needs to self-actualization.

▶ People vary in how they rank their needs at any given moment.

▶ Needs satisfaction can be altered by illness, significant relationships, self-concept, and developmental levels.

▶ A knowledge of human needs helps nurses understand behavior, can provide a framework for applying parts of the nursing process, and can help nurses relieve distress and help people develop and grow.

▶ Definitions and a clear understanding of the terms *care* and *caring* are being developed. The major theorists involved to date are Leininger, Watson, and Benner.

▶ Many theories, other than nursing theories, also have an impact on nursing practice. Included are theories about health and wellness, change theory, stress and adaptation theory, growth and development theories, general systems theory, problem-solving and decision-making theory, and perception theory.

LEARNING ACTIVITIES

■ After reviewing the brief outlines of the theorists contained in this chapter, consider your own definitions of the key concepts in nursing theory. Based on professional knowledge and experience and personal values and beliefs, define the terms *client, nursing, environment,* and *health*. How would you describe the relationship between these concepts based on your definitions? What assumptions are you making in your definitions? With which major theorist are your beliefs most consistent? How consistent is your nursing practice with your concept definitions and their interrelationships?

■ Using one or more of the anthologies of nursing theorists listed below, choose a theorist consistent with your beliefs and summarize that person's metaparadigm of nursing.

Fitzpatrick, J. J. and Whall, A. L. 1989. *Conceptual models of nursing: analysis and application.* 2d ed. Norwalk, Conn.: Appleton & Lange.

George, J. B. 1985. *Nursing theories: the base for professional nursing practice.* 2d ed. Englewood Cliffs, N.J.: Prentice-Hall.

Tomey-Marriner, A. 1989. *Nursing theorists and their work.* St. Louis: C. V. Mosby C.

READINGS AND REFERENCES

SUGGESTED READINGS

Storch, J. L. January 1986. In defense of nursing theory. *Canadian Nurse* 82:16–20.

    Storch suggests that nursing theory may be the key to meeting the changing needs of health consumers. She discusses how theory can make a significant difference in the quality of client care.

RELATED RESEARCH

Baer, E. D., and Lowery, B. J. September/October 1987. Patient and situational factors that affect nursing students' like or dislike of caring for patients. *Nursing Research* 36:298–302.

Benner, P., and Tanner, C. January 1987. Clinical judgment: How expert nurses use intuition. *American Journal of Nursing* 87:23–31.

Slevin, A. P., and Harter, M. O. November/December 1987. The teaching of caring: A survey report. *Nurse Educator* 12:23–26.

SELECTED REFERENCES

Andres, H. A., and Roy, C. 1986. *Essentials of the Roy Adaptation Model.* Norwalk, Conn.: Appleton-Century-Crofts.

Austin, J. K., and Champion, V. L., 1983. King's theory for nursing: Explication and evaluation. In Chinn, P. L., editor. *Advances in nursing theory development.* Rockville, Md.: Aspen Systems Corporation.

Benner, P. 1984. *From novice to expert: Excellence and power in clinical nursing practice.* Menlo Park, Calif.: Addison-Wesley Publishing Co.

Benner, P., and Tanner, C. January 1987. How expert nurses use intuition. *American Journal of Nursing* 87:23–31.

Benner, P. and Wrubel, J. 1989. *The primacy of caring: Stress and coping in health and illness.* Menlo Park, Calif.: Addison-Wesley Publishing Co.

Canadian Nurses' Association. 1984. *A definition of nursing practice: Standards for nursing practice.* Ottawa: Canadian Nurses' Association.

DeYoung, L. 1985. *Dynamics of nursing.* 5th ed. St. Louis: C. V. Mosby Co.

Dunn, H. H. November 1958. What high level wellness means. *Canadian Journal of Public Health* 50:447–57.

Fawcett, J. 1984. *Analysis and evaluation of conceptual models of nursing.* Philadelphia: F. A. Davis Co.

Gaut, D. 1984. A theoretic description of caring as action. In Leininger, M. pp. 27–28. *Care: The essence of nursing and health.* Thorofare, N.J.: Charles B. Slack.

George, J. B., editor. 1985 *Nursing theories: The base for professional nursing practice.* 2d ed. Englewood Cliffs, N.J.: Prentice-Hall.

Goble, F. G. 1970. *The third force: The psychology of Abraham Maslow.* Richmond Hill, Ontario: Simon and Schuster.

Henderson, V. 1966. *The nature of nursing: A definition and its implications for practice, research, and education.* New York: Macmillan Co.

———. October 1969. Excellence in nursing. *American Journal of Nursing* 69:2133–37.

Johnson, D. E. 1980. The behavioral system model for nursing. In Riehl, J. P., and Roy, C., editors. pp. 207–16. *Conceptual models for nursing practice.* 2d ed. New York: Appleton-Century-Crofts.

Jourard, S. 1963. *Personality adjustment.* 2d ed. New York: Macmillan Co.

Kalish, R. A. 1977. *The psychology of human behavior.* 4th ed. Belmont, Calif.: Wadsworth.

King I. M. 1971. *Toward a theory for nursing: General concepts of human behavior.* New York: John Wiley and Sons.

———. 1978. The "why" of theory development. In *Theory development: What, why, how?* New York: National League for Nursing.

———. 1981. *A theory for nursing: Systems, concepts, process.* New York: John Wiley and Sons.

———. 1987. King's theory of goal attainment. In Parse, R. R., editor. *Nursing science: Major paradigms, theories, and critiques.* Philadelphia: W. B. Saunders Co.

Krieger, D. 1981. *Foundations for holistic health nursing practices: The Renaissance nurse.* Philadelphia: J. B. Lippincott Co.

La Monica, E. L. 1985. *The humanistic nursing process.* Monterey, Calif.: Wadsworth Health Sciences.

Leddy, S., and Pepper, J. M. 1989. *Conceptual bases of professional nursing.* 2d ed. Philadelphia: J. B. Lippincott Co.

Leininger, M. 1984. *Care: The essence of nursing and health.* Thorofare, N.J.: Charles B. Slack.

Levine, M. E. January 1969. The pursuit of wholeness. *American Journal of Nursing* 69:93–98.

———. 1973. *Introduction to clinical nursing.* 2d ed. Philadelphia: F. A. Davis Co.

Malinski, V. M. 1986. Explorations on Martha Rogers' science of unitary human beings. Norwalk, Conn.: Appleton-Century-Crofts.

Mariner-Tomey, A. 1989. *Nursing theorists and their work.* 2d ed. St. Louis: C. V. Mosby Co.

Maslow, A. H. 1968. *Toward a psychology of being.* 2d ed. New York: Van Nostrand Reinhold Co.

———. 1970. *Motivation and personality.* 2d ed. New York: Harper and Row.

———. 1971. *The farther reaches of human nature.* New York: Penguin Books.

Mayeroff, M. 1971. *On caring.* New York: Harper and Row.

Mitchell, G. J., Pilkington, B. Summer 1990. Theoretical approaches in nursing practice: A comparison of Roy and Parse. *Nursing Science Quarterly* 3:81–7.

Neuman, B. 1974. The Betty Neuman health-care systems model: A total person approach to patient problems. In

Riehl, J. P., and Roy, C., editors. *Conceptual models for nursing practice.* New York: Appleton-Century-Crofts.

———. 1980. The Betty Neuman health-care systems model: A total person approach to patient problems. In Riehl, J. P., and Roy, C., editors. *Conceptual models for nursing practice.* 2d ed. New York: Appleton-Century-Crofts.

———. 1982. *The Neuman systems model: Applications to nursing education and practice.* New York: Appleton-Century-Crofts.

Newman, M. A. Spring 1990. Newman's theory of health as praxis. *Nursing Science Quarterly* 3:37–41.

Orem, D. E. 1971. *Nursing: Concepts of practice.* New York: McGraw-Hill.

———. 1980. *Nursing: Concepts of practice.* 2d ed. New York: McGraw-Hill.

———. 1985. *Nursing: Concepts of practice.* 3d ed. New York: McGraw-Hill.

Orlando, I. J. 1961. *The dynamic nurse-patient relationship: Function, process and principles.* New York: G. P. Putnam's Sons.

Parse, R. R. 1987. *Nursing science: Major paradigms, theories, and critiques.* Philadelphia: W. B. Saunders Co.

Ray, M. A. Spring 1990. Critical reflective analysis of Parse's and Newman's research. *Nursing Science Quarterly* 3:44–6.

Rogers, M. E. 1970. *An introduction to the theoretical basis of nursing.* Philadelphia: F. A. Davis Co.

———. 1980. Nursing: A science of unitary man. In Riehl, J. P., and Roy, C., editors. *Conceptual models for nursing practice.* 2d ed. New York: Appleton-Century-Crofts.

———. 1986. Science of unitary human beings. In Malinski, V. M. pp. 3–8. *Exploration on Martha Rogers' science of unitary human beings.* Norwalk, Conn.: Appleton-Century-Crofts.

Roy, C. 1976. *Introduction to nursing: An adaptation model.* Englewood Cliffs, N. J.: Prentice-Hall.

———. 1980. The Roy adaptation model. In Riehl, J. P., and Roy, C., editors. *Conceptual models for nursing practice.* 2d ed. New York: Appleton-Century-Crofts.

———. 1984. *Introduction to nursing: An adaptation model.* 2d ed. Englewood Cliffs, N. J.: Prentice-Hall.

———. 1987. Roy's adaptation model. In Parse, R. pp. 35–45. *Nursing science: Major paradigms, theories, and critiques.* Philadelphia: W. B. Saunders Co.

Roy, C., and Roberts, S. L. 1981. *Theory construction in nursing: An adaptation model.* Englewood Cliffs, N. J.: Prentice-Hall.

Schaefer, J. October 1974. The interrelatedness of decision making and the nursing process. *American Journal of Nursing* 74:1852–55.

Slevin, A., and Harter, M. November/December 1987. The Teaching of Caring: A Survey Report. *Nurse Educator.* 12:23–26.

Smith, M. P. August 1984. The new frontier. *RNABC* (Registered Nurses Association of British Columbia) *News* 16:5.

Smuts, J. 1926. *Holism and evolution.* New York: Macmillan Co.

Styles, M. M. 1982. *On nursing: Toward a new endowment.* St. Louis: C. V. Mosby Co.

von Bertalanffy, L. 1969. *General system theory.* New York: George Braziller.

Watson, J. 1979. *Nursing: The philosophy and science of caring.* Boston: Little, Brown and Co.

———. 1988. *Nursing: Human science and human care.* A theory of nursing. National League for Nursing Pub. no. 15–2236. New York: National League for Nursing.

Research in Nursing

Holly S. Wilson

CONTENTS

WHAT IS NURSING RESEARCH?

Most people recognize medicine's highly visible role in research. The public knows the role of medical research in discovering viruses, such as that responsible for acquired immune deficiency syndrome (AIDS); in facilitating surgical transplant of body organs; and in identifying habits, such as cigarette smoking, that endanger health. Until recently, however, the important impact of nursing research was not generally recognized by the public.

The history of nursing research begins in 1923 when the Committee for the Study of Nursing Education studied the educational preparation of nurse teachers, administrators, and public health nurses, and the clinical experiences of nursing students (Polit and Hungler 1991). Most nursing research during these early years was concerned with the education of nurses. It wasn't until the 1950s that nurse researchers began to examine clinical practice questions. Some historians point out that Florence Nightingale changed health care with her carefully researched case studies and detailed statistical accounts of the Crimea (Chenitz 1985).

Nursing research is more than just scientific investigations conducted by a person educated and credentialed as a nurse. It refers instead to research directed toward building a body of nursing knowledge about "human responses to actual or potential health problems" (ANA 1980, p. 9) and to the effects of nursing action on such human responses. The human responses of people may be (a) reactions of individuals, groups, or families to actual health problems, for example, the burden a family experiences when they must care for an elderly relative with Alzheimer's disease; and (b) concerns of individuals and groups about potential health problems, such as accident prevention or stress management in an industrial setting. The purpose of nursing research is to improve health care while reflecting the traditional nursing perspective. In this perspective, the client is seen as a whole person, with physiologic, psychologic, social, cultural, and economic components.

RESEARCH NOTE

What Are the Trends in Nursing Research?

The findings of a 1985 study by Maxine S. Loomis clearly document the 10-year-long trend in nursing dissertation work toward clinical research and a declining emphasis on social issues. For this analysis, Loomis obtained dissertation abstracts from 25 nursing doctoral programs admitting students in the fall of 1982. She identifies distinct patterns within programs, and, happily, gives abundant evidence of active mentor relationships between faculty and students.

Implications: Loomis suggests that certain deficits still exist in the body of nursing research as a whole. Subcategories of cultural/environmental stressors, sociocultural human response systems, and the various aspects of clinical decision making all warrant more attention by researchers, in her view. Study findings also indicate that nursing research has been increasingly successful in integrating the biologic, social, and cultural domains of nursing knowledge.

Source: M. E. Loomis, An analysis of dissertation abstracts and titles: 1976–1982. *Nursing Research,* March/April 1985, 34(2):113–119.

For example, when a person has a head injury, the nurse needs to understand the body's processes for dealing with the increased pressure within the head and the changes this brings about in the patient's condition. At the same time, the nurse focuses on care that can maintain the person's cognitive, that is, thinking and feeling, processes. A nurse also would examine the person's life patterns that could lead to other head injuries. (Roy 1985)

In addition to reflecting concern for the whole person, a nursing perspective implies 24-hour-a-day responsibility. Thus, this perspective encompasses all of the factors in a client's environment, such as fatigue, noise, sensory deprivation, nutrition, and positioning, that might influence coping patterns. Diers (1979) enumerates three distinguishing properties of nursing research:

1. The final focus of nursing research must be on a difference that matters for improving client care.
2. Nursing research has the potential for contributing to theory development and the body of scientific nursing knowledge.
3. A research problem is a nursing research problem when nurses have access to and control over phenomena being studied.

Nursing Research or Research in Nursing

Some authors make a distinction between nursing research (that is, research that focuses on human responses, clinical problems, and processes of care encountered in the practice of nursing) and *research in nursing* (the broader study of the nursing profession including historical, ethical, and political studies. However, the American Nurses' Association Cabinet on Nursing Research (1985) identified the following as priorities for nursing research:

1. Promote the health, well-being, and ability to care for oneself among all age, social, and cultural groups.
2. Minimize or prevent behaviorally and environmentally induced health problems that compromise the quality of life and reduce productivity.
3. Minimize the negative effects of new health technologies on the adaptive abilities of individuals and families experiencing acute and chronic problems.
4. Ensure that the care needs of particularly vulnerable groups, such as the elderly, children with congenital health problems, individuals from diverse cultures,

mentally ill people, and the poor, are met in effective and acceptable ways.

5. Classify nursing practice phenomena.

6. Ensure that principles of ethics guide nursing research.

7. Develop instruments to measure nursing outcomes.

8. Develop integrative methodologies for the holistic study of human beings as they relate to their families and life-styles.

9. Design and evaluate alternative models for delivering health care and for administering health care systems so that nurses will be able to balance high quality and cost-effectiveness in meeting the nursing needs of identified populations.

10. Evaluate the effectiveness of alternative approaches to nursing education for the kind of practice that requires broad knowledge and a wide repertoire of skills, and for the kind of practice that requires specialized knowledge and a focused set of skills.

11. Identify and analyze historic and contemporary factors that influence the shaping of nursing professionals' involvement in national health policy development.

The establishment of the National Center for Nursing Research in 1986 has meant additional federal support for professional growth.

Some Illustrations of Nursing Studies

The examples in Table 5–1 give an idea of the diverse subjects, topics, and settings of actual nursing studies. The sample of contemporary nursing studies in this table only begins to show the diversity of fascinating and ultimately valuable research projects being conducted in the field of nursing. The reader can glance quickly at the table of contents in any of the major journals expressly devoted to nursing research for a fuller notion of its scope.

Finding Nursing Studies

The results of nursing research studies can be found in a variety of sources. Abstracts or reviews of nursing research may be incorporated into textbooks. However, because of the publication time requirements for most textbooks, nursing journals are a more current source of research findings. Nursing journals that focus primarily on nursing research are:

Nursing Research
Advances in Nursing Science
Applied Nursing Research
Research in Nursing and Health
Western Journal of Nursing Research

Additional journals that publish research findings include *Heart and Lung; Nursing Forum; Journal of Advanced Nursing; Journal of Obstetrics, Gynecologic, and Neonatal Nursing; Oncology Nursing Forum; Journal of Emergency Nursing; Journal of Gerontological Nursing;* and *Public Health Nursing.* Non-nursing journals also accept reports of nursing research, e.g., *The American Journal of Public Health.*

The *Cumulative Index to Nursing and Allied Health Literature,* the *International Nursing Index,* and the *Cumulative Medical Index* are excellent resources for locating research published on a topic or problem of interest. Computerized literature searches, such as Medline and MEDLARS, are available through most school libraries. They, too, are helpful in finding relevant study re-

TABLE 5–1 *Examples of Nursing Studies*

Baker et al. (1983) reported on the use of therapeutic touch by nurses to increase the range of motion of joints and to decrease pain in persons with arthritis.

Baker et al. (1984) studied the effect of types of thermometer and length of time inserted on oral temperature measurements of afebrile subjects.

Dufault (1983) used observation, interviews, and case studies to conduct a descriptive, longitudinal field study that identified themes and patterns of hope in elderly cancer patients.

Fehring (1983) compared the effects of a particular relaxation technique with the effects of the same technique augmented with biofeedback on the symptoms of psychologic stress among healthy college students.

Itano et al. (1983) conducted a study in which they correlated factors such as locus of control, self-esteem, anxiety, client's understanding of the illness, client's perception of the severity of the symptoms, and client's perception of the nurse's care and concern plus several demographic factors to compliance to therapy among clients with cancer.

Norbeck and Sheiner (1982) used a social support scale to identify sources of social support related to single-parent functioning.

ports. Since 1983, research on a variety of topics has been collected in yet another valuable source, *The Annual Review of Nursing Research*. Each volume is an excellent compilation of primary sources and references.

WHY IS NURSING RESEARCH FUNDAMENTAL?

In the information revolution transforming the present and shaping the future, reading and understanding nursing research is as fundamental to professional practice as knowledge of asepsis, application of the nursing process, and communication skills are. The ability to access, evaluate, and interpret findings from nursing studies is a source of power in clinical decision making and a strategy for achieving excellence in the delivery of care.

Research in nursing is not only a tool for discovering solutions to clinical practice problems but also a political tool. "Research provides knowledge necessary to improve practice and achieve professional status. Through research, nursing can improve the care of persons in need of health service and affect policy that directs the way health services are provided. Political wisdom is an integral part of the research act" (Chenitz 1985, p. 314).

Ways of Knowing

Do most elderly clients know the names of medications they are taking? What nursing interventions are effective in alleviating backache associated with pregnancy? Is there a circadian rhythm of intracranial pressure that can help a nurse identify the client's time of greatest vulnerability after a head injury? Should clients on oral oxygen have their temperatures taken with an oral thermometer? Does warming infant formulas increase the likelihood of gastrointestinal infection? How can the nurse teach breast self-examination most effectively to Middle Eastern immigrant women? Nurses rely on a diverse array of ways of knowing when confronted with such day-to-day clinical questions. Some may:

- Retreat to established tradition and authority as reflected in a procedure book or established protocol
- Use trial and error combined with their own common sense or past experience
- Consult an expert
- Attempt to arrive at a logically reasoned decision

The Scientific Way of Knowing

The way of knowing that is the focus of this chapter is *scientific inquiry* as evidenced in nursing research. The scientific approach is a process of learning about truth by systematically collecting and comparing observable, verifiable data through the senses to describe, explain, and/or predict events and phenomena. The scientific approach as reflected in nursing research has two characteristics that other usual ways of knowing in nursing do not: (a) It has a built-in system of checks to ensure objectivity and the potential for self-correction and (b) it relies on sensory evidence or empirical data that are collected in a systematic, carefully prescribed manner (Wilson 1989; Wilson and Hutchinson 1986).

A system of checks and balances to minimize bias is applied to knowledge generated through the research process. Nurse scientists who find that one particular hypothesis is supported also check whether alternative hypotheses are supported as well, perhaps more strongly. For instance, if data from normal volunteers indicate that receiving oral or nasal oxygen does not alter oral temperature readings significantly, a nurse researcher determines if this finding is also true of other populations, such as febrile clients. The research methods and conclusions drawn from a study's findings must always be open to the criticism of others. Following the steps in the research process is one way of determining whether a study complies with accepted conventions for conducting credible research studies.

Steps in the Research Process

The truly important discoveries made in the health care field have not been made by scientists who think in dogmatic, mechanical fashion, who focus on knowledge of irrefutable facts without interpretation, or who forget that research is most often a process that moves back and forth between ideas, hunches, existing knowledge, and carefully made observations. Yet, for the sake of clarity, the *research process* is generally conceptualized as a series of steps or phases. Although these phases are dynamic, flexible, and expandable, they can be formalized as follows:

Step 1. Stating a Research Question or Problem An investigator's initial task is narrowing a broad area of interest to a circumscribed problem that specifies exactly what she or he intends to study. Most investigators try to define a research problem as precisely as possible. A problem is often stated in the form of a question. Here are some examples from published nursing research studies:

- How many different treatments for pressure sores are advocated by nurses, and what rationales are given for their use?
- How do different postoperative activity schedules affect the recovery of physical fitness among athletes?
- What is the relationship between types of care given to clients with indwelling urethral catheters and the incidence of urinary tract infection?
- What is the optimal time needed to obtain an accurate oral temperature with a glass thermometer?
- What is the effect of low-frequency auditory and kinesthetic stimulation on the neurologic functioning of the premature infant?

If a study problem is too broad or vague, proceeding to subsequent stages of the process becomes confusing. A research question, according to Brink and Wood (1983, p. 2), "is an explicit query about a problem or issue that can be challenged, examined, analyzed, and will yield useful new information."

Step 2. Defining the Purpose of a Study
The second step is sometimes called defining the rationale of the study. It is the researcher's statement of why the question is important and what use the answer will serve. It lets the reader or funding agency know what to expect from the study. An excellent example of the statement of a study's purpose is the report of Kathryn Barnard's (1973) classic research on the effects of environmental stimulation on the sleep of premature infants:

> Previous work with full-term neonates and older infants supports the general notion that particular kinds of stimulation assist in the regulation of sleep and arousal status. Given this evidence and the increasing evidence that quiet sleep in the immature infant can improve neurological development . . . the purpose of the current investigation was to study the effect of regular, controlled stimulation on the neurological functioning in the infant born prematurely. (p. 15)

Step 3. Reviewing Related Literature
If researchers want their study to build on, confirm, or even transcend the existing knowledge in a discipline and thereby qualify as a real contribution to science, they must know what has already been done. A review of the literature provides the researcher with a framework of background ideas. A theoretical framework is an essay in which the investigator relates the existing concepts, theories, research methods, and findings to his or her study question and purpose (Brink and Wood 1983). At the least, constructing such a framework provides relevant concepts for the research; at best, it gives the researcher a full awareness of facts, issues, prior findings, theories, and instruments that might be related to the study question.

Step 4. Formulating Hypotheses and Defining Variables
Hypotheses are statements of the relationship between two or more concepts, or variables. Some studies are intended to develop hypotheses (exploratory, descriptive, and grounded theory studies), and others are intended to test hypotheses using statistical procedures. Stating hypotheses requires not only sufficient knowledge about a topic to predict the outcome of the study but also definitions that specify the variables under investigation in measurable terms. Finally, the investigator must articulate the relationships among the variables. Hypotheses can be explicitly stated, as Sitzman and her colleagues (1983, p. 219) did in their study of biofeedback training:

> Hypothesis (H_1): Emphysema and chronic bronchitic clients who receive a biofeedback training program to decrease their respiratory rate will have a significantly decreased respiratory rate at the end of the training program and at 1-month follow-up.
>
> Hypothesis (H_2): Emphysema and chronic bronchitic clients who decreased their respiratory rate by the end of the biofeedback training program will have significantly increased their tidal volume at the end of the training program and at 1-month follow-up.

Hypothesis (H) may be stated as null hypotheses (H_0), which essentially test the premise that there are no significant differences in the outcome (dependent variable) other than those that can be attributed to chance. To formulate hypotheses, the investigator must specify the concepts being studied; thus, it is important at this point to determine how to define these variables for the purpose of measuring them. For example, social support might be defined as a score on a written self-report scale, or inventory. This step is called operationally defining the variables. If one does a convincing job, the study is said to have *construct* (or concept) *validity*.

Step 5. Selecting the Research Design
A research design is a well-formulated, systematic, and controlled plan for finding answers to study questions. The design is a road map or blueprint for organizing a study.

Everything from methods of data collection through methods of data analysis should be spelled out in the research design.

Step 6. Selecting the Population, Sample, and Setting

After narrowing a general area of interest to a specific study question, reviewing the literature, and deciding on a research design, the researcher must choose a study population, select a sample, and decide on a setting where the sample can be located. The *population* is the group to be studied. To whom do the findings apply? Some recent studies, for instance, have focused on these populations: divorced fathers, older persons, hospitalized children, disadvantaged minorities, depressed women, nursing mothers, clients with cancer, people with AIDS, clients who have had surgery, and nursing students. The *sample* is that segment of a population from whom data will be collected. Findings from the sample are generalized to the population.

Step 7. Conducting a Pilot Study

A pilot study helps the researcher discover the strengths and weaknesses of the intended design, sample size, and data-collection instrument of the larger project. Pilot studies strengthen nursing studies by weeding out problems in advance; many funding agencies do not approve study proposals unless a pilot study has been conducted.

Step 8. Collecting the Data

The scientific method is characterized by a reliance on *empirical data:* information collected from the observable world. These data are used to make statements about what is true. Any study that goes beyond armchair speculation eventually requires the researcher to collect data. Data sources may be people, documents, or laboratory materials. Data-collection instruments include interviews, questionnaires, physiologic tests, and psychologic tests. The basic point, however, is that by moving either from observation to idea (called *inductive theory*) or from idea to observation (called *deductive theory*), the scientific method relies on empirical data to discover or test knowledge. The researcher uses the senses and measurement tools to collect data relevant to the variables being studied. The time and energy required for this step vary according to the research design. Field studies, historic research, surveys, and most experiments are time-consuming and demanding.

Step 9. Analyzing the Data

The next step in the research process is reorganizing the collected data to relate them to the study question, research objectives, or stated hypotheses. The most important part of this step is to have a procedural plan in mind, have the requisite skills for analysis (such as knowledge of statistics), and realize that analysis provides the answers to the original research questions.

Step 10. Communicating Conclusions and Implications

The researcher's challenge at the final stage is to explain the results of the investigation and link them to the existing body of knowledge in the discipline. Whether results are published or reported verbally, the study's contribution cannot be judged unless the conclusions are communicated to colleagues and critics. Communicating the conclusions, interpreting the meaning and implications of the findings, recognizing the study's limitations, and suggesting directions for future study culminate the research process. In these activities, investigators can synthesize their imaginative, insightful, and engaged style with their rigorous, systematic, and analytic one (Wilson 1989; Wilson and Hutchinson 1986).

The steps of the research process provide the tools with which scientists achieve their major aims or goals. These basic aims are: (a) to develop theories, or explanations of the world (see Chapter 4) and (b) to find solutions to practical problems.

THE RESEARCH–PRACTICE GAP

Bridging the *research-practice gap*, that is, bringing research into the clinical practice arena, is a key strategy in uniting the scholarly, scientific, and caring aspects of nursing in the future. Table 5–2 summarizes this position in the ANA's "Guidelines for the Investigative Function of Nurses" (1981a), which specify the generally expected research competencies of nurses with associate, bachelor's, master's, and doctoral degrees.

It is apparent that nurse leaders want to make nursing practice a more frequent focus of nursing research and to increase the application of valid research findings in clinical work. Yet progress toward achieving these goals is often slowed by several barriers.

Lack of Cumulative Order in the Literature

A scientist from another discipline, according to Gortner (1980), would probably characterize most nursing research as "discrete, nonaggregated studies of isolated

TABLE 5-2 *Investigative Functions of a Nurse at Various Educational Levels*

Associate Degree in Nursing	Master's Degree in Nursing	Doctoral Degree in Nursing or a Related Discipline
1. Demonstrates awareness of the value or relevance of research in nursing	1. Analyzes and reformulates nursing practice problems so that scientific knowledge and scientific methods can be used to find solutions	**Graduate of a Practice-Oriented Doctoral Program**
2. Assists in identifying problem areas in nursing practice		1. Provides leadership for the integration of scientific knowledge with other sources of knowledge for the advancement of practice
3. Assists in collecting data within an established, structured format	2. Enhances the quality and clinical relevance of nursing research by providing expertise in clinical problems and by providing knowledge about the way in which these clinical services are delivered	2. Conducts investigations to evaluate the contribution of nursing activities to the well-being of clients
Baccalaureate Degree in Nursing		3. Develops methods to monitor the quality of the practice of nursing in a clinical setting and to evaluate contributions of nursing activities to the well-being of clients
1. Reads, interprets, and evaluates research for applicability to nursing practice	3. Facilitates investigations of problems in clinical settings through such activities as contributing to a climate supportive of investigative activities, collaborating with others in investigations, and enhancing nursing's access to clients and data	**Graduate of a Research-Oriented Doctoral Program**
2. Identifies nursing problems that need to be investigated and participates in the implementation of scientific studies		1. Develops theoretical explanations of phenomena relevant to nursing by empirical research and analytical processes
3. Uses nursing practice as a means of gathering data to refine and extending practice	4. Conducts investigations for the purpose of monitoring the quality of the practice of nursing in a clinical setting	2. Uses analytical and empirical methods to discover ways to modify or extend existing scientific knowledge so that it is relevant to nursing
4. Applies established findings of nursing and other health-related research to nursing practice	5. Assists others to apply scientific knowledge in nursing practice	3. Develops methods for scientific inquiry of phenomena relevant to nursing
5. Shares research findings with colleagues		

Source: American Nurses' Association, Commission on Nursing Research, *Guidelines for the investigative function of nurses* (Kansas City, Mo.: American Nurses' Association, 1981). Reprinted with permission.

empirical phenomena for which the explanatory theory is not yet well known or defined." It would be much easier for nurse generalists and clinicians with no specialized research training to apply research findings to their practice if nursing research were organized into well-defined programs that would yield cumulative discoveries. In selected instances, this pattern has been more successfully attained than in others. Walike and Walike (1977) conducted a series of studies on the undesirable effects of lactose intolerance in clients receiving tube feedings. As a result of their work, lactose has been eliminated from the formulas, and tube-fed clients with lactose intolerance need no longer experience the nausea,

abdominal cramps, and distention caused by their inability to digest milk sugar. Similarly, Barnard (1973) carried out studies for more than a decade that enabled her to specify special treatment and environmental conditions that simulate prenatal womb life and can positively affect the sleep behavior, weight gain, and development of premature infants. Because of research done by Martinson (1977) with families of leukemic children in Minnesota, hundreds of children can now remain at home with their families during the terminal phase of their illness. Other nurse scientists are striving to develop organized programs of collaborative research on clinically relevant questions such as these.

Insufficient Preparation by Nurses

Building a cumulative, organized, scientific knowledge base to replace traditions, habits, and trial and error as the basis for practice decisions is not enough. Nurses must be motivated and competent to read, understand, evaluate, and interpret this body of work. Reports of research findings are not always easy to locate through the professional media or in the most widely read journals. Once reports are located, nurses may find their traditional scientific format and esoteric language difficult or intimidating. To read and interpret them, nurses need to become astute and active consumers of research findings.

Service Organization Structure

A third obstacle to bridging the research-practice gap is the fact that, until recently, the structure of most service settings rarely encouraged clinical nurses to make changes in interventions based on systematic appraisals or participation in nursing research. Here are some successful strategies for introducing a research orientation into an institution whose focus is the delivery of client care:

- Legitimize the research activities of clinical nurses by granting release time for research and recognizing nursing research through the institution's formal reward system.

- Form a research reference group for clinical nurses. Such a group would bring together nurses who value research, raise research consciousness among nurses, and allow members to exchange formal and informal knowledge about research.

- Help clinical nurse investigators explore the researcher role. In particular, give nurses access to clients for research purposes and help nurses discover differences in the rhythm of research work and clinical work. Clinical nurses are accustomed to a large volume of work that must be accomplished in a short time. Learning how much scholarly and research work to expect from oneself in a specific time represents a major shift for most clinical nurses, who must spend more time in the sedentary activities of prolonged reading and thinking. (Davis 1981)

Nurses must overcome these obstacles if they are to incorporate nursing research into the practice arena and make research a fundamental area of nursing skill and expertise. The following sections address the nurse generalist's investigative roles in more detail.

PROTECTING THE RIGHTS OF HUMAN SUBJECTS

Because nursing research usually focuses on humans, a major nursing responsibility is to be aware of and advocate clients' rights. All clients must be informed about the consequences of consenting to serve as research subjects. The client needs to be able to assess whether an appropriate balance exists between the risks of participating in a study and the potential benefits, either to the client or to the development of knowledge.

Research ethics not only protect the *rights of human subjects* but also encompass a broader list of characteristics. Most of these characteristics are reflected in the ANA's "Human Rights Guidelines for Nursing in Clinical and Other Research." These guidelines are based on historic documents, such as the Nuremberg Code, the Declaration of Helsinki, and United States federal regulations, all of which set standards governing the conduct of research involving human subjects. The ANA Guidelines are presented in Table 5–3.

The Nurse's Role in Protecting Subjects' Rights

All nurses who practice in settings where research is being conducted with human subjects or who participate in such research as data collectors or collaborators play an important role in safeguarding the following rights:

Right Not to Be Harmed The Department of Health and Human Services defines *risk of harm* to a research subject as exposure to the possibility of injury going beyond everyday situations. The risk can be physical, emotional, legal, financial, or social. For instance, withholding standard care from a client in labor so as to study the course of natural childbirth clearly poses a potential physical danger. Risks can be less overt and involve psychologic factors, such as exposure to stress or anxiety, or social factors, such as loss of confidentiality, loss of privacy, and the like.

Right to Full Disclosure Even though it may be possible to collect data about a client as part of everyday care without the client's particular knowledge or consent, to do so is considered unethical. *Full disclosure* is a basic right. It means that deception, either by withholding information about a client's participation in a study, or by giving the client false or misleading infor-

TABLE 5-3   ANA Human Rights Guidelines for Nurses in Clinical and Other Research

The guidelines in this table attempt to specify several important entities: (1) the type of activities that are involved, (2) the rights that are to be protected, (3) the persons to be safeguarded, and (4) the mechanisms necessary to ensure that protection is adequate.

Guideline 1: Employment in Settings Where Research Is Conducted

Conditions of employment in settings in which clinical or other research is in progress need to be spelled out in detail for all potential workers. . . . Anyone employed in work that carries the potential of risk to others needs to be advised as to the types of risks involved, the ways of recognizing when risk is present, and the proper actions to take to counteract harmful effects and unnecessary danger.

Guideline 2: Nurses' Responsibilities for Vigilant Protection of Human Subjects' Rights

In all instances the prospective subject must be given all relevant information prior to participation in activities that go beyond established and accepted procedures necessary to meet his personal needs. . . . Nurses must be increasingly vigilant in their concern for subjects and patients who by reason of their situation and/or illness are not able to protect themselves effectively from externally imposed threat or injury. They must be sensitive to the tendency toward exploitation of "captive" populations such as students, patients in institutions and prisoners. All proposals to be used need to be discussed with the prospective subject and with any worker who is expected to participate as a subject or data collector or both. Special mechanisms must be developed to safeguard the confidentiality of information and protect human dignity.

Guideline 3: Scope of Application

The persons to whom these human rights guidelines apply include all individuals involved in research activities and include the following groups: patients, donors of organs and tissue, informants, normal volunteers including students, and vulnerable populations that are "captive" audiences, such as the mentally disordered, mentally retarded, and prisoners.

Guideline 4: Nurses' Responsibility to Support the Accrual of Knowledge

Just as nurses have an obligation to protect the human rights of patients, so do they also have an obligation to support the accrual of knowledge that broadens the scientific underpinnings of nursing practice and the delivery of nursing services.

Guideline 5: Informed Consent

To safeguard the basic rights of self-determination, nurses must obtain consent from the prospective subject or his legal representative to participate in research or unusual clinical activities. The subject needs to receive:

- A description of any benefit to the subject or the development of new knowledge that might be expected
- An offer to discuss or answer any questions about the study
- A clear statement to the subject that he is free to discontinue participation at any time he wishes to do so
- Full freedom from direct or indirect coercion and deception

Guideline 6: Representation on Human Subjects Committee

There is increasing public support for systematic accountability to ensure that individual rights are not denied to human subjects who participate in research studies. In most instances, the protective mechanism takes place through a committee judged competent to review studies and other investigative activities that involve human subjects. The profession of nursing has an obligation to publicly support the inclusion of nurses as regular members of institutional review committees of this kind.

Source: Adapted and summarized with permission from the American Nurses' Association, *Human rights guidelines for nurses in clinical and other research* (ANA Publication No. D-46 5M 7/75, 1975). Also found in ANA, *Guidelines in nursing research* (Kansas City, Mo.: ANA, 1975).

mation about what participating in the study will involve, will not occur. Full disclosure involves informing study subjects about the following aspects of any study:

- The nature, duration, and purposes of the study

- The methods, procedures, and processes by which data will be collected, expressed in lay language

rather than technical terms (for example, teaspoons of blood to be drawn, rather than milliliters)

- The use to which the findings will be put and any benefits that could be derived

- Any and all inconveniences, potential harms, or discomforts that might be expected, including commitment of unreimbursed time

- Any possible results or side-effects that might follow, including being sent more questionnaires
- The client's alternatives to participating in the study
- The right to refuse to participate or to withdraw at any point
- The identities of the investigators and how to contact them

Right of Self-Determination

Many clients in dependent positions, such as people in nursing homes, feel pressured to participate in studies. They feel that they must please those doctors and nurses who are responsible for their treatment and care. The right of *self-determination* means that subjects should feel free from constraints, coercion, or any undue influence to participate in a study. Masked inducements, for instance, suggesting that they might become famous by making an important contribution to science or get special attention by taking part in the study, must be strictly avoided. Nurses must be assertive in advocating this essential right.

Right of Privacy and Confidentiality

Privacy enables a client to participate without worrying about later embarrassment. The *anonymity* of a study is ensured if even the investigator cannot link a specific subject to the information reported. *Confidentiality* means that any information a subject relates will not be made public or available to others. Investigators must inform research subjects about the measures that provide for these rights. Such measures may include using pseu-donyms, using code numbers, or reporting only aggregate or group data in published research.

Nurses who participate in scientific investigations that involve human subjects are in a key position to serve as advocates for research subjects. All of the study topics in Table 5–4 could put human subjects at risk of loss of privacy.

Vulnerable Subjects

Certain subjects, including children, fetuses, the mentally disabled, the elderly, captives, the dying, and the sedated or unconscious, are considered particularly *vulnerable subjects*. The guiding principle in these cases is that the less a subject is able to give informed consent, the greater the nurse's responsibility to protect the client's rights.

The Principles of Ethical Research

The desire for scientific knowledge must be compatible with the need to preserve the dignity and rights of individuals and social groups. The following principles of ethical research (Wilson 1989) are worth remembering:

1. (S) Scientific objectivity. Objectivity ensures that the research is conducted without bias, misconduct, or fraud.

2. (C) Cooperation with duly authorized review groups, agencies, and institutional review boards (IRB). These committees are charged with reviewing provisions for protecting the rights of human subjects and interpreting law and ethics.

3. (I) Integrity in representing the research study. Integrity means that the researchers do not deceive subjects about the risks, discomforts, or potential benefits of participating as a research subject.

4. (E) Equitability in acknowledging the contributions of others. The researcher should acknowledge coauthors, research associates, and clinical nurses who provided access to clients and participated in data collection.

5. (N) Nobility in the application of processes and procedures to protect the rights of human subjects. Subjects' rights should never be compromised to facilitate the research.

6. (T) Truthfulness about a study's purpose, methods, and findings. "Undercover research" is no longer considered ethical.

7. (I) Impeccability in the use of privileges associated with the researcher's role. Researchers often have

---

TABLE 5–4   Research Studies with Ethical Issues at Stake

1. A nurse who had worked for 6 years on a unit for non-viable clients was concerned about the tendency for nurses to avoid certain clients. She decided to conduct a study of how nurses care for nonviable clients.

2. In a study of unprofessional behavior, several nurse informants revealed some very personal and damaging information about themselves, but this was only a pilot study and they had not signed a consent form.

3. In a study of care of mentally retarded children, the researcher found that there were some glaring deficiencies in the care of these children. For example, children were often left in uncomfortable positions for hours at a time, were rarely offered fluids, and received diaper changes infrequently.

---

access to privileged, private information. This information must be kept confidential and anonymous. All nurse researchers must be as discreet about clients as nurse clinicians are.

8. (F) Forthrightness about a study's funding sources and sponsorship. Any published research must disclose all sources of financial support and any special sponsorship.

9. (I) Illumination of knowledge through contributions to publications and presentations of research findings. Nurse clinicians need to be assured that efforts by nurse researchers will be available to them.

10. (C) Courage to clarify publicly any distortions or misinterpretations of research findings.

As the list acronym (SCIENTIFIC) suggests, following these principles of ethical research makes the scientific ethical (Wilson 1989).

FINDING RESEARCHABLE PROBLEMS IN CLINICAL PRACTICE

Protecting the rights of human research subjects and advocating ethical research are crucial investigative roles for all nurses. Another important role is to identify, in the course of giving nursing care, problems and questions that call for research-based explanations. Identifying problem areas in nursing practice is an investigative skill that all nurses need to master if the interplay between research and practice urged by the ANA is to be achieved (ANA 1981b).

Sources of Research Problems

For the nurse with observation skills and an inquiring mind, each bed bath, back rub, or dressing change is not only a way to meet the client's needs for hygiene and comfort but also an opportunity to recognize discrepancies between what is (existing nursing practice or client status) and what is desirable. Every discrepancy is a potential source of research problems. Valid sources of researchable topics include one's own clinical experience, patterns or trends in someone else's observations or research, and one's own intellectual and scientific interests. Standards of nursing practice developed by the American Nurses' Association and specialty nursing organizations must be evaluated for their application to nursing practice. It has been suggested that nursing diagnoses be used as a framework for clinical research

(Jones, Lepley, and Baker 1984). Consider these examples:

- A staff nurse in a medical setting reads about the hypnotic effects of a dietary amino acid, L-tryptophan, on clients who have recently experienced a myocardial infarction. The nurse wonders if the effects of the amino acid could be approximated by serving certain amounts of dairy products and some meats to these clients (McEnany 1989).

- A surgical nurse battles postoperative infections and is perplexed by the various methods used in different hospitals to change subclavian line dressings. She wishes she knew which method was most effective (McEnany 1989).

- An outpatient clinic nurse who does physical assessments on elderly clients wonders if a program of daily hydration would improve their orientation and decrease their confusion.

Nonresearchable Problems

These examples might give the impression that a constant parade of researchable problems passes before each nurse during daily clinical work. But not all questions that are clinically relevant, important, or even interesting are necessarily researchable ones. A *researchable problem* is one that can be investigated using the steps of the *research process* (Wilson 1989). Two types of questions that are generally *not* researchable (unless they are reformulated) are "should" questions and "yes/no" questions:

- Should a baby be bathed before or after feeding?
- Should nurses wear white uniforms on pediatric units?
- Should clients be ambulated within 24 hours after surgery?

Nonresearchable questions may shed light on the facts bearing on a specific problem, but they do not address a relationship that might shed light on a broader theoretical problem applicable in other circumstances. As such, nonresearchable questions remain relevant to the problem-solving process in a specific nursing care situation, but they are not nursing research problems. "Should the nurse take a blood pressure immediately after a client has exercised?" must be reformulated into "Among healthy adult males, what differences exist between blood pressure readings taken immediately after exercise and after periods of rest?" Likewise, the "yes/no" question "Is normal breathing silent?" can be restated as a researchable question: "What is the relationship between abnormal breathing sounds, such as wheezing, stridor, and rales, and airway constriction or fluid in the lungs?" These restatements transform clinical nursing questions into questions for clinical research. Questions of value, opinion, or policy and accumulations of specific facts and information can be very valuable to clinical problem solving. However, only questions that produce generalizable information for guiding practice under other conditions can turn a nursing care problem into a nursing research problem.

Changing a Clinical Nursing Problem to a Researchable One

Research questions usually begin with *who, what, when, where,* or *why.* Some researchers have sorted questions into different levels, suggesting that some questions are most appropriate when the existing knowledge is at a certain level. For example, if very little is known about a certain topic, it makes sense to ask a *what, who,* or *where* question to acquire descriptive information:

- What are the unmet mental health needs of the frail elderly?
- Where would people prefer to die?
- Who should assume responsibility for preoperative teaching?

When more is known about a topic, it is appropriate to ask *how* or *why* questions:

- How do nurses decide when to initiate protective asepsis?
- Why do clients fail to comply with drug therapy?

Research problems come from a variety of sources. In one's own clinical practice they may come from gripes, wishes, observed patterns of needs, conventions or traditions in nursing care, and the like. Changing a clinical nursing problem into a researchable one can involve four straightforward steps:

1. State the wish, gripe, or the like.
2. Identify the constraints that contribute to the discrepancy between what is going on and what should occur.
3. From the brainstormed list generated in step 2, select the most likely explanation for the discrepancy.
4. Rephrase the problem in conceptual terms so that solutions are not applicable to one case alone but rather can be generalized to clients with similar characteristics and in similar circumstances.

A researchable problem is stated clearly and unambiguously as either a question or a statement, for example:

- What are indicators of reduced respiratory efficiency related to aging?
- The problem in this research is to determine the maximum extent to which exercise can strengthen weakened muscles of clients of age 50 or younger.

Probably the most important point to keep in mind when developing the skills to recognize researchable nursing problems is that much of the tradition of nursing practice is based on just that—tradition—rather than on carefully controlled research. Cardiac precautions, temperature-taking techniques, and oxygenation practices, for example, are all open to investigation through nursing research.

In the near future, nursing research will focus on the interaction of psychologic and psychosocial mechanisms in human experiences of coping with health and illness, the evaluation of nursing interventions, the application of research findings in practice, and underserved and high-risk groups, such as the elderly and minority groups. The nurse of tomorrow will be directly involved in the conduct and application of research.

BECOMING AN INTELLIGENT RESEARCH CONSUMER

Clinical nursing research is the answer to the dilemmas that routinely face the practicing nurse, even when the questions begin with "how do I," "what if," and "what is the best way?" Before clinical nurses can evaluate the worth of a research report, however, they have to understand it. This goal is an ongoing one throughout one's nursing education, but beginning steps include: (a) understanding the format of a research journal article, (b) translating the vocabulary of scientific research, and (c) evaluating the credibility of a scientific presentation of findings.

The Format of a Research Report

Almost all reports of research findings have a standardized format. The nursing student who becomes familiar with it gets the most out of time spent reading the report; it is easier to grasp the meaning of unfamiliar terminology if one understands the context in which the information is being presented. The typical research article is organized in the following way:

1. Abstract
2. Introduction
   a. Review of related literature (including theoretical framework)
   b. Statement of the purpose or specific goals of the study (including hypotheses)
3. Methodology
   a. Procedure for selecting the study sample
   b. Study design
   c. Data collection tools or strategies
   d. Data analysis procedures
4. Results or findings
5. Discussion and implications
6. References

Once the nurse has a general idea of how a research report is organized, she or he must read it with understanding. This involves developing the skill to "come to terms with research terminology" (Wilson 1989, p. 106).

Research Terminology

Concepts, Constructs, and Theory   Nurses work with concepts all the time. *Infection, bonding, self-care level, elimination, loss, comfort, stress, burn-out, decentralization, infection,* and *deinstitutionalization* are all terms for categories of phenomena that share certain characteristics. Some phenomena, such as temperature elevation, can be measured directly with instruments. Others, because they are more abstract, call for proxy measures. For example, anxiety may be measured by a score on an anxiety scale alone or by the combination of an anxiety scale score and some physiologic measures, such as respiration and pulse rate. Certain abstract concepts are often called constructs. Examples of constructs from various theories are *social class* from sociology, *locus of control* from psychology, and *leadership style* from management theory.

Science is concerned with identifying, refining, and explaining relationships among concepts by comparing them to empirical observations. For this reason, deciding whether a study uses appropriate, valid, and believable measures for concepts and constructs is an important step in judging the credibility of a nursing research study. Theories are systems that interrelate concepts and constructs. Most nursing students are familiar with the theories of relativity, gravity, and evolution as well as psychoanalytic theory and learning theory. Nursing theories are discussed in detail in Chapter 4.

Independent and Dependent Variables

The term *variable* refers to anything that varies. The *dependent variables* (DV) in a study may also be called the output, outcome, or criterion variables. Change or the lack of it presumably depends on causes or conditions that the investigator can manipulate. In most cases, the dependent variable (sense of well-being, absence of infection, accuracy of temperature measurement, etc.) is what the researcher is trying to study. The *independent variables* (IV) are *existing* conditions or causes or those variables that the researcher manipulates to affect the dependent variable. It is possible to have multiple independent and dependent variables. Most research is designed to illuminate the relationships among them. The ability to recognize the dependent and independent variables in a study is an important step in grasping a study's potential meaning and significance.

Uncontrolled Variables   Determining the dependent and independent variables in a research study is usually straightforward. Interpreting the study's findings, however, is more complicated. The researcher must take into consideration all the other relevant variables, other than the identified IV, that might affect the DV. Sometimes these other variables relate to how standardized and unbiased the data-collection procedures are, and sometimes they relate to characteristics of the subjects in the sample or how they were chosen. Sometimes, unwanted variables may be introduced through the passage of time or through unforeseen events in the course of conducting the study. A well-designed study specifies the precise steps the researcher must take to be as certain as possible that the results or findings are not a result of *uncontrolled* (*extraneous* or *confounding*) variables. If such variables cannot be controlled through sampling procedures or analysis procedures, the researcher should report their possible influence on the findings and list them as a limitation of the study. When one reads the results of a study, it is important to ask what else could have accounted for the study findings or have influenced them in one way or another. A good practice when one is in doubt about the credibility of a research study's findings is to refer to a research critique (see, for example, Wilson 1989, Chapters 6 and 7).

Data   *Data* is a plural noun meaning information, in this case the information that a nurse researcher collects from the subjects of a research study. Data may be physiologic measurements, such as blood pressure readings, pulse readings, or ratings of pressure sores; psychologic measures, such as scores on intelligence, personality, or other mental measurement scales; or sociologic measures, such as social class reflected by such factors as educational preparation, occupation, income, and the like. Data are obtained from subjects through instruments (or tools). Many instruments are used in nursing studies, including interviews, questionnaires, intelligence tests, rating scales, and such biologic measures as body temperature or serum albumin.

Validity and Reliability

Among the most important concerns of the reader evaluating the worth of instruments used to measure variables in a nursing study are their *validity* and *reliability*. A valid instrument measures what it is supposed to measure. A reliable measure produces consistent results or data on repeated use because the researcher has established a carefully standardized procedure for administering it. If blood pressure readings are taken several times on the same subject under unchanging conditions and the results are consistent, the measure (the procedure for taking the reading) is reliable.

Populations and Samples

The population for a study (N) is the total possible membership of the group being studied. Because it is not always possible or feasible to study everybody in a population, a microcosm of the population, called a sample (n) of participants or respondents, is usually used. When reading a study, the research consumer must attempt to determine if the findings were obtained from a sample that is representative of the study population. A *random sample* is one in which all members of a population have an equal chance of being included in the study sample.

Tables and Graphs

It is beyond the scope of this text to teach the reader how to evaluate whether qualitative or statistical analysis procedures in a nursing study were appropriate. However, a research consumer must learn to read and comprehend findings that customarily are presented in tables and graphs. The following guidelines should prove helpful:

- Try to spot trends.
- Decide if the researcher has picked the correct measure of central tendency. It can be the mean (the total divided by the number of cases); the median (the midpoint between the upper and lower halves); or the mode (the case that is most common). The consumer must determine which is the best way to describe the central tendency for any particular study question.
- Pay attention to the range of numbers in charts and graphs. The range can reveal how typical the dominant response was.
- Look for exceptions. Sometimes these are missing data or "outlyers": instances, observations, or scores that don't fall into the typical pattern.
- Compare findings presented in the text of a research article against data presented in tables, charts, and their captions, keeping alert for any inconsistencies.
- Look up unfamiliar statistical procedures in a good basic statistics book (for example, Triola 1989).

The word *criticism,* in everyday language, has negative connotations. When the nurse is analyzing, reviewing, carefully dissecting, evaluating, and even judging the merits of a research report, criticism becomes a professional responsibility. In fact, the word as Aristotle used it meant a standard for "judging well." A thoughtful research critique requires more than just following the steps of a process that begins with the question, "Is the problem clearly stated?" The research consumer must learn the standards against which to judge research reports. What are the qualities of good problem statements? How does one judge the credibility of evidence, the adequacy of explanations, the reliability and validity of a study's instruments and design? It is the professional responsibility of nurses to acquire the investigative skills that will be required of all nurses in the future.

CHAPTER HIGHLIGHTS

▸ Nursing research refers to research directed toward building a body of nursing knowledge about "human responses to actual or potential health problems."

▸ The *Cumulative Index to Nursing and Allied Health Literature,* the *International Nursing Index,* and the

Cumulative Medical Index are excellent resources for locating research that has been published on a topic or problem of interest.

▸ In the information revolution transforming the present and shaping the future, reading and understanding nursing research are as fundamental to professional practice as knowledge of asepsis, application of the nursing process, and communication skills are.

▶ The ability to access, evaluate, and interpret findings from nursing studies is a source of power in clinical decision making and a strategy for achieving excellence in the delivery of care.

▶ The scientific approach is a process of learning about truth by systematically collecting and comparing observable, verifiable data through the senses to describe, explain, and/or predict events and phenomena.

▶ The scientific approach as reflected in nursing research has two characteristics that the major ways of knowing in nursing do not: (a) It has a built-in system of checks to ensure objectivity and the potential for self-correction and (b) it relies on sensory evidence or empirical data that are collected in a systematic, carefully prescribed manner.

▶ The research process is generally conceptualized as a series of steps or phases, which, however, are dynamic, flexible, and expandable.

▶ The steps of the research process provide the tools with which scientists achieve their major aims or goals. These basic aims are to develop explanations of the world called theories and to find solutions to practical problems.

▶ If nursing is to emerge as a socially significant, credible, scientific, and learned profession with a commitment to high-quality client care, then research (for all nurses) is a necessity.

▶ If nursing is to develop as a research-based practice, the clinical nurse must know the process and language

of research, be sensitive to protecting the rights of human subjects, participate in the identification of significant researchable problems, and be a discriminating consumer of research findings.

▶ Bridging the research-practice gap, that is, bringing research into the clinical practice arena, is a key strategy in uniting the scholarly, scientific, and caring aspects of nursing in the future.

▶ All nurses who practice in settings where research is being conducted with human subjects or who participate in such research as data collectors or collaborators play an important role in safeguarding the rights of human subjects.

▶ Certain subjects, including children, fetuses, the mentally disabled, the elderly, captives, the dying, and the sedated or unconscious, are considered particularly vulnerable.

▶ Identifying problem areas in nursing practice is an investigative skill that all nurses need to master if the interplay between research and practice urged by the ANA is to be achieved.

▶ A researchable problem is one that can be investigated using the steps of the research process.

▶ Valid sources of researchable topics include one's own clinical experience, patterns or trends in someone else's observations or research, and one's own intellectual and scientific interests.

▶ Criticism is a professional responsibility of readers of nursing research.

LEARNING ACTIVITIES

■ Identify a problem area in your nursing practice. Following the guidelines provided on page 82, develop a researchable question related to the problem. How would you go about identifying existing research related to the problem?

■ Visit a university, college, or medical library and identify the resources for obtaining literature related to the problem. Explore computerized reference systems with a library assistant.

■ Review one or more nursing journals, perhaps one in your specialty area. How many of the articles purport to be research articles? Read the research reports and evaluate the applicability of the findings to your area of nursing practice. Are there findings you would like to implement in your nursing practice?

READINGS AND REFERENCES

SUGGESTED READINGS

Benner, P. 1984. *From novice to expert: Excellence and power in clinical nursing practice*. Menlo Park, Calif.: Addison-Wesley Publishing Co.

This book reports descriptive research based on levels of competency identified by practicing nurses themselves through interviews and questionnaires. It is an excellent example of nursing research conducted to discover what nurse clinicians learn from their own clinical practice.

Werley, H. H., and Fitzpatrick, J. J. 1983. *Annual review of nursing research*. Vol. 1. New York: Springer Publishing Co.

Since the publication of volume 1 in 1983, the *Annual Review of Nursing Research* has offered a yearly integrative review of research on selected topics. These reviews are designed to help readers identify what has been done, what has been done well, what the gaps are, and what the suggested directions for research are. Each review includes parts devoted to research on nursing practice and nursing care delivery. The first volume reviewed research that pertained to five areas of human development along the life span, from infants to the elderly and the dying.

Wilson, H. S., and Hutchinson, S. A. 1986. *Applying research in nursing*. Menlo Park, Calif.: Addison-Wesley Publishing Co.

This resource book gives practical tools for understanding and using nursing research in everyday practice. It offers thoughtfully selected information, examples, guided activities, and resources to help the reader become an informed consumer of research and a participant in clinical nursing studies.

SELECTED REFERENCES

American Nurses' Association. 1975. *Human rights guidelines for nurses in clinical and other research*. Kansas City, Mo.: American Nurses' Association.

———. 1980. *Nursing: A social policy statement*. Kansas City, Mo.: American Nurses' Association.

———. Commission of Nursing Research. 1981a. *ANA guidelines for investigative functions of nurses*. Kansas City, Mo.: American Nurses' Association.

———. Commission on Nursing Research. 1981b. *Priorities for the 1980s*. Kansas City, Mo.: American Nurses' Association.

———. Cabinet on Nursing Research. 1985. *Directions for nursing research: Toward the twenty-first century*. Kansas City, Mo.: American Nurses' Association.

Baker, N., Carter, M. A., and Harrison, O. A. 1983. An experimental trial of therapeutic touch in the treatment of arthritis. *Western Journal of Nursing Research* 5(3):56.

———. April 1984. The effect of type of thermometer and length of time inserted on oral temperature measurements of afebrile subjects. *Nursing Research* 33:109–11.

Barnard, K. E. 1973. The effect of stimulation on the sleep behavior of the premature infant. *Community Nursing Research* 6:12–33.

Brink, P. J., and Wood, M. J. 1983. *Basic steps in planning nursing research*. Belmont, Calif.: Wadsworth, 1983.

Chenitz, C. 1985. The politics of nursing research. In Mason, D. J., and Talbott, S. W. *Political action handbook for nurses*. Menlo Park, Calif.: Addison-Wesley Publishing Co.

Davis, M. March 1981. Promoting nursing research in the clinical setting. *The Journal of Nursing Administration* 122–27.

Diers, D. 1979. *Research in nursing practice*. Philadelphia: J. B. Lippincott Co.

Dufault, K. 1983. Process of hope in elderly cancer patients. *Western Journal of Nursing Research* 5(3):72.

Fehring, R. J. 1983. Effects of biofeedback relaxation on the psychological stress symptoms of college students. *Nursing Research* 32(6):362–66.

Gortner, S. July/August 1980. Out of the past and into the future. *Nursing Research* 29:204–7.

Itano, J., et al. 1983. Compliance of cancer patients to therapy. *Western Journal of Nursing Research* 5(3):15–25.

Jones, D., Lepley, M., and Baker, B. 1984. *Health assessment across the life span*. New York: McGraw-Hill.

Loomis, M. E. March/April 1985. An analysis of dissertation abstracts and titles: 1976–1982. *Nursing Research* 34(2):113–19.

Martinson, I. M. 1977. When the patient is dying: Home care for the child. *American Journal of Nursing* 77:1815–17.

McEnany, G. 1989. *Instructor's guide to research in nursing*. Menlo Park, Calif.: Addison-Wesley Publishing Co.

Norbeck, J. S., and Sheiner, M. 1982. Sources of social support related to single-parent functioning. *Research in Nursing and Health* 5:3–12.

Polit, D. F., and Hungler, B. P. 1991. *Nursing research: principles and methods*. 4th ed. Philadelphia: J. B. Lippincott Co.

Roy, C. 1985. "Nursing research makes a difference." *Nurses' Educational Funds Newsletter* 4(1):2–3.

Sitzman, J., et al. July/August 1983. Biofeedback training for reduced respiratory rate in chronic obstructive pulmonary disease: A preliminary study. *Nursing Research* 32(6):218–23.

Starzomski, R. October 1983. The place of research in nursing. *The Canadian Nurse* 34–35.

Triola, M. F. 1989. *Elementary statistics*. 4th ed. Menlo Park, Calif.: Benjamin/Cummings Publishing Co.

Walike, B. C., and Walike, J. W. 1977. A clinical study of tube-fed patients. *Journal of American Medical Association* 238:948–51.

Wilson, H. S. 1985. *Research in nursing*. Menlo Park, Calif.: Addison Wesley Publishing Co.

———. 1989. *Research in nursing*. 2d ed. Redwood City, Calif.: Addison-Wesley Publishing Co.

Wilson, H. S., and Hutchinson, S. A. 1986. *Applying research in nursing*. Menlo Park, Calif.: Addison-Wesley Publishing.

THE NURSING PROCESS

Overview and Assessing

HISTORICAL PERSPECTIVE OF THE NURSING PROCESS

Before the nursing process was developed, nurses tended to provide care that was based on medical orders written by physicians and focused on specific disease conditions rather than on the person being cared for. Nursing practice that was provided independently of the physician was often guided by intuition and experience rather than a scientific method.

The term *nursing process* and the framework it implies are relatively new. In 1955, Hall originated the term *nursing process*. Since then, various nurses have described the process of nursing in different ways. Wiedenbach (1963) described three steps in nursing: obser-

vation, ministration of help, and validation. Later, Knowles (1967, pp. 248–72) suggested "five Ds" necessary for the practice of nursing: discover, delve, decide, do, and discriminate. During the first two stages, the nurse collects data about the client. During the third stage (decide), the nurse determines a plan of action; and during the fourth stage (do), the nurse implements the plan. In the fifth stage (discriminate), the nurse assesses the client's reaction to the nursing actions.

In 1967, the Western Interstate Commission on Higher Education identified a nursing process with five steps: perception, communication, interpretation, intervention, and evaluation. WICHE defined the nursing process as "the interrelationship between a patient and a nurse in a given setting; it incorporates the behaviors of patient and nurse and the resulting interaction" (WICHE 1967). Also in 1967, the nursing faculty of the Catholic University of America proposed four components of the nursing process: assessment, planning, intervention, and evaluation.

The use of the nursing process in clinical practice gained additional legitimacy in 1973 when the American Nurses' Association (ANA) published *Standards of Nursing Practice,* which describes the five steps of the nursing process; assessing, diagnosing, planning, intervention, and evaluation (ANA 1973). Subsequently, a number of states revised their nurse practice acts to reflect these aspects of nursing.

As the nursing process developed both theoretically and clinically, the term *nursing diagnosis* gained considerable recognition in the nursing literature. The concept of a nursing diagnosis, as it evolved in the 1950s and 1960s, applied to the identification of client problems or needs. The term was not easily accepted, although many nursing authors regarded the nursing diagnosis as basic to professional nursing (Durand and Prince 1966; Rothberg 1967). Nearly a decade later, Bloch defined the terms that were crucial in nursing and found that the term diagnosis—in relation to nursing practice—was still quite controversial (Bloch 1974, pp. 689–94).

In 1973, Gebbie and Lavin at St. Louis University School of Nursing helped to form the first national conference on the classification of nursing diagnoses. The participants at this conference defined the nursing diagnosis as the "conclusion or judgment which occurs as a result of nursing assessment" (Gebbie and Lavin 1975, p. 70). Subsequently, conferences have been held every two years and have gained support and interest. In 1982, the conference group accepted the name North Ameri-

TABLE 6-1   *Evolution of the Nursing Process*

Nurse	Selected Contributions	Nurse	Selected Contributions
Peplau, H. 1952	Identified four phases in an interpersonal relationship: orientation, identification, exploitation, and resolution. The phases are sequential and focus on interpersonal therapeutic interaction (George 1985, pp. 60–65).		ing actions (George 1985, pp. 162–68).
		Henderson, V. 1965	Stated that the nursing process was the same as the steps of the scientific method (Henderson 1965, pp. 3–10; Henderson 1980, p. 907).
Hall, L. 1955	Originated the term *nursing process* (George 1985, p. 116).		
Kreuter, F. R. 1957	Described steps in a nursing process as coordinating, planning, and evaluating nursing care and directing the family and the nursing auxiliary as they give nursing care. These were considered to promote the quality of professional practice (Kreuter 1957, p. 302).	Wiedenbach, E. 1963, 1970	Introduced a three-step nursing process model: identify help needed, minister help, validate that help was given.
		Heidgerken, L. 1965	Described steps of professional nursing care as evaluating behavior and situations; recognizing physical symptoms; diagnosing, planning, and meeting nursing needs; and coordinating the client's regimen through all stages of care (Heidgerken 1965, p. 95).
Johnson, D. E. 1959	Saw the nursing process as assessing situations, arriving at decisions, implementing a course of action designed to resolve nursing problems, and evaluating (Johnson 1959, p. 200).		
		McCain, R. A. 1965	Was the first to use the term *assessment* in an article published in 1965. Used the functional abilities of the client as the framework for assessment. Collected and recorded objective and subjective data in assessment (McCain 1965, pp. 82–84).
Orlando, I. J. 1961	Saw the nursing process as interactive (Orlando 1961, p. 29). Stated that the process included three phases: client's behavior, reaction of the nurse, and nurs-		

can Nursing Diagnosis Association (NANDA), thus recognizing the participation and contributions of Canadian nurses. This group has currently established and accepted about 100 diagnostic categories (NANDA 1990).

In 1980, ANA declared that "nursing is the diagnosis and treatment of human responses to actual or potential health problems" (ANA 1980). Clearly, the ANA saw diagnosis as a nursing function even though it was not unusual for some people to believe diagnosis was the prerogative of the physician. In 1982, the National Council of State Boards of Nursing defined and described the five-step nursing process in terms of nursing behaviors: assessing, analyzing, planning, implementing, and evaluating (National Council of State Boards of Nursing 1982). Table 6–1 lists some of the nurses and groups who contributed to the development of the nursing process and nursing diagnosis movements.

COMPONENTS OF THE NURSING PROCESS

A *process* is a series of planned actions or operations directed toward a particular result. The *nursing process* is a systematic, rational method of planning and providing nursing care. Its goal is to identify a client's health status, actual or potential health care problems, to establish plans to meet the identified needs, and to deliver specific nursing interventions to meet those needs. The nursing process is cyclical; that is, the components of the nursing process follow a logical sequence, but more than one component may be involved at any one time. See Figure 6–1.

To carry out the nursing process most effectively and individualize approaches to each person's particular

TABLE 6–1 *(continued)*

Nurse	Selected Contributions	Nurse	Selected Contributions
Knowles, L. 1967	Introduced a process model called the "five Ds"; discover, delve, decide, do, and discriminate. Stated that nurses collected data about the client's health during the first two stages.	ANA Standards of Nursing Practice 1973	Referred to a five-step process: assessing, diagnosing, planning, intervention, and evaluation.
WICHE (Western Interstate Commission on Higher Education) 1967	Listed the steps of the nursing process as perception and communication; interpretation; intervention; and discrimination.	Bloch, D. 1974	Suggested a five-step nursing process that was similar to the four-step model: collection of data, definition of problem, planning of intervention, implementation of the intervention, and evaluation of the intervention (Bloch 1974, p. 693).
Catholic University of America 1967	Proposed four components of the nursing process: assessment, planning, intervention, and evaluation (Yura and Walsh 1988, p. 22).	Gebbie, K., and Lavin, M. A. 1975	Initiated first national conference on the classification of nursing diagnoses in 1973, which led to the use of a five-step nursing process model: assessment, nursing diagnosis, planning, intervention, and evaluation.
Orem, C. 1971	Stated that there were three steps in nursing care: (a) initial and continuing determination of need for nursing care; (b) designing nursing actions for the client that will contribute to the client's achievement of health goals; and (c) the initiating, conducting, and control of assisting actions (Orem 1985, p. 224).	Roy, Sr. C 1976	Used six-step nursing process: assessment of client behaviors, assessment of influencing factors, problem identification, goal setting, intervention, selection of approaches, and evaluation. Advocated the use of the term *nursing diagnosis* (Roy 1976, pp. 23–38).

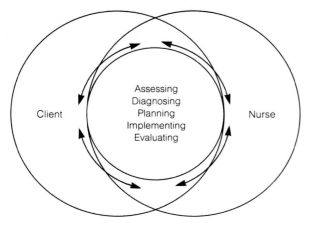

Figure 6-1 The interrelationship of the client, the nurse, and the nursing process.

needs, the nurse must collaborate with the client. An individual, a family, or a community may be considered a client. If the client is unable to take part in the planning and decision-making process, a family member may be asked to participate on the client's behalf. Application of the nursing process requires that the nurse have a variety of skills, including interpersonal, technical, and intellectual. Interpersonal skills include communicating; listening; conveying interest, compassion, knowledge, and information; developing trust and obtaining data in a manner that enhances the individuality of the client, promotes the integrity of the family, and contributes to the viability of the community. Technical skills are manifested in the use of equipment and the performance of procedures. Intellectual skills required by a nurse include problem solving, critical thinking, and making

TABLE 6-2 *Overview of the Purposes and Activities of the Nursing Process*

Component and Purpose(s)	Activities	Component and Purpose(s)	Activities
Assessing			
To establish a database	Obtain health history		Write evaluation goals and outcome criteria in collaboration with client
	Perform physical assessment		Select nursing strategies
	Review records, e.g., laboratory records, other health care records		Consult other health personnel
	Interview support persons		Write nursing orders
	Review literature		Write nursing care plan
	Validate assessment data	*Implementing*	
Diagnosing		To carry out planned nursing interventions to help the client attain goals	Reassess client
To identify the client's health care needs and to prepare diagnostic statements	Organize data		Update database
	Compare data against standards		Review and revise care plan
	Cluster or group data (generate tentative hypotheses)		Perform or delegate planned nursing interventions
	Identify gaps and inconsistencies	*Evaluating*	
	Determine the client's health problems, risks, and strengths	To determine the extent to which goals of nursing care have been achieved	Collect data about the client's response
	Formulate nursing diagnoses statements		Compare the client's response to evaluation (outcome) criteria
Planning			Analyze the reasons for the outcomes
To identify the client's goals and appropriate nursing interventions	Set priorities in collaboration with client		Modify the care plan

nursing judgments. Decision making is involved in every component of the nursing process (Yura and Walsh 1988, p. 108).

The nursing process consists of a series of four or five components or steps. The four-step process is assessing, planning, implementing, and evaluating. In this system, diagnosing is included in the assessing phase. The five-step nursing process is assessing, diagnosing, planning, implementing, and evaluating. Some authorities believe the five-step nursing process gives greater prominence to diagnosing than the four-step process.

Both the four- and five-step nursing processes provide an organizational structure for achieving the goals of the process. In both nursing processes, interaction between the client and the nurse is essential, as illustrated in Figure 6–1.

Nursing theorists may use different terms to describe these steps. In spite of these differences, the activities of the nurse using the process are similar. To avoid misunderstanding, nurses should be familiar with alternate terms that describe steps in the process. For example, *nursing diagnosis* may be called *analysis,* and *implementation (implementing)* may be called *intervention* or *intervening.*

An overview of the five-step nursing process may be found in Table 6–2. Each of the five components of the nursing process is discussed in depth in subsequent chapters of this unit.

The nursing process is an adaptation of problem-solving techniques and systems theory. It can be viewed as parallel to but separate from the medical process. Table 6–3 lists the two processes for comparison. The focus of

TABLE 6-3 *Comparison of the Nursing Process and the Medical Process*

Nursing Process	Medical Process	Nursing Process	Medical Process

1. Assessing
Collection of data from:
  a. Nursing history
  b. Health examination
  c. Review of records
  d. Consultation with other team members
  e. Review of literature
	1. Assessing
	Collection of data from:
	  a. Medical history
	  b. Physical examination
	  c. Diagnostic tests
	  d. Review of literature
		b. Implementation
		  c. Postimplementation strategies: update database, review and revise care plan
			b. Medical therapy
			  c. Referrals

2. Diagnosing
  a. Analysis and synthesis of data
  b. Identification of the health problems
  c. Formulation of nursing diagnosis
	2. Medical diagnosis*
	  a. Organization of data
	  b. Analysis and interpretation of the data
	  c. Formulation of a diagnosis
		5. Evaluating
		  a. Collection of data about the client's response
		  b. Comparison of the data to the established objectives and goals
		  c. Determination of the effectiveness of the nursing plan
		  d. Analysis of variables affecting the outcomes
		  e. Modification of the care plan
			5. Evaluating
			  a. Establishment of the effectiveness of the medical therapy in terms of the goals
			  b. Analysis of variables
			  c. Revision of the plan of therapy as necessary

3. Planning
  a. Establishment of priorities
  b. Establishment of goals
  c. Development of objectives
  d. Written nursing care plan
  e. Delegation of nursing activities
	3. Medical planning
	  a. Establishment of priorities
	  b. Establishment of goals for therapy
	  c. Written plan of therapy		

4. Implementing
  a. Preimplementation interventions
	4. Therapy
	  a. Physician's orders		

*Medical diagnosis has four or five phases:
1. Suspected diagnosis following the patient's initial complaint
2. Tentative diagnosis following the medical history
3. Provisional diagnosis following the physical examination
4. Definitive diagnosis following diagnostic tests
5. Anatomic diagnosis following a postmortem

the medical process is examining, diagnosing, planning, treating or curing disease processes, and evaluating the effectiveness of the treatment. The focus of the nursing process is gathering data, diagnosing (analyzing), planning, implementing, and evaluating the degree to which the client's goals have been met.

Both processes begin with data gathering and analysis and base action (intervention or treatment) on a problem statement (nursing diagnosis or medical diagnosis). Both processes include an evaluative component. Where the focus of the medical process is on the disease process, however, the nursing process is directed toward a client's *response* to illness.

The nurse can be highly creative when using the nursing process. Nurses are not bound by standard responses but may apply problem-solving skills, creativity, critical thinking, and their own knowledge and skills to assist clients. The nursing process is universally applicable. It can be applied in a variety of situations. It can be used with individuals of all ages, groups, and communities.

Characteristics of the Nursing Process

- The system is open, flexible, and dynamic.
- It individualizes the approach to each client's particular needs.
- It is planned.
- It is goal directed.
- It is flexible to meet the unique needs of client, family, or community.
- It permits creativity for the nurse and client in devising ways to solve the stated health problem.
- It is interpersonal. It requires the nurse to communicate directly and consistently with clients to meet their needs.
- It is cyclical. Since all steps are interrelated, there is no absolute beginning or end.
- It emphasizes feedback, which leads either to reassessment of the problem or to revision of the care plan.
- It is universally applicable. The nursing process is used as a framework for nursing care in all types of health care settings, with clients of all age groups.

The five steps of the nursing process are not discrete entities but overlapping, continuing subprocesses. For example, assessing, the first step of the nursing process, may also be carried out during implementing and evaluating. Each step must be continually updated as the situation changes. Just as a client's health is never static but constantly changing, the nursing process, because it is responsive to the client's health, is also dynamic.

Each step or phase of the nursing process affects the others; they are closely interrelated. For example, if an inadequate database is used during assessment, the nursing diagnoses will be incomplete or incorrect; this will be reflected in the planning, implementing, and evaluating phases. Incomplete or incorrect assessment necessarily means equivocal evaluation because the nurse will have incomplete or incorrect criteria against which to evaluate changes in the client and the effectiveness of intervention.

The nursing process individualizes the approach to each client. In the assessment phase, data are collected to determine the habits, routines, and needs of the client. These data about the normal health patterns of the client allow the nurse to write a care plan that incorporates these prior routines whenever possible. The nursing process is also interpersonal. To assure the delivery of quality nursing care, the nurse and client must share concerns and problems and participate in continuous evaluation of the care plan. The success of the nursing process depends on open and meaningful communication and the development of rapport between the client and the nurse. See the box to the left for a summary of the characteristics of the nursing process.

A FRAMEWORK FOR ACCOUNTABILITY

Accountability is the condition of being answerable and responsible to someone for specific behaviors that are part of the nurse's professional role. The nursing process provides a framework for accountability and responsibility in nursing and maximizes accountability and responsibility for standards of care (Law 1983, p. 34). Nurses are accountable to the client (public), to their professional statutory nursing body, to colleagues, to the employing agency, and to themselves. The nursing process provides a framework for accountability in all areas. The professional nurse is accountable for activities in all five phases of the nursing process.

Assessing The nurse is accountable for collecting information, encouraging client participation, and for judging the validity of the collected data. When assessing, the nurse is accountable for gaps in data or conflicting data, inaccurate data, and biased data.

Diagnosing During the second phase, nurses are accountable for the judgments made about the client's health problems, i.e., the diagnostic statements. Is the health problem recognized by the client or only by the nurse? Did the nurse consider the client's values, beliefs, and cultural practices when determining the health problems? When making judgments, nurses are accountable for considering a broad spectrum of client sociocultural backgrounds.

Planning Accountability at the planning stage involves determining priorities, establishing client goals and objectives, predicting outcomes, and planning nursing activities. These are all incorporated into a written nursing care plan available to all involved nurses. In this phase, nurses are also accountable for ensuring that the *clients'* priorities are considered as well as the nurse's.

Implementing Nurses are accountable for all their actions in delivering nursing care. These actions may be performed directly or in collaboration with others, or they may be delegated to another. Even though a nurse delegates an activity to another person, the nurse is still accountable for the delegated action as well as for the act of delegating. The nurse should be able to give reasoned answers as to why the activity was delegated, why the person was chosen to perform the activity, and how the delegated action was carried out. Nursing actions must be charted after being carried out, thereby providing a written record.

Evaluating By establishing the degree to which the goals have been attained, the nurse is accountable for the success or failure of the nursing actions. The nurse must be able to explain why a client goal was not met and what phase or phases of the nursing process require changing and why.

The nursing process provides the framework for nurses to help clients with their health needs and to produce a record of the actions and their effectiveness. The nursing process makes nurses responsible primarily to the client. An implicit part of applying the nursing process is having the knowledge and skills to make the required decisions and to implement the required nursing actions. Therefore, nurses are also accountable to themselves for having the knowledge and skills to use the nursing process in a specific situation.

ASSESSING

Assessing is the first phase of the nursing process. It involves data collection and validation and is necessary before a nursing diagnosis can be made. "Assessment is part of each activity the nurse does for and with the patient" (Atkinson and Murray 1986, p. 11). In effect, assessing is a continuous process carried out during all phases of the nursing process. It may be used during the diagnosis phase to validate a diagnosis. During the planning and implementing stages, data collection may be used before writing a nursing intervention or in obtaining information about a client's response to the nursing strategies. In the evaluation phase, assessment is done to determine the outcomes of the nursing strategies and to evaluate goal achievement. All phases of the nursing process depend on the accurate and complete collection of data (information).

In *Nursing: A Social Policy Statement* (ANA 1980, p. 9), the American Nurses' Association states that nursing is "the diagnosis and treatment of human responses to actual or potential health problems." Thus the focus of assessment is to establish a database about a client's *response* to health concerns or illness in order to determine the client's nursing care needs. Clients' responses include areas of daily living, health, and biophysical, emotional, socioeconomic, cultural, and religious concerns. In contrast to other health professionals, the nurse is concerned with human needs that affect the total person rather than one problem or segment of need fulfillment (Yura and Walsh 1988, p. 110).

A database (baseline data) is all the information about a client; it includes the nursing health history and physical assessment, the physician's history and physical examination, results of laboratory and diagnostic tests, and material contributed by other health personnel. Data collection is the process of gathering information about a client's health status. It must be both systematic and continuous. Systematic data collection can largely prevent the omission of significant data, and continuous data collection maintains the currency of the data, reflecting a client's changing health.

Assessing involves active participation by both the client and the nurse. The client may be one or more individuals, a family, or even a community. Both the nurse and the client enter the relationship with specific knowledge and previous experiences that influence their perceptions and interpretations (see the discussion of perception theory in Chapter 4). It is important for nurses to be aware that their interpretations or assumptions may not be fact. For example, a nurse seeing a man holding his arm to his chest might assume that he is experiencing chest pain when in fact he has a painful hand. Another example of mistaking interpretation for fact is assuming that a client who states that her husband died three weeks ago feels sadness when in fact the death was a great relief.

The acceptance of assumptions as fact is called *premature closure*. To build an accurate database and avoid premature closure, nurses must validate assumptions regarding the client's physical or emotional behavior. In the first of the previous two examples, the nurse should question the client as to why he is holding his arm to his chest. The response of the client may validate the assumptions of the nurse or lead to further questioning. In the second example, the nurse should ask the client how she feels about her husband's death. Failure to validate or verify leads to the acceptance of assumptions as fact, and an inaccurate or incomplete nursing assessment. If the nursing process is to be a successful framework for nursing care, the information gathered during the assessment phase must be complete, factual, and accurate. To collect data accurately, nurses need to be aware of their own biases, values, and beliefs and separate fact from inference.

METHODS OF DATA COLLECTION

The major methods of collecting data are observing, interviewing, and examining. Although these nursing activities are often carried out during the implementing and evaluating phases of the nursing process, they are the main nursing activities during the assessing phase. During assessment, observation occurs whenever the nurse is in contact with the client or support persons. The primary interviewing process during the assessment phase is the nursing health history. Examining during the assessment phase is the major method used in the physical health assessment. Consulting, another nursing activity, is discussed in Chapter 8.

Observing

To *observe* is to gather data by using the five senses. Although nurses observe mainly through sight, all of the senses are engaged during careful observations. Observation has two aspects: (a) noticing the stimuli and (b) selecting, organizing, and interpreting the data, i.e., perceiving them. A nurse who observes that a client's face is flushed must relate that observation to, for example, body temperature, activity, environmental temperature, and blood pressure. Because observation involves selecting, organizing, and interpreting data, there is a possibility of error. For example, a nurse might not notice certain signs simply because they are unexpected in a certain client or situation or because they do not conform to preconceptions about a client's illness. Another source of error is faulty organization and misinterpretation of data. A nurse may interpret a client's wish not to talk as depression when in fact the client is very tired.

Observation is a conscious, deliberate skill that is developed only through effort and with an organized approach. Nurses often need to focus on specific stimuli in a clinical situation; otherwise they are overwhelmed by a multitude of stimuli. Observing, therefore, involves discriminating among stimuli, that is, separating stimuli in a meaningful manner. Nursing observations must also be organized so that nothing significant is missed.

Interviewing

An interview is a planned communication or a conversation with a purpose. Some possible purposes are to gather data, to give information, to identify problems of mutual concern, to evaluate change, to teach, to provide support, and to provide counseling or therapy. Interviewing can be viewed as a process that is applied in most phases of the nursing process. One example of the interview is the nursing health history, which is the primary tool for data collection during the assessment phase of the nursing process.

There are two approaches to interviewing: directive and nondirective. The *direct interview* is highly structured and elicits specific information. The nurse establishes the purpose of the interview and controls the interview, at least at the outset, by asking closed questions (see the next section) that call for a specific amount of data. The client responds to questions but may not have an opportunity to ask questions or discuss concerns. Directive interviews are frequently used to gather and to give information in a limited amount of time. During a nondirective, or rapport building interview, the nurse allows the client to control the purpose, subject matter, and pacing. Rapport is an understanding between two or more people. The nurse encourages communication by using open-ended questions (see the next section) and empathetic responses. Nondirective interviewing is used for problem solving, counseling, and performance appraisal (Stewart and Cash 1988, p. 7).

A combination of directive and nondirective approaches is usually appropriate during the information gathering interview. The goals of the information gathering interview are to collect data and to begin to establish rapport. The nurse begins by using open-ended questions to determine areas of concern for the client. As the interview evolves, the nurse may use closed questions to obtain needed data and to complete the nursing health history. Griffin and Christensen (1986, p. 62) suggest using as little authority or structure as possible to obtain the data needed within the allotted time frame.

Kinds of Interview Questions

Although there are many ways to categorize questions, in this book they are classified as open-ended or closed, and neutral or leading. The type a nurse chooses depends on the needs of the client at the time. For example, the nurse asks closed questions in an emergency or other acute situation when information must be obtained quickly. Closed questions, used in the directive interview, are restrictive and generally require only short answers giving specific information. Thus the amount of information gained is generally limited. Closed questions often begin with "when," "where," "who," "what," "do (did, does)," "is (are, was)" and sometimes "how." Examples of closed questions are: "What medication did you take?" "Are you having pain now? Show me where it is." The highly stressed person and the person who has difficulty communicating will find closed questions easier to answer than open questions.

Open-ended questions, associated with the non-directive interview, are ones that lead or invite clients to explore (elaborate, clarify, or illustrate) their thoughts or feelings. They allow clients the freedom to talk about what they wish. They also place responsibility on clients to explore and to understand themselves, in contrast to receiving advice from another. An open-ended question is broad, specifies only the topic to be discussed, and invites answers longer than one or two words. Such questions give the client the freedom to divulge only information he or she is ready to disclose. The response may also convey attitudes and beliefs the client holds. The chief disadvantage of the open-ended question is that the client may spend time conveying irrelevant information. However the open-ended question is useful at the beginning of an interview or to change topics.

Examples of open-ended questions are: "How have you been feeling lately?" "What brought you to the hospital?" "How do you feel about coming to the hospital?" These questions or statements require more than a "yes" or "no" or other short response, such as "yesterday" or "I don't know." They encourage clients to discover what

their thoughts and feelings truly are. Such questions usually begin with "what" or "how."

The nurse often finds it necessary to use a combination of directive and indirective techniques throughout an interview to accomplish the goals of the interview and obtain needed information. See Table 6–4 for advantages and disadvantages of open and closed questions.

A client can answer a neutral question without direction or pressure from the nurse. Examples are: "How do you feel about that?" "Why do you think you had the operation?" A leading question directs the client's answer. Examples are: "You're stressed about surgery tomorrow aren't you?" "You don't think this illness is fair?" "You will take your medicine, won't you?" The leading question does not give the client an opportunity to decide if the answer is true or not. The interviewer suggests the expected answer by the way the question is asked. Leading questions create problems if the client, in an effort to please the nurse, gives inaccurate responses.

Planning the Interview and Setting

It is important to plan an interview before beginning it. The nurse reviews what information is already available such as a postoperative record, information about the current illness, or literature about the client's health problem. The nurse also reviews the data collection form to make sure that the data to be collected are really needed and will serve some purpose related to the client's care. If a form is not available, most nurses prepare an interview guide to remember areas of information and determine what questions to ask. The guide includes a list of topics and subtopics rather than a series of questions.

Each interview and its setting is influenced by time, place, and seating arrangement. In all instances, the client should be made to feel comfortable and unhurried.

Interviews with clients need to be scheduled for a time when the client is physically comfortable and free of pain, and when interruptions by friends, family, and other health professionals are absent or minimal.

The place of the interview must have adequate privacy to promote communication. A room that is relatively free of noise, movements, and interruptions encourages communication.

A seating arrangement in which the parties sit on two chairs placed at right angles to a desk or table or a few feet apart with no table between creates a less formal atmosphere, and the nurse and client tend to feel on equal terms. Avoid a superior or head-of-the-table position.

Most people feel uncomfortable when talking to someone who is too close or too far away. Generally,

TABLE 6-4 *Selected Advantages and Disadvantages of Open and Closed Questions*

Open Questions		Closed Questions	
Advantages	**Disadvantages**	**Advantages**	**Disadvantages**
1. They let the interviewee do the talking.	1. They take more time.	1. Questions and answers can be controlled more effectively.	1. They may provide too little information and require follow-up questions.
2. The interviewer is able to listen and observe.	2. Only brief answers may be given.	2. They require less effort from the interviewee.	2. They may not reveal how the interviewee feels.
3. They are easy to answer and non-threatening.	3. Valuable information may be withheld.	3. They may be less threatening, since they do not require explanations or justifications.	3. They do not allow the interviewee to volunteer possibly valuable information.
4. They reveal what the interviewee thinks is important.	4. They often elicit more information than necessary.		4. They may inhibit communication and convey lack of interest by the interviewee.
5. They may reveal the interviewee's lack of information, misunderstanding of words, frame of reference, prejudices, or stereotypes.	5. Responses are difficult to document and require skill in recording.	4. They take less time.	5. The interviewer may dominate the interview with questions.
6. They can provide information the interviewer may not ask for.	6. The interviewer requires skill in controlling an open-ended interview.	5. Information can be asked for before the information is volunteered.	
7. They can reveal the interviewee's degree of feeling about an issue.	7. Responses require psychologic insight and sensitivity from the interviewer.	6. Responses are easily documented	
8. They can convey interest and trust because of the freedom they provide.		7. They are easy to use and can be handled by unskilled interviewers.	

Table constructed, with permission, from material on pp. 80–85 of Charles J. Stewart and William B. Cash, Jr., *Interviewing: Principles and practices,* 4th ed. © 1985 Wm. C. Brown Publishers, Dubuque, Iowa. All rights reserved.

people feel comfortable 3 to 4 ft apart during an interview. A distance of 5 to 6 ft encourages a client to talk longer (Davis 1984, p. 66). For additional information, see the discussion of personal space in Chapter 18.

Height also affects communication. By standing and looking down at a client, the nurse may intimidate the client. The client may perceive the nurse who stands during an interview as having greater status.

Stages of an Interview   An interview has three major stages: the opening or introduction, the body or development, and the closing.

The opening   The opening can be the most important part of the interview since what is said and done at that time sets the tone for the remainder of the interview. An inadequate opening can be misleading and create problems during and following the interview. The opening is a two-step process: establishing rapport and orienting the interviewee (Stewart and Cash 1988, p. 39). Either step can come first depending on the situation, the relationship between the two parties, or the interviewer's choice. The rapport and orientation stages may occur at the same time as they are often indistinguishable.

Establishing rapport is a process of creating good will and trust. It can begin with a greeting or a self-introduction accompanied by non-verbal gestures such as a smile, a handshake, and a friendly manner. Next the rapport stage is developed by asking questions about the person and proceeding with some small talk about the weather, sports, families, and the like. The nurse must be careful not to overdo this stage since too much superficial talk can arouse anxiety about what is to follow and may appear insincere.

The orientation step consists of explaining the purpose and nature of the interview, e.g., what information is needed, how long it will take, and what is expected of the client. For instance, the nurse might state that the client has the right not to provide data or might tell the client how the information will be used.

The body   In the body of the interview, the client communicates what he or she thinks, feels, knows, and perceives in response to questions from the nurse. Transition from the opening stage to this stage can often be facilitated by the use of an open-ended question that is related to the stated purpose, is easy to answer, and does not embarrass or place stress on the person. For example: "What brought you to the hospital today?"

Effective development of the interview demands that the nurse use communication techniques that make both parties feel comfortable and serve the purpose of the interview. See communication techniques in Chapter 18. Brief guidelines for communicating during an interview are outlined in the box to the right.

The closing   The interview is usually terminated by the nurse, although in some cases the client terminates it. Nurses normally terminate interviews when they have obtained the information they need. Clients terminate interviews when they decide not to give any more information or are unable to offer more information for some other reason—fatigue, for example. The closing is important in maintaining the rapport and trust established during the interview and in facilitating future interactions. The following ways are commonly used to close an interview (Stewart and Cash 1988, pp. 50–52):

1. Signal that the interview is coming to an end by offering to answer questions. Be sure to allow time for the person to answer, or the offer will be regarded as insincere.

2. Declare completion of the purpose or task by saying "Well, that's about all I need to know for now" or "Well, those are all the questions I have for now."

Preceding a remark with the word *well* generally signals that the end of the interaction is near.

3. State appreciation or satisfaction about what was accomplished: "Well—those are all the questions I have. I really enjoyed meeting you, and I think we accomplished a great deal."

4. Express concern for the person's welfare and future: "I hope all goes well for you. If you run into additional problems, be sure to get in touch with me."

5. Plan for the next meeting, if there is to be one. Include the day, time, place, topic, and purpose.

6. Reveal what will happen next. For example: "I will be responsible for giving you care each Monday, Tuesday, and Wednesday between eight o'clock and noon while you are here. At those times, we can adjust your care if we need to."

7. Signal that the time is up if a time limit was agreed

CLINICAL GUIDELINES
Communicating During an Interview

- Listen attentively, using all your senses, and speak slowly and clearly.

- Use language the client understands and clarify points that are not understood, for instance, by asking the person to describe what a word means to him or her.

- Plan questions to follow a logical sequence.

- Ask only one question at a time. Double questions limit the client to one choice and may confuse both the nurse and the client.

- Allow the client the opportunity to look at things the way they appear to him or her and not the way they appear to the nurse or someone else.

- Do not impose your own values on the client.

- Avoid using personal examples, such as saying, "If I were you . . ."

- Nonverbally convey respect, concern, interest, and acceptance.

- Use and accept silence to help the client search for more thoughts or to organize them.

- Use eye contact and be calm, unhurried and sympathetic.

Source: Adapted from A. Benjamin, *The helping interview,* 3d ed. (Boston: Houghton-Mifflin Co., 1981), pp. 20–55.

upon or explain why the interview must close at that time: "Well, I see our time is up; I'm sorry, but we're going to have to end our discussion.

8. Provide a summary to verify accuracy and agreement. Summarizing serves several purposes: it helps to terminate the interview, it reassures the client that the nurse has listened, it checks the accuracy of the nurse's perceptions, it clears the way for new ideas, and it helps the client to note progress and forward direction (Brammer 1985, p. 74). Sometimes clients may spontaneously offer a summary; at other times the nurse must initiate it or ask the client to do so. Summaries are particularly helpful for clients who are anxious or who have difficulty staying with the topic.

Examining

Physical assessments are necessary to obtain the objective data needed to complete the assessment phase of the nursing process. A complete database of both subjective and objective data allows the nurse to formulate nursing diagnoses, develop client goals, and intervene to promote health and prevent disease.

The physical assessment is carried out systematically. It may be organized according to the examiner's preference, in a head-to-toe approach or as a body systems approach. During the physical assessment, the nurse assesses all body parts and determines anthropometric measurements. Instead of giving a complete examination, the nurse may focus on a specific problem area noted from the nursing assessment, such as the inability to urinate. On occasion, the nurse may find it necessary to resolve a client complaint or problem prior to completing the examination, e.g., if the client appears short of breath. Alternatively, the nurse may perform a screening examination, a brief review of essential functioning of various body parts or systems. Data obtained from this examination are measured against norms or standards, such as ideal height and weight standards or norms for body temperature or blood pressure levels.

STRUCTURING DATA COLLECTION

To obtain data systematically the nurse needs to use an organized assessment framework or structure. This systematic method of collecting desired data about the client is referred to as a nursing health history or, more recently, a nursing assessment. The purpose of the nursing assessment is to gather as much information as possible about the client in order to identify problems for nursing interventions (Yura and Walsh 1988, p. 116). The data collected during the nursing health history between the nurse and client largely constitute a *subjective assessment*. The nurse obtains information about the client,

---

Gordon's Typology of 11 Functional Health Patterns

- *Health-perception–health-management pattern*. Describes client's perceived pattern of health and well-being and how health is managed

- *Nutritional-metabolic pattern*. Describes pattern of food and fluid consumption relative to metabolic need and pattern indicators of local nutrient supply

- *Elimination pattern*. Describes patterns of excretory function (bowel, bladder, and skin)

- *Activity-exercise pattern*. Describes pattern of exercise, activity, leisure, and recreation

- *Cognitive-perceptual pattern*. Describes sensory-perceptual and cognitive pattern

- *Sleep-rest pattern*. Describes patterns of sleep, rest, and relaxation

- *Self-perception–self-concept pattern*. Describes self-concept pattern and perceptions of self (e.g., body comfort, body image, feeling state)

- *Role-relationship pattern*. Describes pattern of role-engagements and relationships

- *Sexuality-reproductive pattern*. Describes client's patterns of satisfaction and dissatisfaction with sexuality; describes reproductive patterns

- *Coping-stress-tolerance pattern*. Describes general coping pattern and effectiveness of the pattern in terms of stress tolerance

- *Value-belief pattern*. Describes patterns of values, beliefs (including spiritual), or goals that guide choices or decisions

Source: M. Gordon, *Nursing diagnosis: Process and application*, 2d ed. (New York: McGraw-Hill, 1987), p. 93.

the client's health, responses to illness, sociocultural factors, health beliefs and practices, coping patterns, and day-to-day activities.

There are many nursing models and frameworks that guide data collection through structured assessment tools. An example is Newman's tool, an assessment/intervention tool that has seven categories: intake summary, stressors as perceived by the client, stressors as perceived by the caregiver, intrapersonal factors, interpersonal factors, extrapersonal factors, and formulation of the problem (Cross 1985, pp. 271–72).

Abdellah (1961) and Henderson (1966) developed earlier frameworks used or adapted in many settings. More recently, Gordon (1987) established a framework of 11 functional health patterns (see the box on page 100). Gordon uses the word *pattern* to signify a sequence of behavior. The nurse collects data about dys-functional as well as functional behavior. Thus, using Gordon's framework to analyze data, nurses are able to discern emerging patterns.

Roy (1984) outlines the data to be collected according to the Roy Adaptation model and classifies observable behavior into four categories: physiologic, self-concept, role function, and interdependence. Orem (1985) delineates eight universal self-care requisites of humans. See Table 6–5.

Other frameworks and models from other disciplines are also helpful for data collection, including Maslow's hierarchy of needs (see Chapter 4), Piaget's assessment of cognitive development, and Selye's stress theory (see Chapter 23). These frameworks are narrower than the model required in nursing; therefore, the nurse usually needs to combine these with other approaches to obtain a complete history.

TABLE 6-5 *Areas of Data Collection Delineated by Dorothea Orem and Sister Callista Roy*

Orem (1985)	Roy (1984)	Orem (1985)	Roy (1984)
Universal self-care requisites	Adaptive modes	7. The prevention of hazards to human life, human functioning, and human well-being	3. Role function
			4. Interdependence
1. The maintenance of a sufficient intake of air	1. Physiologic needs	8. The promotion of human functioning and development within social groups in accord with human potential, known human limitations, and human desire to be normal. (Normalcy is used in the sense of that which is essentially human and that which is in accord with the genetic and constitutional characteristics and the talents of individuals.)	
	a. Exercise and rest		
	b. Nutrition		
2. The maintenance of a sufficient intake of water	c. Elimination		
	d. Fluid and electrolytes		
	e. Oxygen and circulation		
3. The maintenance of a sufficient intake of food	f. Regulation: temperature		
	g. Regulation: the senses		
	h. Regulation: endocrine system		
4. The provision of care associated with elimination processes and excrements	2. Self-concept		
	a. Physical self		
	b. Moral-ethical self		
5. The maintenance of a balance between activity and rest	c. Self-consistency		
	d. Self-ideal and expectancy		
	e. Self-esteem		
6. The maintenance of a balance between solitude and social interaction			

CHAPTER HIGHLIGHTS

▶ The nursing process is a systematic, rational method of planning and providing nursing care. The nursing process is also cyclical, because all steps are interrelated.

▶ The goals of the nursing process are to identify a client's actual or potential health care needs (assessment and diagnosis), to establish plans to meet the identified needs, and to deliver and evaluate specific nursing interventions to meet those needs.

▶ The basic components of the nursing process are assessing, diagnosing, planning, implementing, and evaluating.

▶ Specific nursing activities and responsibilities are associated with each component of the nursing process.

▶ The nursing process can be applied to individuals, families, and communities.

▶ Assessment is the collection, verification, and documentation of subjective and objective data about a client's health status.

▶ Assessing involves active participation by the client and the nurse.

▶ The nursing assessment must be complete and accurate, since nursing diagnosis and interventions are based on this information.

▶ Observation is a conscious, deliberate skill.

▶ The observations of the nurse must be validated; interpretations of client's behavior must not be used as fact.

▶ The nurse often uses a combination of directive and nondirective interviewing approaches to obtain the nursing health history.

▶ Skills required for data collection are communicating, interviewing, observing, and examining.

LEARNING ACTIVITIES

■ Most nurses are adept at assessing client health status utilizing instruments developed by their employer institutions. However, few of these instruments are developed according to a theoretic nursing framework. For this activity, you will organize assessment data obtained from a client in your area of professional practice, utilizing Orem's assessment framework of eight universal self-care requisites (Table 6–5).

■ Reorganize the same data using the framework of Roy's Adaptation Model (Table 6–5).

■ Finally, reorganize the data according to Gordon's typology of 11 functional health patterns (see the box on page 100).

■ What effect do the different organizational frameworks have on the clarity of information about the client? Do the frameworks assist in the prioritization of the data? Do the frameworks assist in the delineation between nursing and nonnursing activities? When utilizing the different frameworks, is there data left over that doesn't seem to fit? Are there components of the frameworks for which no data was obtained? Based on this experience, would you modify your employer's client health assessment instrument in any way?

READINGS AND REFERENCES

SUGGESTED READINGS

Bodnar, B., and Pedersen, S. 1986. The nursing process. In Edelman, C., and Mandle, C., editors. pp. 44–71. *Health promotion throughout the life span*. St. Louis: C. V. Mosby. The authors present the nursing process in a wellness perspective. Theorists who contributed to a health focus for nursing are discussed. An example of an assessment tool for use with healthy clients is included. A modified definition of the nursing process to include wellness is presented, and the need for health-oriented nursing diagnoses is discussed.

Brown, M. D. May 1988. Functional assessment of the elderly. *Journal of Gerontological Nursing* 14:13–17.

With advanced age, the cumulative effects of age and disease have a significant impact on the functional reserve of all organ systems. Comprehensive functional assessment of the elderly is therefore essential. Brown describes the functional assessment protocol used in one geriatric clinical setting.

Capers, C. F., and Kelly, R. May 1987. Neuman nursing process: A model of holistic care. *Holistic Nursing Practice* 1:19–26.

The authors describe the implementation of the three-phase method of the Neuman prescribed nursing process: the diagnosis phase, the goals phase, and the outcome phase. A unique aspect of this model is the detailed comparison of the perceptions of the nurse and the client. The authors provide a sample database detailing five client variables—psychologic, physiologic, developmental, sociocultural, and spiritual. Examples of nursing diagnoses, outcomes, and approaches are also presented.

RELATED RESEARCH

Lenihan, A. A. July/August 1988. Identification of self-care behaviors in the elderly: A nursing assessment tool. *Journal of Professional Nursing* 4:285–88.

Loveridge, C. E., and Heinkeken, J. May 1988. Confirming interactions. *Journal of Gerontological Nursing* 14:27–30, 38–39.

Moss, A. R. September 1988. Determinants of patient care: Nursing process or nursing attitudes? *Journal of Advanced Nursing* 13, 615–20.

SELECTED REFERENCES

Abdellah, F. G., et al. 1961. *Patient-centered approaches to nursing.* New York: Macmillan Co.

Alfaro, R. 1986. *Application of nursing process: A step by step guide.* Philadelphia: J. B. Lippincott Co.

American Nurses' Association. 1980. *Nursing: A social policy statement.* Kansas City, Mo: ANA.

Atkinson, L. D., and Murray, M. E. 1986. *Understanding the nursing process.* 3d ed. New York: Macmillan Co.

Barker, P. November/December 1987. Assembling the pieces: Assessment is like a jigsaw puzzle. *Nursing Times* 83:67–68.

Bloch, D. November 1974. Some crucial terms in nursing: What do they really mean? *Nursing Outlook* 22:689–94.

Brigdon, P., and Todd, M. January 1990. In search of the perfect assessment. *Professional Nurse* 5:181–84.

Carnevali, D. L. 1983. *Nursing care planning: Diagnosis and management.* 3d ed. Philadelphia: J. B. Lippincott Co.

Cross, J. R., and Newman, B. In George, J. B., editor, 1985. pp. 258–86. *Nursing theories: A base for professional practice.* 2d ed. Englewood Cliffs, N.J.: Prentice-Hall.

Durand, M., and Prince, P. 1966. Nursing diagnosis: Process and decision. *Nursing Forum* 5(4):50–64.

Gebbie, K., and Lavin, M. 1975. *Classification of nursing diagnosis.* St. Louis: C. V. Mosby.

George, J. B., editor. 1985. *Nursing theories: The base for professional nursing.* 2d ed. Englewood Cliffs, N.J.: Prentice-Hall.

Gordon, M. 1987. *Nursing diagnosis: Process and application.* 2d ed. New York: McGraw-Hill.

Griffith, J. W., and Christensen, P. J. 1986. *Nursing Process: Application of theories, frameworks, and models.* 2d ed. St. Louis: C. V. Mosby.

Hall, L. June 1955. Quality of nursing care. *Public health news.* Newark, N.J.: State Department of Health.

Hanna, D. V., and Wyman, N. B. November 1987. Assessment + diagnosis = care planning: A tool for coordination. *Nursing Management* 18:106–9.

Hannah, K. J.; Reimer, M.; Mills, W. C.; and Letourneau, S., editors. 1987. *Clinical judgment and decision making: The future with nursing diagnosis.* New York: John Wiley and Sons.

Heidgerken, L. E. 1965. *Teaching and learning in schools of nursing: Principles and methods.* 3d ed. Philadelphia: J. B. Lippincott.

Henderson, V. January/February 1965. The nature of nursing. *International Nursing Review* 12:23–30.

———. 1966. *The nature of nursing.* New York: Macmillan.

———. May 22, 1980. Nursing: Yesterday and tomorrow. *Nursing Times* 76:905–7.

Iyer, P.; Taptich, B.; and Bernocchi-Losey, D. 1986. *Nursing process and nursing diagnosis.* Philadelphia: W. B. Saunders Co.

Johnson, D. E. April 1959. A philosophy of nursing. *Nursing Outlook* 7:198–200.

Knowles, L. 1967. *Decision-making in nursing: A necessity for doing:* ANA Clinical Sessions, 1966. New York: Appleton-Century-Crofts.

Kreuter, F. R. May 1957. What is good nursing care? *Nursing Outlook* 5:302–4.

La Monica, E. L. 1985. *The humanistic nursing process.* Monterey, Calif.: Wadsworth Health Sciences.

Law, G. M. October 5–11, 1983. Accountability in nursing: Providing a framework . . . the nursing process and accountability are inextricably linked. Part 2. *Nursing Times* 79:34–36.

McCain, R. F. April 1965. Nursing by assessment—Not intuition. *American Journal of Nursing* 65:82–84.

McCann-Flynn, J. B., and Heffron, P. B. 1988. *Nursing: From concept to practice.* 2d ed. Bowie, Md.: Robert J. Brady Co.

Merry, J. A. January 1988. Take your assessment all the way down to the toes. *RN* 51:60–63.

National Council of State Boards of Nursing. 1982. *Test plan for the National Council licensure examination for registered nurses.* Chicago: National Council of State Boards of Nursing.

North American Nursing Diagnosis Association. Summer 1988. New diagnosis accepted. *Nursing Diagnosis Newsletter,* 15:1–3.

Orem, D. E. 1971. *Nursing: Concepts of practice.* New York: McGraw-Hill.

———. 1985. *Nursing: Concepts of practice.* 3d ed. New York: McGraw-Hill.

Orlando, I. 1961. *The dynamic nurse-patient relationship.* New York: G. P. Putnam's Sons.

Peplau, H. E. 1952. *Interpersonal relations in nursing.* New York: G. P. Putnam's Sons.

Rothberg, J. May 1967. Why nursing diagnosis? *American Journal of Nursing.* 67:1040–42.

Roy, C. 1976. *Introduction to nursing: An adaptation model.* Englewood Cliffs, N.J.: Prentice-Hall.

———. 1984. *Introduction to nursing: An adaptation model.* 2d ed. Englewood Cliffs, N.J.: Prentice-Hall.

Schamel, K. October 1987. How to assess the patient on long-term care. *RN* 50:65–68.

Schare, B. L.; Gilman, B.; Adams, G.; and Albright, J. C. February 1988. Health assessment skill utilization by sophomore nursing students. *Western Journal of Nursing Research* 10:55–65.

Sherwood, M. J.; Szczech, P. C.; Glasgow, G. M.; and Munoz, C. C. 1988. *Determining diagnosis through assessment.* Baltimore: Williams & Wilkins.

Western Interstate Commission on Higher Education. 1967. *Defining clinical content.* Graduate Nursing Programs, Medical and Surgical Nursing. Boulder, Colo.: Western Interstate Commission on Higher Education.

Wiedenbach, E. November 1963. The helping art of nursing. *American Journal of Nursing.* 63:54.

———. May 1970. Nurses' wisdom in nursing theory. *American Journal of Nursing.* 70:1057–62.

Yura, H., and Walsh, M. B. 1988. *The nursing process: Assessing, planning, implementing, evaluating.* 5th ed. Norwalk, Conn.: Appleton & Lange.

CHAPTER 7

Diagnosing

CONTENTS

NURSING DIAGNOSIS

The identification and development of nursing diagnoses began formally in 1973 when the National Conference Group for the Generation and Classification of Nursing Diagnoses was formed. This group originated through the efforts of two faculty members of Saint Louis University, Kristine Gebbie and Mary Ann Lavin, who perceived a need to identify their roles in an ambulatory care setting. The First National Conference held to identify nursing diagnoses was sponsored by the Saint Louis University School of Nursing and Allied Health Professions in 1973. Since that time, national conferences have been held in 1975, 1978, 1980, 1982, 1984, 1986, 1988, and 1990. The proceedings of the conferences have been published (Gebbie and Lavin 1975; Gebbie 1976; Kim and Moritz 1982; Kim, MacFarland, and McLane

1984; Hurley 1986; McLane 1987). Through the efforts of these groups, much progress has been made in defining, classifying, and describing nursing diagnoses. International recognition was shown by the First Canadian Conference, held in Toronto in 1977, and the International Nursing Conference held in May 1987 in Calgary, Alberta, Canada. In 1982, the conference group accepted the name North American Nursing Diagnosis Association (NANDA), thus recognizing the participation and contributions of nurses in the United States and Canada.

The members of NANDA include staff nurses, clinical specialists, faculty, directors of nursing, deans, theorists, and researchers. The group has currently approved approximately 100 nursing diagnostic categories or labels for clinical use and testing. See the accompanying box.

Approved Nursing Diagnoses

North American Nursing Diagnosis Association (NANDA)
1990 Approved Nursing Diagnostic Categories

Activity intolerance
Activity intolerance: High risk
Adjustment, Impaired
Airway clearance, Ineffective
Anxiety
Aspiration: High risk
Body image disturbance
Body temperature, Altered: High risk
Bowel incontinence
Breast-feeding, Effective (potential for enhanced)[1]
Breast-feeding, Ineffective
Breathing pattern, Ineffective
Cardiac output, Decreased
Communication, Impaired: Verbal
Constipation
Constipation, Colonic
Constipation, Perceived
Coping, Defensive
Coping, Family: Potential for growth
Coping, Ineffective family: Compromised
Coping, Ineffective family: Disabling
Coping, Ineffective individual
Decisional conflict (specify)
Denial, Ineffective
Diarrhea
Disuse syndrome: High risk
Diversional activity deficit
Dysreflexia
Family processes, Altered
Fatigue
Fear
Fluid volume deficit
Fluid volume deficit: High risk
Fluid volume excess
Gas exchange, Impaired
Grieving, Anticipatory
Grieving, Dysfunctional
Growth and development, Altered
High maintenance, Altered
Health maintenance, Altered
Health-seeking behaviors (specify)
Home maintenance management, Impaired
Hopelessness
Hyperthermia
Hypothermia

Infection: High risk
Injury: High risk
Knowledge deficit (specify)
Mobility, Impaired physical
Noncompliance (specify)
Nutrition, Altered: Less than body requirements
Nutrition, Altered: More than body requirements
Nutrition, Altered: High risk for more than body requirements
Oral mucous membrane, Altered
Pain (Acute)
Pain, Chronic
Parental, role conflict
Parenting, Altered
Parenting Altered, High risk
Personal identity disturbance
Poisoning: High risk
Post-trauma response
Powerlessness
Protection, Altered
Rape-trauma syndrome
Rape-trauma syndrome: Compound reaction
Rape-trauma syndrome: Silent reaction
Role performance, Altered
Self-care deficit: Bathing/hygiene
Self-care deficit: Dressing/grooming
Self-care deficit: Feeding
Self-care deficit: Toileting
Self-esteem disturbance
Self-esteem, Low: Chronic
Self-esteem, Low: Situational
Sensory/perceptual alterations: Visual, auditory, kinesthetic, gustatory, tractile, olfactory (specify)
Sexual dysfunction
Sexuality patterns, Altered
Skin integrity, Impaired
Skin integrity, Impaired: High risk
Sleep pattern disturbance
Social interaction, Impaired
Social isolation
Spiritual distress
Suffocation: High risk
Swallowing, Impaired

Definitions

Nursing diagnosis has provided the profession with an appropriate focus on the content and the diagnostic categories that were in the domain of nursing. The term *diagnosis*, according to the dictionary, is derived from the Greek word *diagignoskein,* which means "to distinguish." Definitions include (a) the art of identifying a disease from its signs and symptoms, (b) a statement or conclusion concerning the nature of some phenomenon, and (c) analysis of the course or nature of a condition, situation, or problem. Although the first definition pertains to physicians, diagnosis is not restricted to one particular profession and must be qualified by a professional designation. In fact, anyone who makes a statement or conclusion about the nature of a condition or problem is diagnosing.

The term *nursing diagnosis* refers to both the process of making a diagnosis and to the clinical judgment reached and expressed in a category name or label (Gordon 1987b, p. 7). Several definitions of nursing diagnosis have been stated since the early 1950s. Each has a different emphasis, but all have many similarities. The earliest definition of nursing diagnosis was formulated by Abdellah (1957, p. 4), who stated that it was the "determination of the nature and extent of nursing problems presented by the individual patients or families receiving nursing care."

In 1973, the First National Conference on the Classification of Nursing Diagnosis accepted this definition: A *nursing diagnosis* "is the judgment or conclusion [that] occurs as a result of nursing assessment" (Gebbie and Lavin 1975). To Gordon (1976, p. 1299), *nursing diagnoses,* or clinical diagnoses made by professional nurses, describe a combination of signs and symptoms that indicate actual or potential health problems that nurses by virtue of their education and experience are able, licensed, and accountable to treat. To Edel (1982,

p. 6), a *nursing diagnosis* is the statement of a potential or actual altered health status of a client, which is derived from nursing assessment and which requires intervention from the domain of nursing. Edel's definition emphasizes that the entity to be diagnosed is *health status,* which avoids the negative connotation of problem and allows for positive diagnoses of clients. (Health status is the health of a person at a given time.) The strengths and the problems of the person are considered. To Shoemaker (1984, p. 109), a *nursing diagnosis* is a clinical judgment about an individual family or community that is derived through a deliberate, systematic process of data collection and analysis. The diagnosis is the basis for prescriptions of definitive therapy for which the nurse is accountable. It is expressed concisely and includes the etiology (when known) of the condition.

In March 1990, the Ninth Conference on the Classification of Nursing Diagnoses in Orlando, Florida accepted the working definition of nursing diagnosis shown in the accompanying box.

---

*1990 NANDA Definition of
Nursing Diagnosis*

"Nursing diagnosis is a clinical judgment about individual, family, or community responses to actual and potential health problems/life processes. Nursing diagnoses provide the basis for selection of nursing interventions to achieve outcomes for which the nurse is accountable."

Ninth Conference on the Classification of Nursing Diagnoses, March 17–21, 1990, Orlando, Florida.

Implied in these definitions are the following characteristics:

- Professional nurses (registered nurses) are the persons responsible for making nursing diagnoses. Even though other nursing personnel may contribute data to the process of diagnosing and may implement specified nursing care, the formulation of a diagnostic statement lies within the realm of the professional nurse.

- A health problem is any condition or situation in which a client requires help to promote, maintain, or regain a state of health or to achieve a peaceful death. It does not always refer to an undesirable state but does refer to a situation for which the client needs nursing assistance.

- Nursing diagnoses describe (a) actual health problems (deviations from health), (b) potential health problems (risk factors that predispose persons and families to health problems), and (c) areas of enriched personal growth. Examples of actual health problems are **Ineffective airway clearance, Fluid volume deficit,** and **Knowledge deficit.** Examples of potential health problems are **High risk for infection** and **High risk for injury.** Examples of areas of enriched personal growth are self-development, health maintenance management, and parenting.

- The domain of nursing diagnosis includes only those health states that nurses are able and licensed to treat. For example, nurses are not educated to diagnose or treat diseases such as diabetes mellitus; this task is defined legally as within the practice of medicine. Yet they can diagnose a **Knowledge deficit, Ineffective individual coping, Altered nutrition,** and **High risk for injury,** all of which may accompany diabetes mellitus. These problems are within the nurse's capabilities and the scope of the nurse's licensing laws; thus, the nurse is responsible and accountable for the treatment provided for these nursing diagnoses.

- A nursing diagnosis is a judgment made only after a thorough, systematic process of data collection.

Differentiating Nursing Diagnosis from Medical Diagnosis

To clarify the domain of nursing and make it distinct from the medical profession, nurses had to define the characteristics of a nursing diagnosis. This was accomplished most definitively by Shoemaker (1984). She surveyed 111 experts in the field to determine the essential characteristics of a nursing diagnosis. These findings describe and define a nursing diagnosis and also allow for differentiation from medical diagnoses. For a summary, see Table 7–1. A medical diagnosis describes a specific pathophysiologic response that is fairly uniform from one client to the other. In contrast, a nursing diagnosis describes a client's response to an illness or a potential health problem; this response varies among individuals. Nursing diagnoses are oriented to the individual and change as the client's responses change. For example, two clients with a medical diagnosis of rheumatoid arthritis can have quite similar disease processes but very different responses. A 70-year-old woman may respond with acceptance, viewing her condition as part of the aging process, whereas a 20-year-old woman may respond with anger and hostility because of the changes this condition will make in her personal identity, body image, role performance, and self-esteem.

Medical diagnoses are described in concise phrases of two or three words according to a universally accepted taxonomy (system of classification). For nursing diag-

TABLE 7–1 *Comparison of Nursing and Medical Diagnoses*

Nursing Diagnosis	Medical Diagnosis
Describes an individual's response to a disease process condition or situation	Describes a specific disease process
Is oriented to the individual	Is oriented to pathology
Changes as the client's responses change	Remains constant throughout the duration of illness
Guides independent nursing activities: planning, intervening and evaluating	Guides medical management, some of which may be carried out by the nurse
Is complementary to the medical diagnosis	Is complementary to the nursing diagnosis
Has no universally accepted classification system; such systems are in the process of development	Has a well-developed classification system accepted by the medical profession
Consists of a two-part statement with etiology when known	Consists of two or three words

noses, however, the format is a two-part statement that includes the *etiology* (cause or source) when known. Some nursing diagnoses are long and complex. It is doubtful that nursing diagnoses will ever be as condensed as medical diagnoses. A nursing diagnosis may be complementary to a medical diagnosis but is separate and distinct. A client who has one or more medical diagnoses and medical orders may also have one or more nursing diagnoses and nursing orders. These diagnoses and orders are complementary rather than contradictory.

A nursing diagnosis is a statement of a nursing judgment, and refers to a condition that nurses are licensed to treat. In contrast, a medical diagnosis is made and treated by a physician. Nursing diagnoses refer to physical, sociocultural, psychologic, and spiritual conditions, whereas medical diagnoses refer to disease.

Nursing diagnoses relate to the nurse's independent functions, i.e., the areas of health care that are unique to nursing and are separate and distinct from the care included in medical management. Even though the nurse is obligated to carry out medical orders, i.e. dependent functions, the nurse is also obligated to diagnose and prescribe within the limits of nurse practice acts.

Some of the advantages of using nursing diagnoses are outlined in the accompanying box.

Advantages of Using Nursing Diagnoses

- Nursing diagnoses facilitate communication among nurses and with other health team members. A diagnosis identifies a client's health status, strengths, and health problems.
- They strengthen the nursing process and provide direction for planning independent nursing interventions.
- They help the nurse focus on independent nursing actions.
- They help identify the focus of a nursing activity and thus facilitate peer review and quality assurance programs. Peer review is the appraisal of a nurse's practice, education, or research by co-workers of equal status. Quality assurance is the evaluation of nursing services provided and the results achieved against an established standard.
- They facilitate nursing intervention when a client moves from one hospital unit to another or from hospital to home. The nursing diagnoses guide the planning of the nursing interventions that the client requires after discharge.
- They facilitate comprehensive health care by identifying, validating, and responding to specific health problems (Risner 1986b, p. 151).

THE DIAGNOSTIC PROCESS

Diagnosis is a process of analysis and synthesis. Analysis is the separation into components, i.e., breaking down the whole into its parts. Synthesis is the opposite, i.e., putting together the parts into the whole.

The cognitive skills required for analysis and synthesis are objectivity, critical thinking, decision making, and inductive and deductive reasoning (Risner 1986a, p. 126). Deductive and inductive reasoning and decision making are discussed in Chapter 4. To be objective is to be without bias; i.e., the values and beliefs of the nurse do not affect how data are viewed and analyzed. To be objective, nurses must be aware of their own values and beliefs. *Critical thinking* is a cognitive process during which data are reviewed and explanations considered before an opinion is formed. In this process, nurses use all the subjective and objective data acquired and validated during the assessment phase as well as their knowledge to develop a nursing diagnostic statement.

The diagnostic process is used continuously by most nurses working in hospitals, ambulatory care settings, clients' homes, and long-term care facilities. An experienced nurse may enter a client's room and immediately observe significant data about the client. The nurse is able to do this because of knowledge, skill, and expertise in the practice setting. The outcome of the diagnostic process, the statement of the nursing diagnosis, is recorded in the care plan. This conclusion or statement provides nurse colleagues with a common language and direction for individualized interventions.

Although experienced practitioners are able to perform these mental processes automatically, the novice needs guidelines to understand and formulate diagnoses. The diagnostic process has the following steps:

1. Data processing—interpreting collected data
2. Determining the client's health problems, health risks, and strengths
3. Formulating nursing diagnoses

Data Processing

Data processing, the first aspect of analyzing, is the act of interpreting collected data. It involves the following steps:

1. Organize data
2. Compare data against standards (identify significant cues)
3. Cluster data (generate tentative hypotheses)
4. Identify gaps and inconsistencies

These activities occur continuously rather than sequentially.

Organizing the Data   Once the data are collected, they need to be organized into a usable framework for the nurse and others who may need access to them. As discussed in Chapter 6, theoretical frameworks and conceptual models often guide the format of the assessment tool, thus facilitating the organization of data. The nurse may choose one or more nursing models and develop skill by using them consistently. For further information on nursing models, see Chapter 4.

To illustrate data organization, a summary of the nursing assessment data using a functional health pattern assessment format is shown in the box on the following page.

Comparing Data against Standards   The nurse compares the client's data to a wide range of standards, such as normal health patterns, normal vital signs, laboratory values, basic food groups, growth, and development. The nurse also uses personal knowledge—e.g., of physiology, psychology, and sociology—as well as past experience when comparing the data.

A *standard* or *norm* is a generally accepted rule, model, pattern, or measure. To be used in comparing, however, a standard must be both relevant and reliable. To be relevant, it must be of the same class as the data to which it is compared. Just as oranges cannot be the standard used to judge apples, the ideal breakfast for a teenager cannot be used as a standard for the breakfast of a person over 65 years of age. To be reliable, the standard must be based on data from a sufficiently large sample. For example, to determine the average interests of 12-year-olds, one must survey a large number of teenagers, not just three.

Standards used for comparison include the Daily Food Guides, Erickson's stages of development, and the Metropolitan Life Insurance charts for normal ranges of height and weight. When comparing data against standards, the nurse must know the client's view of "normal," which may differ from that of the nurse. For example, a client may think it is perfectly normal to bathe once a week whereas the nurse may believe once a day is normal. What is considered normal varies according to the client's expectations, culture, values, socioeconomic status, and knowledge. It is important to gather and record useful and specific data. Thus, if the client states, "My urinary elimination is normal," the nurse should ask for clarification: "Can you explain what you mean by normal?" The nurse compares the client data against standards and norms in order to identify significant and relevant cues. A *cue* is a piece of information or data that influences decisions (Gordon 1987b, p. 182). Cues are acquired through the use of the five senses (taste, touch, smell, hearing, and sight). Gordon (1987b, p. 191) suggests the following guidelines to assist in determining significant cues.

1. *Cues that point to change in a client's health status or pattern.* These may be positive or negative. For example the client states: "I have recently experienced shortness of breath while climbing stairs" or "I have not smoked for three months."

2. *Cues that vary from norms of the client population.* The client's pattern may fit within cultural norms but vary from norms of the general society. The client may consider a pattern—for example, eating very small meals and having a poor appetite—to be normal. This pattern, however, may not be productive and may require further exploration.

3. *Cues that indicate a developmental delay.* Changes in health patterns occur as the person grows and develops. By age 9 months, the infant is usually able to sit alone without support, stand while holding on, and turn the wrists to examine objects (James and Mott 1988, p. 96). The infant who has not accomplished these tasks needs further assessment for possible developmental delays. To identify significant cues, the nurse must be aware of normal patterns and changes.

The nurse must always consider the client's interpretation of the situation. Making diagnostic decisions without eliciting the perceptions of the client or family may lead to missed diagnoses or misdiagnoses. The client's perceptions are an important aspect of the decision-making process.

Clustering Data   Clustering or grouping data is a process of determining the relatedness of facts and finding patterns in the facts. This is the beginning of synthesis. Data are examined to determine whether any patterns are present, whether the data represent isolated incidents, and whether the data are significant. The process of data clustering is influenced by the nurse's background of scientific knowledge, past nursing experi-

---

Organization of Data for Mr. Frederick Smith

Health Perception/Health Management

- No energy
- Shortness of breath
- Had left hip replacement 2 years ago
- Eats a good diet
- Does not smoke
- Does not drink

Nutritional/Metabolic

- Has diabetes
- Does not eat sugar
- Lost 5 pounds over past year

Elimination

- Urinates frequently

Activity/Exercise

- Lacks energy to do daily ranch chores
- Moves more slowly since hip surgery

Cognitive/Perceptual

- Slightly hard of hearing
- Wears glasses
- Doesn't read much, prefers to be told how to do things

Roles/Relationships

- Lives with wife and 6 of 13 children
- Family "scared" about his illness
- Cattle rancher and farmer

Self-Perception/Self-Concept

- Too weak to do day work on the farm

Coping/Stress

- Usually too busy to worry about things
- Perceives his son Tom as helpful in talking things over

- Wants family to visit

Value/Belief

- Religion/spirituality is important to him
- Wants to see hospital chaplain

Medication/History

- Tolazamide (Tolinase) 250 mg daily
- Furosemide (Lasix) 20 mg daily
- Slow K 20 mEq daily
- Nitroglycerin 1/150 gr prn for angina

Nursing Physical Assessment

- 81 years old
- Height 171 cm
- Weight 95.3 kg
- TPR 36.5, 80, 16
- Blood pressure 124/80 mm Hg
- Large, slightly obese
- Joint stiffness
- Slight limp
- No pedal edema
- Femoral pulses very strong (R) and bounding (L)
- Popliteal, dorsalis pedis, posterior tibial pulses absent in left leg
- Left leg cooler than right leg
- Heart rhythm is regular
- Loud heart murmur in aortic area
- History of angina (6 months)
- Rales in bases of both lungs cleared by coughing
- Urinary frequency because of Lasix
- No allergies

ences, and concept of nursing. Together, these factors are a mental reference file of facts and principles the nurse uses to verify the significance of the data. The nurse may cluster data inductively by combining data from different assessment areas to form a pattern, or the nurse may begin with a framework, such as Gordon's functional health patterns, and cluster the subjective and objective data into the appropriate categories. The latter is a deductive approach to data clustering, or pattern formation.

To relate and group data, the nurse must consider nursing diagnostic categories or areas of nursing responsibility. Gordon (1987b, p. 20) states that clustering information involves a search in the nurse's memory stores for previously learned meaningful groups of clinical cues that are associated with a diagnostic category. Gordon believes that clustering occurs in conjunction with data collection and interpretation, as evidenced in remarks or thoughts such as, "I'm getting a picture of" or "This cue doesn't fit the picture." The novice nurse does not have the knowledge base or the clinical experience that facilitates the recognition of cues related to diagnostic categories. Thus, the novice must take careful assessment notes, search data for abnormal cues, and use textbook resources for comparing the client's cues with the defining characteristics and etiologic factors of the accepted nursing diagnoses. (A list of accepted nursing diagnostic categories is shown earlier in the chapter.) After comparing the client cues against available resources, the nurse can group data into clusters.

TABLE 7–2 *Formulating Nursing Diagnoses for Mr. Frederick Smith*

Diagnostic Category	Data Clustering/ Grouping Data	Determining Strengths and Health Problems	Formulating Nursing Diagnostic Statements
Activity intolerance	Shortness of breath Lacks energy to do daily chores Does not smoke	Does not smoke (strength) Activity intolerance (problem)	**Activity intolerance** related to shortness of breath and lack of energy secondary to decreased strength of cardiac contraction
Ineffective airway clearance	Rales in bases of both lungs relieved by coughing	Able to expel secretions by coughing (strength) Secretions in lung bases (problem)	**Potential ineffective airway clearance** postoperatively related to chest incision
High risk for injury	Left hip replacement Movement slightly limited Joint stiffness Slight limp	Carries out daily activities independently (strength) Movement slightly limited (problem)	**High risk for injury (trauma)** related to joint stiffness and limp from hip replacement surgery
Altered nutrition	Is diabetic Takes tolazamide (Tolinase) daily "No sugar" in diet "Eats a good diet" Overweight for height Weight loss of 5 pounds in past year	Controls diabetes with Tolinase and "no sugar" (strength) Weight loss of 5 pounds in past year (strength) Overweight (problem)	**Altered nutrition: more than body requirements** related to imbalance of intake versus activity expenditure
Knowledge deficit	Takes furosemide (Lasix) daily Takes Slow K daily Urinates frequently	Complies with medical regime (strength) Does not relate urinary frequency to diuretic (problem)	**Knowledge deficit:** side-effects of diuretic therapy

▶

Data clustering involves making inferences. An *inference* is the nurse's judgment or interpretation of cues. Inferences are made throughout the diagnostic process. During data clustering, the nurse interprets the possible meaning of the cues and labels the cue clusters with tentative diagnostic hypotheses. Data clustering or grouping for Mr. Frederick Smith is illustrated in Table 7–2. The data are clustered according to nursing diagnostic categories.

Identifying Gaps and Inconsistencies in Data

Gaps are missing information needed to determine a data pattern. For example, during the assessment phase, the nurse needs data about a client's definition of health to interpret his statement "I am sick all the time." Data may be completely missing or incomplete. For example, information about a 15-month-old child's mobility may not specify whether the child crawls or walks. This information is essential for establishing the child's developmental stage.

Inconsistencies are conflicting data. Possible sources of conflicting data include: measurement error, expectations, and conflicting or unreliable reports (Gordon, 1987b, p. 259). For example, if the client reports a history of high blood pressure but the nurse obtains a low reading, the nurse should check the equipment and procedure for possible error. All inconsistencies must be clarified before a valid pattern can be established.

TABLE 7–2 *(continued)*

Diagnostic Category	Data Clustering/ Grouping Data	Determining Strengths and Health Problems	Formulating Nursing Diagnostic Statements
Altered peripheral tissue perfusion	Vital signs normal Heart rhythm regular Loud heart murmur (aortic area) Femoral pulses stronger than normal Absent pulses (popliteal, dorsalis pedis, posterior tibial) in left leg Left leg cooler than right leg Integument pink and intact	Vital signs within normal range (strength) Skin intact and of good color (strength) Impaired circulation in left leg (problem)	**Altered peripheral tissue perfusion** (left leg) related to impaired arterial circulation
Fear	Hospitalized for cardiac catheterization and possible aortic valve replacement States family "scared" about illness Wants to see chaplain Wants family to visit Perceives son Tom as helpful Says is usually too busy to worry about things	Perceives family as supportive (strength) Says family anxious about illness. Did not indicate own feelings (problem)	**Fear** related to cardiac catheterization, possible surgery, and its outcome
Pain	History of angina (6 months) Takes nitroglycerin for angina	Has not needed nitroglycerin for 2 months (strength)	**Potential pain (angina)** related to excessive activity or stress

Determining the Client's Health Problems, Health Risks, and Strengths

After data are processed, the nurse and the client can together identify strengths and problems. This is primarily a decision-making process.

Health Problems and Risks   During data processing, the nurse groups data according to categories and labels the clusters with tentative diagnoses. However, for health problems (existing or potential) to have a successful outcome, the client must accept the existence of the problem. The nurse, by contrast, determines whether the client needs help dealing with the problem. The nurse and the client can then make any of the following judgments (Yura and Walsh 1988, pp. 126–129):

1. No problem exists, and the client's health status is confirmed.
2. No problem exists, but there is a potential problem.
3. A problem exists, but the client is coping effectively.
4. A problem exists, and the client needs help in handling it.
5. A problem exists, but the client cannot deal with it at this time.
6. A problem requires further study and diagnosis.
7. A problem is not presently incapacitating but will be at a later date.
8. A problem places heavy demands on the client's ability to cope.
9. A problem is critical to the client.
10. The problem is long term and permanent.

See Table 7–2 for examples of Mr. Frederick Smith's problems.

Strengths   At this stage, the nurse and client also establish the client's strengths, resources, and abilities to cope. Generally, people have a clearer perception of their problems or weaknesses than of their strengths and assets, which are often taken for granted. By taking an inventory of strengths, the client can develop a more well-rounded self-concept and self-image. Strengths can be an aid to mobilizing health and regenerative processes.

A client's strengths might be that his weight is within the normal range for his age and height, thus enabling him to cope better with surgery. In another instance, a client's strengths might be that she is allergy-free and a nonsmoker. The same client's resources could be a supportive family and an ability to cope. Coping is a learned pattern or response that helps an individual deal with crises and stressful events. Nurses must remember, however, that because of the magnitude of an event, the number of stressful events occurring at one time, or the unfamiliarity of the situation, a client may be unable to cope and require assistance of the nurse.

A client's strengths can be found in the nursing assessment record (health, home life, education, recreation, exercise, work, family and friends, religious beliefs, and sense of humor, for example), the health examination, and the client's records. See Table 7–2 for examples of Mr. Frederick Smith's strengths.

FORMULATING NURSING DIAGNOSES

At this final stage, the nurse formulates causal relationships between the health problems and the factors related to them. These factors may be, for example, environmental, sociologic, psychologic, physiologic, or spiritual. More than one factor may be related to one health problem. It is also important to determine at this time that the problem can be resolved by independent nursing interventions. If it cannot, the nurse should refer the client to the appropriate health team member. By including the causal factors in diagnostic statements, the nurse can tailor a plan of care for the client. For example, the diagnosis **Impaired physical mobility** tells the nurse the problem but does not suggest the direction the nursing intervention should take, whereas **Impaired physical mobility related to neuromuscular impairment** suggests a direction for plans and interventions to deal with the problem. Obviously, the causative factor *neuromuscular impairment* suggests a different direction than the factor *fear of falling* would.

Nurses can refer to a list of accepted nursing diagnoses on page 106 to select a diagnostic category. The causal factors are obtained from the data. If no causal factor appears in the data, the nurse may wish to make a tentative diagnosis based on scientific nursing knowledge and experience. The nurse should then review the database for inconsistencies and gaps and the analysis/synthesis for error. Once the causal relationships have been established, the nurse is ready to write the diagnostic statements.

Prior to writing the diagnostic statement in the care

plan, the diagnostician reviews the following checkpoints (Gordon 1987b, p. 257):

1. Do I understand client data, and have I verified any questionable data? Have I been careful and objective regarding my observations?

2. Have I recognized diagnostic cues accurately?

3. Have I processed data and reports accurately? Did I test data with standards and compare data from different sources to ensure accuracy?

4. Have I considered several tentative diagnoses to explain the cues, and ruled out incorrect ones?

5. Have I reviewed all the *major* and *minor* defining characteristics for the tentative diagnostic statements? See *Nursing Diagnosis Format* below. Have I accurately assessed the client for these signs and symptoms?

6. Do I have adequate cues to support the formulation of the nursing diagnoses?

See Table 7–2 for Mr. Frederick Smith's nursing diagnostic statements.

Nursing Diagnosis Format

There are three essential components of nursing diagnostic statements; they are referred to as the **PES format** (Gordon 1976, p. 1299). Nurses need to consider these components when developing new diagnostic categories and writing diagnoses for specific clients. The components are:

1. *The terms describing the problem (P).* This component, referred to as the *diagnostic category label* or *title,* is a description of the client's (individual, family, community) health problem (actual or potential) for which nursing therapy is given. The state of the client is described clearly and concisely in a few words. See the box on page 106 for a list of nursing diagnostic categories adopted by the Ninth National Conference on Classification of Nursing Diagnoses in 1990. To be clinically useful, category labels need to be specific. When the word *specify* follows a category label in the list on the inside backcover, the nurse states the area in which the problem occurs. For example, a knowledge deficit may be in the area of medication prescription, dietary adjustments, or disease process and therapy.

2. *The etiology of the problem (E)* or contributing factors. This component identifies one or more probable causes of the health problem and gives direction to

the required nursing therapy. Etiology may include behaviors of the client, environmental factors, or interactions of the two. For example, the probable causes of alteration in health maintenance include perceptual or cognitive impairment, lack of gross or fine motor skills, lack of material resources, and ineffective individual coping. See Table 7–3. Several authors have identified etiologies for many diagnoses (Carpenito 1989, Gordon 1987a, Kim and McFarland 1989). Differentiating among possible causes in the nursing diagnosis is essential because each may require different nursing therapies.

3. *The defining characteristics or cluster of signs and symptoms (S).* The defining characteristics provide information necessary to arrive at the diagnostic category label (component 1). Each nursing diagnostic category is associated with signs and symptoms that occur as a clinical entity. *Major* signs and symptoms are those that must be present to make a valid diagnosis. *Minor* characteristics may or may not be present. Nursing diagnostic categories are similar to medical diagnostic categories. For example, the medical diagnostic category myocardial infarction (heart attack) is associated with a standard set of signs and symptoms that are universally understood and accepted. Likewise, the nursing diagnostic category **Activity intolerance** is associated with a standard cluster of signs and symptoms. See Table 7–3. For most nursing diagnoses the list of defining characteristics is still being developed and refined. Partial listings have been published to assist nurses in developing and validating nursing diagnoses.

Writing a Diagnostic Statement

A nursing diagnostic statement (nursing diagnosis) is a clear statement about a client's actual or potential health problem that is within the scope of independent nursing intervention. It is the outcome of the diagnostic process: the second phase in the nursing process.

Nurses may write diagnoses as either two-part or three-part statements. The two-part nursing diagnostic statement includes

1. Problem (P)—Statement of the client's response

2. Etiology (E)—Factors contributing to or probable causes of the responses

The two parts are joined by the words *related to* or *associated with* rather than *due to.* The phrase *due to* implies a cause-and-effect relationship; one clause causes or is responsible for the other clause. By contrast, the

TABLE 7-3 Components of a Nursing Diagnostic Category

Diagnosis	Definition	Etiology	Defining Characteristics
Activity intolerance	A state in which an individual has insufficient psysiologic or psychologic energy to endure or complete required or desired daily activities	Sedentary life-style Generalized weakness Prolonged bedrest or immobility Sensory deficits Impaired motor function Fatique Alterations in oxygen transport system Lack of motivation Obesity Acute or chronic pain	*Major* (must be present) Altered response to activity, e.g., Dyspnea, shortness of breath, tachypnea, rapid shallow respirations Weak, thready pulse, tachycardia, irregular pulse, failure to return to resting after 3 minutes, EKG changes during activity Failure of blood pressure to increase with activity, hypotension, increased dialtolic pressure of 15 mm Hg Weakness and fatique *Minor* (may be present) Pallor, cyanosis, vertigo, diaphoresis, confusion

Source: M. J. Kim, G. K. McFarland, and A. M. McLane, editors, *Pocket guide to nursing diagnosis,* 3d ed. St. Louis: C. V. Mosby Co., 1989, p. 2; L. J. Carpenito, *Nursing diagnosis: Application to clinical practice,* 3d ed. Philadelphia: J. B. Lippincott Co., 1989, p. 105; J. R. Lederer, G. L. Marculescu, B. Mocnik, and N. Seaby, *Care planning pocket guide: A nursing diagnosis approach,* 3d ed. Redwood City, California: Addison-Wesley Nursing, 1990), p. 14.

phrases *related to* and *associated with* merely imply a relationship. The phrase *related to* is most commonly used. If one part of the diagnostic statement changes, the other part may change as well. Legal hazards are thus avoided. Here are some examples of nursing diagnoses containing two parts:

- **Ineffective breathing pattern** (problem) related to *pain* (etiology)

- **Self-esteem disturbance** (problem) related to *altered body image* (*loss of arm*) (etiology)

- **Anticipatory grieving** (problem) related to *anticipated loss* (etiology) secondary to *husband's illness* (etiology)

A three-part nursing diagnosis statement includes

1. Problem (P)—Statement of the client's response
2. Etiology (E)—Factors contributing to or probable causes of the response
3. Signs and symptoms (S)—Defining characteristics manifested by the client

The three-part diagnostic statement includes the problem, the etiology, and the observed signs and symptoms (PES). Actual nursing diagnoses can be documented by using the three-part statement (using *related to* and *manifested by*), since the signs and symptoms have been

identified. Several alternatives for writing the PES format have been suggested (Carpenito 1987, Guzzetta 1988).

1. Nurses learning to write diagnoses may find it helpful to list the signs and symptoms before (even though the S is last) or after the two-part diagnostic statement in a care plan format. The defining characteristics may include both objective and subjective data.

2. Signs and symptoms may be written after the diagnostic statement joined by the words *manifested by* or *evidenced by.*

Here are some examples of three-part statements:

- **Self-esteem disturbance** (problem) related to *altered body image* (*loss of arm*) (etiology) manifested by *crying and hostility* (signs and symptoms)

- **Anticipatory grieving** (problem) related to *husband's terminal illness* (etiology) manifested by *anorexia and withdrawn behavior* (signs and symptoms)

- **Altered family processes** (problem) related to *mother's hospitalization* (etiology) as manifested by son's *unmet physical and emotional needs* (signs and symptoms)

Characteristics of a diagnostic statement are summarized in the box on the following page.

Common Diagnostic Errors

Clear, concise, client-centered nursing diagnoses can be written by following the guidelines presented in Table 7–4. Some common errors in writing diagnostic statements are

1. Writing the client's response as a need instead of a problem
2. Using judgmental statements
3. Placing the etiology before the client's response
4. Using statements that provide no specific direction for planning independent nursing interventions
5. Using medical rather than nursing terminology
6. Starting the diagnosis with a nursing intervention
7. Using a single symptom as the client's response

The accuracy of nursing diagnostic statements also depends on a complete database and appropriate data processing. If data are omitted, a diagnosis can be missed. If data are not processed properly, e.g., are not clustered appropriately, a diagnosis can be made prematurely or incorrectly, or be missed. Gordon (1987b, p. 286) categorizes diagnostic errors as (a) errors of omission, i.e., failure to diagnose a problem and (b) errors of commission, i.e., diagnosing a problem when no problem exists. Both errors can occur during data collection, data interpretation, and data clustering.

To avoid such errors during assessment, the nurse needs to ensure that relevant data are not missed and that large quantities of irrelevant data are not obtained. The nurse can prevent data omissions by using an organized assessment plan, striving for accuracy, and drawing on personal knowledge. Collecting irrelevant data can be avoided if the nurse asks appropriate questions. An overload of irrelevant data hinders the nurse's capacity to process information.

Data interpretation errors occur when the meaning of cues is misinterpreted. The nurse can avoid inaccurate

RESEARCH NOTE

Are Nursing Diagnoses Actually Used?

The researchers in this project were interested in determining if the list of nursing diagnoses that was prepared by the North American Nursing Diagnosis Association were actually being used. In particular, they were interested in their use in diagnosing the needs of the elderly.

To examine this, they gathered data from elderly residents in a large long-term care facility in Iowa and compared their findings with the results of four other studies that were done in similar settings.

They discovered that the following nursing diagnoses were used with more than 10% of the patients in these facilities:

- Impaired physical mobility
- Altered thought process
- Impaired skin integrity
- Pain
- Constipation
- Altered nutrition: less than body requirements

These findings indicated that the listings that were developed by NANDA to describe nursing diagnoses were being used and that they were useful in actual practice.

Implications: Studies such as this one bring credibility to NANDA'S efforts to establish professional standards and descriptions of the diagnoses that nurses will use in a variety of health care settings.

M. Hardy, M. Maas, and J. Akins, The prevalence of nursing diagnoses among elderly and long-term care residents: A descriptive study. In R. M. Carroll-Johnson, editor, *Classification of nursing diagnoses, Proceedings of the Eighth Conference* (Philadelphia, J. B. Lippincott, 1989).

interpretation of cues by determining how the client perceives the health problem, its probable cause, and actions taken to remedy it. For example, the nurse observes that a client repeatedly gets out of bed after the physician has ordered complete bed rest. The nurse may interpret this behavior as noncompliance. However, the client may be experiencing diarrhea and may be embarrassed to use the bedpan or may be refusing to accept a dependent sick role. Obviously, inaccurate interpretation of cues leads to diagnostic errors. Another source of

TABLE 7-4 *Guidelines for Writing a Nursing Diagnostic Statement*

Guideline	Correct Statement	Incorrect and/or Ambiguous Statement
1. State in terms of a problem, not a need	**Fluid volume deficit** (problem) related to fever	**Fluid replacement** (need) related to fever
2. State so that it is legally advisable	**Impaired skin integrity** related to immobility (legally acceptable)	**Impaired skin integrity** related to improper positioning (implies legal liability)
3. Use nonjudgmental statements	**Spiritual distress** related to inability to attend church services secondary to immobility (nonjudgmental)	**Spiritual distress** related to strict rules necessitating church attendance (judgmental)
4. Make sure that both elements of the statement do *not* say the same thing	**High risk for impaired skin integrity** related to immobility	**High risk for impaired skin integrity** related to ulceration of sacral area (response and probable cause are the same)
5. Make sure that the client's response precedes the contributing or causal factor	**Noncompliance with diet** (response) related to lack of knowledge (contributing factor)	**Knowledge deficit** (contributing factor) related to noncompliance with diet (response)
6. Use statements that provide guidance for planning independent nursing interventions	**Social isolation** related to loss of speech (loss of speech provides direction for planning alternative communication methods)	**Social isolation** related to laryngectomy (the nurse can do nothing about the laryngectomy)
7. Word diagnosis specifically and precisely to provide direction for planning nursing intervention	**Impaired tissue integrity (oral mucous membrane)** related to decreased salivation secondary to radiation of neck (specific)	**Impaired tissue integrity (oral mucous membrane)** related to noxious agent (vague)
8. Use nursing terminology rather than medical terminology to describe the client's response	**Potential ineffective airway clearance** (nursing terminology)	**Potential pneumonia** (medical terminology)
9. Use nursing terminology rather than medical terminology to describe the probable cause of the client's response	**Potential ineffective airway clearance** related to accumulation of secretions in lungs (nursing terminology)	**Potential ineffective airway clearance** related to emphysema (medical terminology)
10. Do not start the nursing diagnosis with a nursing intervention	**Altered nutrition: less than body requirements** related to inadequate intake of protein (directs but does not state nursing intervention)	Provide high-protein diet because of **Potential altered nutrition** (starts with nursing intervention)
11. Avoid using a symptom such as nausea as the client's response. A symptom does not reflect a pattern and requires additional data collection	Insufficient data for a diagnosis	**Nausea** related to medication

diagnostic errors in data interpretation is overgeneralization from one isolated observation of client behavior. For example, one episode of angry behavior does not mean that the client is hostile.

A diagnosis may be made prematurely, before all relevant data have been considered or collected. For example, a nurse, learning of a client's history of angina and his prescription for nitroglycerin, may write this diagnostic statement: **Pain (anginal).** Additional data, however, reveal that angina has not been a problem since the client had cardiac bypass surgery a year ago and that pain is therefore not a current problem.

Incorrect clustering of data also leads to diagnostic errors. For example, by clustering "urinary frequency" and "has diabetes," the nurse could erroneously begin a diagnostic statement for Mr. Frederick Smith with **Altered urinary elimination pattern.** However, clustering other data such as "takes furosemide (Lasix, a diuretic) daily," "shortness of breath," "no energy," and "aortic valve insufficiency," changes the diagnostic focus from a urinary problem to **Activity intolerance** or **Decreased cardiac output.**

TAXONOMY OF NURSING DIAGNOSES

A **taxonomy** is a classification system of groups, classes, or sets. The first taxonomy of nursing diagnoses was done in 1973, at the First National Conference on the Classification of Nursing Diagnoses. Following the approval of the 31 diagnostic categories, the diagnoses were then grouped alphabetically (Gebbie and Lavin, 1975). The nonhierarchic alphabetical ordering (see page 106) was considered unscientific by some, and a hierarchic structure was sought.

NANDA's Taxonomy I, Revised
In 1978, the Nurse Theorist Group of NANDA proposed the utilization of the "nine patterns of unitary man" as an organizing principle. This proposal was accepted by NANDA in 1982. An initial taxonomic tree was generated. One of the major reasons for classifying and coding nursing diagnosis is to facilitate computer storage and access of information.

In 1984 NANDA renamed the "patterns of unitary man" as "human response patterns." See the box above. In 1986, NANDA accepted the system as *Taxonomy I* (McLane, 1987). In 1988, some refinements and revisions were made after the acceptance of new diagnoses, and the new taxonomy was called *Taxonomy I, Revised.* All nursing diagnoses, once accepted, now become subcategories of these nine human response patterns. For example, the human response pattern *Feeling* includes:

- Anxiety
- Pain or chronic pain
- Grieving (anticipatory, dysfunctional)
- Fear
- High risk for violence (self-directed or directed at others)
- Post-trauma response

Human Response Patterns

1. Exchanging: mutual giving and receiving.
2. Communicating: sending messages
3. Relating: establishing bonds
4. Valuing: assigning relative worth
5. Choosing: selection of alternatives
6. Moving: activity
7. Perceiving: reception of information
8. Knowing: meaning associated with information
9. Feeling: subjective awareness of information

- Rape-trauma syndrome (compound reaction, silent reaction)

The taxonomy is numerically coded and organized from the most abstract (Level I) to the most concrete (Level IV or V). Each of the nine human response patterns constitute Level I concepts, which are the most abstract. Level II concepts refer to alterations in the human response patterns, and subsequent levels refer to more specific responses.

Translating Taxonomy I Revised into ICD Code
To prepare the taxonomy for possible inclusion into the World Health Organization's 10th revision of the *International Classification of Diseases* (ICD 10), the NANDA Taxonomy Committee, in liaison with the American Nurses' Association, made further revisions to conform to the ICD framework (Fitzpatrick et al. 1989, pp. 493–495).

These revisions approved by the NANDA board include:

1. Arranging the nine human response patterns in alphabetical order: choosing, communicating, exchanging, feeling, knowing, moving, perceiving, relating, and valuing.

2. Decreasing the levels of abstraction from four, five, or six levels to only two levels.

3. Modifying the diagnostic coding to meet ICD criteria. A four character code is used: an alphabetical character (Y) is placed first, followed by three numerical characters. For example Y27.1 is the code for **Skin integrity, impaired.**

The box below indicates the proposed ICD-10 version of the first (previously fifth) human response pattern: *Choosing*. Note that there are some changes in wording from previously accepted NANDA diagnostic labels; e.g., the word "ineffective" is changed to "impaired."

Advantages of a Nursing Diagnosis Taxonomy

- *Nursing diagnosis promotes professional accountability and autonomy by defining and describing the independent area of nursing practice.* It provides a standardized terminology for categorizing clusters of signs and symptoms for specific conditions. These category names, such as **Knowledge deficit** or **Self-care deficit** focus the nursing interventions needed to achieve the desired outcomes (Maas and Hardy 1988, p. 13).

- *Nursing diagnoses provide an effective vehicle for communication among nurses and other health care professionals.* Because a nursing diagnosis consolidates a great deal of information into concise state-

ments and includes assessment parameters, it provides a shorthand method of communication. A nurse who knows that a client has a certain nursing diagnosis knows about that client's problem, the causal or contributing factors, and the necessary nursing actions.

- *Nursing diagnoses provide an organizing principle for the building of meaningful research.* A valid nursing diagnosis taxonomy would more clearly define the scope of nursing practice. This ability to access such client data in relation to their nursing diagnoses would provide a framework for testing the validity of nursing interventions and also provide feedback for further development of nursing's unique body of knowledge. In addition, the organization of data in this manner would facilitate retrieval and analysis by computer-based information systems.

Challenges for the Future

The evolution of nursing diagnostic categories is in its early developmental stages, and the list of diagnoses is not to be considered a comprehensive guide for nursing practice. Although some nurses feel constrained and frustrated with the existing list of diagnoses, it is well to remember that disciplines with well-established taxonomies, such as medicine, have taken many decades to develop. Each NANDA publication emphasizes that the existing list is not at all definitive. McLane (1987, p. 469) states that this taxonomy "is an investment by NANDA which can be . . . tested, refined, revised and expanded. A major task of all nurses is to locate diagnoses that are neglected, to test and develop them, and to present them for inclusion in future listings."

A relationship between the nursing diagnosis taxonomy and theoretical frameworks for nursing is yet to be demonstrated. The diagnostic focus of proposed conceptual frameworks for nursing depends on the concepts outlined in the nursing theory. For this reason, such frameworks do not necessarily fit the taxonomy of nursing diagnoses. Dialogue between nursing practitioners and theorists is essential for continued development in this area.

The taxonomy needs to be tested for reliability and validity. Although it has been approved and accepted by participants at the national NANDA conferences, the usefulness of each diagnostic category must still be validated by appropriate research. *Validation* is the determination that the diagnosis accurately reflects the problem of the client, that the methods used for data gathering were valid, and that the conclusion or diagnosis is justified by the data.

Proposed ICD-10 Version of the First Human Response Pattern

Human Response Pattern: Choosing

Y100	Family coping, impaired*
Y00.0	Compromised
Y00.1	Disabled
Y01	[Health-seeking behavior]†
Y01.0–9	Health-seeking behaviors (specify)
Y02	Individual coping, impaired*
Y02.0	Adjustment, impaired
Y02.1	Conflict: decisional
Y02.2	Coping: defensive
Y02.3	Denial, impaired*
Y02.4	Noncompliance

*Denotes change in wording from previously accepted NANDA diagnostic label.
†Item in brackets is not an accepted diagnosis.

Source: J. J. Fitzpatrick, M. E. Kerr, V. K. Saba, L. M. Hoskins, M. L. Hurley, W. C. Mills, B. C. Rottkamp, J. J. Warren, and L. J. Carpenito, Nursing diagnosis: Translating nursing diagnosis into ICD code, *American Journal of Nursing* April 1989, 89:494.

There is some concern that the use of nursing diagnoses may lead to stereotyping by the nurse and lessen the client's role in the decision-making process. Nurses must ensure that the client's perception of the problem is the focus of care. They need to be aware of the problems involved in professional labeling and make every effort to provide individualized client care. Henderson (1987, p. 15) suggests the use of client questionnaires to maintain a consistent approach.

A weakness of the present nursing diagnoses taxonomy is the lack of focus on health promotion and health education. Nationally and internationally there is now an emphasis on consumer education and activities to promote a healthy life-style. However, the present taxonomy of nursing diagnoses is mainly focused on client problems. Assessing the strengths of the client and promoting wellness activities are also important nursing functions and should be more visible in the nursing diagnoses taxonomy.

The development of *Taxonomy I, Revised* based on the nine human response patterns is receiving some criticism. Porter (1986, p. 136) points out that the human response patterns provide a theoretical or conceptual framework for the diagnostic categories rather than a true taxonomic structure that is based on principles of classification. Modifications therefore may need to be made to *Taxonomy I, Revised,* or an alternative taxonomy may have to be developed.

One of the major purposes of nursing diagnoses is to establish a method of validating independent nursing functions that would define nursing's unique role. A major task that is yet to be considered is the development of nursing interventions specific to each nursing diagnosis. Nurses will be accountable for these prescribed interventions. To date, a taxonomy of accepted clinical nursing interventions does not exist. However, lists of independent nursing functions are being developed.

CHAPTER HIGHLIGHTS

▶ A nursing diagnosis is a statement of an actual or potential health problem amenable to independent nursing intervention.

▶ The diagnostic process is one of analysis and synthesis.

▶ The cognitive skills for analysis/synthesis are objectivity, critical thinking, decision making, and deductive and inductive reasoning.

▶ The three phases of the diagnostic process are data processing; determination of the client's health problems, health risks, and strengths; and formulation of nursing diagnoses.

▶ A nursing diagnostic statement should be clear, concise, client-centered, related to one problem, and based on reliable and relevant assessment data.

▶ A nursing diagnostic statement may have two or three parts: A two-part statement includes (a) the client's response and (b) factors contributing to the response or probable causes of the response. A three-part statement includes the defining characteristics of the problem as well.

▶ Nursing diagnoses provide direction for planning independent nursing interventions.

▶ A valid nursing diagnoses taxonomy would define the independent scope of practice, facilitate nursing research, and clarify communication among nurses and other health professionals.

▶ The development of a taxonomy of nursing diagnoses is an ongoing process.

LEARNING ACTIVITIES

■ Review the NANDA list of Approved Nursing Diagnoses on page 106. Do the listed diagnoses meet your needs in describing client problems in your area of nursing practice? If not, what actual or potential client problems occur in your nursing practice that are not included in the current list?

■ Review your list. Are any of your nursing diagnoses medical problems, that is, problems that are only solved by physician intervention? Are all of your nursing diagnoses amenable to nursing intervention? List the interventions for your nursing diagnoses.

READINGS AND REFERENCES

SUGGESTED READINGS

Gordon, M. December 1987. Implementation of nursing diagnoses: An overview. *Nursing Clinics of North America* 22:875–879.

    Gordon discusses some of the forces fueling the diagnosis movement including professional policy and practice changes and the usefulness of diagnosis to communicate and demonstrate nursing's productivity and effectiveness. The history of the North American effort to identify and classify nursing diagnosis is also outlined briefly.

Hutcherson, A. H. July/August 1989. Care plan hints. *Advanced Clinical Care* 4:8–10.

    Examples illustrate the use of defining characteristics. These examples help explain the relationship of the various components of the care plan and the nursing process.

Tribulski, J. December 1988. Nursing diagnosis: Waste of time or valued tool? *RN* 51:30–34.

    Tribulski uses a case study to demonstrate the importance and practical use of nursing diagnosis. The common complaints related to using nursing diagnosis are presented and challenged, and guidelines are offered for writing diagnoses and developing a plan of care.

RELATED RESEARCH

Brunckhorst, L.; Placzek, L.; Payne, J.; McInerney, J.; and Parzuchowski, J. February 1989. Who's using nursing diagnoses? *American Journal of Nursing* 89:267–268.

Hardy, M., Maas, M., and Akins, J. 1989. The prevalence of nursing diagnoses among the elderly and long-term care residents: A descriptive study. In R. M. Carroll-Johnson, editor. *Classification of nursing diagnoses, Proceedings of the eighth national conference.* Philadelphia: J. B. Lippincott Co., 1989.

Johnson, C. F., and Hales, L. W. January/February 1989. Nursing diagnosis anyone? Do staff nurses use nursing diagnoses effectively? *Journal of Continuing Education in Nursing* 20:30–35.

Levin, R. F.; Krainovitch, B. C.; Bahrenburg, E.; and Mitchell, C. A. Spring 1989. Diagnostic content validity of nursing diagnoses. *Image: Journal of Nursing Scholarship* 21:40–44.

SELECTED REFERENCES

Alfaro, R. 1990. *Applying Nursing Process and Diagnosis: A step-by-step guide.* 2nd ed. Philadelphia: J. B. Lippincott Co.

Baretich, D. M., and Anderson, L. B. September 1987. Diagnostics. Should we diagnose strengths? No—stick to the problem. *American Journal of Nursing* 87:1211–1212.

Carpenito, L. J. 1991. *Nursing diagnosis: Application to clinical practice.* 4th ed. Philadelphia: J. B. Lippincott Co.

———. 1991. *Handbook of Nursing Diagnosis 1990–1991.* Philadelphia: J. B. Lippincott Co.

Derdiarian, A. March 1988. A valid profession needs valid diagnoses. *Nursing and Health Care.* 9:136–140.

Edel, M. 1982. The nature of nursing diagnosis. In Carlson, J. H., Craft, C. A., and McGuire, A. D. *Nursing diagnosis.* Philadelphia: W. B. Saunders Co.

Fitzpatrick, J. J., Kerr, M. E., Saba, V. K., Hoskins, L. M., Hurley, M. E., Mills, W. C., Rottkamp, B. C., Warren, J. J., and Carpenito, L. J. April 1989. Translating nursing diagnosis into ICD code. *American Journal of Nursing* 89: 493–495.

Gebbie, K. M. 1976. *Classification of nursing diagnoses: Summary of the second national conference.* St. Louis: C. V. Mosby Co.

Gebbie, K. M., and Lavin, M. A., editors. 1975. *Classification of nursing diagnoses:* Proceedings of the First National Conference. St. Louis: C. V. Mosby Co.

Gordon, M. August 1976. Nursing diagnosis and the diagnostic process. *American Journal of Nursing.* 76:1298–300.

———. 1987a. *Manual of nursing diagnosis.* New York: McGraw Hill.

———. 1987b. *Nursing diagnosis: Process and application.* 2d. ed. New York: McGraw-Hill.

———. December 1987c. Implementation of nursing diagnoses. An overview. *Nursing Clinics of North America.* 22:875–879.

Griffith, J. W., and Christensen, P. J., editors. 1986. *Nursing process: Application of theories, frameworks, and models.* 2d ed. St. Louis: C. V. Mosby Co.

Guzzetta, C. 1988. Nursing diagnosis. In McCann Flynn, J. B., and Burroughs Heffron, P. *Nursing: From concept to practice.* 2d ed. Norwalk, Conn: Appleton & Lange.

Guzzetta, C.; Bunton, S.; Prinkey, L.; Sherer, A.; and Seifert, P. 1989. *Clinical assessment tools for use with nursing diagnosis.* St. Louis: C. V. Mosby Co.

Hannah, K. J.; Reimer, M.; Mills, W. C.; and Letourneau, S., editors. 1987. *Clinical judgment and decision making: The future with nursing diagnosis.* New York: John Wiley and Sons.

Henderson, V. May 1987. Nursing process—A critique. *Holistic Nursing Practice* 1:7–18.

Hurley, M. E., editor. 1986. *Classification of nursing diagnoses. Proceedings of the sixth conference. North American Nursing Diagnosis Association.* St. Louis: C. V. Mosby Co.

James, S., and Mott, S. 1988. *Child Health Nursing.* Menlo Park, Calif. Addison-Wesley Publishing Co.

Kim, M. J., McFarland, G. K., and McLane, A. M. 1989. *Pocket guide to nursing diagnoses,* 3d ed. St. Louis: C. V. Mosby Co.

Kim, M. J., McFarland, G. K., and McLane, A. M., editors. 1984. *Classification of nursing diagnoses: Proceedings of the Fifth National Conference.* St. Louis: C. V. Mosby Co.

Kim, M. J., and Moritz, D. A., editors. 1982. *Classification of nursing diagnosis: Proceedings of the Third and Fourth National Conferences.* New York: McGraw-Hill.

Lederer, J. R.; Marculescu, G.; Mocnik, B.; and Seaby, N. 1990. *Care planning pocket guide: A nursing diagnosis approach.* 3d ed. Redwood City, Calif.: Addison-Wesley Nursing.

Maas, M., and Hardy, M. March 1988. Focus: Nursing diagnosis. A challenge for the future. *Journal of Gerontological Nursing* 14:8–13.

McLane, A. M., editor. 1987. *Classification of nursing diagnoses: Proceedings of the Seventh Conference.* St. Louis, C. V. Mosby Co.

North American Nursing Diagnosis Association. Summer 1988. NANDA approved nursing diagnostic categories for clinical use and testing. *Nursing Diagnoses Newsletter* 15:1–3. St. Louis, MO.

Popkess-Vawter, S., and Pinnell, N. September 1987. Diagnostics. Should we diagnose strengths? Yes: Accentuate the positive. *American Journal of Nursing.* 87:1211, 1216.

Porter, E. J. Winter 1986. Critical analysis of NANDA nursing diagnosis taxonomy I. *Image: Journal of Nursing Scholarship* 18:136–139.

Risner, P. B. Analysis and Synthesis. 1986a. In Griffith, J. W., and Christensen, P. J., editors. pp. 124–150. *Nursing process: Application of theories, frameworks, and models.* St. Louis: C. V. Mosby Co.

———. 1986b. Nursing diagnosis. In Griffith, J. W., and Christensen, P. J., editors. pp. 151–168. *Nursing process: Application of theories, frameworks, and models.* St. Louis: C. V. Mosby Co.

Shoemaker, J. 1984. *Essential features of nursing diagnoses.* In Kim, M. J., McFarland, G. K., and McLane, A. M., editors. pp. 104–115. *Classification of nursing diagnoses: Proceedings of the Fifth National Conference.* St. Louis: . V. Mosby Co.

Turkoski, B. May/June 1988. Nursing diagnosis in print, 1950–1985. *Nursing Outlook* 36:142–144.

Woolley, N. January 1990. Nursing diagnosis: Exploring the factors which may influence the reasoning process. *Journal of Advanced Nursing* 15:110–7.

Yura, H., and Walsh, M. B. 1988. *The nursing process: Assessing, planning, implementing, evaluating.* 5th ed. Norwalk, Conn. Appleton & Lange.

Planning and Implementing

CONTENTS

DEFINITION AND PROCESS

In general, planning is designing or arranging the parts of something to achieve an end or goal. In nursing, planning is the third step of the nursing process. In this context, **planning** is the process of designing the nursing strategies or interventions required to prevent, reduce, or eliminate those client health problems identified and validated during the diagnostic phase. The following people can be involved in planning nursing strategies: one or more nurses; the client, family members, support persons, and/or caregivers; and sometimes members of other health professions. Although the planning process is basically the responsibility of the nurse, input from the client and support persons is essential if a plan is to be effective. It is no longer sufficient that nurses plan *for* the client; whenever possible, the client must participate actively.

For a client in a home setting, the home health care nurse needs to involve the client, if the client's health permits, as well as the client's support persons and/or the caregiver. With the nurse's guidance, these people can implement the plan of care; thus, its effectiveness depends largely on them. They can also provide information about problems previously unknown to the nurse.

When a client is admitted to the hospital or long-term care setting, it is important for the nurse to know if the person required care at home prior to admission. If care was necessary, input from the family and other caregivers assists the nursing staff in continuing to implement appropriate interventions and thus provide the client optimum continuity of care.

Planning is a deliberative, systematic process that is critical to the attainment of quality nursing care. It is a process in which decision making and problem solving are carried out. The planning process uses (a) data obtained during assessing and (b) the diagnostic statements that present the client's health problems (potential and actual). Accurate nursing diagnoses provide direction for determining client goals and developing a plan of care.

COMPONENTS OF PLANNING

The six components of planning are:

1. Setting priorities
2. Establishing client goals and outcome criteria
3. Planning nursing strategies
4. Writing nursing orders
5. Writing the nursing care plan
6. Consulting

Setting Priorities

Priority setting is the process of establishing a preferential order for nursing strategies. To set priorities, the nurse and the client first order the nursing diagnoses preferentially, i.e., they decide which deserves attention first, which second, and so on. Diagnoses can be grouped as having high, medium, or low priority. This priority setting, however, does not mean that all the high-priority diagnoses must be resolved before any others are considered. A high-priority diagnosis may be dealt with partially, and then a diagnosis of lesser priority may be dealt with. In addition, the nurse may address more than one diagnosis at a time. Because client problems are usually multiple, this is often the case. See Table 8–1 for the assignment of priorities to the diagnostic statements for Mr. Frederick Smith.

Setting priorities is made easier by using a framework such as a nursing model or theory. One frequently used framework is Maslow's hierarchy of needs. See Figure 4–1. Maslow's physiologic needs, such as air, food, and water, are basic to life and receive higher priority than the need for security or activity.

Life-threatening problems, such as loss of respiratory or cardiac functioning, have the highest priority. Health-threatening problems, either actual or potential, such as acute illness and decreased coping ability, may result in delayed development or impaired functioning. Health-threatening problems usually have medium priority. Growth needs, such as self-esteem, are not necessary for sustaining life. Thus, when the nurse plans care for a client with unmet physiologic needs and unmet growth needs, the basic or physiologic needs are the first priority.

The importance of the client's involvement in setting priorities cannot be overemphasized. Although a nurse may believe she or he knows a client, the client's values may be different than the nurse supposes, and the client may set priorities differently. For example, one nursing diagnosis may relate to smoking and another to nutrition. The nurse may give the smoking problem a higher priority than the problem of obesity, but the client may see the problem of obesity as more important. When there is such a difference of opinion, the client and nurse should discuss it openly or resolve the conflict. However, in a life-threatening situation, the nurse needs to take the initiative.

The priorities assigned to problems should not remain fixed. Nursing priorities must change as a client's health problems and therapy change.

Client's Health Values and Beliefs   Values concerning health may be very important to the nurse but not to the client. For example, a client may see attendance at school or being home for the children as more urgent than a health problem.

Client's Priorities   Offering the client the opportunity to set priorities allows client participation in care planning and enhances cooperation between the nurse and client. Sometimes, however, the client's perception of what is important conflicts with the nurse's knowledge of potential future problems or complications. For example, an elderly female may not regard ambulation or turning and repositioning every 2 hours as important, preferring to be undisturbed. The nurse, however, aware of the potential complications of prolonged bed rest (e.g., muscle weakness and decubitus ulcers), needs to inform the client and implement necessary interventions to prevent such debilitating effects.

Resources Available to the Nurse and Client   If money, equipment, or personnel are scarce, then a health problem may be given a lower priority than usual. Nurses in a home setting, for example, do not

TABLE 8-1 *Assigning Priorities to Diagnostic Statements for Mr. Frederick Smith (before cardiac catheterization)*

Diagnostic Statement List	Priority Rating	Rationale
Activity intolerance related to shortness of breath and lack of energy secondary to decreased strength of cardiac contractions	Medium priority	Lack of energy is the client's stated major concern. Too much activity can create excessive cardiac demands, resulting in further decreased cardiac output with lowered blood pressure and inadequate circulation. However, because Mr. Smith is able to handle basic activities of daily living, strategies to deal with this diagnostic statement can be deferred until after cardiac catheterization and/or cardiac surgery.
Potential ineffective airway clearance postoperatively related to chest incision	Low priority	Until surgery is performed, ineffective airway clearance is not likely since he is currently able to clear his airways by coughing.
High risk for injury (trauma) related to joint stiffness and limp from hip replacement surgery	High priority	The client is independent and moves slowly to accommodate his limitations. However, new surroundings and a sedative given before cardiac catheterization increase his risk of injury.
Knowledge deficit: side effects of diuretic therapy	Medium priority	Although the client complies with his medical regime, he does not seem to understand the side-effects of the prescribed diuretic, e.g., its relation to increased urination.
Altered peripheral tissue perfusion (left leg) related to impaired arterial circulation	High priority	Decreased circulation and tissue perfusion to the client's left leg can result in damage to the tissues of the limb.
Fear related to cardiac catheterization, possible heart surgery, and its outcome	High priority	Extreme fear could impair his coping capacity.
Potential pain (angina) related to excessive activity or stress	Medium priority	Angina has not been a problem for 2 months, but it could recur with the stress of hospitalization and planned treatments.

have the resources of a hospital; therefore, if the resources needed for specific nursing strategies are not available, the solution of that problem might need to be postponed, or the client may need referral.

Client resources, such as finances or coping abilities, may also influence the setting of priorities. For example, a client who is unemployed may defer dental treatment; a client whose husband is terminally ill and dependent on her may consider nutritional guidance directed toward weight loss as too much to handle.

Time Needed for the Nursing Strategies
Each client feels comfortable with a certain pace of action. Some clients may want to discuss the problem with family members or think about it overnight. Others may want "to get on with it." The nurse must allow adequate

time for the necessary nursing strategies resulting from the nursing diagnosis.

Urgency of the Health Problem
Life-threatening situations require that the nurse establish priorities quickly. This also applies to situations that affect the integrity of the client, i.e., that could have a negative or destructive effect on the client. Such health problems as drug abuse and radical alteration of self-concept due to amputation can be destructive not only to the individual but also to the family. These health problems should receive high priority.

Medical Treatment Plan
The priorities for treating health problems must be congruent with treatment by other health professionals. For example, a high

priority for the client might be to become ambulatory; however, if the physician's therapeutic regimen calls for extended bed rest, then ambulation must assume a lower priority in the nursing strategy plan. In such a case, however, the nurse can provide or teach exercises to facilitate ambulation later, provided the client's health permits. The diagnostic statement related to ambulation is not ignored; it is merely deferred.

Establishing Client Goals and Outcome Criteria

Goals   A *client goal* is a desired outcome or change in client behavior in the direction of health. Goal attainment reflects the resolution of the client concern or health problem that is specified in the nursing diagnosis. The nursing diagnosis guides the type of goal statement: goals may reflect health restoration, health maintenance, or health promotion (Christensen 1986, p. 173).

In the past, nursing goals were often written to direct care. For example, a nursing goal might have been stated as follows: "Increase the client's exercise," or "Teach client about diabetic diet." From these nursing goals, specific nursing activities were derived, such as ambulating the client at specified intervals, offering instruction about needed dietary adjustments, and ensuring that the correct diet was provided. Recently, however, nurses have begun to state goals in terms of desired *client behavior,* not in terms of nursing activities. The term *outcome* means the result of an activity rather than the activity itself.

The concept of goals varies in nursing literature. In nursing education, goals are often referred to as objectives. In nursing process literature, some nurses separate goals from objectives; others use the terms synony-

mously. Still others use the term *outcomes* or *outcome criteria* synonymously with objectives. In this book, the terms *goal* and *outcome criteria* are differentiated, whereas *outcome criteria* and *behavioral objectives* are used synonymously. Goals are broadly stated and require further specification. Outcome criteria are specific and measurable.

A *client goal,* then, is a broad statement about the expected or desired change in the status of the client after he or she receives nursing interventions. Since goals are broad indicators of performance, the use of such verbs as *increase, decrease, maintain, improve, develop,* and *restore* is appropriate. See examples of client goals in the accompanying box.

The purpose of client goals is to:

1. Provide direction for planning nursing interventions that will achieve the anticipated changes in the client.

2. Provide direction for establishing evaluation criteria to measure the effectiveness of the interventions.

Relationship of goals to the nursing diagnosis

Client goals are derived from the first clause of the nursing diagnosis, i.e., from the identified client response. For example, if the first clause of the nursing diagnosis or problem (P) is **Feeding self-care deficit,** the goal might be stated as follows: "Client will demonstrate increased ability to feed self." See establishing goals from nursing diagnosis in the box on the facing page. More specific client outcomes (criteria) are then set from this goal; these criteria form the basis of evaluation. For example, if the goal is "The client will demonstrate increased ability to feed self," two criteria might be, "Will drink from a glass through a straw" and "Will feed self using utensils with sponge-wrapped handles." See the section on outcome criteria next in this chapter.

Long-term and short-term goals

Goals may be short term or long term. A short-term goal might be, "Client will raise right arm to shoulder height by Friday." In the same context, a long-term goal might be, "Client will regain full use of right arm in 6 weeks." Because a great deal of the nurse's time is focused on the immediate needs of the client, most goals are short term. In addition, the nurse is better able to evaluate the client's progress or lack of it with short-term goals.

Long-term goals are often used for clients living at home and having chronic health problems or clients in nursing homes, extended care facilities, and rehabilitation centers. Short-term goals are useful (a) for clients who require health care for only a short time and (b) for persons who are frustrated by long-term goals that seem

---

Examples of Client Goals

The client/clients will:

- Increase activity tolerance
- Maintain urinary elimination pattern
- Restore fluid volume
- Decrease potential for injury
- Develop coping abilities
- Improve nutritional pattern
- Increase parenting knowledge
- Establish change in family roles

For example, if the nursing diagnosis is **High Risk for impaired skin integrity** related to imposed bed rest, and the client goal is, "Maintain intact skin, particularly over bony prominences," the outcome criteria might be as follows. The client:

- Demonstrates correct technique for positioning and turning, and the use of pillows to prevent pressure, within two days.
- Discusses two methods for reducing pressure over bony prominences, within two days.
- Has an absence of redness or irritation to skin when discharged from the hospital.

Generally, three to six outcome criteria are needed for each goal. Some nurses consider outcome criteria to be part of goals and add criteria directly to the goal statement, as follows: "Client's hydration status will be maintained (goal) as evidenced by (outcome criteria): (a) fluid intake of at least 2500 ml daily, (b) urinary output in balance with fluid intake, (c) normal skin turgor, (d) moist mucous membranes." Other nurses find this method cumbersome and separate the goal statement from the criteria statements.

Whichever method is used, the process of developing outcome criteria is the same. The nurse needs to ask two questions:

1. How will the client look or behave if the desired goal is achieved?
2. What must the client do and how well must the client do it before the goal is attained?

Characteristics of well-stated outcome criteria are shown in the box below.

difficult to attain and who need the satisfaction of achieving a short-term goal.

Outcome Criteria

Outcome criteria or objectives are needed to add specificity to the broad goal statements. A *criterion* is a standard or model that can be used in judging. *Outcome criteria* are statements that describe specific, observable, and measurable responses of the client. They determine whether the stated goals have been achieved and are therefore essential to the evaluation phase of the nursing process.

Outcome criteria serve four purposes:

1. They provide direction for nursing interventions.
2. They provide a time span for planned activities.
3. They serve as criteria for evaluation of progress toward goal achievement.
4. They enable the client and nurse to determine when the problem has been resolved.

Relationship of outcome criteria to client goals

Outcome criteria are derived from and relate to the client goals. Client goals, as described previously, are derived from the first clause of the nursing diagnosis.

Components of outcome criteria Outcome criteria generally have all or some of the following four components:

1. *Subject.* The subject, a noun, is the client, any part of the client, or some attribute of the client, such as the client's pulse or urinary output. Often, the subject is omitted in nursing care plan goals; it is assumed that the subject is the client unless indicated otherwise.

2. *Verb.* The verb denotes an action the client is to perform, e.g., what the client is to do, learn, or experience. Verbs that denote directly observable behaviors, such as *administer, demonstrate, show, walk, drink, tell, list, state,* etc., are used.

3. *Conditions or modifiers.* Conditions or modifiers may be added to the verb to explain the circumstances under which the behavior is to be performed. They explain what, where, when, or how. For example:

   Walks *with the help of a walker* (how)

   After attending two group diabetes classes, lists signs and symptoms of diabetes (when)

   When at home, maintains weight at existing level (where)

   Discusses *four food groups and recommended daily servings* (what)

   Conditions need not be included if the standard of performance clearly indicates what is expected.

4. *Criterion of desired performance.* The criterion indicates the standard by which a performance is evaluated or the level at which the client will perform the specified behavior. These criteria may specify time or speed, accuracy, distance, and quality. To establish a time-achievement criterion, the nurse needs to ask "how long?" To establish an accuracy criterion, the nurse asks "how well?" Similarly, the nurse asks "how far?" and "what is the expected standard?" to establish distance and quality criteria, respectively. Examples are:

Weighs 75 kg *by April* (time)

Lists *five out of six* signs of diabetes (accuracy)

Walks *one block per day* (time and distance)

Administers insulin *using aseptic technique* (quality)

See Table 8–2 for other examples of outcome criteria.

Guidelines for Writing Goals and Outcome Criteria

The following guidelines can help nurses write goals and outcome criteria:

1. Write goals and outcome criteria in terms of client behavior. Begin each goal and outcome criteria with "the client." This helps to focus on what the client will be able to do when the outcome criteria are achieved. Outcome criteria should focus on what the client will accomplish, *not what the nurse will do*. For example, a postoperative client may have the following goal (and outcome criteria): The client will maintain clear, open airways (goal) and manifest normal breath sounds (e.g., no wheezing or rales), normal rate of respirations, and absence of dyspnea and cyanosis (outcome criteria).

   Avoid statements that start with *enable, facilitate,*

TABLE 8–2 *Components of Outcome Criteria*

Subject	Verb	Conditions/Modifiers	Desired Performance Standard
Client	drinks	2500 ml of fluid	daily (time)
Client	administers	correct insulin dose	using aseptic technique (quality standard)
Client	lists	three hazards of smoking (after reading literature)	(accuracy indicated by number of hazards)
Client	recalls	five symptoms of diabetes before discharge	(accuracy indicated by number of symptoms)
Client	walks	the length of the hall without a walker	by date of discharge (time)
Client's ankle	measures	less than 10 inches in circumference	in 48 hours (time)
Client	carries out	leg ROM exercises as taught	every 8 hours (time)
Client	identifies	foods high in salt from a prepared list	before discharge (time)
Client	states	the purposes of his medications	before discharge (time)

allow, let, permit, or similar verbs followed by the word *client* (Carnevali 1983, p. 191). These verbs indicate what the nurse hopes to accomplish, not what the client will do. For example, the statement "assist the client to deep breathe and cough every two hours" is a nursing action, not an observable behavior.

2. Make sure the goal statement is appropriate for the nursing diagnoses and that the outcome criteria are appropriate for the goal. Validate the outcomes. If the outcomes are accomplished, will the goal be achieved? Validate the goal statement. If the goal is accomplished, will the client's nursing diagnosis be resolved?

3. Make sure that the outcome criteria are realistic for the client's capabilities, internal and external limitations, and designated time span, if it is indicated. *Internal limitations* refer to the person's physical and mental health status and coping mechanisms. *External limitations* refer to finances, equipment, family support, social services, and time. For example, the goal "The client will walk with crutches on level surfaces and on stairs" may be unrealistic for an elderly woman with a heavy leg cast. "The client will walk with crutches from bed to bathroom with assistance" may be more realistic. The goal "Measures insulin accurately" may be unrealistic for a client who has poor vision due to cataracts.

4. Make sure the client considers the goals important and values them. Outcomes are value decisions (Gordon 1987, p. 309). Some outcomes, such as those for problems related to self-esteem, parenting, and communication, involve choices that are best made by the client or in collaboration with the client. Whenever possible, clients should be given information that will allow them to make informed choices with regard to goals.

    Some clients may know what they wish to accomplish with regard to their health problem. For instance, the client's goal may be "relief of pain." Other clients may not know all the outcome possibilities for their specific problem. The nurse must actively listen to the client to determine personal values, goals, and desired outcomes in relation to current health concerns. Then, discuss the nursing diagnosis and goals to determine if the client agrees with the stated problem and goals. Clients are usually motivated and expend the necessary energy to reach a goal if they consider it important.

5. Ensure that the goals and outcome criteria are compatible with the work and therapies of other professionals. The goal "Increase the client's activity tolerance" and the attending criterion "Will increase the time spent out of bed by 15 minutes each day" are not compatible with a physician's prescribed therapy of bed rest for 3 days.

6. Make sure that each *goal* is derived from only one nursing diagnosis. For example, the goal "The client will increase the amount of nutrients ingested and show progress in the ability to feed self" is derived from two nursing diagnoses: **Feeding self-care deficit** related to neuromuscular impairment and **Altered nutrition: less than body requirements** related to anorexia. Keeping the goal statement related to only one diagnosis ensures that outcome criteria and planned nursing interventions are clearly related to the diagnosis.

7. When writing *outcome criteria,* use observable, measurable terms; avoid words that are vague and require interpretation or judgment by the observer. For example, such phrases as "increase daily exercise," "increase participation in social activities," and "improve knowledge of nutrition" can mean different things to different people. If used in criteria, these phrases can lead to disagreements about whether the criterion was met. These phrases may be suitable for a broad client goal but are not sufficiently clear and specific for use in outcome criteria used to evaluate the client's response. Examples of client goals and outcome criteria associated with the diagnostic statements for Mr. Frederick Smith are shown in Table 8–3. Note that the diagnostic statements have been reordered according to established priorities.

Planning Nursing Strategies

Nursing strategies, or interventions, are nursing actions chosen to treat a specific nursing diagnosis in order to achieve client goals. The specific strategies chosen for actual nursing diagnoses should focus on eliminating or reducing the cause of the nursing diagnosis, which is the second clause of the diagnostic statement. When nurses determine strategies for *potential* nursing diagnosis, the interventions should focus on measures to reduce the client's contributing factors, i.e., signs and symptoms.

The correct identification of the etiology during the nursing assessment provides the framework for choosing successful nursing interventions. For example, **Activity intolerance** may have several etiologies—pain, weakness, sedentary life-style, anxiety, or cardiac arrhythmias. The interventions will vary depending on the cause of the problem.

TABLE 8-3 *Goals and Outcome Criteria for Mr. Frederick Smith (before cardiac catheterization)*

Diagnostic Statement*	Client Goals	Outcome Criteria
1. **Fear** related to cardiac catheterization, possible heart surgery, and its outcome	Experience increased emotional comfort and feelings of control	Verbalizes specific concerns
		Communicates thoughts clearly and logically
		Facial expressions, voice tone, and body posture correspond to verbal expressions of increased emotional comfort or feelings of control
		After instruction, describes the cardiac catheterization procedure and what is expected of him before and after the procedure
2. **Altered peripheral tissue perfusion (left leg)** related to impaired arterial circulation	Improve circulation to left leg and foot	Skin intact, pink, and moist
		Skin temperature warm (as other foot)
		Left dorsalis pedis, posterior tibial, and popliteal pulses palpable and of same strength as corresponding right pulses
		Verbalizes factors that improve and inhibit peripheral circulation
		Capillary refill of left toenails within 1 to 3 seconds
3. **High risk for injury (trauma)** related to joint stiffness and limp from hip replacement surgery	Prevent injury	Moves in and out of bed and ambulates without falling or injuring self
4. **Activity intolerance** related to shortness of breath and lack of energy secondary to decreased strength of cardiac contraction	Avoid performance of activities causing shortness of breath and excessive cardiac workload	Rests after meals
		No shortness of breath during activities
		Pulse and blood pressure remain stable at 80 beats per minute and 124/80 mm Hg

*Note new order of diagnostic statements to reflect highest priorities.

Selecting nursing strategies is a decision-making process. Planning nursing strategies involves generating a number of alternative nursing actions likely to solve the client's problem, considering the consequences of each alternative action, and choosing one or more nursing strategies.

Generating Alternative Nursing Strategies

The client and nurse can use several methods of generating alternative nursing strategies at this stage: brainstorming, hypothesizing, and extrapolating.

Brainstorming is a technique used by more than one person, usually a group of people. In this process, one person's idea elicits an idea from another, and so forth. The ideas should not be evaluated while they are being generated. An idea is expressed, developed by another,

modified by another, and so on, until a solution acceptable to all is established. The results of this process are often creative solutions.

Hypothesizing is a technique of predicting which actions will solve a problem or meet a goal. Hypothesized alternatives are the result of knowledge and experience, and each of the proposed alternatives is likely to be effective. Hypothesizing is *not* guessing because the alternatives have been tried successfully in the past.

Extrapolating is inferring facts or data from known facts or data. In this technique, the individual suggests an action because everything that is known about the problem suggests the action will be effective.

Often, the nurse and the client can establish a number of nursing strategies for each problem statement. Too many alternatives can be confusing. Usually three to five alternative nursing strategies for each health problem are satisfactory. See Table 8–4.

Considering the Consequences of Each Strategy

The next step is to consider the consequences of each action, including the risks. Often, each action will have more than one consequence. For example, the strategy "Provide accurate information" could result in the following client behaviors:

1. Increased anxiety
2. Decreased anxiety
3. Wish to talk with the physician
4. Desire to leave hospital
5. Relaxation

Establishing the consequences of each strategy requires nursing knowledge and experience. The nurse's experience may suggest that providing information before the client's bedtime may increase the client's worry and tension and that maintaining the usual rituals before sleep is more effective. Perhaps some alternative nursing actions should be implemented during the day to facilitate sleep at night, e.g., providing accurate information during the day and increasing daytime activity.

Choosing Nursing Strategies

After considering the consequences of the alternative nursing strategies, the nurse chooses one or more that are likely to be most effective. Although the nurse bases this decision on knowledge and experience, the client's input is very important. For example, a client may say: "I always have a sandwich and glass of milk before going to bed when I am home. I know I'll sleep if I can have that." Maintaining the client's routine may indeed help the client sleep, and this action might be the first choice as a nursing strategy.

The following criteria can help the nurse choose the best nursing strategy. The planned action must be:

1. Safe and appropriate for the individual's age, health, and so on.
2. Achievable with the resources available (e.g, in the previous example, sandwiches and milk must be available).
3. Congruent with the client's values and beliefs.
4. Congruent with other therapies (e.g., if the client is not permitted food, the strategy of an evening snack must be deferred until health permits).
5. Based on nursing knowledge and experience or knowledge from relevant sciences. Example:

TABLE 8-4 *Developing Alternative Nursing Strategies*

Diagnostic Statement	Client Goal	Alternative Nursing Strategies
Sleep pattern disturbance related to anxiety	Obtain 6 to 9 hours of sleep	Provide warm milk and a snack in the evening
		Provide more activity during daytime
		Encourage client to decrease activity 2 hours before bedtime
		Assess diet for stimulants, i.e., caffeine
		Provide soft music
		Encourage verbalization of worries

Client's Diagnosis
High risk for impaired skin integrity related to immobility

Nursing Strategies
Assess skin integrity over bony prominences q2h.
Turn and change position q30 minutes.
Pad pressure points.
Use egg crate mattress on bed.

Rationale
Continuous pressure on a body area compresses tissue, obstructs blood flow to and from an area, and can result in damaged tissue.

6. Within established standards of care as determined by state laws, professional associations (American Nurses' Association, Canadian Nurses' Association), and the policies of the institution.

Each state has nurse practice acts that govern the scope of nursing practice. What nurses can do varies somewhat from state to state. Nurses should know the laws of the state where they practice and remain aware of current changes.

Selecting Nursing Activities for Hospitalized Clients

This study was conducted to investigate how important 50 selected nursing activities were to elderly hospitalized clients and their nurses and how much agreement there was between nurses and clients about their importance. The areas of nursing activities studied included: physical and psychosocial care, discharge planning, and the implementation of doctor's orders. A random sample of 50 pairs of nurses and their clients at a private southwestern hospital responded independently to a five-point questionnaire. The possible responses ranged from 1 (the intervention had no importance) to 5 (the intervention was extremely important).

The results revealed that nurses and clients agreed that interventions related to physical activities and the implementing of doctor's orders were extremely important. Areas of disagreement included nursing interventions related to psychosocial care and discharge planning. The nurses perceived psychosocial care activities as of significant importance, whereas the clients did not. The clients, by contrast, perceived interventions related to discharge planning as very important, whereas the nurses saw them as less important.

Implications: The results of this study suggest that (a) nurses need to educate clients of their capability to manage psychosocial aspects of care and (b) nurses need to be aware of the importance of discharge planning activities to the elderly, who may have multiple health problems that need to be managed at home.

J. E. Johnson. Selecting nursing activities for hospitalized clients. *Journal of Gerontological Nursing,* October 1987, 13:29–33.

Many agencies have policies to guide nursing activities and the activities of other health professionals. Policies are usually intended to safeguard clients, e.g., rules for visiting hours, procedures to follow when a client has cardiac arrest, and so on. If a policy does not benefit clients, nurses have a responsibility to bring this to the attention of the appropriate people.

Writing Nursing Orders

Carnevali (1983, p. 222) says the term *nursing order* is preferable to the terms *approaches, activities, actions,* and *interventions* because *order* connotes a sense of accountability for the nurse who gives the order and for the nurse who carries it out.

The degree of detail included in the nursing orders depends to some degree on the health personnel who will carry out the order. It is advisable, however, to be exact in writing orders.

Nursing orders should include the following five components (Carnevali 1983, p. 222):

- Date when they are written.
- Precise action verb to start the order (e.g., *Explain* [to the client] the action of insulin). Two examples of imprecise verbs (Carnevali 1983, p.233) are shown in the box below.
- Content area, or the *where* and *what* of the order (e.g., Apply *spiral bandage* to the *left lower leg*).
- Time element (e.g., Assist client to change position every *2 hrs between 0700 and 2100 hrs*).
- Signature of the nurse prescribing the order.

Orders for *nursing therapy* include those activities that maintain or restore the client's usual patterns, alleviate symptoms, and prevent additional problems. These make up the majority of orders.

The *collection of additional data* is often necessary to define a nursing diagnosis better or to learn how to manage a problem. For example, if the nurse notices that a client appears withdrawn, worried, and tense, the nurse needs additional data from the client to clarify the contributing causes of this behavior. The nurse may write a tentative nursing diagnosis of **Anxiety** and then write nursing orders that guide interventions toward confirm-

---

Examples of Imprecise Action Verbs

Imprecise verbs	*Suggested alternatives*
Have the client	Ask the client if he will ___
	Request the client to ___
	Remind the client to ___
Reassure the client	Inform the client of ___
	Listen to the client ___
	Stay with the client ___

ing the cause. For example, a nursing order may state, "Talk with client to determine cause of anxiety."

If the nurse needs information about *how to manage a problem*, data may be collected from many sources. One example is the order "RN to consult physician about method of cleaning ulcer." The nurse may consult with a pharmacist about the side-effects of a medication, a dietitian about the foods allowed on a certain diet, a physical therapist about appropriate exercise, and so on. See *Consulting* later in this chapter.

Nursing orders may specify the need to distribute information about continuing management of a problem to the client's support persons or other health team members. For example, a family member may need to learn how to help the client manage a long-term illness, or a visiting nurse association may need information about follow-up nursing care requirements for a client who is being discharged.

Writing the Nursing Care Plan

The nursing care plan organizes information about a client's health into a meaningful whole; it focuses on the actions nurses must take to address the client's identified nursing diagnoses and meet the stated goals. It is also referred to as the *client care plan,* since its focus is the client.

The purposes of a written care plan are:

1. To provide direction for *individualized care* of the client. The plan is organized according to each client's unique nursing care needs.

2. To provide for *continuity of care.* The written plan is a means of communicating and organizing the actions of a constantly changing nursing staff.

3. To provide *direction about what needs to be documented* on the client's progress notes.

4. To serve as a *guide for assigning staff* to care for the client. Certain aspects of the client's care may need to be delegated to someone who can make necessary judgments about the client's responses.

5. To serve as a *guide for reimbursement* from medical insurance companies (third-party reimbursement). The medical record is used by the insurance companies to determine what they will pay in relation to the hospital care received by the client. If nursing care has not been documented precisely in the care plan, the nurse has no way to prove that it was done, and the insurers will not pay for care that is not documented.

Format   Although formats differ from agency to agency, the plan is generally organized into four columns or categories: (a) nursing diagnoses or problem list, (b) goals, (c) nursing strategies/interventions/nursing orders, and (d) outcome or evaluation criteria. See Table 8–5. Some agencies have a five-column plan that includes a column for assessment data before the nursing diagnoses column. Others use a three-column plan that subsumes the evaluation (outcome criteria) column under the goal column.

Nursing students are required to write care plans to demonstrate their ability to apply their knowledge to client situations. For this reason, educators often modify the standard care plan by adding a column headed "Rationale" after the nursing intervention column. A rationale is the scientific reason for selecting a specific nursing action. Students may also be required to cite supporting literature for this stated rationale. These care plans are called instructional care plans and differ in purpose from the care plans developed by practicing nurses.

Many agencies use a nursing Kardex or Rand system for organizing and storing nursing care plans. Some agencies have adopted 8½-by-11-inch nursing care plan records that correspond to the standard chart size and require that the plan be written in ink so that it can be retained as part of the client's permanent legal record. In other agencies, problem-oriented medical records (POMR) are used; in this situation, the nursing care plan is documented in a SOAP format. In still other agencies, medical orders are not included on the nursing care plan.

Guidelines for Writing Nursing Care Plans

In addition to following the earlier suggestions for writing nursing orders, the nurse can use the following guidelines when writing nursing care plans:

1. Date and sign the plan. The date the plan is written is essential for evaluation, review, and future planning.

2. Indicate that goals are met or revised by a signature or some other method specified by the agency.

3. List the nursing orders for each goal in order of priority.

4. Use standardized medical or English symbols and key words rather than complete sentences to communicate your ideas.

5. Refer to procedure books or other sources of information rather than including all the steps on a written plan. For example, write: "See unit procedure

TABLE 8–5 *Nursing Orders for Mr. Frederick Smith*

Diagnostic Statement	Goals	Nursing Orders	Outcome Criteria
1. **Fear** related to cardiac catheterization, possible heart surgery, and its outcome	Experience increased emotional comfort and feelings of control	Establish a trusting relationship with the client and family Encourage client and family to express feelings and concerns Discuss the cardiac catheterization procedure and what is expected of him before and after the procedure Encourage conversation with another client who has recuperated from similar surgery	Verbalizes specific concerns Communicates thoughts clearly and logically Facial expressions, voice tone, and body posture correspond to verbal expressions of increased emotional comfort or feelings of control After instruction, describes the cardiac catheterization procedure and what is expected of him before and after the procedure
2. **Altered peripheral tissue perfusion (left leg)** related to impaired arterial circulation	Improve circulation to left leg and foot	Consult with physician about exercise program, such as walking and range-of-motion exercises to hip, knee, and ankle Keep the extremity in a *dependent* position (i.e., lower than the heart) Use Doppler ultrasound stethoscope (DUS) to assess blood flow in left dorsal pedis, posterior tibial, and popliteal arteries q2h Instruct client to keep his leg warm, e.g., wear warm socks but discourage use of external heat sources	Skin intact, pink, and moist Skin temperature warm (as other foot) Left dorsalis, posterior tibial, and popliteal pulses palpable and of same strength as corresponding right pulses Capillary refill of left toenail within 1 to 3 seconds
3. **High risk for injury (trauma)** related to joint stiffness and limp from hip replacement surgery	Prevent injury	Closely assess ambulation and transfers during first few days Keep bed at lowest level Encourage to request assistance to ambulate during the night Closely attend or put side rails up when client is sedated	Moves in and out of bed and ambulates without falling or injuring self
4. **Activity intolerance** related to shortness of breath and lack of energy secondary to decreased strength of cardiac contraction	Avoid performance of activities causing shortness of breath and excessive cardiac workload	Organize client care and provide undisturbed rest periods Discuss energy conservation methods such as taking periodic rest periods Tell the client to reduce the intensity, duration, and frequency of activity if he experiences chest pain, shortness of breath, dizziness, or abnormal pulse and blood pressure after activity Monitor vital signs q2h and report decreasing blood pressure, increasing heart rate, or increasing respiratory rate	Rests after meals No shortness of breath during activities Pulse and blood pressure remain stable at 80 beats per minute and 124/80 mm Hg

book for tracheostomy care," or attach a standard nursing plan about such procedures as radiation-implantation care and preoperative or postoperative care.

6. Tailor the plan to the unique characteristics of the client by ensuring that the client's choices, such as preferences about the times of care and the methods used, are included. This reinforces the client's individuality and sense of control.

7. Ensure that the nursing plan incorporates *preventive* and health maintenance aspects as well as restorative aspects.

8. Include collaborative and coordination activities in the plan.

9. Include plans for the client's discharge and home care needs. It is often necessary to consult and make arrangements with the community health nurse, social worker, and specific agencies that supply client information and needed equipment.

Consulting

Consulting is deliberating between two people. Nurses consult a variety of personnel, including other nurses, throughout the nursing process. Consulting implies that the nurse involved in the care seeks advice or clarification regarding client goals. Also, the nurse may serve as a resource to provide assistance in health- or client-related issues. Increasingly nurses consult with other nurses within the agency about a variety of specialized nursing practice areas. Nurses may also consult with other health care personnel including physicians, nutritionists, physical therapists, and social workers. Some agencies have a protocol to be followed by those consulting a health professional not presently involved in the client's care. For example, if a nurse wants to discuss a client's depression with an agency psychiatrist, the nurse may need to send a form to the psychiatrist requesting a consultation. However, many consultations are done on an informal basis. For example, the nurse may discuss a client's skin problem with the physician during the physician's rounds.

Nurses generally consult to verify findings, implement change, and obtain additional knowledge. Nurses frequently ask other nurses to verify assessment data, such as extremely low blood pressure or exceptionally fast pulse, when their findings are unexpected or they are uncertain about them. Sometimes nurses discuss a client's care plan with another nurse, often to make sure the best possible plan has been arranged, or to implement change in the plan. A second person's ideas can

often generate new approaches to the client's care. Consultation to obtain knowledge is desirable. No nurse can know everything about nursing, and another nurse may have knowledge and experience about a particular problem.

The consulting process has seven steps: (1) identify the problem, (2) collect pertinent data about the client, (3) select the consultant, (4) communicate the problem and pertinent information, (5) discuss the recommendations with the consultant, and (6) include the recommendations in the client's nursing care plan.

Identify the Problem Before consulting another person, the nurse must have the problem clearly in mind, including circumstances surrounding the problem. For example, a nursing student is unsure how to place the dressings on a draining wound to catch all the drainage because the student did not see the previous dressing before the physician removed it. The problem is clearly described, i.e., how to place the dressing, and the circumstances include the site of the source of the drainage, the amount of drainage, and the present absence of a correct dressing.

Collect Pertinent Data About the Client When planning to consult a health professional who is unfamiliar with the client, collect all the data relevant to the problem.

Select the Consultant The nurse who has identified a problem regarding nursing care should consult a recognized health professional who has the skills or knowledge required—a nurse with special knowledge and skills.

Communicate the Problem and Pertinent Information This information often varies with each client and each problem. However, it is important to convey information about the client's strengths and problems. Convey the information clearly and objectively so that the consultant does not become biased yet obtains a clear picture of the situation. Make sure the data provided are factual and not interpretive.

Discuss the Recommendations with the Consultant The consultant may provide recommendations at the time the nurse describes the problem, or a later meeting may be necessary.

Include the Recommendations in the Client's Nursing Care Plan Once recorded, the recommendations become part of the client's record and are available to all health professionals involved in the client's care. After implementing the recommendations, the nurse needs to evaluate their effectiveness and to record these. If they are not effective, it may be necessary to see the consultant again and make further adjustments in the client's nursing plan.

DISCHARGE PLANNING

Because the average client stay in acute care hospitals has become shorter due to cost-containment efforts, people are sometimes discharged still needing care. Such care is increasingly being delivered in the home. *Discharge planning,* the process of anticipating and planning for needs after discharge from a hospital or other facility, is becoming a crucial part of comprehensive health care and should be addressed in each client's care plan. Effective discharge planning begins with the admission of the person and continues with ongoing assessment of both client and family needs, until discharge. It involves a comprehensive assessment not only of physical care needs but also of the availability of family and friend caregivers, the home environment as described by the client and family, client and family resources, and community resources.

Some large hospitals have *discharge planners,* nurses whose primary responsibility is to assess anticipated needs after discharge. In most settings, however, staff, head nurses, and clinicians, with the help of social workers, are doing discharge planning. To facilitate collecting the assessment data needed for effective discharge planning, hospital staff may establish liaisons with community-based nurses who can visit the home before the client's discharge, thereby having the opportunity to anticipate needs and plan with the family in advance of discharge.

Effective two-way communication is obviously essential for the coordination of information and planning. The nurse can be effective in helping family members think through their typical day and week and process the changes they can anticipate when the ill person is at home. Thinking through "what-if" situations (e.g., What if the client falls? What if there is an emergency? What if the caregiver needs to go to the store or do other essential errands?) helps families to confront what is happening to them at their own pace and in their own style and to plan for anticipated problems, thereby experiencing a sense of control and confidence (McCorkle and Germino 1984). It also provides the nurse an opportunity to identify the learning needs of clients and families. These learning needs can be met by individualized teaching

prior to discharge or, if necessary, after discharge by the home health nurse. (See Chapter 19.)

When possible, referrals and other actions should be initiated before the day of discharge so that preparations for the client's return home are complete when he or she arrives. In this way, the client's and family's anxiety about the return is kept to a minimum. Referrals of a hospitalized client for home care are often initiated and implemented by the nurses caring for that client, but signed physician's orders for care are required if care is to be reimbursed by third-party payment. The physician may order treatments, medications, adjunctive therapies (e.g., physical, occupational, or speech therapy), and skilled nursing care.

IMPLEMENTING DEFINED

Implementing, also called intervening, is putting the nursing strategies listed in the nursing care plan into action; it is the nursing action taken to attain the desired outcome of the client's goals. According to Marriner (1983), implementing involves carrying out nursing orders *and* physician's orders. Within the context of the nursing process, Bulechek and McCloskey (1985, p. 8) define nursing intervention (implementation) as "an autonomous action based on scientific rationale that is executed to benefit the client in a predicted way related to the nursing diagnosis and stated goals." By this definition, nursing interventions *do not* include those strategies resulting from a physician's order.

The client is always the primary participant in implementing the nursing care plan, although the nurse may act on the client's behalf, e.g., referring the client to a community health nurse for home care. The client's degree of participation often depends on the client's health status. For example, because an unconscious man is unable to participate in his care, he needs to have care given to him. By contrast, an ambulatory client may require very little care from the nurse and carry out health care activities independently. The nurse or nurses, other health professionals, support persons, and/or caregivers can all be involved in implementing nursing.

TYPES OF NURSING ACTIONS

The terms *independent, dependent,* and *collaborative* (interdependent) are often used to describe nursing actions. An action, in this context, is an activity appropriate to a person's role. It is also called a nursing strategy. An *independent nursing action* is an activity that the nurse initiates as a result of the nurse's own knowledge and skills. Mundinger prefers the term *autonomous nursing practice* to *independent nursing practice*. She states, "Knowing why, when, and how to position clients and doing it skillfully makes the function an autonomous therapy" (Mundinger 1980, p. 4). In this instance, the nurse determines that the client requires certain nursing interventions, either carries these out or delegates them to other nursing personnel, and is accountable for the decision and the actions. To be accountable is to be an-swerable. Independent nursing actions are receiving increasing attention from nurses today.

Bulechek and McCloskey (1987) have identified a taxonomy of independent nursing interventions. A *taxonomy* is a set of classifications that are ordered and arranged on the basis of a single principle or consistent set of principles (Bloom 1956, p. 10). See Table 8–6 for a beginning taxonomy of nursing interventions.

Dependent nursing actions are those activities carried out on the order of the physician, under the physician's supervision, or according to specified routines. The de-

TABLE 8-6 *Beginning Taxonomy of Nursing Interventions*

Most Abstract Level 1	Level 2	Level 3	Most Concrete Level Nth
Stress management	Relaxation training Cognitive reappraisal Music therapy		Nursing orders
Life-style alteration	Self-modification Patient contracting Counseling Nutritional counseling Sexual counseling Reminiscence therapy Role supplementation Patient teaching Values clarification Support groups Exercise programs Group psychotherapy Assertiveness training		
Acute care management	Preparatory sensory information Crisis intervention Preoperative teaching Surveillance Presence		
Self-care assistance	Ambulation Bathing Bladder training Bowel training Feeding Oral hygiene Positioning Skin care		
Communication	Active listening Advocacy Cultural brokerage Truth telling Discharge planning		

Source: Reprinted from *Holistic Nursing Practice*, Vol. 1, No. 3, p. 38, with permission of Aspen Publishers, Inc., © May 1987.

pendent activity in nursing practice is usually directly related to the client's disease, and its importance should not be minimized. In addition to the task of carrying out the physician's order, the nurse who performs a dependent nursing action also conducts the appropriate nursing activities associated with the order, e.g., monitoring the client for signs of improvement.

Collaborative nursing actions are those activities performed either jointly with another member of the health care team or as a result of a joint decision by the nurse and another health care team member. Collaborative nursing activities sometimes illustrate the overlapping responsibilities of health personnel and reflect the collegial relationship between health professionals. For example, a nurse and a respiratory therapist together may decide on a schedule of breathing exercises for a woman. The therapist may initially teach the exercises to the client, and the nurse reinforces the learned behavior and assists the client in the therapist's absence.

A social policy statement by the American Nurses' Association (ANA) describes collaboration as "true partnership, in which the power on both sides is valued by both, with recognition and acceptance of separate and combined spheres of activity and responsibility, mutual safeguarding of legitimate interests of each party, and a commonality of goals that is recognized by both parties" (ANA 1980, p. 7). To achieve effective collaborative nursing practice, nurses must have clinical competence, feel confident of their knowledge and skills, and assume responsibility for their own actions.

The amount of time that the nurse spends in an independent versus a collaborative or dependent role will vary according to the clinical area, type of institution, and specific position of the nurse. Guzzetta (1987, p. 634) estimates that the critical care nurse spends only about 10% of the day functioning in the independent nursing role. In other settings, e.g., home health care, nurses may find that they function independently 50% of the time. Clinical nurse specialists may work independently 100% of the time. Often, so many activities are integrated into a clinical day that it is difficult for many nurses to assess how much of their time is spent in an independent practice role.

PROCESS OF IMPLEMENTING

The process of implementing normally includes reassessing the client, validating the nursing care plan, determining the need for nursing assistance, implementing the nursing strategies, and communicating the nursing actions. Reassessing the client and validating the nursing care plan are subprocesses that operate continuously throughout the implementing phase.

Reassessing the Client

As was mentioned in Chapter 6, assessing or reassessing is carried out throughout the nursing process, i.e., during assessing, implementing, and evaluating—in fact, whenever the nurse has contact with the client. While providing care, nurses must continue to collect data about changes (subtle or acute) in the client's level of wellness, i.e., health problems as well as reactions, feelings, and strengths.

Following an extensive assessment during the first phase of the nursing process, reassessing in later phases usually focuses on more specific needs or responses of the client, i.e., fluid intake, pain, pulse rate, and urine output. Through this mechanism, nurses are able to determine whether planned nursing strategies are currently appropriate for the client.

It should never be assumed that once nursing strategies are established or ordered they must be implemented without assessing the client first. New data may, in the nurse's judgment, indicate a need to change the priorities of care or the nursing strategies. For example, a nurse begins to teach a client, Miss Eves, who has diabetes, how to give herself insulin injections. Shortly after beginning the teaching, the nurse realizes that Miss Eves is not concentrating on the lesson. Subsequent discussion reveals that she is worried about her eyesight and fears she is going blind. The nurse ends the lesson because the client's level of stress is interfering with her learning and makes arrangement for a physician to examine the client's eyes. The nurse also provides supportive communication to alleviate the client's stress and revises the nursing care plan appropriately.

Validating the Nursing Care Plan

A nursing care plan cannot be fixed; it must be a flexible tool. When new data are collected, they should be compared with the database. Sometimes, the new data are incongruent with baseline data. The nurse must judge the value of the new data and determine whether the nursing care plan is still valid. When a client's health status changes, i.e., when physical or psychosocial responses change, the nursing care plan needs to be adjusted.

If the data regarding the client's health status are unchanged, the nurse proceeds with the implementing process. For information on modifying or changing the nursing care plan, see Chapter 9.

Determining the Need for Assistance

When implementing some nursing strategies, the nurse may require assistance for one of the following reasons: The nurse is unable to implement the nursing strategies safely alone (e.g., turning an obese client in bed) and to reduce stress upon a client (e.g., turning a person who has acute pain when moved). In addition, nurses should obtain assistance if they lack the knowledge or skills to implement a particular nursing activity. For example, a nurse who is not familiar with a particular model of oxygen mask needs assistance the first time it is applied.

Implementing Nursing Strategies

Nursing strategies are implemented to help the client meet his or her health goals.

There are four primary areas of nursing practice: health promotion, health maintenance, health restoration, and care of the dying. Nursing actions in each of these areas can be independent, dependent, or collaborative.

Six important considerations for implementing nursing strategies are

1. The client's individuality. Individualized actions are needed, while care is taken not to violate the scientific basis of the activity. For example, a client may prefer to have an oral medication after meals rather than before. However, this might not be justified if the medication will not act in the stomach in the presence of food.

2. The client's need for involvement. Some clients want to be totally involved in their care, while others prefer little involvement. The amount of desired involvement is often related to the client's energy, severity of illness; number of stressors, fear, understanding of the illness, and understanding of the intervention.

3. Prevention of complications. When changing a sterile dressing, for example, the nurse must observe sterile technique to prevent the complication of infection.

4. Preservation of the body's defenses. For example, when turning a client, the nurse protects the client's skin from abrasions, which could permit microorganisms to enter the body and establish an infection.

5. Provision of comfort and support to the client.

6. Accurate and careful implementation of all nursing activities. The nurse takes care to administer the correct dosage of a medication by the ordered route, for example.

Communicating Nursing Actions

Nursing actions are often communicated verbally as well as in writing. When a client's health is changing rapidly, the charge nurse and/or the physician may want to be kept up to date with verbal reports. Verbal reports are given to another nurse or other health professionals. Nurses often give verbal reports regarding clients at a change of shift and upon a client's discharge to another unit or health agency.

CHAPTER HIGHLIGHTS

▶ Planning is the process of designing nursing strategies required to prevent, reduce, or eliminate a client's health problems.

▶ Planning can involve the nurse, the client, support persons, and caregivers.

▶ Nursing strategies are planned around a client's diagnostic statements and goals.

▶ Six components of planning are setting priorities, establishing client goals, planning nursing strategies, writing nursing orders, writing a nursing care plan, and consulting.

▶ Nursing diagnoses are assigned high, medium, and low priorities in consultation with the client, if health permits.

▶ Client goals are used to plan nursing strategies that will achieve anticipated changes in the client.

▶ Client goals are derived from the *first* clause of the nursing diagnosis.

▶ Outcome criteria describe specific and measurable client responses and help the nurse evaluate the effectiveness of the nursing intervention.

▶

CHAPTER HIGHLIGHTS *(continued)*

▸ Goal statements and outcome criteria are written in terms of the client's behavior.

▸ Nursing strategies are focused on the etiology or *second* clause of the nursing diagnosis.

▸ Nursing strategies can be generated by brainstorming, hypothesizing, and extrapolating.

▸ Establishing the consequences of each nursing strategy requires nursing knowledge and experience.

▸ The nurse consults with other nurses or health professionals to verify information, implement changes, or obtain additional knowledge to aid in client goals.

▸ Shorter acute care hospitalizations necessitate careful discharge planning.

▸ Implementing is putting planned nursing strategies into action.

▸ Reassessing and validating the nursing care plan occur continuously during the implementing phase.

▸ Caring and communicating are essential for all nursing activities and for establishing relationships.

▸ The implementing phase of the nursing process is terminated with the documentation of the nursing activities.

LEARNING ACTIVITIES

■ Review your own area of nursing practice. Do references exist providing standardized care plans for clients in your specialty area? If standardized care plans are used in your unit, review them for currency. Develop a plan to update existing care plans as necessary.

 If there are no standardized care plans available, are there client problems that occur with sufficient frequency to warrant the development of standardized care plans? Develop a standardized care plan to meet a recurrent client problem in your specialty area. What would be required to individualize this care plan for a specific client's situation?

■ Review your nursing practice for one day. List your nursing actions. What percentage of your nursing actions are independent? What percentage are dependent? What percentage are collaborative? Ask one of your nursing colleagues on a different nursing unit to review his or her nursing practice. Compare the data.

READINGS AND REFERENCES

SUGGESTED READINGS

Bulechek, G. M. and McCloskey, J. C. May 1987. Nursing interventions: What they are and how to choose them. *Holistic Nursing Practice* 1:36–44.
 The authors discuss the role and development of independent nursing interventions and offer a beginning list or ordering of the levels of nursing interventions. Five guidelines for choosing nursing interventions for diagnosis are presented, and problems related to implementation and evaluation are discussed.

McElroy, D., and Herbelin, K. February 1988. Writing a better patient care plan. *Nursing 88* 18:50–51.
 The authors present the basic reasons for writing a good care plan: assuring quality nursing care, documenting in case of lawsuits, and validating care for reimbursement purposes. The purpose and parts of the care plan are reviewed, and a sample care plan is presented for examination.

RELATED RESEARCH

Aasen, N. June 1987. Interventions to facilitate personal control: The nursing home experience. *Journal of Gerontological Nursing* 13:20–28.

Becker, H., and Sands, D. May 1988. The relationship of empathy to clinical experience among male and female nursing students. *Journal of Nursing Education* 27:198–203.

Brett, J. L. L. November/December 1987. Use of nursing practice research findings. *Nursing Research* 36:344–49.

McCorkle, R. and Germino, B. 1984. What nurses need to know about home care. *Oncology Nursing Forum* 11(6):63–69.

Petrucci, K. E.; McCormick, K. A.; and Scheve, A. A. S. November 1987. Documenting patient care needs: Do nurses do it? *Journal of Gerontological Nursing* 13:34–38, 46–48.

SELECTED REFERENCES

American Nurses' Association. 1980. *Nursing: A social policy statement*. Kansas City, Mo.: A.N.A. Pub. no. NP–63 35M 12/80.

Atkinson, L. D., and Murray, M. E. 1986. *Understanding the nursing process*. 3d ed. New York: Macmillan Co.

Bloom, B.S. (editor) 1956. *Taxonomy of Educational Objectives*. New York: David McKay Company.

Breyerman, K. L. Summer 1988. Consultation roles of the clinical nurse specialist: A case study. *Clinical Nurse Specialist* 2:91–95.

Bulechek, G. M., and McCloskey, J. C. May 1987. Nursing interventions: What they are and how to choose them. *Holistic Nursing Practice* 1:36–44.

Carnevali, D. L. 1983. *Nursing care planning: Diagnosis and management*. 3d ed. Philadelphia: J. B. Lippincott Co.

Christensen, P. J. 1986. Planning: Priorities, goals and objectives. In Griffith, J. W., and Christensen, P. J., editors. pp. 169–182. *Nursing Process: Application of theories, frameworks, and models*. St. Louis: C. V. Mosby Co.

Gordon, M. 1987. *Nursing diagnosis: Process and application*. 2d ed. New York: McGraw-Hill.

Griffith, J. W., and Christensen, P. J. 1986. *Nursing Process: Application of theories, frameworks, and models*. 2d ed. St. Louis: C. V. Mosby Co.

Guzzetta, C. E. November 1987. Nursing diagnoses in nursing education: Effect on the profession. Part 1. *Heart and Lung*. 16:629–35.

Hanna, D. V., and Wyman, N. B. November 1987. Assessment + diagnosis = care planning: A tool for coordination. *Nursing Management* 18:106–9.

La Monica, E. L. 1985. *The humanistic nursing process*. Monterey, Calif.: Wadsworth Health Sciences.

Lederer, J. R.; Marculescu, G. L.; Mocnik, B.; and Seaby, N. 1990. *Care planning pocket guide: A nursing diagnosis approach*. 3d ed. Redwood City, Calif.: Addison-Wesley Nursing.

MacLeod, E., and MacTavish, M. Spring 1988. Solving the nursing care plan dilemma: Nursing diagnosis makes the difference. *Journal of Nursing Staff Development*. 4:70–73.

Marriner, A. 1983. *The nursing process: A scientific approach to nursing care*. 2d ed. St. Louis: C.V. Mosby Co.

Yura, H., and Walsh, M. B. 1988. *The nursing process: Assessing, planning, implementing, evaluating* 5th ed. Norwalk, Conn.: Appleton & Lange.

Evaluating

CONTENTS

DEFINITION OF EVALUATION

To evaluate is to judge or to appraise. In the context of the nursing process, evaluation is the fifth and last phase. Here, to evaluate means to identify whether or to what degree the client's goals have been met. Evaluation is an exceedingly important aspect of the nursing process because conclusions drawn from the evaluation determine whether the nursing interventions can be terminated or must be reviewed or changed.

Evaluating is a concurrent and a terminal process. It is concurrent in that the nurse normally evaluates during the implementing phase of the process. How is the client reacting to this nursing action? Is the reaction expected or unexpected? At this stage, the nurse may change a nursing action to help the client meet the planned goals. It is a terminal process because after completing the nursing activity, the nurse evaluates whether the client's goals have been met. Often the time frame (if stated) in the outcome criteria is used.

Evaluating is a purposeful and organized activity. Through evaluating, nurses accept responsibility for their actions, indicate interest in the results of the nursing actions, and demonstrate a desire not to perpetuate ineffective actions but to adopt more effective ones.

PROCESS OF EVALUATING

The evaluation process has six components:

1. Identifying the outcome criteria (standards for measuring success) that will be used to measure achievement of the goals

2. Collecting data related to the identified criteria
3. Comparing the data collected with the identified criteria and judging whether the goals have been attained
4. Relating nursing actions to client outcomes
5. Reexamining the client's care plan
6. Modifying the care plan

Identifying Outcome Criteria

The identification of outcome criteria used to evaluate the client's response to nursing care is discussed in Chapter 8. See Table 8–3. Criteria serve two purposes: They establish the kind of evaluative data that need to be collected, and they provide a standard against which the data are judged. Criteria that are clearly stated, precise, and measurable guide the next step of the evaluation process: data collection.

Collecting Data

Data are collected so that conclusions can be drawn about whether goals have been reached. The nurse collects data in relation to the specified criteria, either by observation, direct communication, and purposeful listening or from reports of other health professionals.

Collection of both objective and subjective data may be necessary. Objective, measurable data are preferred for evaluation purposes; for example, "Respirations increased from 12 to 16 breaths per minute, and pulse rate increased from 70 to 90 beats per minute after client walked around the corridor." However, the nurse often needs to collect subjective data and some objective data that require interpretation. Examples of objective data requiring interpretation are the degree of tissue turgor of a dehydrated client or the degree of restlessness of a client with pain. Examples of subjective data include complaints of nausea or pain by the client.

When objective data require interpretation, the nurse may obtain the views of one or more other nurses to substantiate changes. When subjective data are required, the nurse must rely upon either (a) the client's statements (e.g., "My pain is worse now than it was after breakfast") or (b) objective indicators of the subjective data, even though these indicators may require interpretation (e.g., decreased restlessness, decreased pulse and respiratory rates, and relaxed facial muscles as indicators of pain relief). Data collected must be recorded concisely and accurately to facilitate the third part of the evaluating process. Flowsheets and problem-

oriented medical records in the SOAP format are recording aids.

Judging Goal Achievement

If the first two parts of the evaluation process have been carried out effectively, determining whether a goal has been achieved is relatively simple. Both the nurse and the client play active roles in this. The data collected are compared with established criteria. There are three possible outcomes of evaluation:

1. The goal was met; i.e., the client responded as expected.
2. The goal was partially met; i.e., a short-term goal was achieved, but the long-term goal was not; or, some, but not all, of the outcome criteria were attained.
3. The goal was not met.

See Table 9–1 on page 148 for evaluation examples of Mr. Frederick Smith's outcome criteria.

Relating Nursing Actions to Client Outcomes

The fourth aspect of the evaluating process is determining whether the nursing actions had any relation to the outcomes. It should never be assumed that a nursing action was the cause of or the only factor in meeting, partially meeting, or not meeting a goal. For example, Mrs. Sophi Ringdale was obese and needed to lose 14 kg (30 lb). When the nurse and client drew up a care plan, one outcome criterion was "Lose 1.4 kg (3 lb) by 4/7/91." A nursing strategy in the care plan was "Explain how to plan and prepare a 900-calorie diet." On 4/7/91, the client weighed herself and had lost 1.8kg (4 lb). The goal had been met, in fact, exceeded. It is easy to assume that the nursing strategy was highly effective. However, it is important to collect more data before drawing that conclusion. Upon questioning the client, the nurse could find any of the following: (a) the client planned a 900-calorie diet and prepared and ate the food; (b) the client planned a 900-calorie diet but did not prepare the correct food; (c) the client did not understand how to plan a 900-calorie diet, so she did not bother with it. If the first possibility is found to be true, the nurse can safely judge that the nursing strategy "Explain how to plan and prepare a 900-calorie diet" was effective in helping the client lose weight. However, if the nurse learns that either the second or third possibility actually happened, then it must be assumed that the nursing strategy did not affect the outcome. The next step for the nurse is to collect data about what the client actually did to lose weight. It is important to establish the relationship (or lack thereof) of the nursing actions to the outcomes.

Reexamining the Client's Care Plan

Evaluating goal achievement provides the feedback necessary to determine if the care plan was effective in resolving, reducing, or preventing the client's problems. It is then necessary for the nurse to reexamine all aspects of the care plan, whether or not the goals have been met. Reexamining is a process of reassessing and replanning. See Table 9–1, for an example of evaluating goal achievement for Mr. Frederick Smith.

When Goals Are Met
If a goal or goals have been met, one of the following decisions may be made:

- The nurse may decide that the problem stated in the diagnosis no longer exists. In this instance, the nurse must document that the goal was met and that the care planned to meet this goal is discontinued.
- The nurse may decide that the problem still exists even though the goal was met. For example, if the criterion is "Client will ingest 3000 ml of fluid daily," and the goal is "Client's state of hydration will be maintained," nursing interventions need to continue even though the goal and criterion have been met.

When Goals Are Not Met
When goals are not met or only partially met, the nurse needs to reexamine the client's database, nursing diagnoses statements, goal statements, and nursing strategies.

Database
An incomplete or incorrect database influences all subsequent steps of the nursing process and care plan. In some instances, new data may invalidate the database, necessitating new nursing diagnoses, new goals, and new nursing actions.

Diagnostic statements
If the database is incomplete, new diagnostic statements are required. If the database is complete, the nurse needs to analyze whether the problem was identified correctly and whether the nursing diagnoses are relevant to that database.

Goal statements
If the nursing diagnostic statement is inaccurate and requires correcting, it is obvious that the goal statement needs revision. If the nursing di-agnostic statement is appropriate, the nurse then checks that the goal statements are realistic and attainable. Unrealistic, unattainable goals require correction. The nurse should also determine whether priorities have changed and whether the client and nurse still agree on the priorities. For example, a priority for the nurse may be to increase the client's fluid intake, but a priority for the client may be to decrease intake because of nausea.

Nursing strategies
Last, the nurse investigates whether the nursing strategies are related to the goals and whether the best nursing strategies were selected. Even when the diagnoses and goals are appropriate, the nursing strategies selected may not have been the best ones to achieve the goal. Before selecting new strategies, the nurse should check whether the ordered nursing actions have been carried out. Other personnel may not have carried them out, either because the orders were unclear or because the orders were unreasonable in terms of such external constraints such as money, staff, and equipment.

Modifying the Care Plan

When it is determined that the care plan needs revising, the nurse follows five steps:

1. Change the data in the assessment column to reflect the more recent findings. The new data should be dated and flagged in some way to indicate they are new. Follow agency practice: Some nurses use ink of a different color; others put a colored tab at the edge of the paper.
2. Revise the nursing diagnoses to reflect the new data. The new nursing diagnoses are also dated.
3. Revise the client's priorities, goals, and outcome criteria to reflect the new nursing diagnoses. These are also dated.
4. Establish new nursing strategies to correspond to the new nursing diagnoses. New nursing strategies may reflect increased or decreased need of the client for nursing care, scheduling changes, and rearrangement of nursing activities to group similar activities or to permit longer rest or activity periods for the client.
5. Change the outcome criteria to reflect the other changes in the plan. These changes should project the desired level of wellness indicated by the client. Criteria that apply to outdated nursing diagnoses should be deleted. See Table 9–2 on page 150.

TABLE 9-1 *Evaluating Goal Achievement for Mr. Frederick Smith*

Assessment Data	Diagnostic Statement	Goal
Hospitalized for cardiac catheterization and possible aortic valve replacement States family scared about illness Wants to see chaplain Wants family to visit Perceives son Tom as helpful Says is usually too busy to worry about things	**Fear** related to cardiac catheterization, possible heart surgery, and its outcome	Experience increased emotional comfort and feelings of control
Vital signs normal Heart rhythm regular Loud heart murmur (aortic area) Femoral pulses stronger than normal Absent pulses (popliteal, dorsalis pedis, posterior tibial) in left leg Left leg cooler than right leg Integument pink and intact	**Altered peripheral tissue perfusion (left leg)** related to impaired arterial circulation	Improve circulation to left leg and foot
Left hip replacement Movement slightly limited Joint stiffness Slight limp	**High risk for injury (trauma)** related to joint stiffness and limp from hip replacement surgery	Prevent injury
Shortness of breath Lacks energy to do daily chores Does not smoke	**Activity intolerance** related to shortness of breath and lack of energy secondary to decreased strength of cardiac contraction	Avoid performance of activities causing shortness of breath and excessive cardiac workload

TABLE 9-1   *(continued)*

Nursing Orders	Outcome Criteria	Evaluation
		Goal met
Establish a trusting relationship with the client and family	Verbalizes specific concerns	Verbalized concerns: "I'm worried about how my wife will support the family especially if anything bad happens during surgery."
Encourage client and family to express feelings and concerns	Communicates thoughts clearly and logically	Asked questions about cardiac catheterization and surgery
Discuss what the cardiac catheterization procedure entails and what is expected of him before and after the procedure	Facial expressions, voice tone, and body posture correspond to verbal expressions of increased emotional comfort or feelings of control	Nonverbal and verbal communication are congruent
Encourage conversation with another client who has recuperated from similar surgery	After instruction, describes the cardiac catheterization procedure and what is expected of him before and after the procedure	Described what to expect and what is expected of him before and after the cardiac catheterization procedure, e.g., "I know I will be taking a pill to help me relax before the procedure."
		Goal partially met
Consult with physician about exercise program, such as walking and range-of-motion exercises to hip, knee, and ankle	Demonstrates intact, pink, and moist skin	Skin of left foot and ankle intact but pale
Keep the extremity in a dependent position (i.e., lower than the heart)	Exhibits warm skin temperature (as other foot)	Skin temperature still cooler in left than right foot
Use Doppler ultrasound stethoscope (DUS) to assess blood flow in left dorsalis pedis, posterior tibial, and popliteal arteries q2h	Demonstrates palpable left dorsalis pedis, posterior tibial, and popliteal pulses of same strength as corresponding right pulses	Left popliteal pulse palpable but weak
		Left dorsalis pedis and posterior tibial pulses not palpable
	Verbalizes factors that improve and inhibit peripheral circulation	Blood flow evident only by DUS
Instruct client to keep his legs warm, e.g., by wearing warm socks, but discourage use of external heat	Demonstrates capillary refill of left toenails within 1 to 3 seconds	Capillary refill in left toenails within 7 seconds
		Goal met
Closely assess ambulation and transfers during first few days	Moves in and out of bed and ambulates without falling or injuring self	Ambulated and moved in and out of bed safely
Keep bed at lowest level		
Encourage client to request assistance to ambulate during the night		
Closely attend client or put side rails up when client is sedated		
		Goal met
Organize client care and provide undisturbed rest periods	Rests after meals	Rested after meals and activities
Discuss energy conservation methods, such as taking periodic rests	No shortness of breath during activities	Experienced no shortness of breath while performing ADLs
Tell the client to reduce the intensity, duration, and frequency of activity if he experiences chest pain, shortness of breath, dizziness, or abnormal pulse and blood pressure after activity	Shows stable pulse rate and blood pressure at 80 bpm and 124/80 mm Hg	Pulse rate and blood pressure remained stable at 80 bpm and 124/80 mm Hg
Monitor vital signs q2h and report decreasing blood pressure, increasing heart rate, or increasing respiratory rate		

TABLE 9–2 *Modified Care Plan for Mr. Frederick Smith after Cardiac Surgery (selected examples only)*

Assessment Data	Diagnostic Statement	Goal
Rales in bases of both lungs relieved by coughing before surgery Painful chest incision	**Potential ineffective airway clearance** related to chest incision	Maintain a clear airway
Aortic valve replacement (7/15) Heart rhythm regular at rest Pulse: 80 beats per minute (bpm) BP: 110/80 mm Hg	**Potential decreased cardiac output** related to physical exertion and/or shock	Maintain cardiac output and blood volume
Left dorsalis pedis pulse and posterior tibial artery not palpable Skin of left extremity cool and pale	**Altered tissue perfusion** related to impaired arterial circulation	Improve arterial circulation
Aortic valve replacement	**High risk for activity intolerance** related to reduced strength of cardiac contraction	Increase activity tolerance

TABLE 9–2 *(continued)*

Nursing Orders	Rationale	Outcome Criteria
Administer analgesics q4h during first 48 hours	Pain relief makes coughing less uncomfortable and more effective	Normal breath sounds auscultated in all areas of both lungs
Splint incision with pillows or hands during coughing	Splinting minimizes pain	
Turn q2h during first 48 hours	Turning prevents the accumulation of secretions in one lung area	
Assist with deep breathing and coughing (DB & C) exercises q2h	DB & C exercises help to move and expel secretions	
Assess vital signs q1h for first 24 hours, q2h if stable for next 48 hours, and q4h thereafter if stable	A lowered blood pressure and rapid pulse indicate lowered blood volume or inadequate cardiac output	Stable vital signs Pulse: 80–100 bpm BP: not less than 110/80 mm Hg
Assess apical pulse and heart rhythm, not radial pulse		Respirations not more than 15 breaths per minute
Report an increase in resting pulse rate above 110 bpm and a BP below 100 mm Hg		
Keep client's legs warm (especially left leg) with blankets or socks	Warmth increases circulation	Left posterior tibial and dorsalis pedis pulses palpable and of same strength as corresponding right pulses
Assess blood flow in left dorsalis pedis artery and posterior tibial artery q2h using DUS	The DUS detects and indicates movement of blood through the arteries	Skin warm, intact, pink
Keep left leg in dependent position	A dependent position facilitates arterial blood flow by gravity	Capillary refill of left toenails within 1 to 3 seconds
Consult physician about a schedule for increasing activity	A gradual increase in activity helps the heart muscle and new valve accommodate increased demands	After activity, heart rate remains below 110 bpm and within 6 bpm of resting pulse after 3 minutes
Monitor and later show the client how to monitor his response to increased activity by: 1. Taking a resting pulse before activity 2. Taking pulse immediately after activity 3. Taking pulse 3 minutes after activity 4. Noting rate decreases, rates about 110, rates not within 6 bpm of resting pulse after 3 minutes	Pulse rate monitoring provides awareness of activities that do not overly exert the heart	
Monitor blood pressure after activity	A drop in blood pressure indicates a reduction in cardiac output	
Starting on 7/19, discuss factors contributing to increased cardiac workload, such as stress, excessive weight, overactivity, large meals	Knowledge of factors contributing to increased cardiac workload may facilitate necessary life-style changes, such as eating smaller meals, losing weight, and altering activity patterns	
Starting on 7/19, discuss the effects of reduced cardiac output such as shortness of breath, pain, fatigue, edema	Knowledge of the effects of reduced cardiac output may motivate him to avoid excessive activity	

EVALUATING THE QUALITY OF NURSING CARE

Over the past 30 years, there has been considerable work on the evaluation of the quality of nursing care to determine what good care is, whether the care nurses give is appropriate and effective, and whether the quality of care provided is good. Evaluating the quality of nursing care is an essential part of professional accountability. Other terms used for this measurement are quality assessment and quality assurance. Quality assessment is an examination of services only; quality assurance implies that efforts are made to evaluate *and* ensure quality health care.

Historical Perspective

Evaluation of the quality of care is not a new concept. Florence Nightingale's *Notes on Hospitals,* published in 1859, included an evaluation of medical and nursing care. Since that time, evaluation has progressed through a number of stages. Initially, it focused on the environment, e.g., whether equipment was available at the time it was needed. Later, organizational standards in agencies were developed. For example, the ratio of nurses to clients was studied and evaluated in terms of clients' needs. Since 1952, the Joint Commission on Accreditation of Hospitals (JCAH), a voluntary organization, has surveyed hospitals. Objective criteria were applied to evaluate a client's record after discharge from the hospital. This was called a retrospective audit. A nursing audit is a review of clients' charts to evaluate nursing competence or performance.

In 1972 and 1973, the JCAH revised its standards to include the requirement that hospitals be subjected to medical and nursing audits before receiving accreditation. The maximum length of accreditation is three years, with reports submitted periodically to determine the institution's progress toward the recommendations submitted by the surveyors at the last visit.

In 1972, the United States government enacted legislation to control health care costs and evaluate the quality of health care services received by Medicare and Medicaid patients. Since that time a national and statewide system of professional review organizations (PROs) has been developed (Gordon 1987). The purposes of the PROs include developing standards and monitoring the quality of, cost of, and access to care. Hospitals are required to contract with a PRO for utilization review. The objective of these procedures is to ensure that the care given under federal programs was necessary and that the appropriate facilities were chosen to provide the care. Once problems are identified, an education process may be suggested to facilitate the correction of unacceptable staff practices, or penalties may be imposed on noncompliant care providers.

The PROs are based on the concept of peer review, an encounter between two persons equal in education, abilities, and qualifications, during which one person critically reviews the practices that the other has documented in a client's record. These evaluative processes may be concurrent audits, that is, reviews of present practices.

Approaches to Quality Evaluation

Three aspects of care—structure, process, and outcome—can be evaluated. Standards of care for each type of evaluation have been developed based on nursing and health-related research and expert opinion.

The Structure in Which Client Care Takes Place
Structure evaluation focuses on the organization of the client care system, for instance, administrative and financial procedures that direct the provision of care, staffing patterns, management styles, availability of equipment, and physical facilities. Information about these support structures can be obtained easily. All of these factors indirectly influence care. For example, the hospital administration determines the number of nursing positions that the hospital can afford. Quality care cannot be delivered without adequate staff and resources. However, adequate staffing patterns and adequate facilities do not ensure quality care.

The Process of Care
The focus of process evaluation is the activities of the nurse i.e., the performance of the caregiver in relation to the client's needs. This approach may be the most effective in determining the quality of care provided. The care given by the nurse is evaluated by talking with the client, auditing the client's record, and observing the nursing activities. Evaluators may seek answers to questions such as these: Are medications recorded properly? Was client teaching documented? Is the care plan complete? This type of evaluation is time consuming and requires the judgment of expert practitioners. The American Nurses' Association (ANA) *Standards of Practice* (1973) are process standards that provide the nursing profession with a framework for the delivery and evaluation of care.

Outcomes of the Care The focus of outcome evaluation is the client's health status, welfare, and satisfaction, or the results of care in terms of changes in the client. Its advantage is that outcomes may be easily observed, especially in relation to medical care, which focuses on disease entities. In nursing, however, outcomes are more difficult to determine, since nursing takes a holistic view of the client. Defining emotional, social, and behavioral outcomes is more complex than defining medical outcomes. In addition, client outcomes cannot be wholly attributed to nursing care. The client's own physical and psychologic mechanisms and contributions by family and other health professionals collectively produce outcomes. Outcome evaluation can focus on the client's change in behavior toward goal achievement prior to discharge (concurrent audit), or the client's record may be reviewed after discharge for evidence of goal attainment (retrospective audit).

Tools and Methods for Measuring Quality Care

Measuring the quality of care is a complex task. Development of tools involves four steps (Wright 1984, pp. 457–61):

1. Defining and clarifying the nature of nursing.

2. Deciding what approach to take (structure, process, outcome).

3. Developing standards and criteria. *Standards* are optimum levels of care against which actual performance is compared. *Criteria* are predetermined indicators of measures of health care, the presence, absence, and completeness of which indicate the quality of services (Meisenheimer 1985, p. 333, 338). Here is an example of a standard and its criteria:
   Standard IV: Each client has a written nursing care plan.
   Criteria: The nursing care plan is initiated within 8 hours of admission. It is based on information from the nursing health history and physical assessment. Goals are mutually set with the client and family, and the nursing care plan is evaluated and modified according to the client's needs.

4. Testing the criteria. Criteria must be valid and reliable. A valid criterion measures what it is intended to. A reliable criterion produces consistent results when used by the same person over time or by a different person.

RESEARCH NOTE

What Nursing Care Behaviors Predict Client Satisfaction?

The purpose of this study was to (a) determine how satisfied hospitalized clients were with nursing care behaviors and (b) predict which nursing behaviors were associated with client satisfaction. Client satisfaction was based on how closely the care the client received (actual) approached the care the client would have liked to receive (ideal). A patient satisfaction instrument (PSI) measured three nursing care variables: trust, patient education, and professional technical aspects. The subjects included 24 women and 26 men with a mean age of 60.36 years. Some nursing care behaviors associated with client satisfaction included being friendly, spending time talking to the client, following through with directions, explaining the diagnosis, and showing the client how to carry out physicians' orders. The subjects were least satisfied with the amount and type of information the nurse gave them.

Implications: This study suggests (a) that placing an emphasis on meeting the emotional and psychologic needs of clients and (b) providing more information to clients about themselves and their situation would increase client satisfaction. Clients need more information to take an active part in health care decisions.

M. M. M. Bader, Nursing care behaviors that predict patient satisfaction, *Journal of Nursing Quality Assurance,* May 1988, 2:11–17.

Several established tools are available for measuring the quality of care. Some are process tools, some are outcome tools, and others are process-outcome tools. Each tool consists of standards and criteria. Developing effective quality care evaluation tools is a challenge for the nursing profession. Much work is continuing even on established tools.

Methods of using these tools also vary. Some evaluate by retrospective audits of nursing records using nursing audit committees. Others evaluate using a concurrent audit of process, i.e., direct observation of the nurse or nurses providing the nursing care by educated observers or by peers. Data may also be obtained by questioning and observing clients, questioning the family, and observing the client's environment and the general environment. The time period for measurement also varies. Some tools are designed for use over a 2-hour period; some are designed to evaluate the whole process of care given to the client from admission to discharge.

Scoring systems differ among tools. Levels of care may be rated as *excellent, good, incomplete, poor,* and *unsafe.* Some tools require only simple *yes* or *no* responses. Nurses' performances may be rated on a scale of 5 (best nurse) to 1 (worst nurse).

CHAPTER HIGHLIGHTS

▸ Evaluation determines whether or to what degree the client goals have been met.

▸ Evaluating is both a concurrent and terminal process.

▸ Evaluating is purposeful and organized.

▸ Identifying outcome criteria is the first aspect of evaluating.

▸ Outcome criteria determine the evaluative data that must be collected to judge whether the goals have been met.

▸ Outcome criteria must be measurable and precise.

▸ Reexamining the client care plan is a process of reassessing and replanning.

▸ Evaluating the quality of nursing care is an essential aspect of professional accountability.

LEARNING ACTIVITIES

▪ Identify your health care organization's method for evaluating quality of care. Spend a day with the quality assurance coordinator (often a nurse). Based on the experience, how would you change your nursing practice?

READINGS AND REFERENCES

SUGGESTED READINGS

Porter, A. L. September 1988. Assuring quality through staff nurse performance. *Nursing Clinics of North America* 23:649–655.

The author describes the importance of a quality nursing staff to ensure quality patient care. The nurse must have the basic educational and personal credentials and then demonstrate quality performance as determined by preestablished standards. Clinical standards and performance appraisal methods must be clearly stated and effectively designed. Continuing education is suggested as a method to assist the nursing staff to refine and improve ineffective behaviors.

Smeltzer, C. H. August, 1988. Evaluating a successful quality assurance program: The process. *Journal of Nursing Quality Assurance* 2:1–9.

For a quality assurance program to benefit the nursing profession, it must be understood by all departments, implemented in a timely and appropriate manner, and include an ongoing evaluation component to determine effectiveness. Smeltzer presents and examines criteria for a successful quality assurance program that will provide a systematic method for evaluation of quality professional practice.

RELATED RESEARCH

Bader, M. M. M. May 1988. Nursing care behaviors that predict patient satisfaction. *Journal of Nursing Quality Assurance* 2:11–17.

Fink, A., Siu, A. L., and Brook, R. H. October 9, 1987. Assuring the quality of health care for older persons: an expert panel's priorities. *Journal of the American Medical Association* 258:1905–8.

Smeltzer, C. H., Hinshaw, A. S., and Feltman, B. May 1987. The benefits of staff nurse involvement in monitoring the quality of patient care. *Journal of Nursing Quality Assurance* 1:1–7.

SELECTED REFERENCES

American Nurses' Association. 1973. *Standards of nursing practice.* Kansas City, MO.

Bachrach, M. K.; Ballesteros, P.; and Black, A. N. Winter, 1988. Using patient outcomes to define nursing practice. *Nursing Administration Quarterly* 12:45–51.

Gordon, M. 1987. *Nursing diagnosis: Process and application.* 2d ed. New York: McGraw Hill.

Joint Commission on Accreditation of Health Organizations. 1989. *Accreditation Manual for Hospitals.* Chicago: Joint Commission on Accreditation of Health Organizations, Nursing Services.

Latreille, D. D.; Roth, M. J.; and Burgoyne, J. A. January 1988. Quality assurance. *Journal of Psychosocial Nursing and Mental Health Services* 26:28–31, 36, 38.

Lieske, A. 1985. Standards: The basis of a quality assurance program. In Meisenheimer, C., editor. *Quality assurance: A complete guide to effective programs.* Rockville, Md.: Aspen Systems Corporation.

Marker, C. G. S. May 1987. The Marker Umbrella model for quality assurance: Monitoring and evaluating professional practice. *Journal of Nursing Quality Assurance* 1:52–63.

Meisenheimer, C. 1985. *Quality assurance: A complete guide to effective programs.* Rockville, Md.: Aspen Systems Corporation.

O'Brien, B. November 1988. QA: A commitment to excellence. *Nursing Management* 19:33–34, 38–40.

Patterson, C. H. September 1988. Standards of patient care: The Joint Commission focus on nursing quality assurance. *Nursing Clinics of North America* 23:625–638.

Porter, A. L. September 1988. Assuring quality through staff nurse performance. *Nursing Clinics of North America* 23:649–655.

Rinke, L. 1987. *Outcome measures in home care.* Vol. 1. New York: National League for Nursing (Pub. no. 21-2194).

Rinke, L., and Wilson, A. 1987. *Outcome measures in home care.* Vol. 2. New York: National League for Nursing (Pub. no 21-2195).

Westfall, U. E. February 1987. Standards of practice: Nursing values made visible. *Journal of Nursing Quality Assurance* 1:21–30.

Whittaker, A. and McCanless, L. February 1988. Nursing peer review: Monitoring the appropriateness and outcome of nursing care. *Journal of Nursing Quality Assurance* 2:24–31.

Wright, D. September 1984. An introduction to the evaluation of nursing care: A review of the literature. *Journal of Advanced Nursing* 9:457–67.

Yura, H., and Walsh, M. B. 1988. *The nursing process: Assessing, planning, implementing, evaluating.* 5th ed. Norwalk, Conn.: Appleton & Lange.

PROFESSIONAL ACCOUNTABILITY AND ADVOCACY

Legal Dimensions of Nursing

CONTENTS

GENERAL LEGAL CONCEPTS

Nursing practice is governed by many legal concepts. It is important for nurses to know the basics of legal concepts because nurses are accountable for their professional judgments and actions. Accountability is an essential concept of professional nursing practice and the law. Knowledge of laws that regulate and affect nursing practice is needed for three reasons:

1. To ensure that the nurse's decisions and actions are consistent with current legal principles

2. To ensure public safety and the protection of individual rights

3 To protect the nurse from liability

Law can be defined as "a system of principles and processes by which people, who live in a society, attempt to control human conduct in an effort to minimize the use of force as a means of resolving conflicting interests" (Rhodes and Miller 1984, p. 1).

Functions of the Law in Nursing

The law serves a number of functions in nursing:

- It provides a framework for establishing which nursing actions in the care of clients are legal.
- It differentiates the nurse's responsibilities from those of other health professionals.
- It helps to establish the boundaries of independent nursing action.
- It assists in maintaining a standard of nursing practice by making nurses accountable under the law.
- It protects the public safety by establishing rules and regulations under which nurses are permitted to practice.

Sources of Law

The legal systems in both the United States and Canada have their origins in the English common law system. Three primary sources of law are constitutions, statutes, and decisions of courts (common law).

Constitutions   The Constitution of the United States and the Constitution of Canada are the supreme laws of each country. They establish the general organization of the federal governments, grant certain powers to them, and place limits on what federal and state or provincial governments may do. Constitutions create legal rights and responsibilities and are the foundation for a system of justice. The rights created, however, do not relate directly to the nurse-client relationship.

Constitutions have due process and equal protection clauses. The due process clause applies to state or provincial and local agencies, including public hospitals, and to actions that deprive a person of life, liberty, or property. *Due process* has two primary elements:

1. The rules being applied must be reasonable and not vague.

2. Fair procedures must be followed when enforcing the rules.

Equal protection means that like persons must be dealt with in like fashion.

Legislation (Statutes)   Laws enacted by any legislative body are called *statutory laws*. When there is a conflict between federal and state or provincial laws, federal law supersedes. Likewise, state or provincial laws supersede local laws.

The regulation of nursing is a function of state or provincial law. State or provincial legislatures pass statutes that define and regulate nursing, i.e., nurse practice acts. These acts, however, must be consistent with constitutional and federal provisions. Nurses practice acts, Good Samaritan laws, and adult or child abuse laws are examples of statutes that affect nurses.

Legislatures delegate responsibility and power to implement various laws to many administrative agencies who have the time and the expertise to address complex issues. State or provincial administrative agencies oversee the practice of the professions and regulate various aspects of commerce and public welfare. Examples pertinent to nurses are the state boards of nursing and provincial nursing associations, which implement and enforce nurse practice acts.

Common Law   The body of principles that evolves from court decisions is referred to as *common law,* or decisional laws. Although courts are called upon to interpret and apply constitutional or statutory law, they also are asked to resolve disputes between two parties. In such disputes, statutory and constitutional laws cannot support the case. Common law is continually being adapted and expanded. In deciding specific controversies, courts generally adhere to the doctrine of *stare decisis*—"to stand by things decided"—usually referred to as "following precedent." In other words, in a current case, the court applies the same rules and principles as applied in similar cases decided previously and arrives at the same ruling. Courts may depart from precedent when slight differences are noted between cases or when it is thought that a particular common-law rule no longer applies to the needs of society.

Types of Laws

Laws govern the relationship of private individuals with government and with each other.

Public law refers to the body of law that deals with relationships between individuals and the government and governmental agencies. An important segment of public law is *criminal law,* which deals with actions against the safety and welfare of the public. Examples

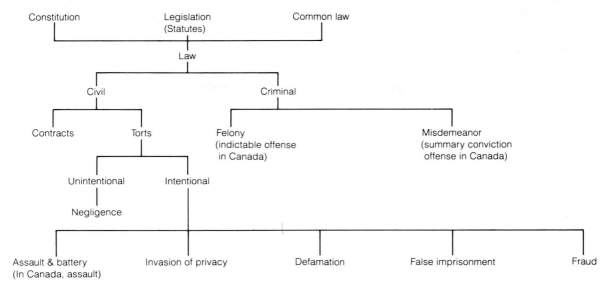

Figure 10-1 Categories of law pertinent to nurses.

are homicide, manslaughter, and theft. Crimes are classified as felonies or misdemeanors in the United States or as indictable offenses or summary conviction offenses in Canada. See the discussion of crimes and torts later in this chapter. Public law also includes numerous regulations designed to enhance societal objectives. Private individuals and organizations are required to follow specified courses of action in their activities. Noncompliance with these regulations can lead to criminal penalties.

Private law, or civil law, is the body of law that deals with relationships between private individuals. It is categorized as contract law and tort law. *Contract law* involves the enforcement of agreements among private individuals or the payment of compensation for failure to fulfill the agreements. *Tort law* defines and enforces duties and rights among private individuals that are not based on contractual agreements. The word *tort* comes from the Latin word *tortus,* meaning twisted. Loosely translated, it means "wrong" or "bad." Some examples of tort laws applicable to nurses are negligence and malpractice, invasion of privacy, and assault and battery. See Figure 10–1 and also Table 10–1 for selected categories of law affecting nurses.

Principles of Law

The system of law rests on four simple principles that are often cloaked in complex terminology (Fenner 1980 p. 84):

1. *Law is based on a concern for justice and fairness.* The law seeks to protect the rights of one party from the transgressions of another by setting guidelines for conduct and mechanisms to enforce those guidelines.

2. *Law is characterized by change.* Social and technologic changes occur rapidly and often without predictions of problems to follow. In response to these changes, the legal system also must change. Often the legal system reacts rather than acts. For example, after technologic devices such as respirators were developed to prolong life, it became necessary for the law to change its guidelines about indications of death—from cessation of heart function to absence of electric currents from the brain for at least 24 hours.

3. *Actions are judged on the basis of a universal standard of what a similarly educated, reasonable, and prudent person would have done under similar circumstances.* All nurses are expected to function the same way that another nurse with similar education and experience would function. This rule of reasonable and prudent conduct is the basis for evaluating a person's actions, e.g., for judging whether or not actions were negligent (see the discussion of negligence and malpractice later in this chapter).

4. *Each individual has rights and responsibilities. Rights* are privileges or fundamental powers that in-

TABLE 10-1 *Selected Categories of Laws Affecting Nurses*

Category	Examples
Constitutional	Due process
	Equal protection
Statutory (legislative)	Nurse practice acts
	Good Samaritan acts
	Child and adult abuse laws
	Living wills
Criminal (public)	Homicide, manslaughter
	Theft
	Arson
	Active euthanasia
	Rape
	Illegal possession of controlled drugs
Contracts (private/civil)	Nurse and client
	Nurse and employer
	Nurse and insurance
	Client and agency
Torts (private/civil)	Negligence
	Libel and slander
	Invasion of privacy
	Assault and battery
	False imprisonment

Source: American Nurses Association. *Standards of Nursing Practice.* (Kansas City, Mo.: ANA, 1973). Used by permission.

dividuals possess unless they are revoked by law or given up voluntarily; *responsibilities* are the obligations associated with these rights. Failure to meet one's responsibilities can endanger one's rights. For example, a registered nurse has the right to practice nursing within the constraints of the law (nurse practice acts). If the nurse fails to observe these constraints (e.g., prescribes medications or conducts a surgical procedure), the behavior is considered irresponsible, and the right to practice can be revoked.

Kinds of Legal Actions

There are two kinds of legal actions: civil or private actions and criminal actions. *Civil actions* deal with the relationships between individuals in society; for example, a man may file a suit against a person who he believes cheated him. Civil actions that are of concern to nurses

include the torts and contracts listed in Table 10–1. Other civil actions that might be of concern to nurses include those relating to wills and the estates of deceased persons. These cases are known as *probate proceedings. Criminal actions* deal with disputes between an individual and the society as a whole; for example, if a man shoots a person, society brings him to trial.

The Civil Judicial Process

The judicial process primarily functions to settle disputes peacefully and in accordance with the law. A lawsuit has strict procedural rules. There are generally five steps:

1. A document called a *complaint* is filed by a person referred to as the *plaintiff,* who claims that the person's legal rights have been infringed upon by one or more persons, referred to as *defendants.*

2. A written response, called an *answer,* is made by the defendants.

3. Both parties engage in pretrial activities, referred to as *discovery,* in an effort to gain all the facts of the situation.

4. In the *trial* of the case, all the relevant facts are presented to a jury or a judge.

5. The judge renders a *decision,* or the jury renders a *verdict.* If the outcome is not acceptable to one of the parties, an appeal can be made for another trial.

During a trial, a plaintiff must offer evidence of the defendant's wrongdoing. This duty of proving an assertion is called the *burden of proof.* An additional aspect of this burden of proof is that the plaintiff must have a greater amount of convincing evidence than the defendant if the plaintiff is to prevail.

Nurses as Expert Witnesses

When called into court as a witness, the nurse has a duty to assist justice as far as possible. An *expert witness* is one who, by education or experience, possesses knowledge and skill needed to understand the matter about which the person is to testify (Rhodes and Miller 1984, p. 18). Such a witness is usually called to help a judge or jury understand evidence pertaining to the extent of damage and the standard of care.

A nurse may be called to testify in a legal action for a variety of reasons. She may be a defendant in a malpractice or negligence action or she may have been a member of the health team that provided care to the plaintiff. It is advisable that the nurse seek the advice of an attorney before providing testimony. In most cases, the attorney for the institution will provide support and counsel during the legal case. However, if the nurse is a defendant she should retain an attorney to protect her own interests.

A testifying nurse should always respond directly and truthfully to the questions. The nurse is not expected to volunteer additional information, nor is the nurse expected to remember completely all the details of a situation that may have occurred months or even years prior to the legal action. The nurse may ask to refer to the client record or to personal notes related to the incident. If the nurse does not remember the details of the incident, it is advisable to state such rather than to attempt an inaccurate recollection.

In any case, it is the nurse's professional responsibility to provide accurate testimony both during the pre-trial discovery phase and the trial phase of a legal action.

Privileged Communication

A *privileged communication* is information given to a professional person who is forbidden by law from disclosing the information in a court without the consent of the person who provided it.

Legislation regarding privileged communications is highly complicated. A nurse would be unwise to encourage disclosures or advise a client about the subject. The privileged communication law is for the benefit of the client; a nurse who is given confidential information should be prepared to answer questions fully and honestly if required to testify in a court of law. Many states with statutes granting privileged communications between the client and various health care providers do not extend the privilege to nurse-client communication.

The matter of privileged communications is referred to in the ANA's *Code for Nurses* (1976). It advises the nurse to seek legal counsel in regard to a privileged communication and to become familiar with the rights and privileges of the client and the nurse.

In Canada, confidentiality of information is incorporated as an ethic in the legislation on nursing practice. Failure to maintain confidentiality can result in disciplinary action against the nurse.

LEGAL ASPECTS OF NURSING

Nurse Practice Acts

Each state in the United States has nurse practice acts, and each province in Canada has a nurse practice act or an act for professional nursing practice. Nurse practice acts protect the nurse's professional capacity and legally control nursing practice through licensing. Nurse practice acts legally define and describe the scope of nursing practice, which the law seeks to regulate, thereby protecting the public as well. Because of the number of acts there are many definitions and descriptions of nursing. In 1981, the ANA described nursing practice as including but not limited to "administration, teaching, counseling, supervision, delegation, and evaluation of practice and execution of the medical regimen, including the administration of medications and treatments prescribed by any person authorized by state law to prescribe" (ANA 1981, p. 6).

Many states have an additional clause that pertains to actions that may be performed only by certain nurses with education beyond the minimum required for licensure under the act. For example, many of the clauses address the practice of nurse-midwives or nurse-anesthetists. Some address the nurse-practitioner role. These clauses conflict with the ANA policy, which advises against legal regulation of advanced or specialty nursing practice. The ANA's position is that it is the function of the professional association, not the law, to establish the scope and desirable qualifications required for each specialized area of practice (Snyder and Labar 1984, p. 7).

Credentialing

Credentialing is the process of determining and maintaining competence in nursing practice. The credentialing process is one way in which the nursing profession maintains standards of practice and is accountable for the educational preparation of members. Credentialing includes licensure, registration, certification, and accreditation.

The ANA enumerated the principles of credentialing; these principles reflect the belief that credentialing exists primarily to protect and benefit the public. See Table 10–2.

Licensure and Registration   *Licenses* are legal permits granted by a government agency to individuals to engage in the practice of a profession and to use a particular title. A particular jurisdiction or area is covered by the license. For a profession or occupation to obtain the right to license its members, it generally must meet three criteria:

1. There is a need to protect the public's safety or welfare.

2. The occupation is clearly delineated as a separate, distinct area of work.

3. There is an organization suitable in ability to assume the obligations of the licensing process.

In the United States, nurses are issued a license by the state board of nursing or by an administrative governmental agency that is empowered by government to

TABLE 10-2 *Principles of Credentialing*

1. In addition to benefiting and protecting the public, credentialing also benefits those who are credentialed.

2. The legitimate interests of the involved occupation or institution and of the general public should be reflected in each credentialing mechanism.

3. Accountability should be an essential component of any credentialing process.

4. A system of checks and balances within the credentialing system should assure equitable treatment for all parties involved.

5. Periodic assessments with the potential for sanction are essential components of an effective credentialing mechanism.

6. Objective standards and criteria and persons competent in their use are essential to the credentialing process.

7. Representation in credentialing systems of the community of interests directly affected by credentialing mechanisms should assure consideration of the legitimate concerns of each group.

8. Professional identity and responsibility should evolve from the credentialing process.

9. An effective system of role delineation is fundamental to any credentialing mechanism for individuals.

10. An effective system of program identification is fundamental to any credentialing mechanism for institutions.

11. Coordination of credentialing mechanisms should lead to efficiency and cost effectiveness and avoid duplication.

12. Geographic, including interstate, mobility should be improved by the credentialing of the individual.

13. Widely accepted definitions and terminology are basic to an effective credentialing system.

14. Communications and understanding between health care providers and society should be facilitated through the credentialing process.

Source: Report of the Committee for the Study of Credentialing in Nursing, American Nurses' Association. *American Journal of Nursing* April 1979, 79:674. Used by permission.

grant licenses. Licenses are issued to registered nurses who have (a) successfully completed a course of studies in a school of nursing accredited by the state board, (b) passed the national qualifying examinations with a score that is acceptable to the board, and (c) paid the required fee. A state board may also grant a license to a nurse who holds an active practicing license in another state, through a process of endorsement, without the candidate having to rewrite examinations. The candidate, however, must have attained a passing score on the national examinations that is equal to, or above, that considered acceptable in the state in which the nurse wishes to practice.

In Canada, nurses are not licensed except in the province of Quebec. They are, however, registered by their provincial nursing association and by the College of Nurses of Ontario. Nurses in the United States are also registered but must in addition be granted a license to practice. Nurses who are registered are permitted to use the title "Registered Nurse." To be registered, the nurse must have completed a basic course of nursing studies in a program approved by the registering body and have passed the national qualifying examinations with an acceptable grade. Canada has a national comprehensive registered nurse examination, offered in both French and English. All state boards of nursing consider the same score an acceptable passing grade. Nurses from other provinces in Canada and from other countries may be granted registration by endorsement provided they meet the requirements of the registering body. Both licensure and registration must be renewed on an annual basis (in some states every 2 years) to be valid.

There are two types of licensure/registration: mandatory and permissive. Under mandatory licensure/registration, anyone who practices nursing must be licensed or, in Canada, registered. The only exceptions are: (a) practice in an emergency, (b) practice by nursing students as part of their education, and (c) practice by nurses employed by the federal government (nurses who practice in Veterans Administration hospitals and in public health must be currently licensed in some jurisdictions but not necessarily where the facility is located). Under permissive licensure/registration, the title RN is reserved for licensed or, in Canada, registered practitioners, but the practice of nursing is not prohibited to others who are not licensed or registered.

Registration is mandatory in most provinces of Canada. In the United States, nursing licensure is mandatory in all states. There is a strong movement underway in Canada to make registration mandatory in all provinces.

In each state and province there is a mechanism by which licenses (or registration in Canada) can be revoked for just cause, e.g., incompetent nursing practice; professional misconduct; conviction of a crime such as using illegal drugs or selling drugs illegally; obtaining a license through deception, falsifying school records, or hiding a criminal history; and, in some areas, aiding in a criminal abortion. In each situation, all the facts are generally reviewed by a committee at a hearing. Nurses are entitled to be represented by legal counsel at such a hearing. If the nurse's license is revoked as a result of the hearing, an appeal can be made to a court, or, in some states, an agency is designated to review the decision before any court action is initiated.

Certification

Certification is the voluntary practice of validating that an individual nurse has met minimum standards of nursing competence in specialty areas, such as maternal-child health, pediatrics, mental health, gerontology, and school nursing. Certification programs are conducted by the ANA and by specialty nursing organizations. Certification is a professional credential, not a legal obligation. A certification program has not yet been established in Canada, but the CNA is currently considering the establishment of a certification program for nurses in specialized fields of nursing.

Accreditation/Approval of Basic Nursing Education Programs

Accreditation is a process by which a voluntary organization (e.g., the NLN) or governmental agency (e.g., the state board of nursing) appraises and grants accredited status to institutions and/or programs or services that meet predetermined structure, process, and outcome criteria (ANA 1979). Minimum standards for basic nursing education programs are established in each state of the United States and in each province in Canada. State accreditation or provincial approval is granted to schools of nursing meeting the minimum criteria. NLN accreditation is concerned with optimum, rather than minimum, standards. In other words, accreditation by the NLN certifies that an educational program not only meets minimum standards but also is considered "good" by national standards. It is not a legal requirement as is state or provincial accreditation.

Standards of Practice

Another way the nursing profession attempts to ensure that its practitioners are competent and safe to practice is through the establishment of standards of practice (see Chapter 1). These standards are often used to evaluate the quality of care provided by nurses. In addition to this basic set of standards, which are applicable in any practice setting, the ANA has developed standards of nursing practice for specific areas such as maternal-child, medical-surgical, geriatric, psychiatric, and community health nursing.

CONTRACTUAL ARRANGEMENTS IN NURSING

A contract is the basis of the relationship between a nurse and an employer—for example, a nurse and a hospital or a nurse and a physician. A *contract* is an agreement between two or more competent persons, upon sufficient consideration (remuneration), to do or not to do some lawful act. A contract may be written or oral; however, a written contract cannot be changed legally by an oral agreement. If two people wish to change some aspect of a written contract, the change must be written into the contract, because one party cannot hold the other to an oral agreement that differs from the written one.

A contract is considered to be *expressed* when the two parties discuss and agree orally or in writing to its terms, e.g., that a nurse will work at a hospital for a stated length of time and under stated conditions. An *implied* contract is one in which there has been no discussion between the parties, but the law considers that a contract exists. In the contractual relationship between nurse and client, clients have the right to expect that nurses caring for them have the competence to meet their needs. This *implies* that the nurse has a responsibility to remain competent. The nurse has the associated right to expect the client to provide accurate information as required.

Contract law requires that four elements be met to make a contract valid (Fenner 1980, p. 94):

1. The act contracted for must be legal. The nurse's employment must be legal, and the duties to be performed and services provided must be within the law. For example, the nurse cannot be required to provide services that are not permitted in the nurse practice act.

2. The parties to the contract must be of legal age (majority) and competent (free of mental impairment) to enter a binding agreement.

3. There must be mutual agreement about the service to be contracted for. A contract becomes invalid, for example, if the nurse does not accept an offer of hire.

4. There must be compensation (or promise of it) for the service to be provided.

These four elements are also required for contracts made by clients (with nurses, other health professionals, or health care institutions) to be valid. For example, the activity contracted for between a client and a hospital is health care, which is legal. Clients who are minors are not usually admitted for care without consent from their parents or legal guardians. The parties agree to the terms of the contract when the client gives informed consent for care and the hospital offers care. The client promises to reimburse the hospital for its services through insurance coverage or other means.

Legal Roles of Nurses

Nurses have three separate, interdependent legal roles, each with rights and associated responsibilities:

1. *Provider of service.* The nurse is expected to provide safe and competent care so that harm (physical, psychologic, or material) to the recipient of the service is prevented. Implicit in this role are several legal concepts: liability, standards of care, and contractual obligations.

   Liability is the quality or state of being legally responsible to account for one's obligations and actions and to make financial restitution for wrongful acts. A primary nurse or team leader, for example, has an obligation to practice and direct the practice of others under supervision so that harm or injury to the client is prevented and standards of care are maintained. Even when a nurse is directed by a physician, the responsibility for nursing activity is the nurse's. When a nurse is requested to carry out an activity that the nurse believes will be injurious to the client, the nurse's responsibility is to refuse to carry out the order and report this to the nurse in charge.

   The *standards of care* by which a nurse acts or fails to act are legally defined by nurse practice acts and by the rule of reasonable and prudent action—what a reasonable and prudent professional with similar preparation and experience would do in similar circumstances. A nurse, for example, would be acting illegally in diagnosing a medical condition or treating a client for a tumor because these functions are within the scope of the physician's practice, and nurses are constrained from engaging in them. *Contractual obligations* refer to the nurse's duty of care, that is, duty to render care, established by the presence of an expressed or implied contract discussed earlier.

2. *Employee or contractor for service.* A nurse who is employed by a hospital works as an agent of the hos-

pital, and the nurse's contract with clients is an implied one. However, a nurse who is employed directly by a client, for example, a private nurse, may have a written contract with that client in which the nurse agrees to provide professional services for a certain fee. If the client is dying, the nurse can be protected by a written contract that allows collection of the fee from the client's estate. A nurse might be prevented from carrying out the terms of the contract because of illness or death. However, personal inconvenience and personal problems, such as the nurse's car failure, are not legitimate reasons for failing to fulfill a contract.

Contractual relationships vary among practice settings. An independent nurse practitioner is a contractor for service, whose contractual relationship with the client is an independent one. The nurse employed by a hospital functions within an employer-employee relationship, in which the nurse represents and acts for the hospital and therefore must function within the policies of the employing agency. This type of legal relationship creates the ancient legal doctrine known as *respondeat superior* ("let the master answer"). In other words, the master (employer) assumes responsibility for the conduct of the servant (employee) and can also be held responsible for malpractice by the employee. By virtue of the employee role, therefore, the nurse's conduct is the hospital's responsibility.

This doctrine does not imply that the nurse cannot be held liable as an individual. Nor does it imply that the doctrine will prevail if the employee's actions are extraordinarily inappropriate, i.e., beyond those expected or foreseen by the employer. For example, if the nurse hits a client in the face, the employer could disclaim responsibility, since this behavior is beyond the bounds of expected behavior. Criminal acts, such as assisting with criminal abortions or taking tranquilizers from a client's supply for personal use, would also be considered extraordinarily inappropriate behavior. Nurses can be held liable for failure to act as well. For example, if a nurse sees another nurse hitting a client and fails to do anything to protect the client, the observer may also be considered negligent.

The nurse in the role of employee or contractor for service has obligations to the employer, the client, and other personnel. The nursing care provided must be within the limitations and terms specified. The nurse has an obligation to contract only for those responsibilities that the nurse is competent to discharge. As an employee, the nurse is expected to uphold the good name of the employer and therefore should not criticize the employer unjustifiably. The employer, in turn, is obligated to provide adequate working conditions, e.g., a safe, functional employment setting.

The nurse is expected to respect the rights and responsibilities of other health care participants. For example, although the nurse has responsibility to explain nursing activities to a client, the nurse does not have the right to comment on medical practice in a way that disturbs the client or causes problems for the physician. At the same time, the nurse has the right to expect reasonable and prudent conduct from other health care providers.

3. *Citizen.* The rights and responsibilities of the nurse in the role of citizen are the same as those of any individual under the legal system. Rights of citizenship protect clients from harm and ensure consideration for their personal property rights, rights to privacy, confidentiality, and other rights discussed later in this chapter and in Chapter 14. These same rights apply to nurses. For example, nurses have the right to physical safety and need not perform functions that are considered to pose an unreasonable risk.

Nurses move in and out of these roles when carrying out professional and personal responsibilities. An understanding of these roles and the rights and responsi-

bilities associated with them promotes legally responsible conduct and practice by nurses. See Table 10–3 for examples of the responsibilities and rights associated with each role.

Collective Bargaining

Collective bargaining is a formal decision-making process between management and labor representatives concerning salaries, work environment, and conditions of employment (Crawford et al. 1985, p. 155). Through a written agreement, both employer and employees legally commit themselves to observe the terms and conditions of employment. Collective bargaining is a controversial issue among nurses. Some nurses argue against collective bargaining on the grounds that it is contrary to the nature of professionalism, it is not necessary, it fosters discord, and it undermines the nurse-administrator's role (McClelland 1983, p. 36). Others argue that collective bargaining is necessary to obtain control of nursing practice and economic security.

The collective bargaining process involves the recognition of a certified bargaining agent for the employees. This agent, which can be a union, a trade association, or a professional organization, represents the employees in negotiating a contract with management. The American Nurses' Association through their state affiliates has

TABLE 10-3 *Nurses' Legal Roles, Rights, and Responsibilities*

Role	Responsibilities	Rights
Provider of service	To provide safe and competent care commensurate with the nurse's preparation, experience, and circumstances	Right to adequate and qualified assistance as necessary
	To inform clients of the consequences of various alternatives and outcomes of care	Right to reasonable and prudent conduct from clients, e.g., provision of accurate information as required
	To provide adequate supervision and evaluation of subordinates for whom the nurse is responsible	
	To remain competent	
Employee or contractor for service	To fulfill the obligations of contracted service with the employer	Right to adequate working conditions, e.g., safe equipment and facilities
		Right to compensation for services rendered
	To respect the rights and responsibilities of other health care participants	Right to reasonable and prudent conduct by other health care givers
Citizen	To protect the rights of the recipients of care	Right to respect by others of the nurse's own rights and responsibilities

TABLE 10-4 *Categories and Examples of Grievances*

Category	Examples
Contract violations	Shift or weekend work is assigned inequitably.
	A nurse is dismissed without cause.
Violations of federal and state law	A female nurse is paid less than a male nurse for the same work.
	Appropriate payment is not given for overtime work.
	Minority group nurses are not promoted.
Management responsibilities	Appropriate locker room facilities are not provided.
	Safe client care is jeopardized by inadequate staffing.
Violation of agency rules	Performance evaluations are conducted only at termination of employment, but the contract requires annual evaluations.
	A vacation period is assigned without the nurse's agreement, as required in personnel policies.

Source: American Nurses Association, *The grievance procedure* (Kansas City, Mo.: ANA, 1985), pp. 2–4. Used by permission.

served as the collective bargaining agent for some nurse employee groups since 1946. According to Ellis and Hartley (1988, p. 297) the ANA represents more nurses than all the other organizations put together.

When collective bargaining breaks down because an agreement cannot be reached, the employees usually call a *strike*. A strike is an organized work stoppage by a group of employees to express a grievance, enforce a demand for changes in conditions of employment, or solve a dispute with management (Crawford et al. 1985, p. 162). A strike is the last resort used when all attempts at negotiation have failed. The union is required by law to give 10 days notice prior to a strike.

Because nursing practice is a service to people, striking presents a moral dilemma to many nurses. Actions taken by nurses can affect the safety of clients. When faced with a strike, each nurse must make an individual decision to cross or not to cross a picket line. The ANA supports striking as a means of achieving economic and general welfare.

Collective bargaining is more than the negotiation of salary terms and hours of work; it is a continuous process in which day-to-day working problems and relationships can be handled in an orderly and democratic manner. Day-to-day difficulties or grievances are handled through the grievance procedure: A formal plan established in the contract that outlines the channels for handling and settling grievances through progressively higher levels of administration. A *grievance* is any dispute, difference, controversy, or disagreement arising out of the terms and conditions of employment. Grievances fall into four main categories, outlined in Table 10–4.

It is important for the nurse to understand the collective bargaining process whether as a nurse manager or as a staff member. It is especially important for mid-level nurse managers working with a collective bargaining unit to understand their relationship with the unit, i.e., whether they are considered "in unit" (a member of the bargaining unit) or "out of unit" (a member of management). This knowledge can impact upon their relationship with participants in labor disputes.

AREAS OF POTENTIAL LIABILITY IN NURSING

Crimes and Torts

A *crime* is an act committed in violation of public (criminal) law and punishable by a fine and/or imprisonment. A crime does *not* have to be intended in order to be a crime. For example, a nurse may accidentally give a client an additional and lethal dose of a narcotic to relieve discomfort.

Crimes are classified as either felonies (or in Canada, indictable offenses) or misdemeanors (or in Canada, summary conviction offenses). A *felony* is a crime of a serious nature, such as murder, punishable by a term in prison. In some areas, second-degree murder is called *manslaughter*. A nurse who accidentally gives an additional and lethal dose of a narcotic can be accused of manslaughter. Other examples of felonies are arson and armed robbery.

Crimes are punished through criminal action by the state or province against an individual. A *misdemeanor* is an offense of a less serious nature and is usually punishable by a fine or short-term jail sentence, or both. A nurse who slaps a client's face could be charged with a misdemeanor.

A *tort* is a civil wrong committed against a person or a person's property. Torts are usually litigated in court by civil action between individuals. In other words, the person or persons claimed to be responsible for the tort are sued for damages. Tort liability almost always is based on fault, i.e., something was done incorrectly (an unreasonable act of commission) or something that should have been done was not done (act of omission).

Torts may be classified as intentional or unintentional. Intentional torts include fraud, invasion of privacy, libel and slander, assault and battery, and false imprisonment. *Fraud* is the false presentation of some fact with the intention that it will be acted upon by another person. For example, it is fraud for a nurse applying to a hospital for employment to fail to list two past employers for deceptive reasons when asked to list the previous five employers.

The right to privacy is the right of individuals to withhold themselves and their lives from public scrutiny. Invasion of privacy is a direct wrong of a personal nature. It injures the feelings of the person and does not take into account the effect of revealed information on the standing of the person in the community. The right to privacy can also be described as the right to be left alone. Liability can result if the nurse breaches confidentiality by passing along confidential client information to others or intrudes into the client's private domain.

In this context, there is a delicate balance between the need of a number of people to contribute to the diagnosis and treatment of a client and the client's right to confidentiality. In most situations, necessary discussion about a client's medical condition is considered appropriate, but unnecessary discussions and gossip are considered a breach of confidentiality. Necessary discussion involves only those engaged in the client's care.

Most jurisdictions of the country have a variety of statutes that impose a duty to report certain confidential client information. Four major categories are (a) vital statistics: e.g., births and deaths, (b) infections and communicable diseases, e.g., diphtheria, syphilis, and typhoid fever, (c) child or elder abuse, and (d) violent incidents, e.g., gunshot wounds and knife wounds.

Both libel and slander are wrongful actions that come under the heading of defamation. *Defamation* is communication that is false, or made with a careless disregard for the truth, and results in injury to the reputation of a person. *Libel* is defamation by means of print, writing, or pictures. *Slander* is defamation by the spoken word, stating unprivileged (not legally protected) or false words by which a reputation is damaged. A nurse has a qualified privilege to make statements that could be considered invasions of a client's privacy, both orally and in writing, but only as a part of nursing practice and only to a physician or another health team member caring directly for the client.

In the United States, the terms *assault* and *battery* are often heard together, but each has its own meaning. *Assault* can be described as an attempt or threat to touch another person unjustifiably. Assault precedes battery; it is the act that causes the person to believe a battery is about to occur. For example, the person who threatens someone by making a menacing gesture with a club or a closed fist is guilty of assault. In nursing, a client may perceive that a nurse is *about* to administer an injection without the client's consent.

Battery is the willful touching of a person (or the person's clothes or even something the person is carrying), which may or may not cause harm. To be actionable at law, however, the touching must be wrong in some way, e.g., done without permission, embarrassing, or causing injury. For example, the nurse who administers a hypodermic injection to a client or ambulates a client without the client's consent could be held liable for battery. Liability applies even though the physician ordered the medication or the activity and even if the client benefits from the nurse's action.

In Canada, the term *battery* is not used. Instead assault is classified into three categories: assault with intention to injure (for example, threatening someone by making a menacing gesture with a knife), assault causing bodily injury, and sexual assault. *False imprisonment* is unjustifiable detention that deprives a person of personal liberty for any length of time. For example, a nurse who locks a client in a room unjustifiably is guilty of false imprisonment. False imprisonment accompanied by forceful restraint or threat of restraint is assault (Creighton 1986, p. 197).

Although nurses may suggest under certain circumstances that a client remain in the room or in bed, the client must not be detained against the client's will. The client has a right to insist upon leaving even though it may be detrimental to health. In this instance, the client can leave by signing an AWA (absence without authority) or an AMA (against medical advice) form.

Negligence and malpractice are examples of unintentional torts that may occur in health care settings. *Negligence* is "the omission to do something that a reasonable person, guided by those ordinary considerations which ordinarily regulate human affairs, would do, or doing something which a reasonable and prudent person would not do" (Creighton 1986, p. 141). *Malpractice* is that part of the law of negligence applied to the pro-

TABLE 10–5 *Comparison of Intentional and Unintentional Torts*

Intentional	Unintentional (Negligence)
1. They involve the commission of a prohibited act.	1. They can result from either an act of commission or an act of omission.
2. The act in question is willful and deliberate (intentional).	2. The wrong results from failure to use due care.
3. They involve certain specific types of conduct listed as "wrong."	3. They are not spelled out in an all-inclusive list.

fessional person: It is, in effect, any professional misconduct or unreasonable lack of professional skill. A nurse could be liable for malpractice if the nurse injured a client while performing a procedure differently from the way other nurses would have done it.

Nurses are responsible for their own actions whether they are independent practitioners or employees of a health agency. The descriptions of negligence and malpractice do not mention good intentions; it is not pertinent that the nurse did not intend to be negligent. If a nurse administers an incorrect medication, even in good faith, the fact that the nurse failed to read the label correctly indicates malpractice if all of the elements of negligence are met.

Another significant aspect of negligence and malpractice is that both omissions and commissions are included. That is, a person can be negligent by forgetting to give a medication as well as by giving the wrong medication. See Table 10–5 for a summary of the differences between intentional and unintentional torts.

Potential Malpractice Situations in Nursing

If a nurse wishes to avoid charges of malpractice, it is helpful to recognize those nursing situations in which negligent actions are most likely to occur and to take measures to prevent them. The most common situation is the *medication error*. Because of the large number of medications on the market today and the variety of methods of administration, these errors may be on the increase. Nursing errors include failing to read the medication label, misreading or incorrectly calculating the dosage, failing to identify the client correctly, preparing the wrong concentration, or administering a medication by the wrong route (e.g., intravenously instead of orally). Some medication errors are very serious and can result in death. For example, administering dicumarol to a client recently returned from surgery could cause the client to have a hemorrhage. Nurses always need to check medications very carefully. Even after checking, the nurse is wise to recheck the medication order and the medication before administering it if the client states, for example, that the client "did not have a green pill before."

Sponges or other small items can be left inside a client during an operation because the nurse either failed to count them before the surgeon closed the incision or counted them incorrectly. In either case, the nurse responsible for the *sponge count* can be held liable for malpractice.

A relatively frequent malpractice action attributed to nurses is *burning a client*. Burns may be caused by hot water bottles, heating pads, and solutions that are too hot for application. Elderly, comatose, or diabetic people are particularly vulnerable to burns due to their decreased sensitivity. Hot objects can burn these people before they notice it. A nurse may also be held negligent for leaving a client without taking precautions (giving warnings or providing protections), for example, when using a steam vaporizer.

Clients often fall accidentally, sometimes with resultant injury. Some falls can be prevented by elevating the side rails on the cribs, beds, and stretchers of babies and small children, and of adults when necessary. If a nurse leaves the rails down or leaves a baby unattended on a bath table, that nurse is guilty of malpractice if the *client falls* and is injured as a direct result of not placing the siderails up or leaving the child unattended. Most hospitals and nursing homes have policies regarding the use of safety devices such as side rails and restraints. The nurse needs to be familiar with these policies and to take indicated precautions to prevent accidents.

In some instances, nurses are found guilty of malpractice by ignoring a client's complaints. This type of malpractice is termed *failure to observe and take appropriate action*. The nurse who does not report a client's complaint of acute abdominal pain is negligent and may be found guilty of malpractice for ensuing appendix rupture and death. By failing to take the blood pressure and pulse and to check the dressing of a client who has just had a kidney removed, a nurse omits important assessments. If the client hemorrhages and dies, the nurse may be held responsible for the death as a result of this malpractice.

Incorrectly identifying clients is a problem, particularly in busy hospital units. Nurses have prepared the wrong client for an operation with unfortunate results such as a healthy gallbladder being removed from the wrong person. Cases of *mistaken identity* are costly to the client and render the nurse liable for malpractice.

Client property, such as jewelry, money, and dentures, is a constant concern to hospital personnel. Today, agencies are taking less responsibility for property and are generally requesting clients to sign a waiver on admission relieving the hospital and its employees of any responsibility for property. There are, however, situations in which the client cannot sign a waiver, and the nursing staff must follow prescribed policies for safeguarding the client's property. In hospital units, dentures are often a major problem; they can be lost in bedding or left on a meal tray. Nurses are expected to take reasonable precautions to safeguard a client's property, and they can be held liable for its *loss or damage* if they do not exercise reasonable care.

Reporting Crimes, Torts, and Unsafe Practices

Nurses may need to report nursing colleagues or other health professionals for practices that endanger the health and safety of clients. For instance, alcohol and drug use, theft from a client or agency, and unsafe nursing practice should be reported. Reporting a colleague is not easy. The person reporting may feel disloyal, incur the disapproval of others, or endanger chances for promotion. When reporting an incident or series of incidents, the nurse must be careful to describe observed behavior only and not make inferences as to what might be happening. The accompanying box outlines guidelines for reporting a crime, tort, or unsafe practice. In cases of substance abuse, states such as California have established voluntary programs that allow nurses to receive help in resolving their problems without losing their licenses to practice.

IMPAIRED NURSES

The high stress of modern nursing practice has contributed to the problem of substance abuse. Professional factors, such as staffing shortages, increased client acuity, frequent shift changes, and the occurrence of more complex ethical problems, combined with the personal demands of family and societal obligations often result in feelings of frustration, anxiety, and depression. Alco-

---

> ### *Guidelines for Reporting a Crime, Tort, or Unsafe Practice*
>
> - Write a clear description of the situation you believe you should report.
> - Make sure that your statements are accurate.
> - Make sure you are credible.
> - Obtain support from at least one trustworthy person before filing the report.
> - Report the matter starting at the lowest possible level in the agency hierarchy.
> - Assume responsibility for reporting the individual by being open about it. Sign your name to the letter.
> - See the problem through once you have reported it.
>
> *Source:* D. M. Price and P. Murphy, How—and when—to blow the whistle on unsafe practices, *Nursing Life,* January/February 1983, 3:50–54.

---

hol is readily available and controlled drugs are easily obtained by the nurse.

The term *impaired nurse* is used to describe the nurse who is attempting to provide nursing care while under the influence of alcohol, drugs, or other chemical substances. Further, such action is interfering with the nurse's ability to carry out safe practice. In 1984 it was estimated that approximately 6–8% of nurses in the United States had a problem with substance abuse (ANA 1984). The majority of nurses involved in disciplinary hearings by State Boards of Nursing in 1985 were practicing nursing under the influence of alcohol or other chemical substances (Sullivan, Bissell, and Williams 1988).

The American Nurses' Association appointed a Task Force on Addiction and Psychological Disturbance in 1981 to develop guidelines for the State Nurses' Associations for the treatment and assistance of nurses whose practice is impaired by alcoholism, drug abuse, or psychologic disturbance. The purpose of these guidelines is 1) to assist the nurse in the recovery process, and 2) to protect the public from unsafe nursing practice.

Behaviors that may indicate impairment include unkempt appearance, excessive absence, excessive errors, inability to meet schedules, decreased ability to concentrate, unclear or sloppy charting, frequent medication errors and erratic arrival and departure times. Changes in behavior or personality or mood swings, slurred speech, and unsteady gait may also indicate substance abuse. Client complaints of little or no relief from pain when under the care of a particular nurse may indicate that the nurse is substituting sterile water or saline for medication, and taking the medication herself.

When a nurse is suspected of substance abuse, it is important to have accurate and complete documentation of the suspicious behaviors or incidents prior to confrontation. Confrontation of the nurse is usually done by the nurse's superior in the presence of a third person, usually a nurse who has observed the suspicious behaviors. Being the "friend" of a chemically impaired nurse obligates the friend to report the abuse and help the friend seek treatment, not to cover up for the friend. Many nurses have friends who were protected who then became totally incapacitated or died or who injured a client because of their unsafe practice.

In many states, the State Board of Nursing has developed intervention programs to assist the recovery of impaired nurses.

SELECTED LEGAL FACETS OF NURSING PRACTICE

Informed Consent

Informed consent is an agreement by a client to accept a course of treatment or a procedure after complete information, including the risks of treatment and facts relating to it, has been provided by the physician. Informed consent, then, is an exchange between a client and a physician. Usually the client signs a form provided by the agency. The form is a record of the informed consent, not the informed consent itself.

Obtaining informed consent is the responsibility of a physician. Although this responsibility is delegated to nurses in some agencies, the practice is highly undesirable. The nurse's responsibility is often to witness the giving of informed consent. This involves the following:

- Witnessing the exchange between the client and the physician
- Witnessing the client's signature
- Establishing that the client really did understand, i.e., was really informed

If a nurse witnesses only the client's signature and not the exchange between the client and the physician, the nurse should write "witnessing signature only" on the form (Northrop 1984, p. 223). If the nurse finds that the client really does not understand the physician's explanation, then it is important that the physician be notified.

Northrop (1984, p. 223) describes three major elements of informed consent:

1. The consent must be given voluntarily.
2. The consent must be given by an individual with the capacity and competence to understand.
3. The client must be given enough information to be the ultimate decision maker.

To give informed consent voluntarily, the client must not feel coerced. Sometimes fear of disapproval by a health professional can be the motivation for giving consent; such consent is not voluntarily given.

To give informed consent, the client must receive sufficient information to make a decision; otherwise, the client's right to decide has been usurped. Information needs to include benefits, risks, and alternative procedures. It is also important that the client understand. Technical words and language barriers can inhibit understanding. If a client cannot read, the consent form must be read to the client before it is signed. If the client does not speak the same language as the health professional who is providing the information, an interpreter must be acquired.

If given sufficient information, the client can make decisions regarding health. To do so, the client must be competent and an adult. A competent adult is a person over 18 years of age who is conscious and oriented. A person under 18 years who is considered "an emancipated minor," i.e., self-supporting or married, can also give consent. A client who is confused, disoriented, or sedated is not considered functionally competent at that time.

There are three groups of people who cannot provide consent. The *first* is minors. In most areas, consent must be given by a parent or guardian before minors can obtain treatment. The same is true of an adult who has the mental capacity of a child if a guardian has been appointed. In some states, however, minors are allowed to give consent for such procedures as blood donations, treatment for drug dependency and sexually transmitted disease, and procedures for obstetric care. The *second* group is persons who are unconscious or injured in such a way that they are unable to give consent. In these situations, consent is usually obtained from the closest adult relative if existing statutes permit. In an emergency, if consent cannot be obtained from the client or a relative, then the law generally agrees that consent is assumed. The *third* group is mentally ill persons who have been judged to be incompetent. State and provincial mental health acts or similar statutes generally provide definitions of mental illness and specify the rights of the mentally ill under the law as well as the rights of the staff caring for such clients.

Recordkeeping

The client's medical record is a legal document and can be produced in court as evidence. Often the record is used to remind a witness of events surrounding a lawsuit, since it usually takes several months or years for the suit to go to trial. The effectiveness of a witness's testimony can depend on the accuracy of such records. Nurses, therefore, need to keep accurate and complete records of nursing care provided to clients. Failure to keep proper records can constitute negligence and be the basis for tort liability. Insufficient or inaccurate assessments and documentation can hinder proper diagnosis and treatment and result in injury to the client.

Controlled Substances

United States and Canadian laws regulate the distribution and use of controlled substances such as narcotics, depressants, stimulants, and hallucinogens. Misuse of controlled substances leads to criminal penalties. Controlled substances are kept in securely locked drawers or cupboards, and only authorized personnel have access to them.

The Incident Report

An incident report is an agency record of an accident or incident. This report is used to make all the facts about an accident available to agency personnel, to contribute to statistical data about accidents or incidents, and to help health personnel prevent future accidents. All accidents are usually reported on incident forms. Some agencies also report other incidents, e.g., the occurrence of client infection or the loss of personal effects. The box above lists the information to be included in an incident report. The report should be completed as soon as possible, always within 24 hours of the incident.

Incident reports are often viewed by an agency committee, which decides whether to investigate the incident further. The nurse may be required upon further investigation to answer such questions as: Why do you believe the accident occurred? How could it have been prevented? Should any equipment be adjusted? Nurses who believe they may be dismissed or that suit may be

Information to Include in an Incident Report

- Identify the client by name, initials, and hospital or identification number.

- Give the date, time, and place of the incident.

- Describe the facts of the incident. Avoid any conclusions or blame. Describe the incident as you saw it even if your impressions differ from those of others.

- Identify all witnesses to the incident.

- Identify any equipment by number and any medication by name and number.

- Document any circumstance surrounding the incident, e.g., another client (Mrs. Losas) was experiencing cardiac arrest.

brought should obtain legal advice. Even if the agency clears the nurse of responsibility, the client or the client's family may file suit. The plaintiff, however, bears the burden of proof that the accident occurred because reasonable care was not taken. Even if the accepted standard of care was not given, the plaintiff must prove that the accident was the direct result of unacceptable standards of care and that the accident caused physical, emotional, or financial injury.

When an accident occurs, the nurse should first assess the client and intervene to prevent injury. If a client is injured, nurses must take steps to protect the client, themselves, and their employer. Most agencies have policies regarding accidents. It is important to follow these policies and not to assume one is negligent. Although this may be the case, accidents do happen even when every precaution has been taken to prevent them.

Wills

A *will* is a declaration by a person about how the person's property is to be disposed of after death. In order for a will to be valid the following conditions must be met:

- The person making the will must be of sound mind, that is, able to understand and retain mentally the general nature and extent of the person's property, the relationship of the beneficiaries and of relatives to whom the estate will be left, and the disposition being made of the property. A person, therefore, who is se-

When Do Incidents Occur in a Health Care Facility?

A study of all incident reports in five special-care homes of various resident capacities in Saskatchewan revealed that (a) the incidents per client day increased inversely with the size of the facility, (b) all facilities reported fewer incidents on the 2300 to 0700 hour shift, (c) in two facilities the evening shift had more incidents than the day shift, (d) in one facility there were more incidents during the day shift than the evening shift, and (e) falls accounted for the largest percentage of incidents.

Implications: In practice, nurses can help prevent accidents to clients by being alert to when and why accidents are likely to occur.

Source: V. Wasiatu, Reporting incidents: How many is too many? *Dimensions in Health Service,* September 1982, 59:16–18.

riously ill and unable to carry out usual roles may be still able to direct preparation of a will.

- The person must not be unduly influenced by anyone else. Sometimes a client may be persuaded by someone who is close at that particular time to make that person a beneficiary. Clients sometimes are persuaded to leave their estates to persons looking after them rather than to their relatives. Frequently, the relatives contest the will in such situations and take the matter to court, claiming undue influence.

Nurses may be requested from time to time to witness a will, although most agencies have policies that nurses not do so. In most states and provinces, a will must be signed in the presence of two witnesses. In some situations, a mark can suffice if the person making the will cannot write a signature. If a nurse is a witness to a will, the nurse should note on the client's chart the fact that a will was made and the nurse's perception of the physical and mental condition of the client. This record provides the nurse with accurate information if the nurse is called as a witness later. The record may also be helpful if the will is contested. If a nurse does not wish to act as a witness—for example, if in the nurse's opinion undue influence has been brought on the client—then it is the nurse's right to refuse to act in this capacity.

Do Not Resuscitate Orders

Physicians may order "no code" or "slow code" for clients who are in a stage of terminal, irreversible illness or expected death. No-code orders may also be written as *"no heroics"* or *DNR* (do not resuscitate or do not make resuscitative efforts). Slow-code orders are frequently unwritten orders and are conveyed in an informal manner (i.e., the physician issuing the order does *not* want it to be written as a verbal or telephone order) and are *not* legally acceptable. The legality of no-code and slow-code orders is not well established in most settings. New York state has a law that permits adults and minors (through a parent or guardian) to consent to a DNR order. It applies only to CPR, not to the withholding or withdrawing of other medical treatment. The statute also permits a competent adult to designate a surrogate to direct that CPR be withheld if the individual becomes incompetent (Bellocq 1988, p. 313).

The American Heart Association (AHA) has issued "Standards and Guidelines for Cardiopulmonary Resuscitation and Emergency Cardiac Care" outlining the medicolegal considerations and offering recommendations about DNR orders for physicians (AHA 1986, p. 2880). Although these standards, like those of any professional organization, are not legally binding, they are persuasive to a judge and jury. They indicate that CPR is intended to prevent *unexpected* death and that its intent is not to continue life when death is *expected.* The implications of the AHA no-code standards mean that the nurse must:

- Ensure that the DNR order is written on the client's order sheet and progress notes. Verbal orders can be easily misunderstood and disclaimed.

- If the physician refuses to write such an order, follow agency policies and procedures. Some agencies have established formal protocols for nurses to follow. Because such procedures are usually carefully reviewed by legal counsel, they can minimize the risk of legal liability substantially.

- If the agency does not have a well-established procedure, seek a legal opinion through the agency attorney or state or provincial nursing association.

- If none of the above steps provides the nurse with sufficient guidelines, the nurse must make a personal decision based on moral values and sense of humanity. Even when there are appropriate guidelines, the guidelines may conflict with the nurse's personal ethics. Thus, DNR orders may create an ethical dilemma as well as a legal dilemma for the nurse.

Death and Related Issues

Legal issues surrounding death include the death certificate, labeling of the deceased, autopsy, organ donation, and inquest. By law, a death certificate must be made out when a person dies.

Nurses have a duty to handle the deceased with dignity and label the corpse appropriately. Mishandling can cause emotional distress to survivors. Mislabeling can create legal problems if the body is inappropriately identified and prepared incorrectly for burial or a funeral.

An *autopsy* or *postmortem examination* is performed only in certain cases. The law describes under what circumstances an autopsy must be performed, e.g., when death is sudden or when it occurs within 48 hours of admission to a hospital. The organs and tissues of the body are examined to establish the exact cause of death, to learn more about a disease, and to assist in the accumulation of statistical data.

It is the responsibility of the physician or, in some instances, of a designated person in the hospital to obtain consent for autopsy. Consent must be given by the decedent (before death) or by the next of kin. Laws in many states and provinces prioritize the family members who can provide consent as follows: surviving spouse, adult children, parents, siblings. After autopsy, hospitals cannot retain any tissues or organs without the permission of the person who consented to the autopsy.

Organ Donation Under the Uniform Anatomical Gift Act in the United States or the Human Tissue Act in Canada, any person 18 years or older and of sound mind may make a gift of all or any part of the body for the following purposes: for medical or dental education, research, advancement of medical or dental science, therapy, or transplantation (Annas et al. 1981, p. 227). The donation can be made by a provision in a will or by signing a cardlike form in the presence of two witnesses. This card is usually carried at all times by the person who signed it. In most states and provinces, the gift can be revoked either by destroying the card or by an oral revocation in the presence of two witnesses. Nurses may serve as witnesses for persons consenting to donate organs. In some states (e.g., California) health care workers are required to ask survivors for consent to donate the deceased's organs.

Inquest An *inquest* is a legal inquiry into the cause or manner of a death. When a death is the result of an accident, for example, an inquest is held into the circumstances of the accident to determine any blame. The inquest is conducted under the jurisdiction of a coroner or medical examiner. A *coroner* is a public official, not necessarily a physician, appointed or elected to inquire into the causes of death, when appropriate. A *medical examiner* is a physician who usually has advanced education in pathology or forensic medicine. Agency policy dictates who is responsible for reporting deaths to the coroner or medical examiner.

LEGAL PROTECTIONS FOR NURSES

Good Samaritan Acts

Good Samaritan acts are laws designed to protect health care providers who provide assistance at the scene of an emergency against claims of malpractice unless it can be shown that there was a gross departure from the normal standard of care or willful wrongdoing on their part. Gross negligence usually involves further injury or harm to the person.

In the United States, most state statutes do not require citizens to render aid to people in distress. Such assistance is considered more of an *ethical* than a *legal* duty. A few states, however, have enacted legislation that requires people educated in health care to stop and aid the injured. To encourage citizens to be good Samaritans, most states have now enacted legislation releasing the good Samaritan from legal liability for injuries caused under such circumstances.

In Canada, some provinces specify in traffic acts that it is the responsibility of people to give aid at the scene of an accident. Alberta is the only province that exempts physicians and nurses from liability unless gross negligence is proved. However, lawsuits against good Samaritans are rarely successful.

It is generally believed that a person who renders help in an emergency, at the level of helping that would be provided by any reasonably prudent person under similar circumstances, cannot be held liable. The same reasoning applies to nurses, who may be the people best prepared to help at the scene of an accident. If the level of care a nurse provides is of the caliber that would have been provided by any other nurse, then the nurse will not be held liable.

Professional Liability Insurance

Because of the increase in the number of malpractice lawsuits against health professionals, nurses are advised in many areas to carry their own liability insurance. Most hospitals have liability insurance that covers all employees, including all nurses. However, some smaller facilities, such as "walk-in" clinics, may not. Thus the nurse should always check with the employer at the time of hiring to see what coverage the facility provides. A physician or a hospital can be sued because of the negligent conduct of a nurse, and the nurse can also be sued and held liable for negligence or malpractice. Because hospitals have been known to countersue nurses when they have been found negligent and the hospital was required to pay, nurses are advised to provide their own insurance coverage and not rely on hospital-provided insurance.

Liability insurance coverage usually defrays all costs of defending a nurse, including the costs of retaining an attorney. The insurance also covers all costs incurred by the nurse up to the face value of the policy, including a settlement made out of court. In return, the insurance company may have the right to make the decisions about the claim and the settlement.

Nursing faculty and nursing students are also vulnerable to lawsuits. In hospital nursing education programs, instructors and students are often specifically covered for liability by the hospital. An instructor, however, can still be sued by a hospital in cases of negligence and malpractice.

Students and teachers of nursing employed by community colleges and universities are less likely to be covered by the insurance carried by hospitals and health agencies. It is advisable for these people to check with their school about the coverage that applies to them. Increasingly, instructors are carrying their own malpractice insurance in both the United States and Canada. In the United States, insurance can be obtained through the ANA or private insurance companies; in Canada, it can usually be obtained through provincial nurses' associations. Registered nurse students may be required by their school to carry personal liability insurance during clinical courses. It is advised to check the school policy regarding insurance coverage.

LEGAL RESPONSIBILITIES IN NURSING PRACTICE

Carrying Out Physician's Orders

Nurses are expected to know basic information about procedures and medications ordered by the physician. It is the nurse's responsibility to seek clarification of am-biguous or seemingly erroneous orders from the prescribing physician. Clarification from any other source is unacceptable and regarded as a departure from competent nursing practice.

If the order is neither ambiguous nor apparently erroneous, the nurse is responsible for carrying it out. For example, if the physician orders oxygen to be administered at 4 liters per minute, the nurse must administer oxygen at that rate, and not at 2 or 6 liters per minute. If the orders state that the client is not to have solid food after a bowel resection, the nurse must ensure that no solid food is given to the client. Nurses also have a responsibility to check for changes in orders from previous shifts of duty.

Becker (1983, pp. 21–23) outlines four orders that nurses must question to protect themselves legally:

1. Question any order a client questions. For example, if a client who has been receiving an intramuscular injection tells the nurse that the doctor changed the order from an injectable to an oral medication, the nurse should recheck the order before giving the medication.

2. Question any order if the client's condition has changed. The nurse is considered responsible for notifying the physician of any significant changes in the client's condition, whether the physician requests notification or not. For example, if a client who is receiving an intravenous infusion suddenly develops a rapid pulse, chest pain, and a cough, the nurse must notify the physician immediately and question continuance of the ordered rate of infusion. If a client who is receiving morphine for pain develops severely depressed respirations, the nurse must withhold the medication and notify the physician.

3. Question and record verbal orders to avoid miscommunications. In addition to recording the time, the date, the physician's name, and the orders, the nurse documents the circumstances that occasioned the call to the physician, reads the orders back to the physician, and documents that the physician confirmed the orders as the nurse read them back.

4. Question standing orders, especially if the nurse is inexperienced. *Standing orders* give the nurse added responsibility to exercise appropriate judgment when implementing them. The nurse is delegated the authority to, for example, adjust the amount of a medication or other substances and make decisions about when a medication is needed. Nurses need to take the same precautions when implementing these orders as when implementing any other orders. In

addition, the nurse who does not feel confident about exercising discretionary judgment should request specific guidelines from the physician or assistance from a more experienced nurse. In some states, standing orders are not allowed except in intensive care or coronary care units.

Implementing Delegated and Independent Nursing Interventions

Nurses implementing care need to take the following precautions (Grane 1983, pp. 17–20; Rhodes and Miller 1984, pp. 153–60):

- Know their job description. This enables nurses to function within the scope of the description and know what is and what is not expected. Job descriptions vary from agency to agency.

- Follow the policies and procedures of the agency in which they are working.

- Always identify clients, particularly before initiating major interventions, e.g., surgical or other invasive procedures, or when administering blood transfusions.

- Make sure the correct medications are given in the correct dose, by the right route, at the scheduled time, and to the right client.

- Perform procedures appropriately. Negligent incidents during procedures generally relate to equipment failure, improper technique, and improper performance of the procedure. For instance, the nurse must know how to safeguard the client in the event that a respirator or other equipment fails.

- Promptly and accurately document all assessments and care given. Records must show that the nurse provided and supervised the client's care daily.

- Report all incidents involving clients. Prompt reports enable those responsible to attend to the client's well-being, to analyze why the incident occurred, and to prevent recurrences.

- Build and maintain good rapport with clients. Keeping clients informed about diagnostic and treatment plans, giving feedback on their progress, and showing concern for the outcome of their care prevent a sense of powerlessness and a build-up of hostility in the client.

- Maintain clinical competence in their area of practice. This means continued study, including maintaining and updating clinical knowledge and skills.

CLINICAL GUIDELINES
Legal Precautions for Nurses

- Function within the scope of your education, job description, and area nurse practice act.
- Follow the procedures and policies of the employing agency.
- Observe and monitor the client accurately.
- Communicate and record significant changes in the client's condition to the physician.
- Check any orders that a client questions.
- Identify clients before initiating any interventions.
- Protect clients from falls and preventable injuries.
- Document all nursing assessments and interventions accurately.
- Ask for assistance and supervision in situations for which you feel inadequately prepared.
- Delegate tasks to persons with the knowledge and skill to carry them out.
- Build and maintain good rapport with clients.

- Know their own strengths and weaknesses. For example, nurses who recognize that they have difficulty calculating medication dosages should always ask someone to check the calculations before proceeding.

- When delegating nursing responsibilities, make sure that the person who is delegated a task understands what to do and that the person has the required knowledge and skill. The delegating nurse can be held liable for harm caused by the person to whom the care was delegated.

- Be alert when implementing nursing interventions and give each task their full attention and skill.

Ways nurses can protect themselves legally are summarized in the accompanying Clinical Guidelines box.

LEGAL RESPONSIBILITIES OF STUDENTS

Nursing students are responsible for their own actions and liable for their own acts of negligence committed during the course of clinical experiences. When they perform duties that are within the scope of professional nursing, such as administering an injection, they are legally held to the same standard of skill and competence as a registered professional nurse (Creighton 1986, p. 128). Lower standards are *not* applied to the actions of nursing students.

In cases arising from negligent acts by nursing students, the student has traditionally been treated as an employee of the hospital, which was held liable under the doctrine of *respondeat superior*. Today, associate degree and baccalaureate nursing students are not usually considered employees of the agencies in which they receive clinical experience, since these nursing programs contract with agencies to provide clinical experiences for students. Today's students are more likely considered employees of the college or university and that institution is potentially liable for negligent actions by its students.

Students in clinical situations must be assigned activity within their capabilities and be given reasonable guidance and supervision. Nursing instructors are responsible for assigning students to the care of clients and for providing reasonable supervision. Failure to provide reasonable supervison and/or the assignment of a client to a student who is not prepared and competent can be a basis for liability.

Students who work as part-time or temporary nursing assistants or aides must also remember that *legally* they can perform only those tasks that appear in the job description of a nurse's aide or assistant. Even though a student may have received instruction and acquired competence in more advanced practices, such as administering injections or suctioning a tracheostomy tube, the student should not be asked to perform these tasks while employed as an aide or assistant.

CHAPTER HIGHLIGHTS

▶ Accountability is an essential concept of professional nursing practice under the law.

▶ Nurses need to understand laws that regulate and affect nursing practice to ensure that the nurses' actions are consistent with current legal principles and to protect the nurse from liability.

▶ Nurse practice acts legally define and describe the scope of nursing practice that the law seeks to regulate.

▶ Competence in nursing practice is determined and maintained by various credentialing methods, such as licensure, registration, certification, and accreditation, which protect the public's welfare and safety.

▶ Standards of practice published by national and state or provincial nursing associations and agency policies, procedures, and job descriptions further delineate the scope of a nurse's practice.

▶ The nurse has specific legal obligations and responsibilities to clients and employers. As a citizen, the nurse has the rights and responsibilities shared by all individuals in the society.

▶ Collective bargaining is one way nurses can improve their working conditions and economic welfare.

▶ Nurses can be held liable for intentional torts, such as fraud, invasion of privacy, defamation, assault and battery, and false imprisonment; and for unintentional torts, or negligence.

▶ Negligence or malpractice of nurses can be established when (a) the nurse (defendant) owed a duty to the client, (b) the nurse failed to carry out that duty, (c) the client (plaintiff) was injured, and (d) the client's injury was caused by the nurse's failure to carry out that duty.

▶ The problem of chemical dependency in nursing has occurred in response to the professional and personal stresses on today's nurse. State nursing organizations have developed intervention programs for the chemically impaired nurse.

▶ The nurse is responsible for ensuring that the physician obtains informed consents from clients (or from the closest relative in emergencies or from parents or guardians when the client is a minor) before treatment regimens and procedures begin.

▶ Informed consent implies that (a) the consent was given voluntarily; (b) the client was of age and had the capacity and competence to understand; and (c) the ▶

CHAPTER HIGHLIGHTS *(continued)*

client was given enough information on which to make an informed decision.

▶ When a client is accidentally injured or involved in an unusual situation, the nurse's first responsibility is to take steps to protect the client and then to notify appropriate agency personnel.

▶ The legality of no-code and slow-code orders is not well established; nurses are advised to follow the state law for no-code orders.

▶ Nurses must be knowledgeable about their responsibilities in regard to legal issues surrounding death: death certificate, labeling of the deceased, autopsy, organ donation, and inquest.

▶ Good Samaritan acts protect health professionals from claims of malpractice when they offer assistance at the scene of an emergency, provided there is no willful wrongdoing or gross departure from normal standards of care.

▶ Practicing nurses who are not covered by liability insurance in their employing agency can obtain liability insurance through professional nursing associations.

▶ Nursing students need to make sure they are prepared to provide the necessary care to assigned clients and to ask for help or supervision in situations for which they feel inadequately prepared.

LEARNING ACTIVITIES

■ Attend a medical legal action trial in a court of law. Observe the roles of the different actors in the trial (defendant, plaintiff, attorneys, jury, and judge). Especially observe the nurse witnesses: Were they articulate? Did they present a professional image?

   Would you find for the plaintiff or the defendant? Why?

■ Review the nurse practice act of your state or province. What is the legal definition of nursing practice? Is the nursing process defined? How does the nurse practice act impact on nursing eduction, nursing administration, and nursing practice? What penalties are provided for failure to comply with the nurse practice act? Does the nurse practice act address the impaired nurse? Does the nurse practice act establish a Board of Nursing? What is the composition of the Board of Nursing? What is its purpose?

■ Attend a State Board of Nursing Disciplinary Hearing (if permitted). In most states these are open hearings. Observe the nature of the disciplinary actions. What are the penalties imposed? How might nurses assist each other to assure safe nursing practice and decrease job-related stress?

READINGS AND REFERENCES

SUGGESTED READINGS

Arbeiter, J. S. October 1988. Are you merely a witness to the patient's consent? *RN* 51:53–57.

   Arbeiter writes about the approaches of two panelists to the issue of informed consent. According to one panelist, about 99% of the responsibility for obtaining informed consent is the physician's. The issue of when a client is not fully informed is discussed. A questionnaire regarding witnessing a consent is also described. The alternatives open to a nurse who refuses to witness an informed consent are also described.

Rabinow, J. February 1989. Where you stand in the eyes of the law. *Nursing 89* 19:34–42.

   Rabinow explains that there may be 2000 nurses sued by 1989. She describes a number of nursing and legal trends, such as expanding nursing responsibilities and their legal implications. The legal process is diagrammed in the article, and incident reports are discussed.

RELATED RESEARCH

Wasiuta, V. September 1982. Reporting incidents: How many is too many? *Dimensions in Health Service* 59:16–18.

SELECTED REFERENCES

American Heart Association. June 6, 1986. Standards and guidelines for cardiopulmonary resuscitation and emergency cardiac care. *Journal of the American Medical Association*. 255:2841–3044.

American Nurses Association. July 1973. ANA issues statement on diploma graduates. *American Journal of Nursing* 73:1135.

———. 1976. *The code for nurses*. Kansas City, Mo.: ANA.

———. April 1979. Credentialing in nursing. A new approach. Report of the Committee for the study of Credentialing in Nursing. *American Journal of Nursing* 79:674–83.

———. 1981. The nursing practice act: Suggested state legislation. Kansas City, Mo.: ANA.

———. 1985. *The grievance procedure*. Kansas City, Mo.: ANA.

———. 1984. *Addictions and psychological dysfunctions in nursing: The profession's response to the problem*. Kansas City, Mo.: ANA Publications.

Annas, G. J.; Glantz, L. H.; and Katz, B. F. 1981. *The right of doctors, nurses and allied health professionals*. New York: Avon Books.

Barbash, J. 1980. Collective bargaining: Contemporary American experience—A commentary. In Sommers, G. H., editor. *Collective bargaining: Contemporary American experience*. Madison, Wis.: Industrial Relations Research Association.

Becker, M. January/February 1983. Five orders you must question to protect yourself legally. *Nursing Life* 3:21–23.

Bellocq, J. A. September/October 1988. Legal and ethical issues: Changing attitudes about death. *Journal of Professional Nursing* 4:313.

Brill, J. M. April 1990. Informed consent may entail risk. *American Nurse* 22:42.

Crawford, M.; Fisher, M.; and Kilbane, N. 1985. Collective bargaining in nursing. In DeYoung, L. *Dynamics of nursing*. 5th ed. St. Louis: C. V. Mosby Co.

Creighton, H. November 1985. Law for the nurse manager. Relatives sue for putting patient on life support. *Nursing Management* 16:56, 60.

Ecklund, V. Winter 1986. Is there a chemically dependent nurse on your staff? *Professional Nurses Quarterly* 1:22.

Ellis, J. F., and Hartley, C. L. 1988. *Nursing in today's world: Challenges, issues, and trends*. 3d ed. Philadelphia: J. B. Lippincott Co.

Fenner, K. 1980. *Ethics and the law in nursing*. New York: D. Van Nostrand Co.

Gaskin, J. April 1986. Nurses in trouble. *Canadian Nurse* 82:31–34.

Grane, N. B. January/February 1983. How to reduce your risk of a lawsuit. *Nursing Life* 3:17–20.

Green, P. 1989. The chemically dependent nurse. In *Nursing Clinics of North America*. Vol. 24, No. 1: 81–94.

Jefferson, L. V. and Ensor, B. E. April 1982. Confronting a chemically impaired colleague. *American Journal of Nursing* 82:574–576.

Lachman, V. D. April 1986. Why we must take care of our own—drug and alcohol abusers in our own profession. *Nursing* 86:44.

McClelland, J. Q. November 1983. Professionalism and collective bargaining: A new reality for nurses and management. *Journal of Nursing Administration* 13:36–38.

Moylan, L. B. June 1988. Implications of the National Labor Relations Act. *Nursing Management* 19:80.

Northrop, C. 1988. Legal aspects of nursing. In McCann Flynn, J. B., and Heffron, P. B. *Nursing: From concept to practice*. 2d ed. East Norwalk, Conn: Appleton & Lange.

Pettengill, M. M. September/October 1985. Multilateral collective bargaining and the health care industry: Implications for nursing. *Journal of Professional Nursing* 1:275–82.

Price, D. M., and Murphy, P. January/February 1983. How—and when—to blow the whistle on unsafe practices. *Nursing Life* 3:50–54.

Rhodes, A. M., and Miller, R. D. 1984. *Nursing and the Law*. 4th ed. Rockville, Md.: Aspen Systems Corporation.

Smith, G. R. July/August 1985. Unionization for nurses: An issue for the 1980's. *Journal of Professional Nursing* 1:192–201.

Snyder, M. E., and LaBar, C. 1984. *Issues in professional nursing practice 1. Nursing: Legal authority for practice*. Kansas City, Mo.: American Nurses' Association.

Snyder, R., Westerfield, J. June 1990. Should nurses pronounce death? *Nursing 90* 20:41.

Sullivan, E., Bissell, L., and Williams, E. 1988. *Chemical dependence in nursing*. Menlo Park, Calif.: Addison-Wesley Publishing Co.

———. 1982. New ANA Task Force will seek answers for impaired R.N.'s. *American Journal of Nursing* 82:242.

U.S. Department of Labor, 1979. Impact of the 1974 Health Care Amendments to the NLRA on collective bargaining in the health care industry. Washington, D.C.: U.S. GPO.

Ethical Dimensions of Nursing

CONTENTS

VALUES, BELIEFS, ATTITUDES, AND ETHICS DEFINED

Nurses are becoming increasingly aware of the values, beliefs, and attitudes of clients and their support persons and of the ethics involved in nursing practice. Values, beliefs, and attitudes differ from one another but are often interconnected.

A *value* can be defined as something of worth, a belief held dear by a person. A value is an affective disposition toward a person, object, or idea (Steele and Harmon 1983, p. 1). According to Simon et al. (1978), "values are a set of personal beliefs and attitudes about the truth, beauty, worth of any thought, object, or behavior. They are action oriented and give direction and meaning to one's life." Values develop from associations with people, the environment and self; they are derived from life experiences (Steele and Harmon 1983, p. 1). Values form a basis for behavior; a person's real values are shown by consistent patterns of behavior. Once one is aware of one's values, the values become an internal control for behavior. "Values are significant in choice making" (Salladay and McDonnell 1989, p. 544).

Values common to many people are peace, truth, and freedom. Values exist in some relationship to one another within a person. A *value system* is the organization of a person's values along a continuum of relative importance. Values underlie people's purposive behavior.

Purposive behavior refers to actions that are performed "on purpose" with the intention of reaching some goal or bringing about a certain result (Muldary 1983, p. 200). Purposive behavior, then, is based on a person's decisions or choices, and these decisions or choices are based on underlying values.

There are two types of values: intrinsic and extrinsic. An *intrinsic value* relates to the maintenance of life, e.g., food and water have intrinsic value. An *extrinsic value* originates outside the individual and is not necessary for the maintenance of life, e.g., health, holism, and humanism (Steele and Harmon 1983, p. 2).

Values can be either positive or negative. A positive value is a view of what is desirable or how something *should be*. For example, some nurses value a holistic approach to nursing. Negative values, by contrast, are views of what is undesirable or how something *should not be*. For example, talking unkindly about clients is considered by many nurses to be undesirable. Therefore, being unkind is a negative value.

A *belief* (opinion) is something accepted as true by a judgment of probability rather than actuality. It is a special type of attitude whose cognitive (intellectual) component is based more on faith than on fact. People hold beliefs that may be true or that can, with reliable evidence, be proved true. Family traditions and folklore are beliefs passed from one generation to another.

Beliefs may or may not involve values. For example, a client may believe that all nurses are honest. The client has accepted that a relationship exists between "nurse" and "honesty," nurse being the object and honesty the value. The client considers this relationship self-evident. A belief of this type is sometimes called a value judgment.

An *attitude* is a feeling tone directed toward a person, object, or idea. Attitudes have behavioral, cognitive, and affective components. The behavioral component of an attitude is exemplified by the tendency of the person to take action. It reflects the inclination of the individual to act as a result of his or her attitude. For example, a nurse who dislikes a peer's behavior toward a client is inclined to think, "If she speaks that way to Mr. B again, I am going to. . . ." This is the inclination to act, a part of one's attitude toward the peer. The cognitive component of an attitude includes the beliefs and factual information associated with the attitude, e.g., nursing is a high-stress occupation. The affective component may be the central component of an attitude. It is the feelings that are associated with the belief, knowledge, and the target of the attitude. Feelings vary greatly among people; for example, one client may feel very strongly about the sound from a television in the next room, whereas another cli-

ent dismisses it as unimportant. The affective component of one's attitudes is usually rooted in a person's values (Muldary 1983, p. 210).

Attitudes are made up of many beliefs (Steele and Harmon 1983, p. 3). For example, a child may learn such attitudes as cooperation and kindness from parents and in turn exhibit these in behavior. According to values clarification theory, a belief or attitude can become a value only if the belief satisfies seven criteria. See the section on values later in this chapter.

Ethics are the rules or principles that govern right conduct. The word *ethics* is derived from the Greek *ethos,* meaning custom or character. An ethic is "what ought to be." The term *bioethics* is being used increasingly in the health field. *Bioethics* is the ethics concerning life.

In nursing, ethical practice refers to a nurse's moral behavior and decisions regarding ethical dilemmas (Ketefian 1989, p. 509). The nurse must first understand the development of the individual's morality in order to understand how the acquisition of values, beliefs, and attitudes impact on the ethical behavior of both the individual and the society in which the individual resides.

MORAL THEORIES

Moral development, a complex process not fully understood, involves learning what ought to be and what ought not to be done. It is more than imprinting parents' rules and virtues or values upon children. The term *moral* means relating to right and wrong. Distinctions need to be made between the terms morality, moral behavior, and moral development. *Morality* refers to the requirements necessary for people to live together in society; *moral behavior* is the way a person perceives those requirements and responds to them; *moral development* is the pattern of change in moral behavior with age (White 1975). See Table 11–1 for a summary of moral development.

Freud

Freud (1961) believes that the mechanism for right and wrong within the individual is the superego, or conscience. He hypothesizes that a child internalizes and adopts the moral standards and character or character traits of the model parent through the process of identification during resolution of the Oedipus complex. To Freud, children acquire morals unconsciously from parental standards, specifically from the model parent with whom the child identifies. Freud believes moral behav-

TABLE 11-1 *Summary of Moral Development*

Developmental Stage	Moral Development	Examples of Values Developed
Infant (0 to 1 years)	The infant is generally considered not to have values but perceives emotions and the behavior of others. A mother's or caregiver's behavior toward the infant can reflect her or his values.	Parents who communicate love to their infants and convey pleasure in the infant's pleasure teach the infant the values of love and caring.
Toddler (1 to 3 years)	The toddler learns values largely through copying others; i.e., through modeling. Toddlers don't understand the meaning behind a value.	By showing appreciation and saying thank you when others give gifts and when the toddler starts to give the parents toys, objects, or food, parents teach toddlers that "giving" makes others feel good and, in turn, makes one feel good about oneself.
Preschooler (4 to 5 years)	The preschooler learns the right and wrong of singular acts but does not possess a concept of right and wrong.	By pointing out to her son that taking a toy away from a sister or friend is wrong and makes the other person feel as badly as he would if the same happened to him, a mother teaches the child to consider other person's feelings and to treat everyone as you want to be treated.
School-aged child (6 to 12 years)	People with diverse values have contact with school-aged children. Parents who provide alternatives in situations help the school-aged child solve problems, make decisions, and learn the value of self-determination.	Parents who help and encourage a child with a school project teach the child the value of industry and completing projects once started.
Adolescent (12 to 18 years)	Adolescents encounter a multitude of new values. Adolescents learn to identify some of their own significant values. Parents continue to be a major source of values.	Parents who recognize that adolescents and other people have the right to their own tastes and preferences convey to the adolescent the value of respect for others.
Early adulthood	Most young adults can identify many of their own values. Although these may be tested through experience, the young adult establishes these as part of self. Some values may differ from those of the parents.	By moving away from home and through widening experiences, a young adult develops values associated with health, e.g., becomes a vegetarian and exercises daily.
Middle adulthood	Middle-aged adults who are secure and satisfied with their values will experience pleasure and a sense of serenity with each day. People who are dissatisfied and insecure may discard held values.	A man who values youth and helping others spends much of his time with scouts.
Late adulthood	Older adults may see their values challenged in a changing society. Older adults often learn to appreciate differing values of others but at the same time keep their own values.	A woman accepts that her grandson is living with his girlfriend, although she feels that people of the opposite sex should marry before doing so.

ior results from the strength of the superego, which strives to be "supermoral," in conflict with the ego, which strives to be "moral," and the id, which is totally "nonmoral." The strength of the superego depends on the intensity of the child's feelings of aggression and attachment toward the model parent rather than on the actual standards of the parent.

As a psychoanalyst, Freud focuses on human failings, including moral failure and failure to mature. He notes that some people fixate at a certain level and develop a

TABLE 11-2 *Freud's Five Stages of Development*

Stage	Age	Characteristics	Implications
Oral	0 to 1 year	Mouth is the center of pleasure.	Feeding produces pleasure and sense of comfort and safety. Feeding should be pleasurable and provided when required.
Anal	2 and 3 years	Anus and rectum are the centers of pleasure.	Controlling and expelling feces provide pleasure and sense of control. Toilet training should be a pleasurable experience, and appropriate praise can result in a personality that is creative and productive.
Phallic	4 and 5 years	The child's genitals are the center of pleasure.	The child identifies with the parent of the opposite sex and later takes on a love relationship outside the family. Encourage identification.
Latency	6 to 12 years	Energy is directed to physical and intellectual activities.	Encourage child with physical and intellectual pursuits.
Genital	13 years and after	Energy is directed toward attaining a mature heterosexual relationship.	Encourage separation from parents, achievement of independence, and making decisions.

Source: Adapted from Patricia H. Miller, *Theories of developmental psychology.* Copyright © 1983 W. H. Freeman and Company. Used by permission.

fixated character. His theory implies that moral development is completed in childhood and focuses on an emotional component. See Table 11–2. Because, in Freud's view, morals develop unconsciously, there is no rational conscious component in moral development. Through feelings of love or affection for the mother or father and identification with that parent's character traits, the child develops feelings of guilt, self-respect, praise, or blame.

Erikson

Erikson's theory of the development of virtues or unifying strengths of the "good man" suggests that moral development continues throughout life. Erikson (1964) believes that if the conflicts of each psychosocial developmental stage are favorably resolved, then an "ego-strength" or virtue emerges. See Table 11–3. This theory of virtues or moral development focuses on goals that can be achieved at various stages of life. It implies that fidelity, love, care, and wisdom are adult phenomena only.

Kohlberg

Kohlberg suggests three levels of moral development that encompass six stages (Berkowitz and Oser 1985, p. 28). He focuses on the reasons for the making of a

decision, not on the morality of the decision itself. At Kohlberg's first level, called the *premoral* or *preconventional level,* children are responsive to cultural rules and labels of good and bad, right and wrong. However, children interpret these in terms of the physical consequences of their actions, i.e., punishment or reward. At the second level, the *conventional level,* the individual is concerned about maintaining the expectations of the family, group, or nation and sees this as right. The emphasis at this level is conformity and loyalty to one's own expectations as well as society's. Level three is called the *postconventional, autonomous,* or *principled level.* At this level, people make an effort to define valid values and principles without regard to outside authority or to the expectations of others. For additional information about Kohlberg's levels, see Table 11–4 on page 186.

With reference to Kohlberg's six stages, Munhall writes that stage four, the "law and order" orientation, is the dominant stage of most adults (Munhall 1982, p. 14). It is recognized that there is a difference in action between nurses who act at the conventional level (level II) and those who act at the postconventional or principled level (level III). Nurses who are conventional thinkers base perceptions of moral obligations and rights on the maintenance of the social system and loyalty to established institutions and social groups. However, the postconventional nurse understands that societies and social

TABLE 11–3 *Erikson's Virtues or Ego-Strengths*

Stage of Development	Virtue
Trust versus mistrust	*Hope* or *confidence*. Belief that fervent wishes will be attained
Autonomy versus doubt	*Will*. Determination to exercise free choice as well as self-restraint
Initiative versus guilt	*Purpose*. Courage to envisage and pursue valued goals
Industry versus inferiority	*Competence*. Free exercise of dexterity and intelligence in the completion of tasks
Identity versus identity diffusion	*Fidelity*. Ability to sustain loyalties freely pledged in spite of the inevitable contradictions of value systems
Intimacy versus isolation	*Love*. Mutuality of devotion
Generativity versus stagnation or self-absorption	*Care*. Widened concern for what has been generated by love extending to whatever a person generates, creates, produces, or helps to produce
Integrity versus despair	*Wisdom*. Detached concern with life in the face of death

Source: E. H. Erikson, *Insight and responsibility: Lectures on the ethical implications of psychoanalytic insight* (New York: W. W. Norton and Co., 1964).

relationships can be arranged in many ways, and that these different ways can maximize or minimize values (Munhall 1982, p. 13). Therefore, the nurse at level III questions authority and follows social norms as long as they support human values.

Peters

Peters combines aspects of existing theories to arrive at a concept of morality and moral behavior. He proposes a concept of rational morality based on principles. Moral development is usually considered to involve three separate components: *moral emotion* (what one feels), *moral judgment* (how one reasons), and *moral behavior* (how one acts). Various theorists of moral development emphasize one component above the other two. For example, Freud emphasizes the moral emotional component by focusing on the role of one's conscience or ego-strength and feelings such as guilt or self-respect.

Piaget and Kohlberg emphasize the moral judgment or reasoning component. They see moral behavior as resulting from either the feelings or reasoning components, or both. Peters (1981, p. 83) states that much of moral philosophy in the past has not addressed *what* is morally important.

Facets of Moral Life   Peters (1981, p. 69) holds that morality and moral development are complex phenomena and that at least five facets of moral life must be distinguished:

1. Under the concepts of *good, worthwhile,* and *desirable* fall those activities that are thought to be so important that time must be spent on initiating children into them. Examples are poetry, science, engineering, and a variety of games and pastimes. Most of these activities are intimately connected with possible vocations and ideals of life.

2. Under the concepts of *obligation* and *duty* fall ways of behaving connected with social roles. For example, much of a person's moral life is taken up with one's station and its duties, for instance, with what is required of that person as a parent, spouse, and citizen.

3. There are those duties, more prominent in an open society, that are not specifically connected with social roles but that relate to following the general *rules governing conduct* between members of society, e.g., unselfishness, honesty, and fairness. These are personalized as character traits.

4. There are equally wide-ranging goals of life that are personalized in the form of *motives* or *traits of character* thought of as *virtues,* such as honesty, fairness, gratitude, and benevolence, and *vices,* such as meanness, selfishness, greed, and lust. These motives or purposes are not confined to a particular activity or role.

5. Finally, there are those very general traits of character that relate to the *manner in which a person follows rules or pursues purposes,* e.g., integrity, persistence, determination, conscientiousness, and consistency. These are all connected with what people call "the will."

Peters says the reason for spelling out this complexity of moral life is to rid persons of simple-minded views of morality, e.g., morality is just good interpersonal relationships or simply observing rules about stealing, sex, and the like. He believes that getting someone committed to a worthwhile activity is no less a part of morality than is the curbing of selfishness (Peters 1981, p. 70).

TABLE 11–4 Kohlberg's Stages of Moral Development

Level and Stage	Definition	Example
Level I *Preconventional*		
Stage 1: Punishment and obedience orientation	The activity is wrong if one is punished, and the activity is right if one is not punished.	A nurse follows a physician's order so as not to be fired.
Stage 2: Instrumental-relativist orientation	Action is taken to satisfy one's needs.	A client in hospital agrees to stay in bed if the nurse will buy the client a newspaper.
Level II *Conventional*		
Stage 3: Interpersonal concordance (good boy, nice girl)	Action is taken to please another and gain approval.	A nurse gives elderly clients in hospital sedatives at bedtime because the night nurse wants all clients to sleep at night.
Stage 4: Law and order orientation	Right behavior is obeying the law and following the rules.	A nurse does not permit a worried client to phone home because hospital rules stipulate no phone calls after 9:00 P.M.
Level III *Postconventional*		
Stage 5: Social contract, legalistic orientation	Standard of behavior is based on adhering to laws that protect the welfare and rights of others. Personal values and opinions are recognized, and violating the rights of others is avoided.	A nurse arranges for an East Indian client to have privacy for prayer each evening.
Stage 6: Universal-ethical principles	Universal moral principles are internalized. Person respects other humans and believes that relationships are based on mutual trust.	A nurse becomes an advocate for a hospitalized client by reporting to the nursing supervisor a conversation in which a physician threatened to withhold assistance unless the client agreed to surgery.

Source: Adapted from *Moral development: A guide to Piaget and Kohlberg* by Ronald Duska and Mariaellen Whelan. Copyright © 1975 by The Missionary Society of St. Paul the Apostle in the State of New York. Used by permission of Paulist Press.

Hierarchy of Virtues Peters's formulations contrast with Kohlberg's, who maintains that character traits such as honesty are comparatively unimportant in morals and that processes of habit formation by which traits are assumed to be established are of secondary importance. Peters, however, believes that the development of character traits or virtues is an essential aspect of moral development. He believes that virtues or character traits can be learned from others and encouraged by the example of others. For example, Peters states that a child develops concern for others much earlier than a sense of justice or honesty; further, concern for others does not require the same level of conceptual development as

justice and honesty do. In the early stages of their lives, children cannot grasp the principle of justice.

In addition, Peters believes that some virtues can be described as habits because they are in some sense automatic and therefore are performed habitually. Examples are punctuality, politeness, chastity, tidiness, thrift, and honesty (Peters 1981, p. 93). Peters believes that habits need to be established in moral life. A *habit* is a behavior that a person can perform without deliberation or concentration: "Life would be exhausting if, in moral situations, people always had to reflect, deliberate, and make decisions. It would be difficult for people to conduct their social lives if they could not rely on a fair stock of habits such as politeness and punctuality, for example (Peters 1981, p. 98). Kohlberg, by contrast, stresses that the most important features of moral education are cognitive.

Virtues that cannot be classed as habits include compassion, concern for others, caring, justice, tolerance, courage, integrity, perseverance, and consistency. The mind is actively involved in exercising these virtues.

Schulman and Mekler

Schulman and Mekler believe that morality is a measure of how people treat fellow humans and that a moral child is one who strives to be kind and just. Both terms refer to how a person's behavior affects other people. They believe that morality has two components (Schulman and Mekler 1985, p. 6):

1. The intention of the person acting must be good in the sense that the goal of the act is the well-being of one or more people.

2. The person acting must be fair or just in the sense that the person considers the rights of others without prejudice or favoritism. A person's acts may be moral, immoral, or amoral. An act is considered *immoral* if through it a person seeks to harm others or gain an unfair advantage over them. An *amoral* act is not performed specifically to benefit or harm others. Intention is crucial when judging the morality of an act. An act is judged to be *well-intentioned* when the person performs the act without being threatened or coerced and when the primary reward is the well-being of another.

Schulman and Mekler's (1985, pp. 5–9) theory of moral development is based on three foundations, which they believe can be taught:

1. *Internalizing parental standards of right and wrong.* Children internalize parental standards, such as "Share your toys," "Don't hit," and "Consider other people's feelings." Internalization is more than obeying rules to avoid punishment. It is the learning of standards rather than just rules (Schulman and Mekler 1985, p. 21). The child must "define certain actions as *right* or *wrong* based on the parent's rules and learn to apply to him or herself the same words he or she has heard from the parents on how to behave properly" (Schulman and Mekler 1985, p. 8). Internalization is the first stage of self-control over selfish and aggressive impulses and the first step toward an adult conscience. It is accomplished when the child hears the "inner voice" speaking *before* the child acts. It is based primarily on love for parents and the desire to please them.

2. *Developing empathic reactions.* Children need to learn to react with empathy to someone else's feelings, e.g., feeling good about another person's joy and feeling bad about another person's unhappiness. Schulman and Mekler say that empathy appears to be an inborn capacity and is surprisingly common in children. However, the capacity for empathy varies from person to person. Through empathy, children learn that harming others is bad and comforting them is good.

3. *Acquiring personal standards.* The third foundation of morality is the development of personal standards that guide how a person *should* treat fellow human beings and what kind of person the individual wants to be. When individuals develop personal standards, they begin to evaluate parental rules and those of other authorities in relation to the new standards.

Personal standards are not based on the approval of others. Reliance on them depends on the person's confidence in the ability to reason about the long-term consequences of actions. The consequences that keep a person striving to treat others kindly and justly are based on one's personal judgments about whether actions will bring a better world into being. In developing personal moral standards, the child first discerns whether the moral standards acquired from other people, starting with parents, work or not. This process occurs as the child expands relationships and experiences with others. If the moral standards learned earlier seem to bring about a better way of life, the child adopts personal standards learned from others. If the standards do not work, the child formulates new principles and standards.

Gilligan

Carol Gilligan (1982), after more than 10 years of research with women subjects, found that women often considered the dilemmas that Kohlberg used in his research to be irrelevant. Women scored consistently lower on his scale of moral development, in spite of the fact that they approached moral dilemmas with considerable sophistication. Gilligan believed that most frameworks do not include the concepts of caring and responsibility. Yet it is from these frameworks that most research in moral development is done. The result is that male emphasis upon individualism and autonomy is central to most moral development theories.

Gilligan describes three stages in the process of developing an "ethic of care" (Gilligan 1982, p. 74). Each stage ends with a transitional period. A *transitional period* is a time when the individual recognizes a conflict or discomfort with some present behavior and considers new approaches.

Stage 1. Caring for oneself. In this first stage of development, the person is concerned with caring only for the self. The individual feels isolated, alone, and unconnected to others. There is no concern or conflict with the needs of others because the self is the most important. The focus of this stage is survival. The end of this stage occurs when the individual begins to view this approach as selfish. At this time, the person also begins to see a need for relationships and connections with other people.

Stage 2. Caring for others. During this stage, the individual recognizes the selfishness of earlier behavior and begins to understand the need for caring relationships with others. Caring relationships bring with them responsibility. The definition of *responsibility* includes self-sacrifice, where "good" is considered to be "caring for others." The individual now approaches relationships with a focus of not hurting others. This approach causes the individual to be more responsive and submissive to others' needs, excluding any thoughts of meeting one's own. A transition occurs when the individual recognizes that this approach can cause difficulties with relationships because of the lack of balance between caring for oneself and caring for others.

Stage 3. Caring for self and others. During this last stage, a person sees that there is a need for a balance between caring for others and caring for the self. One's concept of responsibility is now defined as including both responsibility for the self and for other people. In this final stage, care still remains the focus on which decisions are made. However, the person now recognizes the interconnections between the self and others and thus realizes that it is important to take care of one's own needs, because if those needs are not met, other people may also suffer.

Gilligan believes women see morality in the integrity of relationships and caring, so that the moral problems they encounter are different from those of men. Men consider what is right to be what is just, whereas for women what is right is taking responsibility for others as a self-chosen decision (Gilligan 1982, p. 140).

Gilligan feels that a blend of perspectives is necessary for a person to reach maturity. The ethic of justice, or fairness, is based on the idea of equality: that everyone should receive the same treatment. This is the development path usually followed by men. It is widely ac-

cepted by the theorists in the field. By contrast, the ethic of care is based on a premise of nonviolence: that no one should be harmed. This is the path typically followed by women. It is an approach that has been given very little attention in the literature.

In the development of maturity, according to Gilligan, both viewpoints blend "in the realization that just as inequality adversely affects both perspectives in an unequal relationship, so too violence is destructive for everyone involved" (Gilligan 1982, p. 174). The blending of these two perspectives could give rise to a new view of human development and a better understanding of human relations.

Gilligan and Murphy, in their studies of postcollege adults, found that these adults began to doubt whether it is possible to construct generalized rules about right and wrong. They found these people evolving a rather new way of thinking in which change and process are primary features of reality. They see contradictions as acceptable and not needing resolution at all costs (Kegan 1982, p. 229).

VALUES

Each person, e.g., nurse, client, and physician, has a personal set of values. A *value set* is the group of values a person holds. Individuals incorporate personal values into their lives as a result of observing the behavior and attitudes of parents and teachers and interacting with their cultural, religious, and social environments. Personal values also reflect experiences and a person's intelligence.

Professional values are a reflection and expansion of personal values (Fromer 1981, p. 15). These values are acquired as a nurse is socialized into the nursing profession.

Acquisition of Values

Raths, Harmin, and Simon (1978) identified seven criteria that must be met for beliefs, attitudes, activities, or feelings to become values:

1. Having been freely chosen without outside pressure
2. Having been chosen from among alternatives
3. Having been chosen after reflection
4. Having been prized and cherished
5. Having been affirmed to others

6. Having been incorporated into actual behavior

7. Having been repeated in one's life (1978, p. 47)

A value must meet the above criteria, i.e., it is a belief put into practice (Thompson and Thompson 1985, p. 78). Values are also hierarchical, i.e., each person has an individual hierarchy of values, ranging from the most important value to the least important value.

Values Transmission

Each person has a relatively small number of values. The origin of these values can be traced to culture, society, institutions, and personality. In addition, these few values guide virtually all aspects of behavior. Values are learned and are greatly influenced by a person's sociocultural environment. For example, Puerto Ricans often value treatment by a folk healer over treatment by a physician. For additional information about cultural and ethnic values relative to health and illness, see Chapter 24.

Values are learned throughout life; however, many values are learned in early childhood. Acquiring values is usually a gradual process of which the individual is unaware. People do not always realize they have a specific set of values or that they base the decisions they make on values. Values are transmitted in a variety of ways. Four approaches are modeling, laissez-faire, moralizing, and responsible choice (Simon et al. 1978, pp. 15–18).

Modeling *Modeling* is a process by which a person engages in ideal behavior to serve as an example to be imitated by other persons (Johnson 1972, p. 189). There are two steps in modeling: (a) one person must engage in the ideal behavior, and (b) the second person must imitate the first person's behavior.

Parents are important models. Young children often want to be like their parents and will copy their parents' behavior. Through modeling, they behave in a manner that they perceive represents ideal values. However, modeling also can transmit socially unacceptable values. For example, a man who repeatedly hits his wife during an argument is modeling a socially unacceptable way to resolve a disagreement.

In clinical nursing settings, nurses are role models for clients and their families. For example, the nurse who smokes will not be as credible when instructing a client to stop smoking as the nurse who does not smoke or who previously quit smoking. Registered nurses are role models for nursing students. Some of the values transmitted to nursing students include attitudes towards clients, physicians, and the nursing profession.

Laissez-faire In this approach, people are left alone "to do their own thing." For example, a child is left free to have new experiences and to form his or her own values without parental guidance. The problem with this approach is that children can become confused when the adults around them do not support any behavior. For young people or people being socialized into roles, e.g., the nursing role, a laissez-faire approach to learning values can result in conflict and frustration.

Moralizing *Moralizing* is a direct method of inculcating values in another person. In some religions, moralizing is the basis of indoctrination into the religion: people are told what is "right" and what is "wrong." People who learn their values through moralizing can have difficulty making responsible choices later in life because they have no experience doing so. Moralizing is a rigid approach to transmitting values: Alternatives are not provided, and the individual has no choice if he or she wishes to do or believe what is "right."

Responsible Choice Values are also transmitted through responsible choice. The individual does not have free choice but is given limited choices. An example is the teenager who is allowed to use the family car only if it is returned by ten o'clock. The teenager has two choices that control behavior: not to use the car or to use it and return it on time. It is questionable, however, whether the teenager in this situation learns any values on which to base future behavior.

Values are also taught, usually by parents and by teachers in school and in religious organizations. For example, a parent will explain to a toddler that he or she should ask for a cookie before taking one, or a father will explain to a son how to be considerate on his first date. People also learn values through experience. For example, a young boy who drinks alcohol and then has an accident with the family car can learn from that experience to value safety and concern for others as well as himself when he drives.

Personal and Professional Values

The nurse enters the profession of nursing with values that guide personal actions. Through the process of socialization into the profession, the nurse may choose additional values. Personal and professional values are closely related and often can be the same. Hall (1973, pp. 23–32) identifies two primary values that are related to and must be in harmony with each other.

1. Self-value, or the idea that one is of worth to others
2. The idea that others are of equal worth

These primary values are not only vital as personal values in North American society but also vital as professional values, since nursing is based on relationships with clients, colleagues, and others.

Nurses' personal values influence client-nurse interactions and the practice of nursing. Steele and Harmon (1983, p. 7) believe that nurses can enact their professional roles with minimal discomfort when their personal and professional values are reasonably congruent. Thompson and Thompson (1985, p. 81) agree that nurses who are comfortable with their professional roles probably experience greater satisfaction and possibly provide better care for clients but question the latter point. Nurses who are comfortable with their roles may not necessarily practice in an ethical manner. For example, a nurse who is comfortable in her role may decide not to "make waves" or may fail to take a stand against a decision that goes against her sense of ethics.

Personal Values   Most people derive some values from the society or subgroup of society in which they live. Values developed by society ensure its continued functioning and enable people to live harmoniously together. Examples of societal values common to Western civilization are shown in the accompanying box. A person may internalize some or all of these values and perceive them as personal values. In addition to internalizing societal values, people have values that are important to them as individuals. Purtilo (1978, p. 71) points out that most people find fulfillment only if they can integrate both societal and personal values into a satisfactory life-style. People need societal values to feel like an accepted part of the society and humankind, and they need personal values to individualize themselves.

Professional Values   Because nursing is a profession based on caring, professional values relate to both competence and compassion. Universal moral values are shown in the box below. Nurses develop these

---

Selected Societal and Personal Values

Societal Values	Personal Values
■ Human life	■ Family unity
■ Individual rights	■ Self-worth
■ Individual autonomy	■ Worth of others
■ Liberty	■ Independence
■ Democracy	■ Religion
■ Equal opportunity	■ Honesty
■ Power	■ Fairness
■ Health	■ Love
■ Wealth	■ Sense of humor
■ Youth	■ Safety
■ Vigor	■ Peace
■ Intelligence	■ Financial security
■ Imagination	■ Material things
■ Education	■ Money
■ Technology	■ Property of self
■ Conformity	■ Property of others
■ Friendship	■ Leisure time
■ Courage	■ Work
■ Compassion	■ Travel
■ Family	■ Plants
	■ Animals
	■ Physical activity
	■ Intellectual activity
	■ Artistic activity
	■ Neatness

Universal Moral Principles Basic to Clinical Nursing Practice

- Respect for persons
- Autonomy (self-determination)
- Beneficence (doing good)
- Nonmaleficence (avoiding harm)
- Veracity (truth telling)
- Confidentiality (respecting privileged information)
- Fidelity (keeping promises)
- Justice (treating people fairly)

Source: American Nurses' Association, *Code for Nurses with Interpretive Statements* (Kansas City, Mo.: American Nurses' Association, 1985).

values during socialization into the profession and from professional codes of ethics, discussed later in this chapter.

Values Clarification

Values clarification is a process by which individuals find their own answers (values) to situations. It is not the transmission of "correct" values or rules, but a process of identifying and developing individual values. The principle of values clarification is that no one set of values is right for everyone.

The process of values clarification was formulated by Louis Raths in 1966, who built on the thinking of John Dewey. Raths was chiefly concerned with the process of valuing, not the content of the values. Valuing is composed of seven processes, which can be placed in three groups (Simon et al. 1978, p. 19):

Prizing one's beliefs and behaviors

1. Prizing and cherishing
2. Publicly affirming beliefs and behaviors when appropriate

Choosing one's beliefs and behaviors

3. Choosing from alternatives
4. Choosing according to consequences
5. Choosing freely

Acting on one's beliefs

6. Acting
7. Acting with a pattern, consistency, and repetition

A belief, attitude, or feeling becomes a value when all seven steps have been satisfied. The individual applies each of the seven steps to an emerging or already formed belief, behavior pattern, or attitude.

By using these seven steps in values clarification, nurses can clarify their own values and enhance their personal growth. These steps also can be applied to client situations; the nurse can help clients identify conflict areas, examine and choose from alternatives, set goals, and act (Coletta 1978, p. 2057).

Steele and Harmon (1983, p. 77) point out that nurses must exhibit ethical behavior to clients whether or not the nurse and client hold the same values. Nurses should, therefore, be "value-neutral"; that is, they should not believe that their own values are right and that a client's values are right or wrong. This attitude permits a nurse to establish an effective relationship with clients who have differing values.

Prizing and Cherishing　Prizing or cherishing is a continuous process in which the individual asks, "Do I cherish or prize my position or belief?" Unprized beliefs may still influence behavior, but they cannot be considered values.

Publicly Affirming When Appropriate
Public affirmation or appropriate sharing is an indication of the quality of a value. Individuals who feel strongly about an issue may publicly stand up and share the value with others. For example, nurses who value the autonomy of clients may refuse to obtain a signed consent form from a client without first assuring the client's complete understanding of the procedure to be performed. Thus the nurses are affirming to others their autonomy.

Choosing from Alternatives　For a belief to be a value, it must be chosen from among other alternatives. Individuals must consider the other options before they commit themselves to one choice.

Choosing After Consideration of Consequences　The individual must be able to consider the consequences of a choice, i.e., the significance of the decision. The person may reject or confirm the choice because of or in spite of the consequences. For example, a nurse may refuse to give a client a medication that the nurse believes may harm the client. The nurse considers the consequences of this behavior in terms of client and of self. The nurse is concerned for the client's welfare, but the refusal could result in disciplinary action. After considering all the alternatives, the nurse may confirm the choice of not giving the medication or select another course of action, e.g., discussing the medication with a physician before making a decision. If an individual's behavior is not the consequence of considering the results of action, it cannot be considered to reflect a value.

Choosing Freely　A value must be chosen freely. Some beliefs are not freely chosen by the individual but are accepted from parents or others without much thought and without choice. These beliefs are not values. Behavior determined by fear or coercion, for example, does not reflect values.

Acting　A value involves action. Therefore, a value must be incorporated into behavior. If it is not, it is not a value but a belief or an attitude.

Acting with a Pattern, Consistency, and Repetition　Behavior must be consistent over a period of time to reflect a value. The behavior is repeated in many aspects of life. For example, a nurse who values health will eat a healthful diet and get enough sleep.

It is important for nurses (a) to examine their own values and clarify them, (b) to recognize the differences in the values of clients and to accept them, and (c) to recognize the differences in the values of peers, other health care professionals, and health care organizations. Nurses need to recognize how such differences can affect them. Often, values represent an ideal; when that ideal is not achievable, some adaptation or compromise has to be made. Awareness of one's own values is a first step. The next step is to learn how to make the best possible compromise of values that circumstances allow.

Advantages of Values Clarification Clarification of values has the following advantages (Steele and Harmon 1983, pp. vii, 13; Thompson and Thompson 1985, p. 78):

- It is a process of discovery that brings to conscious awareness the values that guide one's actions.

- It fosters the making of choices. It is not synonymous with ethical decision-making, however.

- It leads to human growth because it fosters awareness, empathy, and insight.

- It serves as a guide for assessing client values and provides direction for nursing interventions.

- It gives insight into the source of a particular value. This awareness allows the individual to retain or change the value.

Identifying Personal Values

Nurses need to know in particular what values they hold about life, health, illness, and death. To explore personal values, the nurse can begin by answering questions such as (Thompson and Thompson 1985, pp. 77–80): "What ten things do I like to do?" "What ten things do I like about myself?" "What ten things do I dislike about myself?" An awareness of things nurses dislike can lead to thoughts about what they may like to change. After initial exercises, nurses may then list ten values that guide their daily interactions or activities. By comparing their lists with a trusted friend or in a group that fosters trust and mutual respect, nurses can see similarities and differences with others. Resulting discussion often reveals reasons for the items listed. Another strat-

egy for gaining awareness of personal values is to consider individual attitudes to such issues as abortion, unwanted pregnancy, euthanasia, sex-role stereotypes, and sexuality.

Examples of some questions and issues adapted from Corey et al. (1984, pp. 57–94) follow. When considering these issues, ask yourself: "Can I accept this or live with this?" "Why does this bother me?" "What would I do or want done in this situation?"

1. *Sexuality.* What are your attitudes toward?
   a. Teenage sex
   b. Casual sex
   c. Sex as an expression of love and commitment
   d. Group sex

2. *Right to die and the choice of suicide.* See the Learning Activity on page 204.

3. *Abortion.* Indicate whether you agree or disagree with the following statements.
   a. A woman should have the right to choose abortion.
   b. Abortion at any point during gestation is murder.
   c. Abortion is wrong.
   d. Abortion should be performed if the woman's health is endangered.
   e. A mentally handicapped woman should be encouraged to have an abortion.
   f. Abortion should not be performed after 20 weeks' gestation, when a living infant can be borne.
   g. Abortion should be encouraged when parents have genetically transmissible diseases.

4. *Health.* Various definitions of health are proposed in Chapter 13. The nurse who defines and values health as physiologic, emotional, social, cultural, and spiritual well-being does not give the same nursing care as the nurse who defines health as the absence of illness. Remember that values are what the nurse actually puts into practice. Consider whether you agree or disagree with the following:
   a. To be most effective in nursing practice, the nurse must be a role model of health.
   b. An obese nurse can effectively instruct an obese client about nutrition and exercise.
   c. A nurse who smokes can effectively help a client to stop smoking.
   d. The nurse who has been pregnant and delivered an infant is most effective in helping a client through this experience.

5. *Health care.* Aroskar (1982, p. 24) lists four mind-sets about health care that can influence ethical nursing practice. These views are shown in Table 11–5.

TABLE 11-5 Mind-Sets About Health Care and Effects on the Nurse

Health Care Mind-Set	Effects on the Nurse
The medical cure of disease	The nurse is considered primarily accountable to the physician. Medical values dominate.
A commodity to be sold to others	The nurse's major accountability is to the institution. Concerns for the client may conflict with this view.
The client's right to relief from pain and other debilitating conditions	The nurse's obligation is to the clients and their needs as defined by the clients themselves. By supporting the client's autonomy, the nurse abdicates responsibility; needs as defined by the client supersede the nurse's knowledge and experience.
The promotion, maintenance, and restoration of health within a cooperative community	All participants' values are considered in decision making. Both clients and providers have rights and responsibilities.

Source: M. A. Aroskar, Are nurses' mind-sets compatible with ethical nursing practice? Adapted from *Topics in Clinical Nursing,* April 1982, 4:24, with permission of Aspen Publishers, Inc. Copyright © April 1982.

Identifying Client Values

People's values change from time to time as their situation in life changes. State of health greatly influences a person's values. For example, a client with failing eyesight will probably place a high value on the ability to see; a client with failing neuromuscular ability will value the ability to stand or walk; and a client with chronic pain will value comfort. Normally, people take such things for granted. Nurses, therefore, need to identify the major values, beliefs, and behaviors of clients as they influence and relate to a particular health problem.

Reasons for identifying a client's value system include the following: (a) helping a client discover a new and meaningful value system following injury or illness; (b) providing information about the client's responses to injury or illness; (c) helping the client explore alternative goals and intervention strategies when valued goals can-

not be realized; (d) and planning nursing interventions that support the client's cultural and health care beliefs.

There are several ways of learning a client's values (Purtilo 1978, p. 75):

■ Converse with the clients about their jobs, families, pets, hobbies, past achievements, goals, or material possessions.

■ Listen to the client's family and friends. Friends or family members often provide clues through casual remarks, such as "I'll tell you something; he used to be a great concert pianist."

■ Review the client's health records, which can reveal personal values.

Values clarification can be a useful tool to help clients whose unclear or conflicting values are detrimental to their health. Behaviors that may indicate the need for values clarification are listed in the accompanying box.

To help clients clarify their values, the nurse needs to help the clients think about what is and what is not im-

---

Behaviors That May Indicate Unclear Values

Behavior	Example
Ignoring a health professional's advice	A client with heart disease who values hard work ignores advice to exercise regularly
Inconsistent communication or behavior	A pregnant woman says she wants a healthy baby but continues to drink alcohol and smoke tobacco
Numerous admissions to a health agency for the same problem	A middle-aged, obese woman repeatedly seeks help for back pain but does not lose weight
Confusion or uncertainty about which course of action to take	A woman wants to obtain a job to meet financial obligations but also wants to stay at home to care for an ailing husband

portant to them. It is helpful to ask the following questions, each associated with one of the seven steps in values clarification:

1. *List alternatives*. Make sure that the client is aware of all alternative actions and has thought about the consequences of each. Ask: "Are you considering other courses of action?"

2. *Examine possible consequences of choices*. Ask: "What do you think you will gain by doing that?" "What benefits do you foresee from doing that?"

3. *Choose freely*. To determine whether the client chose freely, ask: "Did you have any say in that decision?" "Did you have a choice?"

4. *Feel good about the choice*. To determine how the client feels about a decision or action, ask: "How do you feel about that decision (or action)?" Because some clients may not feel satisfied with their decision and feel badly about a bad choice, a more sensitive question may be: "Some people feel good after a decision is made; others feel bad. How do you feel?"

5. *Affirm the choice*. Ask: "What will you say to others (family, friends) about this?"

6. *Act on the choice*. To determine whether the client is prepared to act on the decision, ask: "Will it be difficult to tell your wife about this?"

7. *Act with a pattern*. Help the client determine whether he or she consistently behaves in a pattern. Ask: "How many times have you done that before?" or "Would you act that way again?"

When implementing these seven steps, the nurse assists the client to think each question through, never imposing personal values. The nurse never offers an opinion, e.g., "It would be better to do it this way," or offers a judgment, e.g., "That's not the right thing to do." The nurse offers an opinion only when the client asks the nurse for it and then only with care.

Value Conflicts

A *value conflict* occurs when two or more values are incongruent. For example, a nurse may value life yet be expected to collaborate with a physician in disconnecting a client from a life support system. Incongruent values may not present a problem until some action must be taken, as in the example above. There is now a value conflict that may confuse the nurse and make it difficult to make a decision.

An ethical or moral *dilemma* is "a situation involving a choice between equally satisfactory or unsatisfactory alternatives or a difficult problem that seems to have no satisfactory solution" (Thompson and Thompson 1985, p. 94). In a moral dilemma there is no right or wrong. For example, a nurse is alone at night on a hospital unit and two clients experience cardiac arrest at almost the same time. What does the nurse do? It may be possible to save one client, but not both. Moral dilemmas are arising with increasing frequency in nursing.

According to Thompson and Thompson (1985, p. 94), for a situation to be a moral dilemma, it must fulfill three criteria:

1. **Awareness of different options.** The individual must be aware of the different options that are open. The awareness may be cognitive, or it may be a feeling that something is wrong.

2. **Moral nature of the dilemma.** Is the dilemma the nurse faces a moral issue? Not all situations that appear confusing to nurses are moral dilemmas, e.g., a conflict between two nurses about how to proceed with specific client care may not be a moral dilemma but simply a differing interpretation of facts or even differing assessments. For example, one nurse may believe that a client's respirations indicate the need for oxygen, while another nurse may believe that the administration of morphine sulfate, as ordered by the physician, will suppress the Hering-Breuer reflex and ease respirations. Both nurses may in fact be right.

3. **Two or more options with true choice.** For a situation to be a moral dilemma, one must have a choice between two or more actions.

For example, a physician tells a client that when he performed the surgery he did all he could. The nurse present at the conversation knows that a resident physician performed the surgery because the client's surgeon could not be reached. The nurse's choices are (a) to tell the client his physician did not perform the surgery, (b) say nothing, (c) report the discussion to the charge nurse, or (d) discuss the conversation with the physician. The nurse in this example has free choice.

ETHICS

Since ethics govern right conduct, they deal with what "should" or "ought to" be done. Ethics are not unlike the law in that each deals with rules of conduct that reflect underlying principles of right and wrong and codes of morality. Ethics are designed to protect the rights of human beings. In nursing, ethics provide professional standards for nursing activities; these standards protect both the nurse and the client.

Although *ethics* and *morals* are often used interchangeably, Jameton differentiates the two. Ethics refers to publicly stated and formal sets of rules or values, while morals are values or principles to which one is personally committed (Jameton 1984, p. 5).

Nursing Codes of Ethics

A *code of ethics* provides a means by which professional standards of practice are established, maintained, and improved. It is essential to a profession. Codes of ethics are formal guidelines for professional action. They are shared by the persons within the profession and should be generally compatible with a professional member's personal values.

A code of ethics gives the members of the profession a frame of reference for judgments in complex nursing situations. No two situations are identical, and nurses are frequently in situations that require judgment about which course of action to take. A code of ethics serves as a guide in many of these situations. It identifies the values and beliefs behind ethical standards (Thompson and Thompson 1985, p. 12).

Codes of ethics are frequently a mixture of creeds and commandments. Benjamin and Curtis (1981) describe a *creed* as an affirmation of professional regard for high ideals of conduct and as a commitment of members of a profession to honor them. An example of a creed is the opening statement of the 1973 *Code for Nurses* of the International Council of Nurses (ICN): "The fundamental responsibility of the nurse is fourfold: to promote health, to prevent illness, to restore health and to alleviate suffering." See Table 11–6. As *commandments*, codes of

---

TABLE 11–6 *International Council of Nurses Code for Nurses*

The fundamental responsibility of the nurse is fourfold: to promote health, to prevent illness, to restore health, and to alleviate suffering.

The need for nursing is universal. Inherent in nursing is respect for life, dignity, and the rights of man. It is unrestricted by considerations of nationality, race, creed, color, age, sex, politics, or social status.

Nurses render health services to the individual, the family, and the community and coordinate their services with those of related groups.

Nurses and People

The nurse's primary responsibility is to those people who require nursing care.

The nurse, in providing care, promotes an environment in which the values, customs, and spiritual beliefs of the individual are respected.

The nurse holds in confidence personal information and uses judgment in sharing this information.

Nurses and Practice

The nurse carries responsibility for nursing practice and for maintaining competence by continual learning. The nurse maintains the highest standards of nursing care possible within the reality of a specific situation.

The nurse uses judgment in relation to individual competence when accepting and delegating responsibilities.

The nurse when acting in a professional capacity should at all times maintain standards of personal conduct which reflect credit upon the profession.

Nurses and Society

The nurse shares with other citizens the responsibility for initiating and supporting action to meet the health and social needs of the public.

Nurses and Coworkers

The nurse sustains a cooperative relationship with coworkers in nursing and other fields. The nurse takes appropriate action to safeguard the individual when his care is endangered by a coworker or any other person.

Nurses and the Profession

The nurse plays the major role in determining and implementing desirable standards of nursing practice and nursing education.

The nurse is active in developing a core of professional knowledge.

The nurse, acting through the professional organization, participates in establishing and maintaining equitable social and economic working conditions in nursing.

Source: International Council of Nurses, *ICN code for nurses: Ethical concepts applied to nursing* (Geneva, Switzerland: Imprimeries Populaires, 1973). Reaffirmed 1989. Reprinted with permission of the ICN.

professional ethics provide prescriptions designed to regulate conduct in more specific situations (Benjamin and Curtis 1981, p. 6). An example of a commandment is this statement in the ICN *Code for Nurses:* "The nurse holds in confidence personal information and uses judgment in sharing this information."

International, national, state, and provincial nursing associations have established codes of ethics. If a nurse violates the code, the association may expel the nurse from membership. Increasingly, professional nursing associations are taking an active part in improving and enforcing standards.

Purposes of ethical nursing codes are as follows:

1. Providing a basis for regulating the relationship between the nurse, the client, coworkers, society, and the profession.

2. Providing a standard basis for excluding the unscrupulous nursing practitioner and for defending a practitioner who is unjustly accused.

3. Serving as a basis for professional curricula and for orienting the new graduate to professional nursing practice.

4. Assisting the public in understanding professional nursing conduct.

In 1953, the International Council of Nurses (ICN) developed and adopted their first code of ethics. This code was revised in 1965 and again in 1973. See Table 11–6. The code should be considered together with the relevant data in each situation; thus it provides assistance in setting priorities and in taking action. For the practitioner of nursing, the code specifically provides assistance in making judgments and in developing attitudes appropriate to nursing.

The American Nurses' Association (ANA) first adopted a code of ethics in 1950, which was revised in 1968, 1976, and 1985. See Table 11–7. This code is designed to provide guidance for nurses by stating principles of ethical concern. In 1988, the ANA published *Ethics in Nursing,* which addresses a wide range of nursing situations that involve ethical action. Nurses have a responsibility to be familiar with the code that governs their nursing practice.

In 1980, the Canadian Nurses' Association adopted a code of ethics. It was revised in 1985. See Table 11–8.

Ethical Issues in Nursing

A discussion of all the ethical issues facing nurses today cannot be complete because of the large number of dilemmas currently encountered in nursing practice. Davis

---

TABLE 11–7 *American Nurses Association Code for Nurses*

1. The nurse provides services with respect for human dignity and the uniqueness of the client unrestricted by considerations of social or economic status, personal attributes, or the nature of health problems.

2. The nurse safeguards the client's right to privacy by judiciously protecting information of a confidential nature.

3. The nurse acts to safeguard the client and the public when health care and safety are affected by the incompetent, unethical, or illegal practice of any person.

4. The nurse assumes responsibility and accountability for individual nursing judgments and actions.

5. The nurse maintains competence in nursing.

6. The nurse exercises informed judgment and uses individual competence and qualifications as criteria in seeking consultation, accepting responsibilities, and delegating nursing activities to others.

7. The nurse participates in activities that contribute to the ongoing development of the profession's body of knowledge.

8. The nurse participates in the profession's efforts to implement and improve standards of nursing.

9. The nurse participates in the profession's effort to establish and maintain conditions of employment conducive to high quality nursing care.

10. The nurse participates in the profession's effort to protect the public from misinformation and misrepresentation and to maintain the integrity of nursing.

11. The nurse collaborates with members of the health professions and other citizens in promoting community and national efforts to meet the health needs of the public.

Source: American Nurses Association, *Code for nurses with interpretive statements* (Kansas City, Mo.: American Nurses' Association, 1985). Reprinted with permission.

TABLE 11-8 *Canadian Nurses' Association Code of Ethics for Nursing**

Clients

I. A nurse is obliged to treat clients with respect for their individual needs and values.

II. Based upon respect for clients and regard for their right to control their own care, nursing care should reflect respect for the right of choice held by clients.

III. The nurse is obliged to hold confidential all information regarding a client learned in the health care setting.

IV. The nurse has an obligation to be guided by consideration for the dignity of clients.

V. The nurse is obligated to provide competent care to clients.

VI. The nurse is obliged to represent the ethics of nursing before colleagues and others.

VII. The nurse is obligated to advocate the client's interest.

VIII. In all professional settings, including education, research, and administration, the nurse retains a commitment to the welfare of clients. The nurse bears an obligation to act in such a fashion as will maintain trust in nurses and nursing.

Health Team

IX. Client care should represent a cooperative effort, drawing upon the expertise of nursing and other health professions. Acknowledging personal or professional limitations, the nurse recognizes the perspective and expertise of colleagues from other disciplines.

X. The nurse, as a member of the health care team, is obliged to take steps to ensure that the client receives competent and ethical care.

The Social Context of Nursing

XI. Conditions of employment should contribute to client care and to the professional satisfaction of nurses. Nurses are obliged to work toward securing and maintaining conditions of employment that satisfy these connected goals.

Responsibilities of the Profession

XII. Professional nurses' organizations recognize a responsibility to clarify, secure, and sustain ethical nursing conduct. The fulfillment of these tasks requires that professional organizations remain responsive to the rights, needs, and legitimate interests of clients and nurses.

*This represents only one element of the code—*values. Standards,* which provide more specific directions for conduct than values, and *limitations,* which describe exceptional circumstances in which a value or standard cannot receive its usual application, are provided with each value in the publication cited above.

Source: Canadian Nurses' Association, February 1985. *Code of ethics for nursing.* Ottawa, Ontario. Reprinted with permission.

(1989, p. 571) attributes the increase in international discussion of nursing ethics to the following: (a) more ethical dilemmas in the health care field have been identified; (b) the general public, policy makers, and health professionals are more aware of these dilemmas; and (c) communication technology has increased our knowledge of how others, including people in other parts of the world, deal with ethical dilemmas.

The changing scope of nursing practice has led to an increasing incidence of conflicts between clients' needs and expectations and nurses' professional values. Some of these areas of conflict are AIDS, abortion, withholding food and fluid, and confidentiality. With the development of sophisticated technology that impacts illness trajectory, the nurse faces more complex ethical decisions.

Acquired Immune Deficiency Syndrome (AIDS) AIDS has had a profound impact upon the whole of society, including the nursing profession. Because of its association with homosexual and bisexual behavior, prostitution, illicit intravenous drug use, and inevitable physical decline and death, it bears enormous social stigma and elicits fear in nurses and all health care personnel. Some nurses have value systems that are incongruent with caring for clients who have AIDS or who test HIV seropositive, yet the profession expects the nurses to care for such clients. Nurses have a responsibility to the clients. There is a moral obligation for a nurse to care for an HIV-infected person (ANA 1988b, p. 8). According to the ANA's *Nursing and the Human Immunodeficiency Virus: A Guide for Nursing's Response to AIDS,* the moral obligation to care for an HIV-infected client cannot be set aside *unless* the risk exceeds the responsibility. The ANA has published a statement regarding risk versus responsibility in providing nursing care to clients who have infectious diseases such as AIDS, Hansen's disease, and typhoid fever.

"Not only must nursing care be readily available to individuals afflicted with communicable or infectious diseases, but nurses must also be advised on the risks and the responsibilities they face in providing care to those individuals. Accepting personal risk which exceeds the limits of duty is not morally obligatory; it is a moral option" (ANA 1988b, p. 31).

In addressing the issue of risk to nurses versus their responsibility to clients, the ANA presents four fundamental criteria to differentiate the nurse's moral duty from the moral option to care for a client:

1. The client is at significant risk of harm, loss, or damage if the nurse does not assist.
2. The nurse's intervention or care is directly relevant to preventing harm.
3. The nurse's care will probably prevent harm, loss, or damage to the client.
4. The benefit the client will gain outweighs any harm the nurse might incur and does not present more than minimal risk to the health care provider (ANA 1988b, p. 32).

When all four of these criteria are met, the nurse is obliged to give care. In most instances, therefore, it is morally obligatory to care for a client with AIDS (ANA 1988b, p. 32). Such care includes acquiring the most current knowledge regarding the provision of care and comfort to the client while minimizing risk to one's self.

Abortion Abortion is a highly publicized issue about which many people, including nurses, feel very strongly. If a nurse cannot be "value-neutral" (Steele and Harmon 1983, p. 77), another nurse should support and care for a client having an abortion.

In most states and provinces, there are provisions in the law known as *conscience clauses*. These clauses permit individual physicians and nurses, as well as institutions, to refuse to assist in performing abortions if doing so violates their religious or moral principles. In these instances, the individual or institution can exercise the right to refuse without fear of reprisal.

Nurses, however, have no right to impose their values on a client. Nurses should, therefore, choose a type of nursing practice that does not conflict with personal values.

Withdrawing or Withholding Food and Fluid Food and fluid are necessary to sustain health and life. It is generally accepted that providing food and fluid is part of nursing practice and, therefore, one of a nurse's moral duties. A nurse is morally obligated, however, to withhold feedings, when it is more harmful to administer than to withhold them (ANA 1988a, p. 2). A clinical example is the withholding of food or fluid preoperatively and postoperatively. In this instance, withholding food and fluid is clearly in the client's best interest despite any resulting discomfort. Ethical dilemmas can occur when it is not clear whether withholding the food or fluid is beneficial or harmful to the client. "It is morally as well as legally permissible for nurses to honor the refusal of food and fluid by competent patients in their care" (ANA 1988a, p. 3). The *Code for Nurses* supports this statement through the nurse's role as a client advocate and through the principle of autonomy, i.e., the moral principle of respect for others. It is important that clients who refuse food and/or fluid understand their situations, the alternatives, and the associated harms and benefits. It is equally important that a nurse establish the client's competency to do this. If a client is not currently competent but has previously expressed a personal preference—e.g., through a living will made when the client was competent—the nurse should respect the client's values. In almost all instances, the giving of fluid and food must be in the client's best interests.

Euthanasia and the Right to Die (Living Wills) *Euthanasia* is the act of painlessly putting to death persons suffering from incurable or distressing disease. It is commonly differentiated as active and passive euthanasia. Active euthanasia is the hastening of death, whereas passive euthanasia is letting a person die, or as it is often described, "letting nature take its course." Regardless of compassion and good intentions or moral convictions, euthanasia is *legally wrong* in both Canada and the United States and can lead to criminal charges of homicide or to a civil lawsuit for withholding treatment or providing an unacceptable standard of care. Because advanced technology has enabled the medical profession to sustain life almost indefinitely, people are increasingly considering the meaning of quality of life. For some people, the withholding of artificial life-support measures or even the withdrawal of life support is a desired and acceptable practice for clients who are terminally ill or who are incurably disabled and believed unable to live their lives with some happiness and meaning.

Voluntary euthanasia refers to situations in which the dying individual desires some control over the time and manner of death. All forms of euthanasia are illegal except in states where right-to-die statutes and living wills exist. Right-to-die statutes legally recognize the client's right to refuse treatment.

Living wills (an individual's signed request to be allowed to die when life can be supported only mechanically or by heroic measures) and right-to-die statutes have received increasing attention in recent years. Most nurses agree that people have a right not to participate in medical treatment or to refuse treatment once it has started. When a person is being maintained on life-sustaining machines, however, a conflict may arise between a physician's ability to prolong life physiologically and the individual's right to die with dignity. Living wills grew out of this conflict. California was the first state to enact legislation, the California Natural Death Act of 1976, that gives legal recognition to a person's desire to control his or her right to die. Since then, 37 other states and the District of Columbia have enacted similar laws (Bellocq 1988, p. 313). Some oppose these laws, contending there is no need for such laws, the laws exclude family from the decision, and the laws hasten death. For a sample living will, see Figure 11–1.

Nurses need to familiarize themselves with statutes that authorize living wills in the state where they practice. Where statutes do exist, policy and procedures are usually detailed specifically. They may include the need to obtain a court order, a medical opinion, the agreement of an ethics or medical committee, family confirmation, or some combination of these. The statutes usually grant civil and criminal immunity to those who carry out living-will requests.

Confidentiality

"The nurse safeguards the clients' right to privacy by judiciously protecting information of a confidential nature" (ANA 1985b, p. 1). Confidentiality dilemmas can arise when clients and their support persons are breaking the law, when clients tell a nurse they have committed a crime, and when a health professional shares information about a client with others not directly involved with the clients' care.

Confidentiality is an aspect of respect for the individual. Nurses must explain to clients that it is often necessary to share pertinent information with others caring for the client. The nurse is not in violation of client trust if the client knows about this sharing (College of Nurses of Ontario 1985, p. 15). The nurse may also find that preventing harm to someone overrides the responsibility of confidentiality. For example, a postoperative client tells

---

To My Family, My Physician, My Lawyer And All Others Whom It May Concern

Death is as much a reality as birth, growth, and aging—it is the one certainty of life. In anticipation of decisions that may have to be made about my own dying and as an expression of my right to refuse treatment, I _____, being of sound
(print name)
mind, make this statement of my wishes and instructions concerning treatment.

By means of this document, which I intend to be legally binding, I direct my physician and other care providers, my family, and any surrogate designated by me or appointed by a court, to carry out my wishes. If I become unable, by reason of physical or mental incapacity, to make decisions about my medical care, let this document provide the guidance and authority needed to make any and all such decisions.

If I am permanently unconscious or there is no reasonable expectation of my recovery from a seriously incapacitating or lethal illness or condition, I do not wish to be kept alive by artificial means. I request that I be given all care necessary to keep me comfortable and free of pain, even if pain-relieving medications may hasten my death, and I direct that no life-sustaining treatment be provided except as I or my surrogate specifically authorize.

This request may appear to place a heavy responsibility upon you, but by making this decision according to my strong convictions, I intend to ease that burden. I am acting after careful consideration and with understanding of the consequences of your carrying out my wishes. *List optional specific provisions in the space below. (See other side)*

Figure 11-1 A sample living will. **Source:** For more information and a complete document, contact: Concern for Dying, 250 W. 57th Street, New York, NY 10107.

---

the nurse in confidence that he is taking amphetamines that a friend brings him while he is in hospital. The nurse tells the client that this information must be shared with the other health professionals because of the possible harmful effect to the client's health.

Termination of Life-Sustaining Treatment

The withdrawal of equipment from clients whose lives are being sustained by artificial means (e.g., ventilators) is a highly complex issue. The Hastings Center (1987, pp. 6–8) has prepared guidelines for the termination of life-sustaining treatment. These guidelines are governed by four values:

1. The client's well-being
2. Client autonomy
3. The integrity of the health professional
4. Justice or equity

A nursing decision in these situations should be based on the four values. If it is the client's wish to die, the nurse must establish the client's competency to make this decision. An agency ethics committee can provide a forum for discussion of this and similar situations.

Safeguarding Client Health and Safety

The *Code of Nurses* states that nurses act as client advocates "to safeguard the client and the public when health care and safety are affected by the incompetent, unethical or illegal practice of any person" (ANA 1985b, p. 1). Each agency should have an established process for reporting and handling practices that jeopardize the health and safety of clients. A nurse's first obligation is to protect a client; in some situations, therefore, it may be necessary to intervene before a client is harmed. For example, a client tells the nurse that he intends to walk out of the hospital even though he is receiving intravenous infusion, has been receiving oxygen, and has a newly sutured abdominal incision. The nurse's judgment is that the client will harm himself if he is permitted to leave his bed. The nurse should follow the agency practices regarding reporting the situation and restraining the client before he is harmed.

Accountability   Nurses are repeatedly faced with conflicting responsibilities. On the one hand, the nurse is frequently employed by and thus responsible to a health agency. On the other hand, the nurse is a professional person with professional ethics. In addition, the nurse is an individual with personal values.

Nurses should be able to identify priorities in their personal value systems. If the nurse perceives a conflict of values between the nurse and a client, the nurse should be able to respect the client's values and provide the necessary care. "The nurse provides services with respect for human dignity and the uniqueness of the client" (ANA 1985b, p. 1). If it is impossible for the nurse to do this, the nurse (or other nursing personnel) should arrange for someone else to carry out the client's care.

RESEARCH NOTE

How Do Nurses Respond to Moral Dilemmas?

At times nurses confront fundamental moral dilemmas arising from their work. Swider, McElmurry, and Yarling examined this and related questions in their study of decisions reported by 775 senior baccalaureate nursing students from 16 midwestern colleges and universities presented with an ethical dilemma in nursing practice. Loyalties to clients, institutions, and physicians were addressed and analyzed. Most of the first decisions out of the chain of decisions to follow were institution-centered. The study revealed, however, that an overall sense of confusion prevails.

Implications: In clinical areas nurses must explore seriously the choices they make in order to practice maturely.

Swider, S. M.; McElmurry, B. J.; and Yarling, R. R. March/April 1985. Ethical decision making in a bureaucratic context by senior nursing students. *Nursing Research* 34:108–12.

Resolving Ethical Dilemmas

To make ethical judgments, one must rely on rational thought, not emotions. Such judgments require conscious, cognitive skills necessary to perceive the client's needs and provide client care (Sigman 1986, p. 21). Every day, nurses make decisions that affect their clients, and these decisions are frequently based on ethics. See the accompanying Research Note.

A number of ethical theories and ethical decision-making models can guide nurses in making ethical decisions. Purtilo and Cassel suggest a four-step process: gather relevant data, identify the dilemma, decide what to do, and complete the action (Purtilo and Cassel 1981, pp. 27–29).

Thompson and Thompson (1981) propose a ten-step bioethical decision model to help nurses examine ethical issues and make a decision. See Table 11–9.

There are three primary ways to approach bioethical issues: teleology, deontology, and intuitionism. *Teleology* is a doctrine that explains phenomena by results; a person who takes a teleologic approach to ethics is concerned with the consequences of ethical decisions. This approach is often summarized in the notion "the end

TABLE 11-9   *A Bioethical Decision Model*

Step One	Review the situation to determine health problems, decision needed, ethical components, and key individuals
Step Two	Gather additional information to clarify situation
Step Three	Identify the ethical issues in the situation
Step Four	Define personal and professional moral positions
Step Five	Identify moral positions of key individuals involved
Step Six	Identify value conflicts, if any
Step Seven	Determine who should make the decision
Step Eight	Identify range of actions with anticipated outcomes
Step Nine	Decide on a course of action and carry it out
Step Ten	Evaluate/review results of decision/action

Source: J. B. Thompson and H. O. Thompson, *Ethics in nursing.* (New York: Macmillan, 1981). Used by permission.

justifies the means." The terms *teleology* and *utilitarianism* are sometimes used interchangeably; however, utilitarianism is also considered a type of teleology, summarized in the ideas "the end justifies the means" and "the greatest good for the greatest number." Many people in medical research support this approach to the ethics of medical problems. For example, Dr. Brown, a surgeon who has had no experience with a particular type of surgery, goes ahead and operates anyway. Although the surgeon recognizes that the surgery may not be successful largely because of his lack of experience, the knowledge he believes he will gain justifies his actions.

Deontology is the theory or study of moral obligation. A simplification of the deontologic approach is that the morality of an ethical decision is completely separate from its consequences. For instance, a nurse might believe it is necessary to tell the truth no matter who is hurt.

The difference in these approaches is shown by applying them to an ethical issue, abortion. A person who takes a teleologic approach to the ethical issue of abortion might consider that saving the mother's life (the end) justifies the abortion (the means). One taking a deontologic approach to abortion might consider any termination of life as morally bad and therefore would not harm the fetus regardless of the consequences. The

approach does not determine the decision, e.g., a person taking a teleologic approach might consider that saving the life of the fetus justifies the death of the mother. The approach, however, guides the steps in the making of ethical decisions.

The third approach to ethical issues is *intuitionism,* summarized as the notion that people inherently know what is right or wrong; it is not a matter of rational thought or of learning. For example, a nurse inherently knows it is wrong to strike a client—this does not need to be taught.

According to Fromer, the four most important principles in a deontologic approach are autonomy, nonmaleficence, beneficence, and justice. *Autonomy* is personal liberty of action; it implies independence, self-reliance, freedom of choice, and the ability to make decisions (Fromer 1986, pp. 82–83).

Nonmaleficence means the duty to do no harm. This principle is the basis of most codes of nursing ethics. Although this would seem to be a simple principle to follow in nursing practice, in reality it is complex. Harm can mean deliberate harm, risk of harm, and harm that occurs during beneficial actions (Fromer 1986, p. 83). In nursing, intentional harm is always unacceptable. However, the risk of harm is not so clear. A client may be at risk of harm during a nursing intervention that is intended to be helpful. For example, a client may react adversely to a medication. Sometimes, the degree to which a risk is morally permissible can be a conflict.

Beneficence means "doing good." Nurses are obligated to "do good," that is, to implement actions that benefit clients and their support persons. However, in an increasingly technologic health care system, "doing good" can also pose a risk of doing harm. For example, a nurse may advise a client about an exercise program to improve general health but should not do so if the client is at risk of a heart attack.

Justice, the fourth principle, is often referred to as fairness. Nurses frequently face decisions in which a sense of justice should prevail. For example, a nurse is alone on a hospital unit, and one client arrives to be admitted at the same time another client requires a medication for pain. Instead of running from one client to the other, the nurse should weigh the facts in the situation and then act based on the principle of justice.

In resolving ethical problems, nurses need to be aware of (a) the ethical theory with which they are most comfortable and (b) their own hierarchy of principles or values in that theory.

Although codes of ethics offer general guidelines for decision making, more specific guidelines are necessary in many cases to resolve the everyday ethical dilemmas encountered by nurses in practice settings. Suggested guidelines for the nurse to resolve these dilemmas are as follows:

1. Establish a sound database.
2. Identify the conflicts presented by the situation.
3. Outline alternative actions to the proposed course of action.
4. Outline the outcomes or consequences of the alternative actions.
5. Determine ownership of the problem and the appropriate decision maker.
6. Define the nurse's obligations.

Establishing the Database

To establish a sound database, the nurse needs to gather as much information as possible about the situation. Aroskar (1980, p. 660) suggests that nurses get answers to the following questions:

1. What persons are involved and what is their involvement in the situation?
2. What is the proposed action?
3. What is the intent of the proposed action?
4. What are the possible consequences of the proposed action?

For example, Mrs. Green, a 67-year-old woman, is hospitalized with multiple fractures and lacerations caused by an automobile accident. Her husband, also in the accident, is admitted to the same hospital and dies. Mrs. Green, who was the driver of the automobile, constantly questions the primary nurse about her husband. The surgeon, Dr. Mario Gonzales, however, has told the nurse not to tell the client about the death of her husband. The nurse is not provided with any reason for such a direction and expresses concern to the charge nurse, who says the surgeon's orders must be followed.

In this example, the database includes

Persons involved: Client (concerned about husband's welfare), husband (deceased), surgeon, charge nurse, and primary nurse.

Proposed action: Withhold information about the husband's death.

Intention of proposed action: Unknown; possibly to protect Mrs. Green from psychologic trauma, overwhelming guilt feelings, and consequent deterioration of her physical condition.

Consequences of proposed action: If information is withheld, the client may become increasingly anxious and angry and may refuse to cooperate with necessary care, delaying recovery.

Identifying Conflicts

A conflict is a clash between opposing elements or ideas. The conflicts for the primary nurse in the example are

- Need to be honest with Mrs. Green without being disloyal to the surgeon and the charge nurse
- Need to be loyal to the surgeon and charge nurse without being dishonest to Mrs. Green
- Conflict about the effects on Mrs. Green's health if she is informed or if she is not informed

Outlining Courses of Action and Outcomes

Alternative courses of action to the proposed action for Mrs. Green and their outcomes might include:

- Follow the surgeon's and charge nurse's advice and do as the surgeon suggests. The outcomes for the nurse would be (a) approval from the charge nurse and surgeon, (b) risk of being seen as nonassertive, (c) violation of own value to be truthful to Mrs. Green, (d) possible benefit to Mrs. Green's health, and (e) possible detriment to her health.
- Discuss the situation further with the charge nurse and surgeon, pointing out Mrs. Green's rights to autonomy and information. The outcomes might be: (a) the surgeon may acknowledge the client's right to be informed and may then inform the client, (b) the surgeon may state that the client's rights have no legal basis and may adhere to the action originally proposed, based on a judgment about the effects of information on Mrs. Green.

Determining Ownership

In some ethical dilemmas, nurses do not make decisions about their own actions but assist clients to make a decision. For example, if a client states he does not want to have an operation, the question of ownership arises. In this example, it is obvious that the client owns the problem and that it is his right to choose this course of action. Associated with ownership, however, is knowledge about the probability and the risk of consequences attending various courses of action. Therefore, the nurse does not abandon the client with this decision. The nurse has the professional knowledge and expertise to ensure that the client makes an informed decision. Thus the client needs information from the professional's frame of reference about the consequences of decisions.

A series of questions that evolve from decision-making theories can help nurses determine who owns a certain problem (Davis and Aroskar 1983, p. 218):

1. Who should be involved in making the decision and why?

2. For whom is the decision being made?

3. What criteria (social, economic, psychologic, physiologic, or legal) should be used in deciding who makes the decision?

4. What degree of consent is needed by the subject (client and other)?

5. What, if any, moral principles (rights, values) are enhanced or negated by the proposed action?

In the example of Mrs. Green, the surgeon obviously believes the decision is his to make for Mrs. Green, and the charge nurse agrees. However, the criteria used to decide who the decision maker should be are not clear. If the criteria were spelled out, perhaps the conflict about the effects on Mrs. Green's health of knowing or not knowing about her husband's death could be resolved. Is it psychologically advantageous for Mrs. Green to know or not to know? Is it physically advantageous? What will the social and economic effects be?

Value systems also influence the decision about problem ownership. The value of Mrs. Green's right to information about her husband will be enhanced if she is told, negated if not. Her right to autonomy will also be affected.

This example shows that there are no clearly defined right or wrong answers to ethical dilemmas. If there were, they would not be ethical dilemmas. To resolve the ethical dilemma about Mrs. Green, it may be necessary for the involved health professionals to confer and clearly establish approaches that will be in Mrs. Green's best interests. Once an approach is agreed on, the nurses and physician can devise consistent continuing methods of support for Mrs. Green. That approach may dictate actions by the nurse that conflict with her or his own value system. However, the action chosen for Mrs. Green's best interest takes precedence.

Defining the Nurse's Obligations When nurses are determining an ethical course of action, Moser and Cox (1980, p. 43) advise them to list their nursing obligations, to assess the conflicts that will arise if all obligations are met, and to determine the alternatives from which the nurse can choose. Examples of obligations are

- To maximize the client's well-being
- To balance the client's need for autonomy and family members' responsibilities for the client's well-being
- To support each family member and enhance the family support system
- To carry out hospital policies
- To protect other clients' well-being
- To protect the nurse's own standards of care

CHAPTER HIGHLIGHTS

▶ There are several theories of moral development, all of which are sequential in nature.

▶ The moral development of an individual will impact upon his values, beliefs, attitudes, and related actions.

▶ Values give direction and meaning to life and guide a person's behavior.

▶ Every individual has a personal set of values influenced by societal standards, parents, teachers, culture, religion, and other life experiences.

▶ Values are freely chosen, prized and cherished, affirmed to others, and consistently incorporated into behavior.

▶ Nurses enter nursing practice with personal sets of values and through socialization acquire additional professional values that influence and guide their actions.

▶ Nursing is a profession based on caring; its professional values relate to both competence and compassion.

▶ Clarification of personal values is important for nurses to identify values that guide one's actions and to facilitate the making of choices.

▶ Values often represent an ideal that is not always achievable; compromises are thus necessary in the practice situation. ▶

CHAPTER HIGHLIGHTS *(continued)*

▸ Value conflicts do not present problems for the nurse until some action must be taken.

▸ Moral dilemmas are situations in which there is no right or wrong choice; the individual must choose between two equally undesirable alternatives.

▸ Professional standards for nursing activities are founded in ethics and designed to protect the rights of clients and nurses.

▸ Ethical issues in nursing may arise because of conflicts between personal values and professional responsibilities or between people involved in client care.

▸ To resolve an ethical dilemma, a nurse must establish a sound database, identify value conflicts, outline courses of action and outcomes, determine who owns the problem, and define the nurse's obligations.

LEARNING ACTIVITIES

■ Values Clarification Strategy: Value Voting
This exercise, adapted from Uustal (1978, p. 2060) and Bernal (1985, p. 174), demonstrates that there are many facets to every issue. How do you determine your position? What factors influence your thoughts and feelings? How will your choice be reflected in your behavior? Talk with some colleagues. Do they feel similarly or differently?

Where do you stand on the following issues? Indicate your responses in the following manner:

SA   strongly agree   D   disagree
A   agree   SD   strongly disagree
U   undecided

Do you believe:

1. ____ Clients have the right to participate in all decisions related to their health care.

2. ____ Clients have a right to refuse extraordinary treatment that is life-sustaining.

3. ____ Refusing life-sustaining treatments is a form of suicide.

4. ____ Clients have a right *not* to be interfered with in a rational act of suicide.

5. ____ Health professionals have a responsibility to assist a client in an act of rational suicide that does not cause injury to others.

6. ____ Comfort measures should always be provided.

7. ____ Health professionals should always do their best to sustain a person's life.

■ Consider your own values and beliefs about:
  ▪ Health, curing, and caring
  ▪ Nursing as a profession
  ▪ Client behaviors such as substance abuse, poor hygiene, homelessness, child or spouse abuse, disability, illiteracy

Are your actions consistent with your values and beliefs? Are your values consistent with the values of those in your work environment: administration, nursing colleagues, physician colleagues?

READINGS AND REFERENCES

SUGGESTED READINGS

Omery, A. June 1989. Values, moral reasoning, and ethics. *Nursing Clinics of North America* 24:499–508.
Omery writes that nurses are facing increasing numbers of moral/ethical dilemmas in professional practice. Values are explained, and moral values as a special kind of values are discussed. In addition, moral reasoning is described using Kohlberg's and Gilligan's models. Ethics is differentiated from values. Omery explains that values and moral reasoning reflect the "is." Moral reasoning is the mental process that nurses use to come to a decision of right or wrong in a moral dilemma. Values are motivational preferences or dispositions. Ethics, according to Omery, is the "ought."

Sheehan, J. July 1985. Ethical considerations in nursing practice. *Journal of Advanced Nursing* 10:331–36.
Some ethical implications for nursing practice are considered in relation to three issues: competence, honesty, and obedience. Sheehan discusses factors that contribute to conformity, obedience, and authoritarianism and suggests

respect for other people as a guiding principle for ethically acceptable conduct.

Yarling, R. R., and McElmurry, B. J. January 1986. The moral foundation of nursing. *Advances in Nursing Science* 8:63–73.

The authors argue that the major predicament facing nurses in their professional practice is their lack of freedom to act morally. It is suggested that two changes are necessary: the emergence of a strong sense of professional autonomy and a change in the locus of accountability from other health professionals to the client. Yarling and McElmurry provide the reader with a historical perspective and present-day realities. They state that nurses have a moral instinct founded on conscience but seldom act on their consciences when their actions are in opposition to the power structure that controls their professional and economic destiny. The authors urge that nursing ethics should be viewed as reform ethics.

RELATED RESEARCH

Crisham, P. March/April 1981. Measuring moral judgment in nursing dilemmas. *Nursing Research* 30:104–110.

Ketefian, S. May/June 1981. Moral reasoning and moral behavior among selected groups of practicing nurses. *Nursing Research* 30:171–76.

Ketefian, S. July/August 1985. Professional and bureaucratic role conceptions and moral behavior among nurses. *Nursing Research* 34:248–53.

SELECTED REFERENCES

American Nurses' Association. 1976, 1985a. *Code for nurses with interpretive statements.* Kansas City, Mo.: ANA.

———. 1985b. *Ethical dilemmas confronting nurses.* Kansas City, Mo.: ANA Committee on Ethics.

———. 1988a. *Ethics in nursing: Position statements and guidelines.* Kansas City, Mo.: ANA.

———. 1988b. *Nursing and the human immunodeficiency virus: A guide for nursing's response to AIDS.* Kansas City, Mo.: ANA

Aroskar, M. A. April 1980. Anatomy of an ethical dilemma. *American Journal of Nursing* 80:658–63.

———. April 1982. Are nurses' mind-sets compatible with ethical nursing practice? *Topics in Clinical Nursing* 4:24–26.

Bandman, E. L., and Bandman, B. 1990. *Nursing ethics through the life span.* 2d ed. Norwalk, Conn.: Appleton & Lange.

Bellocq, J. A. September/October 1988. Legal and ethical issues: Changing attitudes about death. *Journal of Professional Nursing* 4:313.

Benjamin, M., and Curtis, J. 1981. *Ethics in nursing.* New York: Oxford University Press.

Berkowitz, M. W., and Oser, F., editors. 1985. *Moral education: theory and applications.* Hillsdale, N.J.: Lawrence Erlbaum.

Bernal, E. W. April 1985. Values clarification: A critique. *Journal of Nursing Education* 24:174–75.

Chinn, P. L., editor. 1986. *Ethical issues in nursing.* Rockville, Md.: Aspen Publishers.

Coletta, S. S. December 1978. Values clarification in nursing: Why? *American Journal of Nursing* 78:2057.

College of Nurses of Ontario. 1985. *Guidelines for ethical behavior in nursing.* Toronto: The College of Nurses.

Corey, G.; Corey, M. S.; and Callahan, P. 1984. *Issues and ethics in the helping professions.* 2d ed. Monterey, Calif.: Brooks/Cole Publishing Co.

Davis, A. J. June 1989. New developments in international nursing ethics. *Nursing Clinics of North America* 24:571–77.

———. May 1990. Professional obligations, personal values in conflict. *American Nurse* 22:7.

Davis, A. J., and Aroskar, M. A. 1978. *Ethical dilemmas and nursing practice.* New York: Appleton-Century-Crofts.

Erikson, E. H. 1964. *Insight and responsibility: Lectures on the ethical implications of psychoanalytic insight.* New York: W. W. Norton and Co.

Fowler, M. D. M. January 1988. Ethical guidelines. *Heart and Lung* 17:103–4.

———. March 1988. Acquired immunodeficiency syndrome and refusal to provide care. *Heart and Lung* 17:213–15.

Fromer, M. J. 1981. *Ethical issues in health care.* St. Louis: C. V. Mosby.

———. 1986. Solving ethical dilemmas in nursing practice. In Chinn, P. L., editor. *Ethical issues in nursing.* Rockville, Md.: Aspen Publishers.

Freud, S. 1961. The ego and the id and other works (Vol. 19, James Strachney, translator). London: Hogarth Press and the Institute of Psychoanalysis.

Fry, S. T. July 1989. Toward a theory of nursing ethics. *Advances in Nursing Science* 9–22.

Gilligan, C. 1982. *In a different voice: Psychological theory and women's development.* Cambridge, Mass.: Harvard University Press.

Grady, C. February 1989. Acquired immunodeficiency syndrome: The impact on professional nursing practice. *Cancer Nursing* 12:1–9.

———. June 1989. Ethical issues in providing nursing care to human immunodeficiency virus-infected populations. *Nursing Clinics of North America* 24:523–34.

Hall, B. P. 1973. *Value clarification as a learning process.* New York: Paulist Press.

The Hastings Center. 1987. Termination of life-sustaining treatment and care of the dying.

International Council of Nurses. 1973. *ICN code for nurses: Ethical concepts applied to nursing.* Geneva: Imprimeries Populaires.

Jameton, A. 1984. *Nursing practice: The ethical issues.* Englewood Cliffs, N.J.: Prentice-Hall.

Jarczewski, P. H. May/June 1990. What is an ethical decision? Ethics for contemporary nursing practice. *Advancing Clinical Care* 5:28.

Johnson, D. W. 1972. *Reaching out: Interpersonal effectiveness and self-actualization*. Englewood Cliffs, N.J.: Prentice-Hall.

Kegan, R. 1982. *The evolving self: Problem and process in human development*. Cambridge, Mass.: Harvard University Press.

Ketefian, S. June 1989. Moral reasoning and ethical practice in nursing. *Nursing Clinics of North America* 24:509–21.

Lund, M. March/April 1990. Conflict in ethics: Is giving pain relief always right? *Geriatric Nursing* 11:83–4.

Moser, D., and Cox, J. M., editors. May 1980. Perspectives: Resolving an ethical dilemma. *Nursing 80* 10:39–43.

Muldary, T. W. 1983. *Interpersonal relations for health professionals: A social skills approach*. New York: Macmillan Co.

Munhall, P. L. June 1982. Moral development: A prerequisite. *Journal of Nursing Education* 21:11–15.

Murphy, C. P. 1985. *Ethical dilemmas in nursing practice*. Pub. no. NP-68D. Kansas City, Mo.: American Nurses' Association.

Murphy, P. June 1989. The role of the nurse on hospital ethics committees. *Nursing Clinics of North America* 24:551–56.

Peters, R. S. 1981. *Moral development and moral behavior*. London: George Allen and Unwin, Publishers.

Purtilo, R. 1978. *Health professional/patient interaction*. 2d ed. Philadelphia: W. B. Saunders Co.

Purtilo, R. B., and Cassel, C. K. 1981. *Ethical dimensions in the health professions*. Philadelphia: W. B. Saunders Co.

Raths, L. E.; Harmin, M.; and Simon, S. B. 1978. *Values and teaching*. 2d ed. Columbus, Ohio: Charles E. Merrill Books.

Salladay, S. A., and McDonnell, Sr. M. M. June 1989. Spiritual care, ethical choices, and patient advocacy. *Nursing Clinics of North America* 24:543–49.

Schulman, M., and Mekler, E. 1985. *Bringing up a moral child: A new approach for teaching your child to be kind, just, and responsible*. Reading, Mass.: Addison-Wesley Publishing Co.

Sigman, P. 1986. Ethical choice in nursing. In Chinn, P. L. (editor). *Ethical issues in nursing*. Rockville, Md.: Aspen Publishers.

Simon, S. B.; Howe, L. W.; and Kirschenbaum, H. 1978. *Values clarification: A handbook of practical strategies for teachers and students*. Rev. ed. New York: Hart Publishing Co.

Steele, S. M., and Harmon, V. M. 1983. *Values clarification in nursing*. 2d ed. Norwalk, Conn.: Appleton-Century-Crofts.

Swider, S. M.; McElmurry, B. J.; and Yarling, R. R. March/April 1985. Ethical decision making in a bureaucratic context by senior nursing students. *Nursing Research* 34:108–12.

Thompson, J. B., and Thompson, H. O. 1981. *Ethics in nursing*. New York: Macmillan Co.

———. 1985. *Bioethical decision making for nurses*. Norwalk, Conn.: Appleton-Century-Crofts.

Twomey, J. G. Jr. April 1989. Analysis of the claim to distinct nursing ethics: Normative and nonnormative approaches. *Advances in Nursing Science* 11:25–32.

Van Hooft, S. February 1990. Moral education for nursing decisions. *Journal of Advanced Nursing* 15:210–15.

White, R. 1975. *Lives in progress: A study of the natural growth of personality*. 3d ed. New York: Holt, Rinehart and Winston.

CHAPTER

12

Advocacy and Change

CONTENTS

ADVOCACY

An advocate is defined by Webster as one who pleads the cause of another or argues or pleads for a cause or proposal. Advocacy involves concern for and defined actions on behalf of another person or organization to bring about a change. A client advocate is an advocate of clients' rights. According to Disparti (1988, p. 140), advocacy involves promoting what is best for the client, ensuring that the client's needs are met, and protecting the client's rights. Some nurses believe client advocacy is an essential nursing function. Others believe that a client advocate need not be a nurse. All, however, recognize that many clients need an advocate to protect their rights and to help them speak up for themselves. Benner

(1984, p. 212) suggests that clients and their families frequently need the nurse to intervene for them. The client may be fearful or his understanding of explanations may be confused by the health professional's use of technical medical language. "The nurse can interpret patient to doctor and doctor to patient." (Benner 1984)

Kohnke identifies three levels of advocacy: (1) advocacy for self, (2) advocacy for the client, and (3) advocacy for the community of which the nurse is a part. Kohnke postulates that one cannot be an advocate for others if one is unable to advocate for one's self. The nurse needs self-knowledge as well as professional knowledge about nursing and health care or knows where to obtain such knowledge to assist clients in their decision making. Nurses as knowledgeable professionals have an obligation and a right to share their unique knowledge with the community when needed (Kohnke 1982, pp. 8–11). Today's health care crises of AIDS, homelessness, teenage pregnancy, child and spouse abuse, drug and alcohol abuse, and increasing health care costs all demand the nurse to fulfill the role of advocate in the community.

Some people believe that the client advocate should be accountable to the client *and* represent the client. The client advocate should be able to call in qualified consultants, participate actively in hospital committees monitoring the quality of client care, present complaints directly to the hospital director and hospital executive committee, delay discharges, and participate, at the client's request and direction, in discussions of the client's case (Annas 1975, pp. 209, 211). The nurse in the community should be able to advocate for the client in similar ways with agency administrators, inter and intra agency consultants, judicial authorities, and legislators. An advocate can represent a client by presenting the client's point of view and by interpreting and explaining the client's rights.

The role of the advocate involves influencing others. Nurses implement the advocacy role in two supportive ways: acting on behalf of the client, and giving the client full or at least mutual responsibility in decision making (Leddy and Pepper 1985). An example of acting on behalf of a client is asking a physician to talk to the client about the reasons for the immobility of the client's right arm because the client says he always forgets to ask the physician. An example of mutual responsibility for decision making is nurse-client collaboration in planning an exercise schedule.

According to Kohnke, the actions of an advocate are (a) to inform clients about their rights in a particular situation and make sure they have all the necessary information to make an informed decision and (b) to support clients in their decisions. In order to inform, the advocate must either have the information required or know how to get it. The advocate must want the client to have the information, and the client must agree to knowing the information. The knowledge must be presented in a way that is meaningful to the client, and the advocate must be able to deal with the fact that there may be those who do not wish the client to know (Kohnke 1982, p. 5).

Support can involve actions or nonactions (Kohnke 1980, p. 2039). An advocate must know how to support in an objective manner, being careful not to convey approval or disapproval for differing choices. Kohnke further describes the difficulty of advocacy. Advocacy involves accepting and respecting the client's right to make a decision even if in the nurse's professional opinion that decision is wrong. In this role, nurses do not make decisions for clients; clients must make their own decisions freely. For example, Mr. Rae makes a decision not to have further chemotherapy for his malignancy after being fully informed about the chemotherapy treatment, the alternative treatments, and the possible consequences of the available choices. The client advocate informs Mr. Rae of his right to make this decision and supports him in his decision.

Underlying client advocacy are the following beliefs:

- Individuals have the right to select values they deem necessary to sustain their lives.

- Individuals have the right to exercise their judgment of the best course of action to achieve the chosen values.

- Individuals have the right to dispose of values in a way they choose without coercion by others (Donahue 1985, p. 1037).

Guidelines characteristic of responsible advocacy are outlined in the accompanying box.

Nurses who function responsibly as advocates for themselves, their clients, and the community in which they reside are in a position to effect change. Knowledge that the nurse needs as an advocate includes objective understanding of the ethical issues in nursing and health care (see Chapter 11). Further, the nurse needs to have knowledge of the laws and regulations that affect her practice and the health of society (see Chapter 10).

Characteristics of Responsible Advocacy

- Conveying concern for the client's total situation

- Recognizing that what the client really wants may not be what the client verbalizes under stress

- Recognizing the effect a change in a client's situation may have on others

- Balancing the client's needs against others' needs and recognizing that change must come slowly

- Recognizing the importance of good working relationships and communication with others

Source: J. Zusman, Want some good advice? Think twice about being a patient advocate, *Nursing Life,* November/December 1982, 6:49.

CHANGE

Change is all around us. It is a dynamic process and a normal part of people's lives. It is a means by which people grow, develop, and adapt. Change is also an integral aspect of nursing. To be effective and influential in today's world, nurses need to understand change theory and apply its precepts in the workplace, in government and professional organizations, and in the community. Planning and implementing change are professional responsibilities as well as largely unrealized power sources that are vital to the practice of nursing. Some synonyms for change are *alter, transform, modify, convert,* and *vary*. All these terms suggested that a fundamental difference or substitution is the outcome of change.

Brooten, Hayman, and Naylor (1978) define *change* as "the process which leads to alteration in individual or institutional patterns of behavior." Mauksch and Miller define change as "the process by which alterations occur in the function and structure of society." Further, they define *planned change* as a "deliberative and collaborative process including a change agent and a client system," this system being "an individual, group of people, an agency, an organization, or a social institution" (1981, p. 9).

A *change agent* is a person or group who initiates changes or who assists others in making modifications in themselves or in the system (Kemp 1986). Brooten, Hayman, and Naylor (1978) describe a change agent as a professional who relies on a systematic body of knowledge about change to guide the change process.

The promotion of change is an essential component of nursing care. By using the nursing process, the nurse helps the client to propose, implement, and maintain changes (e.g., knowledge, skill, feelings, attitudes) that promote the client's health. Principles and strategies to promote change are integrated into all phases of the nursing process. During the assessment phase, the nurse establishes trust and identifies the client's health status and motivation for change. In the diagnosis phase, problems are specified. In the planning phase, objectives or goals for change are mutually established. In the implementation phase, the change strategies are implemented and maintained. In the evaluation phase, a judgment is made about whether the change process has been successful. On a larger scale, the nurse can be instrumental in promoting change at the institutional, professional, or societal levels.

An effective change agent must be a highly skilled communicator who is able to establish good interpersonal relationships. In addition, change agents must be self-aware and aware of others' attitudes about change and be able to handle disagreements and disappointments (Lancaster and Lancaster 1982, p. 21).

Lancaster and Lancaster describe the functions of a change agent in assisting a group as the following: (a) defining the problem; (b) listing all alternatives and positive and negative consequences; (c) determining the most suitable alternative for the situation and time; (d) organizing a plan to implement the change; (e) providing continuing support and direction; and (f) helping to develop an evaluation format (1982, p. 21).

When assuming the role of change agent, nurses must recognize that they serve as an important link between various components of the change project or people participating in the change project. The change agent should hold a variety of expectations and expect the final outcome to be different from the original plan. It is also important for the change agent to be accessible to all people involved in the change process. The change agent should be honest and straightforward about goals and problems.

A key element is trust. The change agent must trust the participants in the change and they in turn must trust the change agent. One of the greatest risks of change is that the system can become disrupted, even nonfunctional. For example, changing the method of nurse assignments could result in gaps and missed care for some clients. Close observation of the situation during the change process is important to avoid this problem.

A change agent may be formally or informally designated by the system. A *formally designated change agent* is one who has the role and responsibility for change, such as a clinical nurse specialist expected to make changes beneficial to specified clients. This person has the power to plan and implement change. An *informally designated change agent* does not have the authority to make change by virtue of a position but does have the leadership skills and respect of others and therefore can serve an important function in the change process.

Change agents may also be internal or external. An *internal change agent* is a person who is part of the situation or system, e.g., a charge nurse on a hospital unit or a nurse employed on a surgical unit. Internal change agents are familiar with the situation and the organization. However, they may have vested interests in the present system as well as biases. An *external change agent* comes to the situation from the "outside," e.g., a nurse from another state or another hospital. External change agents are able to view the problem and the situation objectively and usually have no biases; however, they are unfamiliar with the situation and the problems. There are advantages and disadvantages to both positions, and it is important for any change agent to be aware of these in each situation.

Change agents who are successful have effective leadership skills. That is, they can influence people in order to attain specified goals. A change agent should be oriented toward changing the group or individual rather than the agency (Kemp 1986).

Mauksch and Miller (1981) list three key characteristics of a change agent:

1. The ability to take risks. This involves the ability to calculate potential risks associated with the change and then to decide whether the risks are worth taking.

2. A commitment to the efficacy of the change. The change agent should investigate the change and be convinced of its value and effectiveness.

3. Comprehensive knowledge of nursing that combines research findings and basic science data; competence in nursing practice, interpersonal relations, and communication skills.

Types of Change

There are many types of change; in fact, change can occur without effort on anyone's part. Change of this type is also referred to as "drift." It occurs as individuals and groups respond to the environment and is usually recognized retrospectively. For example, after the birth of a baby, changes may take place in the parents' lifestyle. They may go out socially less frequently and spend less money. They may become aware of this change only after a period of time, when they realize they have not been going to movies as they were accustomed.

There is also traditional change, which can be approached in five different ways. See Table 12–1. Traditional change is effective in some circumstances and is usually planned. However, most of these approaches have limitations: Anyone wanting to use these strategies to effect change has to be in a position of superior knowledge and power. Today, social scientists recognize that change is not a simple phenomenon but has far-reaching effects involving many people, usually an entire system, e.g., a family or a broader social group.

Other types of change have been described. *Developmental change* refers to the physiopsychosocial changes that occur during the life cycle. This type of change is normally gradual. An example of this is the decreasing physical capability of an elderly person. This kind of change is slow and generally permits the individual time to adapt. *Situational change* occurs without any control by a person or group. An example is the change that occurs as a result of a war or a hurricane. However, not all situational changes are negative; for example, Nurse Smith may be unexpectedly offered a position in a hospital that she has wanted for a long time.

TABLE 12-1 *Traditional Change Strategies*

Strategy	Basis	Application in Nursing
Exposition and propagation	Ideas change the world, and ideas can be responsible for change.	Workshops, client teaching, advertising.
Elite corps	Knowledge is power; people with knowledge in power positions assure change by an elite corps.	The nurse assumes an elitist position in relation to clients and uses this position to convince the client to change.
Psychoanalytic insight	People in power require knowledge, insight, and awareness of psychologic factors operating in a situation. Psychologic insights provide power to effect change.	The nurse uses insights about the client when proposing change.
Scholarly consultation	Experts with special knowledge serve as outside consultants and propose solutions or change.	A nurse acts as a consultant to a client and/or family and uses knowledge to propose changes.
Circulation of ideas to the elite group	Circulating ideas about change to the power group can effect change.	A nurse conveys ideas about change to the nurse in charge, hoping this will result in the desired change.

Changes may also be considered covert or overt. A *covert* change is hidden or occurs without the individual's awareness. For example, a person can become increasingly deaf without being aware of this fact. *Overt* change is change about which a person is aware, for example, the development of abdominal pain or shortness of breath while walking up stairs. People who experience overt change may also experience anxiety. Overt change often necessitates behavioral changes that are at variance with the person's needs or goals. An example is a diagnosis of cancer and the subsequent need for therapy even though it interferes with the person's work and family life.

Change is frequently differentiated as unplanned or planned. *Unplanned change* is usually haphazard, and the results can be unpredictable. *Planned change,* by contrast, involves problem-solving and decision-making skills as well as interpersonal competence (Welch 1979, p. 307). It is deliberate and carried out consciously. According to Lippitt (1973), planned change is an intended,

purposive attempt by an individual, group, organization, or larger social system to influence the status quo of itself, another organism, or a situation. Planned change refers to "changes that are proposed to improve living, working or recreational conditions" (Mauksch and Miller 1981, p. 20). However, according to Bennis, Benne, and Chin (1985, p. 21), not all people want the stated benefits of change.

There are a number of theories of planned change. They all have in common an emphasis less on knowledge than on collaboration among the people involved. Four theories about change of particular value to nurses are those proposed by Lewin, Lippitt, Havelock, and Rogers. See Table 12–2.

Kurt Lewin (1948) originated classical change theory. He saw change as having three basic stages: unfreezing, moving, and refreezing.

During the *unfreezing* stage, the motivation to establish some sort of change occurs. The individual becomes aware of the need for change. This stage is a cognitive

TABLE 12-2 *Theories of Change*

Lewin (1948)	Lippitt (1958)	Havelock (1973)	Rogers (1983)
1. Unfreezing	1. Diagnosing the problem	1. Building a relationship	1. *Knowledge*. The individual, called the decision-making unit, is introduced to change and begins to comprehend it.
	2. Assessing the motivation and the capacity for change	2. Diagnosing the problem	
2. Moving	3. Assessing the change agent's motivation and resources	3. Acquiring relevant resources	2. *Persuasion*. The individual develops an attitude toward the change that may be favorable or unfavorable.
		4. Choosing the solution	
3. Refreezing	4. Selecting progressive change objectives	5. Gaining acceptance	
	5. Choosing an appropriate role for the change agent	6. Stabilization and generating self-renewal	3. *Decision*. The person makes a choice to adopt or not to adopt the change.
	6. Maintaining the change once it has been initiated		4. *Implementation*. The person acts on the choice. At this time, alterations may take place.
	7. Terminating the helping relationship		5. *Confirmation*. The individual looks for confirmation that the choice was right. If the person encounters mixed messages, the choice may be changed.

Sources: K. Lewin, *Field theory in social science* (New York: Harper and Row, 1951); R. Havelock, *The change agent's guide to innovations in education* (Englewood Cliffs, N.J.: Educational Technology Publications, 1973); E. Rogers, *Diffusion of innovations*, 3d ed. (New York: Free Press, 1983); R. Lippitt, Jeanne Watson, and B. Westley: *The Dynamics of Planned Change*. (New York: Harcourt, Brace and World, Inc., 1958).

process in which the person becomes aware of a problem or of a better method of accomplishing a task and hence of the need for change. Having identified this need, the individual must also identify restraining and driving forces. The restraining forces are those that inhibit change, and the driving forces are those that support change. For example, a charge nurse who wants nurses recognized for their nursing excellence may identify the new vice-president of nursing as a driving force but may see nurses on the unit who are resistant to change as restraining forces.

In the second stage, *moving,* the actual change is planned in detail and then started. Information about the problem is gathered from one or several sources. At this stage, it is important that the people involved agree that the status quo is undesirable. In the above example, the charge nurse would help nurses to see the disadvantages of not recognizing clinical excellence and to view the problem from another perspective—i.e., how recognition can be accomplished. The charge nurse could also guide the nurses in their search for information about this problem.

The charge nurse, as a change agent, should provide an environment that is conducive to the change. Rewards may need to be provided to reinforce desired behaviors. An environment that fosters change should be supportive, nonthreatening, and educational (Olson 1979).

In the third stage, *refreezing,* the changes are integrated and stabilized. According to Welch (1979), the individuals involved in the change integrate the idea into their own value system. Thus, in the above example the nurses on the unit would come to value recognition of clinical excellence and would integrate this idea into their own value systems.

Gordon Lippitt (1958) described planned change as having seven phases. See Table 12–2. For a detailed discussion of each of these seven stages, see Welch (1979).

Ronald Havelock (1973) modified Lewin's theory regarding planned change. See Table 12–2. In his theory, the emphasis is on planning the change process, which he believed takes the most time and involves the most significant changes (Welch 1979).

Everett Rogers (1983) viewed people's backgrounds and the environment as important in the process of change. He described change as a five-step process, which he called the *innovation-decision process* (Rogers 1983). See Table 12–2. The individual who undergoes change can also reject the change at a later time. Rogers thus introduced the idea that an adopted change is not necessarily permanent but may be reversed in the future. Rogers emphasized that for successful change, the people involved must be interested in the change and committed to implementing it.

Acceptance of Change

Important aspects of planning change are establishing the likelihood of change being accepted and then identifying the criteria by which it can be identified. Acceptance of change often takes time, particularly when change does not fit into an individual's attitudinal frame of reference; in such a case, change may not occur at all. For example, to stop smoking may not be accepted as a desirable behavior change by an individual who values smoking and does not believe it is harmful. Optimally, this belief changes before the change in behavior is tried. Stages in the acceptance of change are shown in the accompanying box.

Resistance to Change

When a change agent encounters resistance, it is important to determine whether the resistance should be overcome. Sometimes the change is inadvisable, as when there are insufficient resources for making the change.

Stages in the Acceptance of Change

The individual:
1. Becomes aware of the new idea, system, or practice.
2. Seeks more information about the change.
3. Evaluates the information and relates it to the present situation.
4. Mentally tries out the proposed change.
5. Actually tries out the change, on a small scale if possible.
6. Adopts and integrates the change into the present system.

When introducing a change, the nearer the people involved in the change are to the process, the easier the implementation of the change. These stages of acceptance can then naturally evolve.

Source: B. Stevens, Effecting change, *Journal of Nursing Administration,* February 1975, 5:25.

Resistance to change is often greatest when the idea is not concurrent with existing trends, such as trying to change from primary nursing to functional nursing when primary nursing is currently popular. Also, resistance is usually great when the proposed change would alter a situation with which people are comfortable.

Reasons for Resistance

Resistance to change is not merely lack of acceptance but rather behavior intended to maintain the status quo—that is, to prevent the change. However, not all behavior that opposes change is resistance. Sometimes change is opposed for valid, logical reasons. According to New and Couillard (1981), people resist change for one or more of the following reasons: (a) threatened self-interest, (b) inaccurate perceptions, (c) objective disagreement with the change, (d) psychological reactance, and (e) low tolerance for change.

Threatened self-interest as a reason for resistance to change often involves people's perception that the personal costs will be greater than any gains. These costs may occur in time, money, or status, for example. Opposition to a change may be based on *incorrect perceptions* of the change itself. Incomplete or inaccurate information may cause apprehension about the change, resulting in resistance on the part of the people involved. *Objective disagreement* can also cause resistance to a change. In some instances, people may have information that leads them to believe the change will not attain stated objectives. Sometimes individuals have more experience or information than the change agent, and their resistance can result in reconsideration of a planned change and perhaps benefits for the people involved. *Psychologic reactance* is a reaction motivated by perceived loss of freedom to engage in particular behaviors. According to New and Couillard (1981), psychologic reactance is manifested when threatened or eliminated behaviors suddenly assume greater importance than previously, and the person attempts to reestablish eliminated behaviors.

Some people have a *low tolerance* for change. Although they may intellectually understand the change, they are unable to accept it emotionally. This may be due to feelings of low self-esteem, fear of risk, or minimal tolerance for uncertainty.

Stages of Resistance

Stevens (1975) described six stages of resistance to change:

1. Undifferentiated resistance arises from various sources.

2. The sides for and against the change line up and develop their stands.

3. The two sides have direct conflicts. The resistance is either overcome or reduced.

4. The people for the change come into power.

5. The people against the change begin the stages of acceptance.

6. Few opponents are found and most people don't recall that they opposed the change.

Dealing with Resistance

Reinhard (1988) gives the following guidelines for dealing with resistance:

- Communicate with the people who oppose the change and identify the cause of their opposition.

- Clarify information and give accurate feedback.

- Be open to revisions in the plan, but be clear about areas that cannot be changed.

- Induce guilt in the people who oppose the change by, for example, explaining the consequences of their resistance on client care or on available money for care.

- Enhance psychological security and reduce threats to it. This can be done by emphasizing the positive aspects of the change.

- Encourage the people who are resisting to maintain face-to-face contact with supporters. Encourage both sides to empathize with the other: recognize valid objections, and relieve unnecessary fears.

- Maintain a climate of trust, support, and confidence.

Strategies for Change

A nurse can use a number of strategies to implement change. The three categories that follow are described by Bennis, Benne, and Chin (1985):

1. *Power-coercive.* Power-coercive strategies are based on the use of power as a result of legitimate authority or of economic influence. These strategies are particularly valuable when there is a lack of general agreement about a change. The use of this type of strategy may produce considerable resistance to the change and so should not be used without considering the subsequent consequences. A hospital administrator might demonstrate this strategy by establishing a policy that nurses on night shift can take only 15 minutes for a meal break. The administrator has the obvious power to make this decision.

2. *Empirical-rational*. This category of strategies uses knowledge as the basis for change. It assumes that people act in a rational manner. It is also assumed that the change agent has knowledge and has the power to persuade others to accept a change that is desirable for them. An example of this strategy is for a clinical nurse specialist to introduce a new method for recording intravenous infusions that is faster and more accurate than other methods of recordkeeping.

3. *Normative-reeducative*. This category of strategies is based on the assumption that people's actions are guided by sociocultural norms and values. Information is considered to be insufficient to change people's behavior. Therefore, the change must be brought about through skilled interpersonal communication. The change agent collaborates with the others involved in the change process. Normative-reeducative strategies foster personal growth and problem-solving. An example of normative-reeducative change strategy is having a well-known athlete talk to teenagers about the dangers associated with taking drugs. It is hoped that this person's influence will be greater than the peer pressure toward experimentation.

Taking a slightly different approach, Schaller (1972) outlined four general strategies for change: coercion, co-optation, conflict, and cooperation.

Coercion is the application of power to force a change. The individual or group that selects this strategy must gain power before introducing change.

Co-optation means bringing people or a person resisting the change into the prochange group. This may involve making promises of a certain position or money or some type of "buy-off." Co-optation can have the advantage of establishing a group with more diverse points of view; however, the disadvantage is that members may not agree with the promises given in exchange for support.

Conflict or confrontation strategy may clarify issues in the change process, but it may also have a divisive effect and may stimulate resistance that can impede the change (Brooten 1984).

The *cooperative* strategy is widely used in health care institutions. A climate for cooperative change is encouraged by an open exchange of information, opinions, and feelings (Mauksch and Miller 1981). In addition, it requires skills in communication and interpersonal relations. The need for the change must also be based on knowledge and fact.

Steps in the Change Process

The following steps are a model of planned change. The model outlines the actions one must take to plan and control change and make it serve a specific purpose (Spradley 1980).

1. Identify symptoms that indicate something needs changing.

2. Diagnose the problem by reviewing the symptoms and gathering additional data.

3. Explore alternative solutions in terms of their risks, benefits, driving and restraining forces, advantages, disadvantages, and probable outcomes. (An effective technique used by change agents is brainstorming.)

4. Select one course of action from among the identified alternatives.

5. Plan the steps in the change process:
   a. Write measurable objectives.
   b. Determine a timetable.
   c. Plan a budget.
   d. Recruit individuals to carry out each aspect of the plan.
   e. Ensure ability of the change agents to work with the client system.
   f. Evaluate resources (driving forces) and resistance (restraining forces) and plan strategies to manage both.
   g. Design a plan to evaluate the outcomes of the change effort.
   h. Identify measures to refreeze or establish the change within the client system.

6. Implement the change. (Pilot testing a new idea affords one the opportunity to evaluate it on a small scale and to "sell" it to the larger client system.)

7. Evaluate the outcome(s) on the basis of the measurable objectives and make appropriate adjustments.

8. Refreeze the client system so that the changes are seen as standard operating procedures and the system is once again stable.

Examples of Change

It is exciting to realize how effective nurses can be when they determine the need for change and plan strategies to bring it about. The following examples outline changes initiated by nurses who have identified a need to "do something" in each of four spheres of influence: the workplace, organizations, government, and the community.

The Workplace   At each of three shift meetings Mrs. Hawkins, Head Nurse, listened to nurses complain about problems with getting clients' laboratory work done and reported to the unit in a timely manner. She conferred with other head nurses and with the attending and resident physicians on her unit. It appeared that similar complaints were widespread.

At the next head nurse meeting, Mrs. Hawkins described the problem. The group appointed a task force, with Mrs. Hawkins as Chair, and asked it to present a plan to solve the problem at the next meeting. After gathering more data, the task force invited representatives from the attending and resident staff and the laboratory director to meet with them to review the data, consider alternative solutions, and select a plan to solve the problem.

By the next head nurse meeting, a preliminary plan to alter the system of laboratory reporting had been devised, and all concerned were working cooperatively to implement the plan.

The Professional Organization   Nurses on the Education Committee of a district nurses' association recognized the need to make a public policy statement concerning the care of clients with AIDS. Since the Board of Directors had recently expressed interest in promulgating such policy statements, the committee sensed the timing was right and that the board would welcome its draft despite the controversial subject matter.

Members of the committee researched and drafted a statement. The full committee offered a critique and selected an articulate spokesperson to present the statement to the association president and seek support before asking to have the statement presented to the board. Once the president had approved the statement, it was placed on the agenda for the next board meeting.

After making minor additions, the board approved it for distribution to the lay and nursing press and asked the Education Committee to suggest a nurse to present the statement at a local hearing of the City Council Health Committee.

The Government   While the pressure to contain health care costs escalated through the first half of the 1980s, a coalition representing the shared interests of the ANA, the NLN, and the American Association of Colleges of Nursing (AACN) mounted a campaign to convince Congress of the cost-effectiveness of a center for nursing research within the National Institutes of Health (NIH). Despite incredible odds, including a presidential veto and opposition from the American Medical Association, the American Association of Medical Colleges, and the NIH administrations, the proposal was passed by Congress in the fall of 1985. The success of this effort demonstrates the effectiveness of carefully planned change including the collaboration of nursing organizations. It also illustrates the clout organized nurses can wield on any level and in any sphere.

The Community   Every nurse plays several roles besides that of registered nurse. Each resides in a community, and many are parents. Some serve on school boards, belong to the League of Women Voters, or participate in religious, club, or scouting activities. There are numerous opportunities for nurses to contribute to the health and welfare of the communities in which they live. A group of nursing students recognized a health problem within their community and developed a plan to intervene. Many of the students were parents of children in local elementary schools where a high percentage of children were being sent home daily with head lice. Because of previously enacted budget cuts, the district's school nurses were each responsible for between three and five schools. The students volunteered to work with the district nurses to provide screening and health teaching at each of the elementary schools, thereby helping to resolve the community's problem.

All nurses are affected by change; nobody can avoid it. Knowledgeable nurses make rational plans to deal with both opportunities to initiate and guide needed change as well as to respond to change that affects them in the workplace, government, organizations, and the community. To recognize these opportunities for change and respond to the factors that influence nursing from without, it is helpful to consider the history of nursing, current trends in nursing, and present political, social, technological, and economic issues.

EFFECTING PROFESSIONAL CHANGE THROUGH POWER AND POLITICAL ACTION

Nurses are increasingly more knowledgeable about and capable of influencing the development of health care policy and the delivery of client care. Unless nurses develop their individual and collective political skills and use them to be advocates for the health of society and to promote the profession, client care and the nursing profession itself will be jeopardized.

Attitudes and Behaviors Necessary to Overcome Powerlessness

- Power is a positive force in nursing.
- There must be a commitment to continuing education in nursing.
- Professional nursing is a career and not just a job.
- Nursing is intrinsically valuable to society.
- Nurses must be actively involved in the women's movement because the advancement of nursing is tied directly to the advancement of all women's rights.
- Cohesiveness is developed among members of the nursing profession.
- Present nurse leaders are willing to empower the nurse leaders of the future by becoming mentors.
- Nurses support their leaders and regard them as advocates for nursing.
- Nurses are involved politically.
- The nurse's role is defined more clearly to the public.

Source: C. J. Huston and B. Marquis, Ten attitudes and behaviors necessary to overcome powerlessness, *Nursing Connections,* Summer 1988, 1:39–47. Reprinted by permission. Division of Nursing, The Washington Hospital Center, Washington, D.C., publisher.

In the past, nurses have often perceived themselves as powerless to influence nursing and bring about change. However, the sense of powerlessness is increasingly being recognized and overcome, and nurses are using power and political action to improve nursing and working conditions. Attitudes and behaviors necessary to overcome powerlessness are shown in the accompanying box.

Power

Patterns of behavior in groups are greatly influenced by the force of power. *Power* can be defined as the *capacity* to modify the conduct of others in a desired manner, while avoiding having one's own conduct modified in undesired ways by others (Stevens 1980, p. 208). Power is the ability to do or act, to deliver goods and services

on one's own terms, or to be in control or command over others (Ferguson 1985, p. 89).

Many people have a negative concept of power, likening it to control, domination, and even coercion of others by muscle and clout. However, power can be viewed as a vital, positive force that moves people toward the attainment of individual or group goals. The overall purpose of power is to encourage cooperation and collaboration in accomplishing a task.

Often the terms *power, influence,* and *authority* are used interchangeably, but they need to be differentiated. Power is the source of influence, whereas influence is the result of proper use of power. Authority is the official or legitimized right to use a given amount or type of power, i.e., the right to act and the right to command (Claus and Bailey 1977, p. 21). Authority may be either delegated or acquired. Power theorists describe a variety of sources of a person's power. Understanding these sources of power is prerequisite to formulating a plan for developing one's own power and to recognizing it in others.

- *Legitimate* (or positional) *power* is derived from one's formal position or title in an organization. It is associated with the authority that the position gives its holder to make and enforce decisions. The title "Vice President for Nursing" implies that the holder has power by virtue of the position, regardless of who holds that position or how effective that person is.
- *Reward power* is derived from the perception of one's ability to bestow rewards or favors on others.
- *Coercive power,* by contrast, arises from the perception of one's ability to threaten, harm, or punish others.
- *Information power* is associated with persons who are perceived to control key information.

Reward, coercive, and information power all relate to the degree an individual can control the distribution of resources.

- *Referent* (charismatic, or personal) *power* is power derived from an individual's own vision, sense of self, and ability to communicate these so that others regard the person with admiration and are motivated to follow.
- *Connection power* is derived from the perception that one has important contacts or relationships with others. These connections can be an aspect of both formal and informal networks.
- *Expert* (or knowledge) *power* is power derived from one's expertise, talents, and skills. One can include in

this category Benner's (1984) vision of power in caring; i.e., the positive power the nurse brings to the nurse-client relationship. This power enables the nurse to transform the client's life through advocacy and other means of caring.

Politics

What is politics? For many people the word *politics* evokes images of "crooked deals" hatched by men in "smoke-filled rooms," Watergate, the Iran-Contra dealings, bribes, and powerbrokers. More positive examples of political action are legislative initiatives to meet consumer needs and campaigns to elect nurse legislators. Although the words *crafty* and *unscrupulous* are sometimes included in the definition of *political,* a more positive definition is "having practical wisdom." Others describe politics as a means to an end, a process by which one can influence the decisions of others and thus exert control over events (Stevens 1980).

Politics can also be defined as "influencing the allocation of scarce resources" (Talbott and Vance 1981, p. 592). Defined in this way, the word denotes more than action in the governmental arena; it is also applicable to every sphere of life where resources are limited and more than one person or group competes for them (Ehrat 1983). The allocation of scarce resources involves everyone in some way. Consider the following examples:

- A student applying for a college loan or competing with other students for a fair share of a teacher's time and attention

- A client advocate competing for hospital education funds to do more preoperative teaching

- A citizen lobbying against the school board's proposal to divide one RN's time between two large schools

- A member of a professional association seeking association action on a practice issue, such as care of clients with acquired immune deficiency syndrome (AIDS)

Despite nurses' experience with the political realities affecting the allocation of scarce resources, many nurses still harbor negative images of anything associated with the word *politics*. For example, it is not unusual to hear a colleague say, "I like her; she does not play politics." Although this remark is meant as a compliment, apolitical nurses in today's world hinder not only themselves and their colleagues but also the profession. For example, the nursing school dean, the head nurse, and the nurse researcher must all be politically skilled if they are

to influence who gets how much of such scarce resources as funds for nursing education or nursing salaries, space for classrooms or offices, or release time to conduct research.

Why are nurses reluctant to engage in politics? Why do many view political activity as outside the realm of the professional nurse's role and responsibility? There are a number of reasons why nurses, and many women, have avoided becoming involved in political action. Among these are the following:

- There has been minimal recognition of the social activism of many of the profession's early leaders or of the efforts of nurses working together to effect legislative changes on issues relating to nursing and health.

- Prior to the contemporary wave of activism in women's rights, politics was considered an aggressive, men-only endeavor. Even though more women and nurses are becoming involved in governmental politics, many nurses have difficulty viewing the larger world of politics as an appropriate arena in which to participate. Women are socialized differently than men; for this reason, few women exert much influence on the male-dominated world of business and the professions.

- The fact that relatively few nurses know and appreciate their rich heritage also contributes to their discomfort with politics. Nurses who have been leaders and social activists, such as Lavinia Dock, Lillian Wald, Harriet Tubman, and Margaret Sanger, were all skilled politicians. Each was able to make significant contributions to the profession and society because of her political skills. Maybe they had read the wise words of the founder of modern nursing, Florence Nightingale:

    When I entered into service here, I determined that, happen what would, I *never* would intrigue among the Committee. Now I perceive that I do all my business by intrigue. I propose in private to A, B, or C the resolution I think A, B, or C most capable of carrying in Committee, and then leave it to them, and I always win (Huxley 1975, p. 53).

- Associated with the lack of appreciation of nursing history is the sparse education of nursing students, at the undergraduate and graduate level, on how to be politically astute. There is a critical need for students to have the opportunity to work with faculty and other preceptors who are skilled in the art of influencing governmental, organizational, workplace, and community politics.

Thus, a conscious effort needs to be made to educate nurses and nursing students about effective political action. Clearly, for such education to be effective, nurses must examine who they are as women and men and the values that they have been socialized to hold in relation to team play, power, and competition (Vance et al. 1985). This effort can be facilitated by learning more about how nursing leaders historically have used their political skills to bring about change, not only in the profession and health care but also in the values and actions of society as a whole.

Opportunities for Political Action

Government   Most people think of political action in relationship to local, state, or federal government. By voting, responsible citizens convey their opinions to elected and appointed officials on matters of concern. Many women first learn about political action through the educational efforts of the League of Women Voters. Other organizations—including the ANA, CNA, NLN, and NSNA—publish articles on legislative matters and encourage nurses to take action on behalf of health care consumers and the nursing profession. Nursing lobbyists at the state and national level work to influence the development of health policy and legislation, but their success depends on the active support of nurses who back up these paid lobbyists by doing personal lobbying among their own elected officials.

Workplace   Since most nurses work in hospitals and too few nurses derive professional satisfaction from working in these bureaucratic institutions, it seems logical that nurses would work together to change the nature of their workplace. Evidence that hospitals can be rewarding places for delivering quality health care to clients is documented in the American Academy of Nursing's (1983) study of hospitals with a fine record of attracting and retaining professional nurses.

The politics of client care impinges on the practice of every nurse. For example, as the prospective payment system becomes the norm, hospital stays will be cut more drastically in an effort to reduce health care costs (Shaffer 1984, p. 48). The need for nurses to be "faster and smarter" in delivering client care and client education will increase. Nurses are already feeling the pressure to prepare clients for discharge days earlier than before. How can nurses ensure that the quality of nursing care is maintained under the new system? One way is for nurses to collaborate with each other and other providers to eliminate nonnursing tasks, such as answering the telephone, emptying the garbage, and transporting non-

acute clients. Developing a demonstration project that compares cost and quality of care issues under different hospital unit structures can provide the necessary data and generate support from other providers and administrators for changing the role of staff nurses. This sort of "proactive" planning can empower nurses to take charge of nursing practice in ways that benefit clients and health professionals while conserving scarce resources such as money, time, and supplies.

Organizations   Powerful and influential professional associations, such as the ANA and CNA and their affiliated state/province and district associations, provide a collective voice for promoting nursing and quality health care. As such, they exert influence on the individual nurse as well as in the spheres of government, the workplace, the community, and the profession. Associations monitor and influence laws and regulations affecting nursing and health care. Their role in workplace matters ranges from studying practice issues to acting as the collective bargaining agent for nurses. Additionally, the professional nursing organization is often a visible presence in the community because it presents the nursing perspective on health care issues.

Community   The community in which the nurse lives and works can include the local neighborhood, the corporate world, the nation, and the international community. The community encompasses the workplace, professional organizations, and government. Many nurses, including Lillian Wald, founder of the Henry Street Settlement and modern public health nursing, view the community as more than a practice setting. Nurses who live in the community where they work can understand and influence the complex interplay among individuals and groups that compete for scarce resources.

Many communities depend on nurses to help with a wide variety of health and social policy decisions, such as environmental pollution and the feminization of poverty (Archer 1985). For example, a nurse who serves as an elected member of the community school board can influence decisions that affect the health and health care of students, such as the hiring of nurses for the school system. Nurses' opinions on matters of the public health are frequently sought, and the enterprising nurse looks for opportunities to promote a positive image of nursing while serving the community (Frost 1985). The nurse also identifies ways in which fellow citizens can support both consumer health and nursing agendas.

Guiding Principles for Political Action

The following list of "commandments" is designed to help newcomers to political activism consider some ideas to enhance their effectiveness.

1. *Look at the big picture.* Step back and take a look at the larger environment in which you live, work, and study. In the governmental sphere especially, nurses are too often described as concerned only with nursing issues rather than with a broad variety of consumer and health care issues.

   Nurses will not enjoy credibility as health experts unless they become more sensitive to the concerns of others and employ their expertise in all spheres. In the workplace, nurses often focus their attention on their own unit, neglecting to view their position and unit in relationship to the larger organization.

   Astute nurses are aware of the environmental factors that impinge on their work setting. For example, the advent of the prospective payment system has had a major effect on nursing practice and raised many issues regarding the quality of client care. Nurses who make an effort to "take off the blinders" will see and understand the complex forces that affect their practice, the status of the nursing profession, and the nature of health care delivery.

2. *Do your homework.* Homework is not something that ends with graduation. Nurses must take stock of their goals and clarify their personal and professional positions on issues. Taking stock requires setting time aside for reflection. Nurses who use the nursing process as a basis for planning client care can use the same problem-solving approach in their own behalf. For example, developing a strategy to convince the head nurse to support the development of a formal continuing education program for staff nurses requires research and planning and will be most successful if it is based on an understanding of change theory.

3. *Nothing ventured, nothing gained.* Nurses have always been risk takers. Margaret Sanger risked being jailed for promoting birth control. Lavinia Dock and her colleagues chained themselves to the White House fence to call attention to their belief that women should have the vote. Clara Maas lost her life while participating in research on malaria. If you have a dream, an idea, a vision of what might be— make it a reality.

4. *Get a toe in the door.* Incremental changes or actions may have a better chance of success than a major project. Resistance to change is more easily overcome if change is tested by a pilot project. For example, a nursing director is more apt to agree to the introduction of primary nursing on one unit rather than to an overall change in the nursing system of the whole hospital.

5. *"Quid pro quo."* "Something for something." "Scratch my back, and I'll scratch yours." "Everything and everybody has a price." Many nurses are offended by the implications of these aphorisms, believing that they represent a cynical view of human and organizational relationships. Others, however, concede that they represent a realistic view of life. Consider how you relate to your friends and colleagues: Don't you often find yourself making trade-offs?

   When assessing your position within your school of nursing, the clinical area, or among your peers, review your friendships, connections, and pragmatic relationships. Frequently men say, "He owes me one," implying the person has received a favor and will reciprocate. Women and nurses, however, rarely use those words. In fact, they seem uncomfortable with the idea of being "in debt" or owing a favor despite the fact that they participate in give-and-take situations every day. It is important to develop an ease in professional and personal relationships so that one feels connected and supported rather than isolated and resentful.

6. *Walk a mile in another's moccasins.* Nurses learn to evaluate clients, to assess "where they are coming from." But how often do they make similar inquiries of peers, supervisors, or friends? The politically astute nurse who wants to get ahead identifies the goals the head nurse has for the unit and finds ways to support those efforts and get help in meeting personal development goals. Identifying another's agenda can help one plan a win-win situation in which the staff nurse or student meets her or his own needs as well as those of the teacher or head nurse.

7. *Strike while the iron is hot.* Any plan for change must include a timetable that identifies the best time for a particular action. Few people would approach the head nurse to discuss the work schedule while a client is in cardiac arrest, but a surprising number of people give little thought to what might be an opportune time to discuss such a topic. Sometimes an eagerness to take action precludes some important questions: "Is this the best time to do this? Will it be received better now or later?"

8. *Read between the lines.* Some people reveal a lot by the information they choose not to share. Just as nurses listen with a "third ear" to their clients, politically astute nurses attend to colleagues, their bosses, and the work environment for cues that help them achieve some measure of control and influence.

9. *Half a loaf is better than none.* It is human nature to want it all, but the reality is that the world is far from perfect. People often need to learn to share the wealth and settle for less than they would like. One way to adjust to this reality is to develop an ability to identify alternative solutions or outcomes. Rather than setting one's heart on a particular goal, it is prudent to outline acceptable alternatives.

10. *Rome was not built in a day.* Because most nurses work in bureaucratic organizations, they need to accept the fact that change does not occur rapidly. Even in a small, flexible organization, change is often slow because the nature of the change process demands that one proceed only after careful deliberation. While political skills are gained only through practice, nurses who ponder and act on the principles that underlie political action gain the ability to view their efforts in perspective.

CHAPTER HIGHLIGHTS

▶ Client advocacy involves concern for and defined actions on behalf of another person or organization in order to bring about change.

▶ The functions of the nurse advocate are to inform and support.

▶ To be effective and influential in current and future health care delivery systems, nurses need to understand and apply change theory.

▶ Planned change requires problem-solving, decision-making skills, and interpersonal competence.

▶ Nurses frequently act as formal or informal change agents in relation to clients, support systems, and communities.

▶ Resistance to change can have a number of causes, including threatened self-interest, inaccurate perceptions, objective disagreement, psychological reactance, and low tolerance for change.

▶ Nurses who assume a change agent role can implement change using a nursing process framework.

▶ Nurses have been effective in promoting change in the workplace through professional organizations, in the legislative arena, and in the community.

▶ Nurses are actively participating in political processes to promote change within the profession and to be influential in policy-making regarding health issues.

LEARNING ACTIVITIES

■ Review your own ability to advocate for a client. Each of the following situations has several possible solutions. Each requires a change in one or more of the participants' behavior. How would you effect change in each situation? How would you advocate for each client? What information would you require to effectively advocate in each situation?

■ *The client as an individual*
Ronald James, a 58-year-old male, has been told he has terminal cancer of the pancreas. His physician has outlined a plan of treatment that includes chemotherapy to prolong the client's life. The client states that he wishes to refuse treatment and go home to be with his family. Utilizing Kohnke's actions of an advocate, how would you advocate for this client if he continues to refuse treatment? If he changes his mind and elects to follow the treatment plan?

■ *The client as a family*
Maria Rodriguez, a 32-year-old mother of six, confides to you that she does not wish to have any more children. However, she also states that her husband was one of 12 children and believes that a large family is important. She has discussed birth control with her husband and he has refused to consider the practice either for her or for himself. How

would you advocate for this family considering the different wishes of each spouse?

- ■ *The client as community*
The community in which you live has a high rate of pregnancy among unwed teenagers. Many of these teenagers are unable to finish school once they give birth and try to care for their babies. Some of the babies are suffering from abuse or neglect related to poor parenting skills. The School Board is concerned about the problem, but does not want to become involved in birth control counseling. How would you advocate for these teenagers?

READINGS AND REFERENCES

SUGGESTED READINGS

Benner, P. 1984. *From novice to expert: Excellence and power in clinical nursing practice*. Menlo Park, Calif.: Addison-Wesley Publishing Co.

This book is a major contribution to nursing. It provides a lucid description of nursing practice as it is rendered by expert nurses. It provides profound implications for nurses in administration, education, and practice.

Robinson, M. B. 1985. Patient advocacy and the nurse: Is there a conflict of interest? *Nursing Forum* 22:58–63.

Robinson explains that a patient advocate must be able to relate to patients and staff at all levels and must have certain qualities: self-motivation, objectivity, empathy, tact, flexibility, tenacity, a sense of humor, and the ability to cope with stress and pressure. The nurse who becomes a patient advocate should be aware of the possible conflicts of interest and the restrictions of the role. Robinson points out that most hospitals do not have written policies to protect the nurse in the advocacy role.

Welch, L. B. June 1979. Planned change in nursing: The theory. *Nursing Clinics of North America* 14:307–21.

Welch describes the theories of Lewin, Lippitt, Havelock, and Rogers. Welch maintains that planned change is an essential part of nursing intervention and important for quality client care.

RELATED RESEARCH

An examination of the relationship between Medicare prospective payment and the nursing shortage. November/December 1988. *Nursing Economics* 6:317–18.

Feldman, M. J., and Ventura, M. R. May/June 1984. Evaluating changes in using non-interval data. *Nursing Research* 33:182–84.

Heiskanan, T. A. November 1988. Nursing staff's perceptions of work in acute and long-term care hospitals. *Journal of Advanced Nursing* 13:716–24.

SELECTED REFERENCES

American Academy of Nursing. 1983. *Magnet hospitals: Attraction and retention of professional nurses*. Kansas City, Mo.: American Nurses' Association.

Annas, G. J. 1975. *The rights of hospital patients: The basic ACLU guide to a hospital patient's rights*. New York: Avon Books.

Archer, S. E. 1985. Politics and the community. In Mason, D. J., and Talbott, S. W., editors. *The political action handbook for nurses*. Menlo Park, Calif.: Addison-Wesley Publishing Co.

Benner, P. 1984. *From novice to expert: Excellence and power in clinical nursing practice*. Menlo Park, Calif.: Addison-Wesley Publishing Co.

Bennis, W. G., Benne, K. D., Chin, R., editors. 1985. *The planning of change*. 4th ed. New York: Holt, Rinehart & Winston.

Brooten, D. A. 1984. *Managerial leadership in nursing*. Philadelphia: J. B. Lippincott Co.

Brooten, D. A.; Hayman, L.; and Naylor, M. 1978. *Leadership for change: A guide for the frustrated nurse*. Philadelphia: J. B. Lippincott Co.

Canadian Nurses' Association. February 1981. *CNA Position Statements*. Ottawa: CNA.

Claus, K. E., and Bailey, J. T. 1977. *Power and influence in health care: A new approach to leadership*. St. Louis: C. V. Mosby Co.

Disparti, J. 1988. Nutrition and self care. In Caliandro, G., and Judkins, B. L. *Primary nursing practice*. Glenview, Ill.: Scott, Foresman & Co.

Donahue, M. P. 1985. Viewpoints. Euthanasia: An ethical uncertainty. In McCloskey, J. C., and Grace, H. K. *Current issues in nursing*. 2d ed. Boston: Blackwell Scientific Publications.

Ehrat, K. September 1983. A model for politically astute planning and decision making. *Journal of Nursing Administration* 13:29–34.

Ferguson, V. D. 1985. Power in nursing. In Mason, D. J., and Talbott, S. W., editors. *The political action handbook for nurses*. Menlo Park, Calif.: Addison-Wesley Publishing Co.

Frost, A. D. 1985. Working together: Local community action. In Mason, D. J., and Talbott, S. W., editors. *The political action handbook for nurses*. Menlo Park, Calif.: Addison-Wesley Publishing Co.

Havelock, R. 1973. *The change agent's guide to innovations in education*. Englewood Cliffs, N.J.: Educational Technology Publications.

Huxley, E. 1975. *Florence Nightingale*. New York: G. P. Putnam's Sons.

Kanter, F. H. and Goldstein, A. P., editors. *Helping people change: A textbook of methods*. New York: Pergamon Press.

Kemp, V. H. 1986. An overview of change and leadership. In Hein, E. C., and Nicholson, M. J., editors. *Contemporary leadership behavior: Selected readings*. 2d ed. Boston: Little, Brown and Co.

Kohnke, M. F. November 1980. The nurse as advocate. American Journal of Nursing 80:2038–40.

Kohnke, M. F. 1982. *Advocacy: risk and reality*. St. Louis: C. V. Mosby Co.

Kramer, M. 1974. *Reality shock: Why nurses leave nursing*. St. Louis: C. V. Mosby Co.

Lancaster, J., and Lancaster, W. 1982. *Concepts for advanced nursing practice: The nurse as change agent*. St. Louis: C. V. Mosby Co.

Leddy, S. and Pepper, J. M. 1985. *Conceptual bases of professional nursing*. Philadelphia: J. B. Lippincott Co.

Lewin, K. 1951. *Field theory in social science*. New York: Harper and Row.

———. 1948. *Resolving Social Conflicts*. G. W. Lewin, ed. New York: Harper and Brothers.

Lippitt, G. L. 1973. *Visualizing change: Model building and the change process*. La Jolla, Calif.: University Associates.

Lippitt, R., Hooyman, G., Sashkin, M., and Kaplan, J. 1978. *Resourcebook for planned change*. Ann Arbor, Mich.: Human Resource Development Associates of Ann Arbor, Inc.

Lippitt, R., Watson, J., and Westley, B. 1958. *The dynamics of planned change*. New York: Harcourt Brace and Co.

Mason, D. J., and Talbott, S. W., editors. 1985. *The political action handbook for nurses: Changing the workplace, government, organizations, and community*. Menlo Park, Calif.: Addison-Wesley Publishing Co.

McGovern, W. N., and Rodgers, J. A. May 1986. Change theory. *American Journal of Nursing* 86:566–67.

Mauksch, I. G., and Miller, M. H. 1981. *Implementing change in nursing*. St. Louis: C. V. Mosby Co.

New, J. R., and Couillard, N. A. March 1981. Guidelines for introducing change. *Journal of Nursing Administration* 11:17–21.

Olson, E. M. June 1979. Strategies and techniques for the nurse change agent. *Nursing Clinics of North America* 14:323–36.

Reinhard, S. C. 1988. Managing and initiating change. In Sullivan, E. J., and Decker, P. J. *Effective management in nursing*. 2d ed. Redwood City, Calif.: Addison-Wesley Publishing Co.

Rodgers, J. A. 1973. Theoretical considerations involved in the process of change. *Nursing Forum* 12:160.

Rogers, E. 1983. *Diffusion of innovations*. 3d ed. New York: Free Press.

Schaller, L. 1972. *The change agent*. New York: Abingdon Press.

Shaffer, F. (ed.) 1984. *DRG's: Changes and challenges*. New York: National League for Nursing.

Spradley, B. W. 1980. Making change creatively. *Journal of Nursing Administration* 10:32–37.

Stevens, B. February 1975. Effecting change. *Journal of Nursing Administration*. 5:23–25.

Stevens, B. J. November 1980. Power and politics for the nurse executive. *Nursing and Health Care* 1:208–10.

Talbott, S. W., and Vance, C. 1981. Involving nursing in a feminist group—NOW. *Nursing Outlook* 33:281–85.

Vance, C.; Talbott, S. W.; McBride, A. B.; and Mason, D. J. November/December 1985. An uneasy alliance: Nursing and the women's movement. *Nursing Outlook* 33:281–85.

HEALTH PERCEPTIONS AND HEALTH PROMOTION

Health, Wellness, Illness, and Disease

CONCEPTS OF HEALTH, WELLNESS, ILLNESS, AND DISEASE

Defining Health

Health is a changing, evolving concept that is basic to nursing. For centuries, the concept of disease was the yardstick by which health was measured. Until the late 19th century, the major concern of health professionals was the "how" of disease. Recently, there has been an increasing emphasis on health.

There is no consensus about any definition of health. There is knowledge of how to attain a certain level of health, but health itself cannot be measured. In 1947, the World Health Organization (WHO) proposed a broad definition of health: "Health is a state of complete physical, mental, and social well-being, and not merely the absence of disease or infirmity" (WHO 1947, p. 1). At the time, some considered this definition impractical; some view it as a possible goal for all people, while others consider complete well-being unobtainable. However, the WHO definition of health includes three characteristics basic to a positive concept of health:

■ It reflects concern for the individual as a total person rather than as merely the sum of various parts.

- It places health in the context of the environment.
- It equates health with productive and creative living (Pender 1987, p. 17).

In 1953, the [United States] President's Commission on Health Needs of the Nation stated: "Health is not a condition; it is an adjustment. It is not a state but a process. The process adapts the individual not only to our physical, but also our social environment" (President's Commission 1953, p. 4).

Because health is such a complex concept, various researchers have developed models or paradigms to explain health and in some instances its relationship to illness or injury. (A *model* or *paradigm* is an abstract outline or a theoretical depiction of a complex phenomenon.) A number of nurse-theorists have provided nursing-based definitions of health, wellness, and illness, which incorporate elements of certain models. See Table 13–1 for these definitions.

Clinical Model

The narrowest interpretation of health occurs in the clinical model (Smith 1981, p. 47). People are viewed as physiologic systems with related functions, and health is identified by the absence of signs and symptoms of disease or injury. To lay persons, it is considered the state of not being "sick." In this model, the opposite of health is disease or injury. Dunn describes health according to this model as "a relatively passive state of freedom from illness . . . a condition of relative homeostasis" (Dunn 1959b, p. 447).

Many medical practitioners use the clinical model. The focus of many medical practices is the relief of signs and symptoms of disease and the elimination of malfunctioning and pain. When the signs and symptoms of disease are no longer present in a person, the medical practitioner often considers that the individual's health is restored.

Ecologic Model

The ecologic model of health is based on the relationship of humans to their environment. This model has three interactive elements:

1. The host: a person or group who may or may not be at risk of acquiring an illness or disease
2. The agent: any factor in the environment that by its presence or absence can lead to illness or disease
3. The environment, including the extrinsic or intrinsic environment, which may or may not predispose the person to the development of disease (Payne 1983, p. 394)

The three elements of this model interact dynamically, and health is an ever-changing state.

Role Performance Model

Health is defined in terms of the individual's ability to fulfill societal roles, i.e., to perform work. According to this model, people who can fulfill their roles are healthy even if they appear clinically ill. For example, a man who works all day at his job as expected is healthy even though an x-ray film of his lung indicates a tumor. Parsons (1972) views health in this light. Health has also been defined as "the state of optimum capacity of an individual for the effective performance of his roles and tasks" (Parsons 1972, p. 107). An emphasis in this definition is the capacity of the individual rather than a commitment to roles and tasks.

It is assumed in this model that sickness is the inability to perform one's work. A problem with this model is the assumption that a person's most important role is the work role. People usually fulfill several roles, e.g., mother, daughter, friend, and certain individuals may consider nonwork roles paramount in their lives.

Adaptive Model

The focus of the adaptive model is adaptation. This model is derived from the writings of Dubos (1978), who views health as a creative process. Individuals are actively and continually adapting to their environments. In Dubos's view, the individuals must have sufficient knowledge to make informed choices about their health and also the income and resources to act on choices. Dubos believes that complete well-being is unobtainable, thus contradicting the 1947 WHO definition.

In the adaptive model, disease is a failure in adaptation. The aim of treatment is to restore the ability of the person to adapt, i.e., to cope. According to this model, extreme good health is flexible adaptation to the environment and interaction with the environment to maximum advantage (Smith 1981, p. 45). The focus of this model is stability, although there is also an element of growth and change.

Murry and Zentner indicate this growth and change in their definition of health: "a state of well-being in which the person is able to use purposeful, adaptive responses and processes, physically, mentally, emotionally, spiritually, and socially, in response to internal and external stimuli (stressors) in order to maintain relative stability and comfort and to strive for personal objectives and cultural goals" (Murray and Zentner 1985, pp. 4–5).

text continues on p. 229

TABLE 13-1 *Selected Nurse Theorists' Views of Health and Environment**

Nurse Theorist and Theory	Definition/Description	
	Health	Environment
Florence Nightingale (1954, 1969)	Being well and using one's powers to the fullest extent. Health is maintained through prevention of disease via environmental health factors. Disease is a reparative process nature institutes because of some want of attention.	The major concepts for health are ventilation, warmth, light, diet, cleanliness, and noise. Although the environment had social, emotional, and physical aspects, Nightingale emphasized the physical aspects.
Faye G. Abdellah (1960) Twenty-one nursing problems	A state mutually exclusive of illness, defined as a state when the individual has no unmet needs and no anticipated or actual impairments.	Suggests that clients interact with and respond to their environment, the nurse being part of the environment. The environment also includes home and community.
Virginia Henderson (1966, 1978) Definition of nursing	Viewed in terms of the individual's ability to perform 14 components of nursing care unaided (e.g. breathe normally, eat and drink adequately, and so on). Health is a quality of life basic to human functioning and requires independence and interdependence. It is the quality of health rather than life itself that allows a person to work most effectively and to reach his or her highest potential level of satisfaction in life. Individuals will achieve or maintain health if they have the necessary strength, will, or knowledge.	The aggregate of the external conditions and influences affecting the life and development of an organism.
Lydia E. Hall (1969) Core, Care, and Cure Model	Becoming ill is behavioral. Illness is directed by one's feelings-out-of-awareness, which are the root of adjustment difficulties. Healing can be hastened by helping people move in the direction of self-awareness.	
Martha E. Rogers (1970) Unitary human beings	Positive health symbolizes wellness. It is a value term defined by the culture or individual. Health and illness are considered "to denote behaviors that are of high value and low value."	The irreducible, four dimensional energy field identified by pattern and manifesting characteristics different from those of the parts. Each environmental field is specific to its given human field. They are identified by wave patterns manifesting continuous change, and both change continuously and creatively.

*The theorists are listed in chronologic order. See also Table 4-1 for definitions of *nursing* and *client*.

▶

Nurse Theorist and Theory	Definition/Description	
	Health	Environment
Sister Callista Roy (1970, 1976, 1984) Adaptation model	A state and a process of being and becoming an integrated and whole person. Lack of integration represents lack of health.	All the conditions, circumstances, and influences surrounding and affecting the development and behavior of persons or groups; the input into the person as an adaptive system involving both internal and external factors.
Dorothea E. Orem (1971, 1980, 1985) Self-care deficit theory	Health is a *state* that is characterized by soundness or wholeness of developed human structures and of bodily and mental functioning. It includes physical, psychologic, interpersonal, and social aspects. *Well-being* is used in the sense of individuals' perceived condition of existence. Well-being is a state characterized by experiences of contentment, pleasure, and certain kinds of happiness; by spiritual experiences; by movement toward fulfillment of one's self-ideal; and by continuing personalization. Well-being is associated with health, with success in personal endeavors, and with sufficiency of resources.	
Myra Estrine Levine (1973) Four conservation principles	Is socially determined and predetermined by social groups. It is not just an absence of pathologic conditions. The organism maintains its integrity in both internal and external environments through adaptive ability.	The context in which we live our lives. The environment is where we are constantly and actively involved. Each person has his or her own environment.
Dorothy E. Johnson (1980) Behavioral system model	Health is an elusive, dynamic state influenced by biologic, psychologic, and social factors. Health is reflected by the organization, interaction, interdependence, and integration of the subsystems of the behavioral system. Humans attempt to achieve a balance in this system; this balance leads to functional behavior. A lack of balance in the structural or functional requirements of the subsystems leads to poor health.	Consists of all factors that are not part of the individual's behavioral system but that influence the system and some of which can be manipulated by the nurse to achieve the health goal of the client. The individual links to and interacts with the environment.
Imogene King (1981) Goal attainment theory	A dynamic state in the life cycle; illness is an interference in the life cycle. Health implies continuous adaption to stress in the internal and external environment through the use of one's resources to achieve maximum potential for daily living.	Adjustments to life and health are influenced by an individual's interactions with environment. The environment is constantly changing.

▶

TABLE 13-1 *(continued)*

	Definition/Description	
Nurse Theorist and Theory	Health	Environment
Rosemarie Rizzo Parse (1981) Man-Living-Health	Is a lived experience, a synthesis of values, a way of living, and a process of being and becoming. It is not the absence of disease or a state of well-being. It cannot be placed on a continuum or linear entity that can be interrupted or qualified by terms such as good, bad, more or less. It is not man adapting to or coping with the environment.	Man and environment are inseparable—interchanging energy, unfolding together for greater complexity and diversity, influencing one another's rhythmic patterns of relating. Man and environment interchange energy to create what is in the world and man chooses the meaning given to the situation he creates.
Betty Newman (1982) Systems model	Wellness is the condition in which all parts and subparts of an individual are in harmony with the whole system. Wholeness is based on interrelationships of variables that determine the resistance of an individual to any stressor. Illness indicates lack of harmony among the parts and subparts of the system of the individual. Health is viewed as a point along a continuum from wellness to illness; health is dynamic, i.e., constantly subject to change. Optimal wellness or stability indicates that all a person's needs are being met. A reduced state of wellness is the result of unmet systemic needs. The individual is in a dynamic state of wellness-illness, in varying degrees, at any given time.	Both internal and external environments exist and a person maintains varying degrees of harmony and balance between them. It is all factors affecting and affected by the system.
Margaret A. Newman (1986) Theory of expanding consciousness	Encompasses disease and nondisease. It is regarded as the explication of the underlying pattern of the person and the environment. It is a process of developing awareness of self and environment together with increasing ability to perceive alternatives and respond in a variety of ways.	The larger whole; that which is beyond the consciousness of the individual. Consciousness is coextensive in the universe and resides in all matter.

Eudaemonistic Model The eudaemonistic model incorporates the most comprehensive view of health (Smith 1981, p. 44). Health is seen as a condition of actualization or realization of a person's potential. Actualization is the apex of the fully developed personality. (Maslow presents this concept of health. See Chapter 4). In this model, the highest aspiration of people is fulfillment and complete development, i.e., actualization. In the words of Dubos (1978, p. 74), health is primarily a "measure of each person's ability to do what he wants to do and become what he wants to become." It is the same as high-level wellness (see the next section). Illness, in this model, is a condition that prevents self-actualization.

Pender includes stabilizing and actualizing tendencies in her definition of health: "Health is the actualization of inherent and acquired human potential through satisfying relationships with others while adjustments are made as needed to maintain structural integrity and harmony with the environment" (1987, p. 27).

Personal Definitions of Health

Health is a highly individual perception. Meanings and descriptions of health vary considerably. An individual's personal definition of health may not agree with that of health professionals. The following factors influence an individual's definition of health.

- *Developmental status.* The idea of health is frequently related to a person's level of development. The ability to conceptualize a state of health and the ability to respond to changes in health are related directly to age. The nurse's knowledge of an individual's developmental status can facilitate assessment of the appropriateness of the person's behavior and help anticipate future behaviors.

- *Social and cultural influences.* Culture and social interactions also influence a person's notion of health. Each culture has ideas about health, and often these are transmitted from parents to children. For example, in some traditional Chinese families health is defined as a flow of energy (yin and yang). Yin is dark, cold, wet, negative, and female; yang is light, warm, dry, positive, and male. An imbalance of yin and yang results in disease.

RESEARCH NOTE

How Do Adults Define Health?

Do health care professionals and the consumers of health care share the same views about health? In order to make health promotion activities more effective, it is important to know the public's view of health. The purpose of a study done by Colantonio (1988) was to investigate the concept of health in an adult population. One hundred men and women were asked to respond in an interview to the question "What does being healthy mean to you?" Based on the responses, seven categories were identified. The approximate reponse frequencies for each category are as follows:

Being fit (36%):	"able to work," "able to take care of oneself"
Feeling well (16%):	"fresh," "feeling happy"
Not being ill (23%):	"not spending time at the doctor's"
Good health behaviors (12%):	"eating well," "not drinking too much"
Looking well (10%):	"good complexion," "not overweight"
Environment (4%):	"clean air," "having enough money"
Other (10%):	no response

The findings of this study indicate that the most common concept of health refers to feeling fit. This means being able to fulfill those activities of daily living that are both necessary and desirable and being in a positive emotional and physical state. The role of good health habits is considered an important factor in the maintenance of this positive state. Further statistical analysis reveals that there are no significant differences in the perceptions of health concepts between men and women or between younger and older age groups.

Implications: These findings suggest that providers of health care services should be aware that the consumer's concept of health may vary from that of the health care professional.

The results of the study also suggest that (a) health promotion communication should be delivered in positive terms; (b) the information provided may not have to vary for males and females or for different age groups; and (c) indicators of health status may be more useful if they are based on the degree of fitness rather than the degree of illness.

Source: A. Colantonio, Lay concepts of health, *Health Values,* September/October 1988, 12:3–7.

- *Previous experiences.* Experiences with health and illness also affect people's perceptions of health. Some people may consider a pain or dysfunction normal because they have experienced it before. Knowledge gained from these past experiences helps determine people's definitions of health.

- *Expectations of self.* Some people expect to be functioning at a high level physically and psychosocially all the time when they are healthy. They perceive any change in that level of functioning, therefore, as illness. Others expect variations in their level of functioning, and their definitions of health accommodate those variations.

- *Perception of self.* Another factor is how the individual perceives the self generally. These perceptions relate to such aspects of self as esteem, body image, needs, roles, and ability. When there is any threat or perceived threat to these views of self, the individual usually feels some anxiety and may need to reassess health and to redefine health itself. For example, a 75-year-old man who can no longer move large objects as he was accustomed to do may need to examine and redefine his concept of health in view of his age and abilities.

Nurses should be aware of their own personal definitions of health and should appreciate that other people have their own individual definitions as well. The person's definition of health influences behavior related to health and illness. By understanding clients' perceptions of health and illness, nurses can provide more meaningful assistance to help clients regain or attain a state of health. To facilitate development of a personal definition of health, see the accompanying box.

Developing a Personal Definition of Health

The following questions can help nurses develop a personal definition of health.

- Is a person more than a biophysiologic system?
- Is health more than the absence of disease symptoms?
- Is health solely the result of the interaction between host, agent, and environment?
- Is health the ability of an individual to perform work?
- Is health the ability of an individual to adapt to the environment?
- Is health a condition of a person's actualization?
- Is health a state or a process?
- Is health the effective functioning of self-care activities?
- Is health static or changing?
- Are health and wellness the same?
- Are disease and illness different?
- Are there levels of health?
- Are health and illness separate entities or points along a continuum?
- Is health socially determined?
- How do you rate your health and why?

Wellness and Well-Being

Wellness   Some people believe *wellness* and *health* are synonymous, while others believe they differ. Wellness is similar to actualization as defined in the eudaemonistic model of health. In 1959, Dunn differentiated good health from wellness: "Good health can exist as a relatively passive state of freedom from illness in which the individual is at peace with his environment—a condition of relative homeostasis. Wellness is an integrated method of functioning which is oriented toward maximizing the potential of which the individual is capable, within the environment where he is functioning" (Dunn 1959, p. 4).

Wellness can also be defined as an "active process of becoming aware of and making choices toward a higher level of well-being" (Hettler, 1979). These choices are influenced by the individual's self-concept, culture, and environment. Hettler proposes six dimensions of wellness (see Figure 13–1). The *physical dimension* encourages regular physical activity, cardiovascular flexibility and strength, knowledge about food and nutrition, medical self-care, and appropriate use of the medical system. It discourages excessive use of tobacco, drugs, and alcohol.

The *emotional dimension* focuses on the degree to which a person feels positive about the self and enthusiastic about life. It emphasizes awareness and acceptance of one's feelings, the capacity to manage one's feelings, the ability to cope effectively with stress, the ability to maintain satisfying relationships with others, and the assessment and acceptance of one's limitations. The *social dimension* focuses on the interdependence

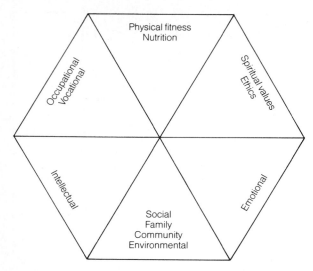

Figure 13-1 Six dimensions of wellness. *Source:* Bill Hettler, M.D., *Six dimensions of wellness* (Stevens Point, Wis.: National Wellness Institute, Inc., South Hall, 1319 Fremont Street, Stevens Point, WI 54481 (715) 346-2172). Used by permission.

with others and nature, development of harmony in the family, and contribution to the welfare of the human and environmental community. The *intellectual dimension* encourages stimulating and creative mental activities and the use of available community resources to expand one's knowledge and increase the potential for sharing with others. The *occupational dimension* focuses on preparation for work that will produce personal satisfaction and enrichment of life. The *spiritual dimension* involves seeking meaning and purpose in human life.

Clark's concept of wellness includes both health and illness. She describes wellness (1986, p. 3) as a process of moving toward greater awareness of oneself and the environment; it is unique to the individual and purposeful in direction. Wellness, health, and illness are dynamic patterns, changing with time and social patterns. Therefore, they must be continuously reevaluated. Ill persons can experience wellness if they have joy in living or a purpose and appreciation of life. The wellness process can be pursued to prevent illness, to assist in rehabilitation, to enhance the quality of life, or to maximize one's potential (Murray and Zentner 1989, p. 570).

In his book about high-level wellness in the individual, Dunn (1973) explores the concept of wellness as it relates to family, community, environment, and society. He believes that family wellness enhances wellness in

individuals. In a well family that offers trust, love, and support, the individual does not have to expend energy to meet basic needs and can move forward on the wellness continuum. By providing effective sanitation and safe water, disposing of sewage safely, and preserving beauty and wildlife, the community enhances both family and individual wellness. Environmental wellness is related to the premise that humans must be at peace with and guard the environment. Societal wellness is significant because the status of the larger social group affects the status of smaller groups. Dunn believes that social wellness must be considered on a worldwide basis.

Well-Being Well-being is a subjective perception of balance, harmony, and vitality (Leddy and Pepper 1989, p. 207). According to Leddy and Pepper, well-being occurs in levels. At the highest levels, a person feels satisfaction and a sense of contributing; such persons might place their state of well-being at the top of a plus-3 scale. At the lowest levels, people see themselves as ill and may place their state of well-being at the bottom of a minus-3 scale. Leddy and Pepper also state that well-being is a state that can be described objectively and therefore can be measured. In contrast, health, which encompasses "well-being, illness, disease and nondisease is an evolving potential that cannot be quantified" (Leddy and Pepper 1989, p. 208).

Illness, Sickness, and Disease

Illness is a highly personal state in which the person feels unhealthy or ill. Illness may or may not be related to disease. An individual could have a disease, for example, a growth in the stomach, and not feel ill. Parsons defines illness as "a state of disturbance in the normal functioning of the total human individual, including both the state of the organism as a biological system, and of his person and social adjustments" (Parsons 1972, p. 107).

Sickness is a status or social entity that is usually associated with disease or illness but can occur independently of them (Twaddle 1977, p. 97). When a person is defined as sick, several dependent behaviors are accepted that otherwise might be considered unacceptable. Bauman (1965, p. 206) found that people use three distinct criteria to determine whether they are ill:

1. The presence of symptoms, such as elevated temperature or pain

2. Their perceptions of how they feel; for example, good, bad, sick

3. Their ability to carry out daily activities, such as a job or schoolwork

Disease can be described as an alteration in body functions resulting in a reduction of capacities or a shortening of the normal life span (Twaddle 1977, p. 97). Disease may further be described as *acute* or *chronic, communicable, congenital, degenerative, functional, malignant, psychosomatic,* or *idiopathic.* Intervention by physicians has the goal of eliminating or ameliorating disease processes. Primitive people thought disease was caused by "forces" or spirits. Later, this belief was replaced by the single-causation theory. Increasingly, a number of factors are considered to interact in causing disease and determining the individual's response to treatment.

The causation of disease is called its etiology. A description of the etiology of a disease includes the identification of all causal factors that act together to bring about the particular disease. For example, the tubercle bacillus is designated as the biologic agent of tuberculosis. However, other etiologic factors, such as age, nutritional status, and even occupation, are involved in the development of tuberculosis and influence the course of infection.

Risk factors are situations, habits, or other phenomena that increase a person's vulnerability to illness or injury. Risk factors can be categorized into five interrelated areas: genetic makeup, age, physiologic factors, lifestyle, and environment: Examples of each follow:

- *Genetic makeup.* A person with a family history of diabetes mellitus or cancer is at risk of developing the disease later in life.

- *Age.* The risk of birth defects and complications of pregnancy increases after age 35; the risk of communicable disease is higher in school-age children; and the risk of cardiovascular disease increases with age for both sexes.

- *Physiologic factors.* Pregnancy places the fetus and mother at increased risk of disease; obesity increases the risk of heart disease.

- *Life-style or health habits.* Overeating increases the risk of heart disease; smoking increases the risk of lung cancer; poor nutrition leads to several deficiencies; promiscuity increases the risk of sexually transmitted disease; excessive use of alcohol increases the risk of accident, liver disease, and disability; unabated stress increases the risk of accidents and illness; and certain activities such as skiing or mountain climbing increase the risk of injury.

- *Environment.* Exposure to specific hazards, such as asbestos, rubber, and plastic, increases the risk of certain kinds of cancer; unclean, overcrowded living conditions predispose people to infections and other communicable diseases; air, water, and noise pollution all increase susceptibility to illness.

All of these risks present challenges to health care workers, especially nurses, in terms of prevention. Measures to enhance health include maintaining ideal body weight; eating regular meals with few snacks; elimination of cigarette smoking; moderation of alcohol consumption; safety measures, such as using seat belts, to prevent accidents and injuries; and periodic screening for such health problems as cancer. See Chapter 15.

In 1974, Marc Lalonde, Canadian minister of national health and welfare, introduced the *health field concept.* In this view, all causes of death and disease have four contributing elements: (a) human biologic factors, such as genetic makeup and age; (b) behavioral factors or unhealthy life-styles; (c) environmental hazards; and (d) inadequacies in the health care system (Canadian Department of National Health and Welfare 1974, pp. 31–34). Using these four elements as a framework, a group of United States experts devised a method to assess the relative contributions of each of these elements to the ten leading causes of death in 1976. The results indicated that approximately 50% of deaths were due to unhealthy behavior or life-style; 20% to human biologic factors; 20% to environmental factors; and 10% to inadequacies in health care (U.S. DHEW 1979, p. 9). These results have implications for nursing; the most important is that a substantial number of deaths could be avoided by efforts directed at health promotion and illness prevention. The leading causes of death in the United States in 1986 are shown in Table 13–2.

Traditionally, medical practitioners have dealt with disease at a subsystem level. Subsystems are those aspects of the body subsumed in the larger system of the whole body. (See systems theory in Chapter 4.) A subsystem may be a cell, an organ, or an organ system. Only recently have medical practitioners started looking at the person as an entity, or whole. Nurses, by contrast, have traditionally viewed the person as an entity, taking a holistic view of people. Nursing practice today is based on the multiple-causation theory of health problems. Unemployment, pollution, life-style, and stressful events, while not disease, may all contribute to illness. These can be considered suprasystem problems, i.e., problems stemming from systems in which the individual is a subsystem. See Figure 13–2. Thus, the concept of illness must include all aspects of the total person as well

TABLE 13-2 *Leading Causes of Death in the United States in 1986*

Cause	Deaths per 100,000 Residents
Diseases of the heart	317.5
Malignant neoplasms	194.7
Cerebrovascular diseases	62.1
Accidents	39.5
Chronic obstructive pulmonary disease	31.8
Pneumonia and influenza	29.0
Diabetes mellitus	15.4
Suicide	12.8
Chronic liver disease and cirrhosis	10.9
Atherosclerosis	9.4
Homicide	9.0

Source: U.S. Center for Health Statistics, U.S. Bureau of the Census, *Monthly vital statistics report,* vol. 37, no. 6 supplement, in *Statistical abstract of the United States,* 109th ed. (Washington D.C.:U.S Government Printing Office, 1989), p. 79, Table 118.

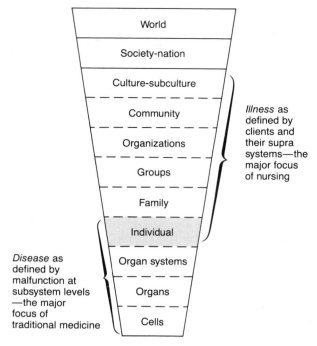

Figure 13-2 A systems hierarchy differentiating illness from disease and nursing from traditional medicine. *Source:* Knopke, H. J., and Diekelmann, N. L., editors, *Approaches to teaching primary health care* (St. Louis: C. V. Mosby Co., 1981). St. Louis, Mosby © 1981. Used with permission.

as the biologic and genetic factors that contribute to disease. Illness, then, is influenced by a person's family, social network, environment, and culture (Kneisl and Ames 1986, p. 18).

The Health-Illness Continuum

Health and illness can be considered either as points along one continuum, as related but separate entities, or as separate entities. (A continuum is a grid or graduated scale.)

Dunn describes a health grid in which a health axis and an environmental axis intersect. The resulting quadrants represent degrees of health and wellness. See Figure 13–3. This grid is intended to demonstrate the interaction of the environment with the continuum from well-being to illness. Jahoda conceptualizes health and illness along separate but coexisting continua (see Figure 13–4). The double continuum reflects the fact that people exhibit health and illness in varying degrees at the same time (Jahoda 1958, p. 75). This approach allows one to view a person's strengths (health) and illnesses at the same time.

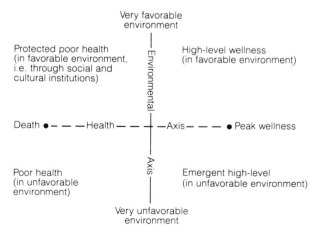

Figure 13-3 Dunn's health grid: its axes and quadrants. *Source:* H. L. Dunn, High-level wellness for man and society, *American Journal of Public Health,* June 1959, 49:788. Reprinted with permission.

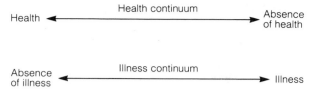

Figure 13-4 Jahoda's coexisting health and illness continua.

The concept of wellness is related to health promotion (see Chapter 15), which places emphasis on the whole person and self-responsibility for health. Ryan and Travis (1981) incorporate this idea in their health-illness continuum ranging from high-level wellness to premature death. They include a treatment model and a wellness model. See Figure 13–5.

HEALTH STATUS, BELIEFS, AND BEHAVIORS

The *health status* (state) of an individual is the health of that person at a given time. In its general meaning, the term may refer to anxiety, depression, or acute illness and thus describes the individual's problem in general. Health status can also describe such specifics as pulse rate and body temperature. The *health beliefs* of an individual are those concepts about health that an individual believes true. Such beliefs may or may not be founded on fact. Some of these are influenced by culture, such as the "hot-cold" system of some Hispanic Americans. In this system, health is viewed as a balance of hot and cold qualities within a person. Citrus fruits

and some fowl are considered cold foods, and meats and bread are hot foods. In this context, hot and cold do not denote temperature or spiciness but innate qualities of the food. For example, a fever is said to be caused by an excess of hot foods. Another example of a culturally related health belief is the belief that health and illness are closely associated with the amount and quality of blood in the body. For example, among some Southern whites and blacks, "high blood," caused by too much blood in the body, causes headaches and dizziness (Mitchell and Loustau 1981, pp. 41–42). For additional information about ethnic views of health and illness, see Chapter 24.

Health behaviors are the actions people take to understand their health state, maintain an optimal state of health, prevent illness and injury, and reach their maximum physical and mental potential. Behaviors such as eating wisely, exercising, paying attention to signs of illness, following treatment advice, and avoiding known health hazards such as smoking are all examples. The ability to relax, emotional maturity, productivity, and self-expression also affect one's health (McCann/Flynn and Heffron 1988, pp. 37–38).

Individual health behaviors may or may not be recommended by health care professionals. For example, an individual who believes that drinking several bottles of beer each day keeps the intestines free of infection may refuse to accept advice against this practice, even in life-threatening situations.

Health behavior is intended to prevent illness or disease or to provide for early detection of disease. Nurses preparing a plan of care with an individual need to consider the person's health beliefs before they attempt to change health behaviors. Otherwise, the individual may reject the nurses' suggestions and become angry because of intrusion into personal habits.

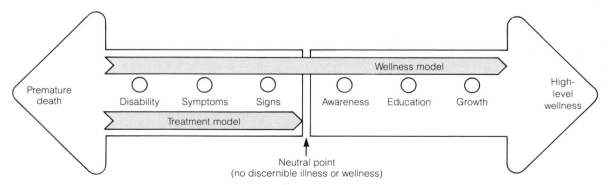

Figure 13-5 Health-illness continuum. Reprinted from Wellness Workbook© 1981, 1988 by John W. Travis M. D. and Sara Regina Ryan, with permission of Ten Speed Press, Berkeley, California.

Variables Affecting Health Status

Multiple variables influence a person's health status. Some of these are internal factors, such as the person's genetic makeup, and others are external, such as the person's culture and physical environment.

Genetic Makeup Genetic makeup influences biologic characteristics, innate temperament, activity level, and intellectual potential. It has been related to susceptibility to specific disease, such as diabetes and breast cancer.

Race Disease distribution is associated with race. For example, blacks have a higher incidence of sickle-cell anemia and hypertension than the general population, and native American Indians have a higher rate of diabetes.

Sex Certain acquired and genetic diseases are more common in one sex than in the other. Disorders more common among females are osteoporosis; autoimmune disease, such as rheumatoid arthritis and systemic lupus erythematosus; anorexia nervosa and bulimia; gallbladder disease; obesity; and thyroid disease. Those more common among males are stomach ulcers, abdominal hernias, respiratory diseases, arteriosclerotic heart disease, hemorrhoids, and tuberculosis. Obviously, diseases that affect reproductive organs, such as testicular or uterine tumors, are sex dependent.

Age and Developmental Level Distribution of disease varies with age. For example, arteriosclerotic heart disease is common in middle-aged males but occurs infrequently in younger persons; such communicable diseases as whooping cough and measles are common in children but are rare in older persons, who have acquired immunity to them. Developmental level is also a significant factor. Capabilities for responding to disease are less during the first few years of life and again near the end of life. Infants lack physiologic and psychologic maturity. Declining physical and sensory-perceptual abilities in older persons limit their ability to respond to environmental hazards and stressors.

Mind-Body Relationship Mind-body relationships—i.e., how emotional responses to stress affect body function and what emotional reactions occur in response to body conditions—also influence health. Emotional distress may increase susceptibility to organic disease or precipitate it. Emotional distress may influence the immune system through central nervous system and endocrine alterations. Alterations in the immune system are related to the incidence of infections, cancer, and autoimmune diseases. Increasing attention is being given to the mind's ability to direct the body's functioning. Relaxation, meditation, and biofeedback techniques are gaining wider recognition by individuals and health care professionals.

Life-Style A person's life-style includes patterns of eating; exercise; use of tobacco, drugs, and alcohol; and methods of coping with stress. Overeating, getting insufficient exercise, and being overweight are closely related to the incidence of heart disease, arteriosclerosis, diabetes, and hypertension. Excessive sugar intake increases the risk of dental caries. Abuse of drugs and alcohol is physically and mentally debilitating. Excessive use of tobacco is clearly implicated in lung cancer, emphysema, and cardiovascular diseases.

Physical Environment The physical environment, including housing and sanitation facilities also affects health. Air, food, and water pollutants are often directly or indirectly related to various types of cancer. Extreme fluctuations in environmental temperature cause temporary disruptions in a person's internal environment, and the person in such an environment must expend more energy to restore physiologic stability. Persons with minimal physical coping responses are more susceptible to the effects of hypothermia and hyperthermia. Seasonal variations also affect health and the incidence of certain illnesses. For example, drownings and insect bites occur more frequently in the summer, whereas allergic reactions occur more frequently when pollen and related allergens are present.

Standards of Living An individual's standard of living (reflecting occupation, income, and education) is related to health, morbidity, and mortality. Hygiene, food habits, and the propensity to seek health care advice and follow health regimens vary among high- and low-income groups. For example, preventing illness may not have as high a priority among the poor as generating and maintaining an income; even when it is a priority, the poor may not be able to afford regular medical examinations, housing, or nutritious foods that promote health. Occupational roles, also predispose people to certain illnesses. For instance, some industrial workers may be exposed to carcinogenic agents. More affluent people may fulfill stressful social or occupational roles that predispose them to stress-related diseases. Such roles may also encourage overeating or social use of drugs or alcohol.

Cultural Beliefs How a person perceives, experiences, and copes with health and illness is partly determined by cultural beliefs. Some people may perceive home remedies or tribal health customs as superior and more dependable than the health care practices of North American society. Cultural rules, values, and beliefs give people a sense of being stable and able to predict outcomes. The challenging of old beliefs and values by second-generation ethnic groups may give rise to conflict, instability, and insecurity, in turn contributing to illness.

Family In addition to transmitting genetic predispositions, the family passes on patterns of daily living and life-styles to offspring. Physical or emotional abuse may cause long-term health problems. Emotional health depends on a social environment that is free of excessive tension and does not isolate the person from others. A climate of open communication, sharing, and love fosters the fulfillment of the person's optimum potential.

Self-Concept How a person feels about the self (the self concept) affects how that person perceives and handles situations. Such attitudes can affect health practices and the times when treatment is sought. A sense of extreme hopelessness, despair, or fear may cause disease and even death. An example is the anorexic woman who deprives herself of needed nutrients because she believes she is too fat even through she is well below an acceptable weight level.

Support Network and Job Satisfaction

Having a support network (family, friends, or a confidant) and job satisfaction helps people avoid illness (Grasser and Craft 1984, p. 210). Support people also help the person confirm that illness exists. Persons with inadequate support networks sometimes allow themselves to become increasingly ill before confirming the illness and seeking therapy. Support people also provide the stimulus for an ill person to become well again. Job satisfaction positively influences both the individual's self-concept and mind-body relationship.

Geography Geography determines climate, and climate affects health. For instance, malaria and malaria-related conditions, e.g., sickle-cell hemoglobin, occur more frequently in tropical than temperate climates (Overfield 1985, p. 84). Multiple sclerosis is more prevalent in northern and central Europe, southern Canada, and the northern United States, for example, than in Asia, Africa, Mexico, and Alaska (Overfield 1985, p. 127).

Factors Influencing Health Behavior

Some factors affecting health status also affect health behavior; cultural and family influences are two examples. However, people can usually control their health behaviors and can choose healthy or unhealthy activities. In contrast, people have little or no choice over their genetic makeup, age, sex, physical environments, culture, or area of residence. This section outlines the factors that affect a person's health beliefs and behavior.

Health Belief Model In the 1950s, Rosenstock (1974) proposed a *health belief model* (HBM) intended to predict which individuals would or would not use such preventive measures as screening for early detection of cancer. Becker (1974) modified the health belief model to include these components: *individual perceptions, modifying factors,* and *variables likely to affect initiating action.*

The health belief model is based on motivational theory. Rosenstock assumed that good health is an objective common to all people. Becker added "positive health motivation" as a consideration. See Figure 13–6.

Individual Perceptions Individual perceptions include the following:

- *Perceived susceptibility.* A family history of a certain disorder, such as diabetes or heart disease, may make the individual feel at high risk.

- *Perceived seriousness.* The question here is: In the perception of the individual, does the illness cause death or have serious consequences? Growing concern about the spread of AIDS (acquired immune deficiency syndrome) reflects the general public's perception of the seriousness of this illness.

- *Perceived threat.* According to Becker, perceived susceptibility and perceived seriousness combine to determine the total perceived threat of an illness to a specific individual. For example, a person who perceives that many individuals in the community have AIDS may not necessarily perceive a threat of the disease; if the person is a drug addict or a homosexual, however, the perceived threat of illness is likely to increase because of the combined susceptibility and seriousness.

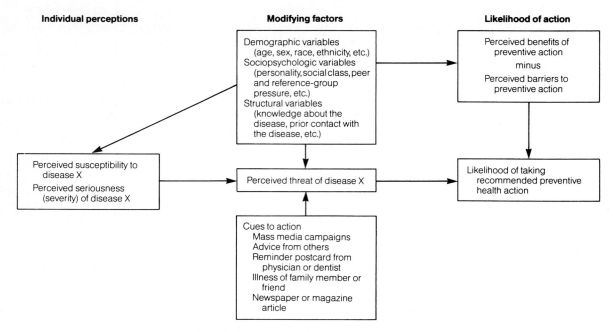

Individual perceptions **Modifying factors** **Likelihood of action**

Demographic variables
(age, sex, race, ethnicity, etc.)
Sociopsychologic variables
(personality, social class, peer
and reference-group
pressure, etc.)
Structural variables
(knowledge about the
disease, prior contact with
the disease, etc.)

Perceived benefits of
preventive action
minus
Perceived barriers to
preventive action

Perceived susceptibility to
disease X
Perceived seriousness
(severity) of disease X

Perceived threat of disease X

Likelihood of taking
recommended preventive
health action

Cues to action
Mass media campaigns
Advice from others
Reminder postcard from
physician or dentist
Illness of family member or
friend
Newspaper or magazine
article

Figure 13-6 The health belief model. *Source:* From Becker, M. H., Haefner, D. P., Kasi, S. V. et al. Selected psychosocial models and correlates of individual health-related behaviors. *Medical Care* 1977. 15:27–46. Used with permission.

Modifying Factors

Factors that modify a person's perceptions include the following:

- *Demographic variables* such as age, sex, race, ethnicity, etc. An infant, for example, does not perceive the importance of a healthy diet; an adolescent may perceive peer approval as more important than family approval and participate as a consequence in hazardous activities or adopt unhealthy eating and sleeping patterns; some ethnic groups consider it inappropriate to seek medical advice unless one is seriously ill.

- *Sociopsychologic variables.* Social pressure or influence from peers or other reference groups (e.g., self-help or vocational groups) may encourage preventive health behaviors even when individual motivation is low. Expectations of others may motivate people, for example, to obtain immunizations for their children, not to drive an automobile after drinking alcohol, to attend dental clinics, and to perform techniques such as breast self-examination for the early detection of cancer.

- *Structural variables* presumed to influence preventive behavior are knowledge about the target disease and prior contact with it. Becker found higher compliance rates with prescribed treatments among mothers whose children had frequent ear infections and occurrences of asthma.

- *Cues to action.* Cues can be either internal or external. Internal cues include feelings of fatigue, uncomfortable symptoms, or thoughts about the condition of an ill person who is close. External cues are listed in Figure 13–6.

Likelihood of Action

The likelihood of a person taking recommended preventive health action depends on the perceived benefits of the action minus the perceived barriers to the action.

- *Perceived benefits of preventive action.* Examples include refraining from smoking to prevent lung cancer and to increase ventilatory capacity; eating nutritious foods and avoiding snacks to maintain slenderness.

- *Perceived barriers to action* can include cost, inconvenience, unpleasantness, and life-style changes.

Pender (1975) adds two further considerations: The importance of health as perceived by the individual and perceived control.

1. *The importance of health to the person.* Behavior indicating that health is perceived as something of value includes providing special foods and vitamins to keep children well, having regular dental checkups, and participating in screening tests for cervical cancer, breast cancer, and cardiovascular disorders.

2. *Perceived control.* People who perceive that they have control over their own health are more likely to use preventive services than people who feel powerless. Control over health can relate to such behaviors as not smoking, maintaining an appropriate weight, using seat belts, or obtaining immunizations for influenza.

Nurses play a major role in helping clients implement healthy behaviors. Nurses help clients monitor health, supply anticipatory guidance, and impart knowledge about health. Nurses can also reduce barriers to action, e.g., by minimizing inconvenience or discomfort, and can support preventive actions. For additional information about nursing activities that promote health and instruments to assess perceptions of health control, see Chapter 15.

Health Care Compliance

Compliance is the extent to which a person's behavior coincides with health practitioners' advice. Clients' compliance with health care advice is of concern to all health professionals. Yoos reports that 86% of studies of compliance report noncompliance in more than 30% of clients (Yoos 1981, p. 27). Compliance can be complete, partial, or nonexistent.

Whether a person complies to a therapeutic regimen depends on many variables, among them age, education, costs, the complexity of the regimen and its convenience, the individual's value of health, and the inconvenience of the illness itself. In 1974, Becker published a sick role model to explain how people react to illness and to predict whether they will comply with health care advice (Becker 1974). See Figure 13–7. Becker's model

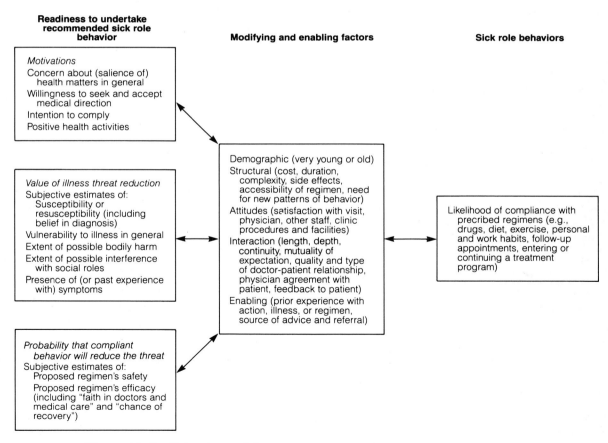

Figure 13-7 Sick role model. ***Source:*** Modified from M. H. Becker, The health belief model and sick role behavior, in M. H. Becker, editor, *The health belief model and personal health behavior* (Thorofare, N.J.: Charles B. Slack, 1974). Reprinted with permission.

indicates that compliance is related to (a) the client's motivation to become well, (b) the value the client places on reducing the threat of illness, and (c) the client's belief that compliance will reduce that threat. Modifying and enabling factors of people's behavior include age, cost, duration, attitudes of health care personnel, interaction with health care personnel, previous health care experiences, and sources of advice.

Researchers have investigated why some people comply with therapeutic regimens and others do not and how to help clients comply with therapeutic regimens. The first step is identifying noncompliance. The nurse can ask the client if the regimen is being followed. If the client is not complying, the nurse needs to find out why and intervene to assist the client in complying. To enhance compliance, nurses can do the following:

- *Demonstrate caring.* The nurse can do so by showing sincere concern about the client's problems and decisions and at the same time accepting the client's right to a course of action. For example, a nurse might tell a client who is not taking his heart medication, "I can appreciate how you feel about this, but I am very concerned about your heart."

- *Encourage healthy behaviors through positive reinforcement.* If the man who is not taking his heart medication is walking every day, the nurse might say, "You are really doing well with your walking."

- *Establish why the client is not following the regimen.* Where indicated, the nurse can provide information, correct misconceptions, attempt to decrease expense, or suggest counseling if psychologic problems are interfering with compliance.

- *Use aids to reinforce teaching.* For instance, the nurse can leave pamphlets for the client to read later or make a "pill calendar," a paper with the date and number of pills to be taken.

- *Establish a therapeutic relationship of freedom, mutual understanding, and mutual responsibility with the client and support persons.* By providing knowledge, skills, and information, the nurse gives clients control over their health and establishes a cooperative relationship, which results in greater compliance (MacElveen-Hoehn 1983, p. 535).

ILLNESS BEHAVIORS

Various scientists have described the stages of illness. By knowing these stages and the illness behaviors that accompany them, nurses can better understand their cli-

ents' behavior and determine ways to assist them. *Illness behavior* is "any activity undertaken by a person who feels ill, to define the state of his health and to discover a suitable remedy" (Igun 1979, p. 445). How people behave when they are ill is affected by many variables, such as age, sex, occupation, socioeconomic status, religion, ethnic origin, psychologic stability, personality, education and modes of coping. Suchman (1972, p. 145) describes five stages of illness:

Symptom Experience Stage
The symptom experience stage is the transition stage during which people come to believe something is wrong. Either a significant person mentions that they look unwell, or people experience some symptoms, which can appear insidiously. The symptom experience stage has three aspects:

- The physical experience of symptoms (e.g., pain or elevated temperature)
- The cognitive aspect (the interpretation of the symptoms in terms that have some meaning to the person)
- The emotional response (e.g., fear or anxiety)

During this stage, unwell persons usually consult others close to them about their symptoms or feelings. People validate with their spouses or support persons that the symptoms are real. At this stage, sick persons sometimes try home remedies, such as laxatives or cough medicines.

Assumption of the Sick Role
The second stage signals acceptance of the illness. At this time, individuals decide that their symptoms or concerns are sufficiently severe to suggest that they are sick. Some people seek professional help quickly; others continue self-treatment, often following the suggestions of family and friends.

In this stage, sick people are usually afraid, but they now accept that they are ill even though they may not be able to accept the possible reasons. In conferring with people close to them, sick people seek not only advice but also support for the decision to give up some activities and, for example, stay home from work.

At the end of this stage, sick people experience one of two outcomes. They may find that the symptoms have changed and that they feel better. If family members support the perceptions of such persons, they are no longer considered or consider themselves sick. Then the recovered persons resume normal obligations, such as returning to work or attending a school concert.

If, however, the symptoms persist or increase and if lack of improvement is validated by the family or significant others, then sick people know they should seek some treatment. The choice of a treatment plan is often affected by the known available alternatives and previous experience.

Medical Care Contact Stage

Sick people seek the advice of a health professional either on their own initiative or at the urging of significant others. When people go for professional advice they are really asking for three types of information:

- Validation of real illness
- Explanation of the symptoms in understandable terms
- Reassurance that they will be all right or prediction of what the outcome will be

If the health professional does not validate illness, people have two recourses: to return to normal activities or to seek other advice. If the symptoms disappear, people often perceive that they really are not ill. If symptoms continue, people usually return to the health professional or go to a second person for care. People who are repeatedly told that they are not ill may seek out quasi-practitioners as a last resort to alleviate the perceived symptoms. Some people will go from health professional to health professional until they find someone who provides a diagnosis that fits their own perceptions.

Most people also want an understandable explanation of their symptoms. When symptoms are not explained, people may assume the health professional does not believe them or perhaps that they are imagining the symptoms. Overly technical explanations, however, often confuse and frighten people.

People often experience anxiety about seeking help with health problems. Even minor symptoms can be construed as serious. Therefore, clients need reassurance that they will be cured. Even when this reassurance cannot be given, most people want to know the likely outcome.

Dependent Patient Role Stage

When a health professional has validated that the person is ill, the individual becomes a client, dependent on the professional for help. During this stage, sick people may or may not be reluctant to accept a professional's recommendations. They may vacillate about what is best for them and alternately accept and reject the professional's suggestions. People vary greatly in the degree of ease with which they can give up their independence, particularly in relation to life and death. Role obligations—such as those of wage earner, father, mother, student, baseball team member, or choir member—complicate the decision to give up independence.

It is also common for the client and the health professional to hold different notions of the nature of the illness, unless complete and open communication exists. During this stage, a nurse can often provide information that may allay some fears and/or provide data that support the person. Misconceptions can result from limited information, which clients interpret in the light of their experiences. For example, a woman may be told by a physician that there is a small encapsulated growth in the right groin and that surgical removal is advised. If the woman's mother died after being told she had a growth in her breast, that person may assume that she also will die.

Most people accept their dependence on the physician, although they retain varying degrees of control over their own lives. For example, some people request precise information about their diseases, their treatment, and the cost of treatment, and they delay the decision to accept treatment until they have all this information. Others prefer that the physician proceed with treatment and do not request additional information.

During this period, sick people often become more passive and accepting. They require a predictable environment in which people are genuinely concerned about them. In addition to being concerned about themselves, some sick people regress to an earlier behavioral stage in their development. As a result, they may have fewer coping mechanisms (physical and emotional adaptive or defensive abilities). Frequently reactions are related to previous experiences and to misconceptions about what will happen.

People have varying dependence needs. For some, illness may meet dependence needs that have never been met and thus provide satisfaction. Other people have minimal dependence needs and do everything possible to return to independent functioning. A few may even try to maintain independence to the detriment of their recovery.

Recovery or Rehabilitation Stage

During the fifth stage, the client learns to give up the sick role and return to former roles and functions. For people with acute illnesses, the time as an ill person is generally short, and recovery is usually rapid. Thus, most find it relatively easy to return to their former life-styles. People who have long-term illnesses and who must make adjustments in life-style may find recovery more difficult. Recovery is particularly difficult for people who have to relearn skills such as walking or talking.

During this stage, readiness for social functioning may not coincide with physical readiness. People may be physically able to go out to dinner but find that functioning socially is still too stressful or they may find that they have the *desire* to perform activities but not the strength. Nurses can help clients function with increasing independence by planning with them those functions they can accomplish by themselves and those with which they need assistance. It is also important for nurses to convey an attitude of hope and to support the client's return to health.

Sick Role Behavior

Sick role behavior is "the activity undertaken by those who consider themselves ill, for the purpose of getting well" (Igun 1979, p. 455). Parsons (1972, pp. 436–37) describes four aspects of the sick role:

1. Clients are not held responsible for their condition.
2. Clients are excused from certain social roles and tasks.
3. Clients are obliged to try to get well as quickly as possible.
4. Clients or their families are obliged to seek competent help.

Many North Americans believe that illness, though undesirable, is beyond a person's control and that individuals are not responsible for incurring an illness. Some subcultures view illness as punishment from God, and therefore consider the infirm responsible for their illnesses, because of their sins. This folk belief persists to some degree in American society. A client may say something like, "What have I done to deserve this?" This remark reflects a sense that illness is a punishment. Today, because of the recognition that life-style contributes to illness and disease, some people—for example, the cardiac client who smokes or the overweight person who develops diabetes—are being held increasingly responsible for developing some illnesses.

Nurses can help clients by providing factual information and by not judging the client. It is important to encourage behaviors that promote health and not to reinforce behaviors that may have helped bring about an illness.

The sick person is usually excused from some normal duties. Social pressures on the sick and people's expectations of the sick usually depend on the prognosis and the severity of the illness. People who are severely ill and whose prognosis is poor or uncertain are permitted more dependence than people who are less seriously ill. People who are not seriously ill and whose prognosis is good are more likely to be encouraged to fulfill personal and social responsibilities. The person with a cold may still be expected to give a scheduled speech or to take an examination. People who are chronically ill may be permanently exempted from some duties or activities by society.

Some people may express feelings of guilt because they are unable to fulfill their normal responsibilities. Nurses can express support to clients who cannot fulfill their perceived roles and help them substitute other appropriate actitivies, when desirable. For example, a young father who cannot play ball with his son may be able to help his son build a model airplane, thereby fulfilling the father's role in another way.

Another aspect of the sick role is the obligation of the person to get well as quickly as possible. The sick role is a dependent one, at least in some respects. The person who fears dependence may be threatened by assuming a sick role and having to seek help. This individual might ignore advice despite the most serious consequences. Some people, however, find dependence gratifying. Some clients find dependence so satisfying that they perpetuate the sick role and do not try to get well or continue to complain of symptoms even after they are physically well. Some people in the dependent stage also find it satisfying to control others through excessive demands. With exceptions, people usually try to get well as quickly as possible.

Nurses can help clients assume a dependence appropriate to their developmental status and health. Part of the nurse's function is to reinforce both dependence and increasing independence at the appropriate times. For example, a man who is acutely ill may have to be shaved by the nurse; however, once he is stronger the nurse can assist him by providing shaving supplies and later complimenting him on his appearance.

An essential aspect of the sick role is seeking competent help. This presupposes that competent help is available to the client. It should also be recognized that the client's notion of competent help may be different from the general population's. For example, a man with a whiplash injury may become dissatisfied with his physician's treatment because of his slow recovery and may go to a healer who uses hypnotism. Or a domineering, talkative woman may reject advice to see a therapist and decide instead to join a cult of young people, considering the members of the cult competent help.

Nurses need to encourage some people to obtain competent help from health professionals. Nurses who are aware of the health facilities available in a community can assist people to obtain care. People may require considerable support before seeking assistance because, for example, they fear the health problem might be serious or they believe competent help might not be available. A nurse's function in these instances is to provide accurate information about available health facilities while recognizing clients' beliefs and their right to hold them.

Effects of Hospitalizaton

Normal patterns of behavior generally change with illness; with hospitalization, the change can be even greater. Hospitalization usually disrupts a person's privacy, autonomy, life-style, roles, and finances.

Loss of Privacy When a client enters a hospital or nursing facility, the loss of privacy is instantly obvious. *Privacy* has been described as a comfortable feeling reflecting a deserved degree of social retreat. Its dimensions and duration are controlled by the individual seeking the privacy. It is a personal internal state that cannot be imposed from without (Schuster 1976, p. 245).

People need varying degrees of privacy and establish boundaries for privacy; when these boundaries are crossed, they feel invaded. Hospital personnel sometimes show little concern for clients' privacy. Clients are asked to provide information that often they consider private; they may share a room with strangers; and their health is frequently discussed with many health professionals.

The boundaries of privacy are highly individual. The adult who lives alone may be used to privacy while eating, sleeping, and reading. A child from a large family may be accustomed to sharing these activities with others. It is important for nurses to ascertain what privacy means to the individual and try to support accustomed practices whenever possible. See also the discussion of territoriality in Chapter 18.

Altered Autonomy *Autonomy* is the state of being independent and self-directed without outside control. People vary in their sense of autonomy; some are accustomed to functioning independently in most of their life activities, while others are more accustomed to direction from others. An example of the former is a writer who lives alone and works independently. By contrast, a wife in a patriarchal home may be accustomed to having decisions made by her husband and receiving direction from him.

Hospitalized people frequently give up much of their autonomy. Decisions about meals, hygienic practices, and sleeping are frequently made for them. This loss of individuality is often difficult to accept, and the client may feel dehumanized into "just a piece of machinery." Nurses have a major responsibility to humanize care by learning about the client as a person and by individualizing nursing care plans.

Altered Life-Style Hospitalization marks a change in life-style. Many hospitals determine when people wake up and when they sleep. The woman who normally rises at 8:00 A.M. and the man who usually works until 11:00 P.M. must change their habits. Food in a hospital is usually mass produced, and individual differences in taste are not always accommodated. Occasionally hospitals have relatively large populations from a particular culture and make special food arrangements, for example, a Chinese menu for traditional Chinese clients or Kosher foods for traditional Jewish clients. However, individual preferences are not always met.

Nurses can help clients adapt to life in a hospital in several ways:

- Providing explanations about hospital routines
- Making arrangements wherever possible to accommodate the client's life-style, such as providing a bath in the evening rather than in the morning
- Encouraging other health professionals to become aware of the person's life-style and to support healthy aspects of that life-style
- Reinforcing desirable changes in practices with a view to making them a permanent part of the client's lifestyle

Economic Burden Hospitalization often places a genuine financial burden on clients and their families. Even though many people have health insurance, it may not reimburse all costs; in addition, many lose wages while they are hospitalized. Nurses can be aware of these costs and provide care that is as economical as is safely possible; for instance, they can use only the minimum supplies necessary for safe care. In some agencies, nurses may initiate referrals to the social service department to assist clients in making arrangements to address the financial burdens imposed by hospitalization. When this is not an independent nursing function, the nurse should consult with the client's physician to obtain such a referral.

Effects of Illness on Family Members

A person's illness affects not only the person who is ill but also the family or significant others. The kind of effect and its extent depend chiefly on three factors: (a) which member of the family is ill, (b) how serious and long the illness is, and (c) what cultural and social customs that family follows.

The changes that can occur in the family include the following:

- Role changes
- Task reassignments
- Increased stress due to anxiety about the outcome of the illness for the client and conflict about unaccustomed responsibilities
- Financial problems
- Loneliness as a result of separation and pending loss
- Change in social customs

Each member of the family is affected differently depending upon which member of the family is ill, because each plays a different role in the family and supports the family in different ways. Parents of young children, for example, have greater family responsibilities than parents of grown children.

The degree of change that family members experience is often related to their dependence on the sick person. For example, when a child is ill, there are few changes other than added responsibilities directly related to the child's illness. When the mother is ill, however, many changes are often necessary because other family members must assume her functions.

Sick Elderly Persons

When an elderly person is ill, a son or daughter often assumes the role of parent to the elderly person, providing housing, meals, and assistance with daily needs over a prolonged time. In other words, the parent-child roles are frequently reversed. This role reversal may be only temporary and may end when the illness ends, or it may become permanent.

The whole family, particularly the spouse of the sick person, experiences stress and concern about the outcome of the illness. Usually, the sick person's spouse feels a pending loss or separation most keenly. After a marriage of 50 or 60 years, elderly people may find it difficult to envisage what life will be like without a husband or wife. Younger persons in the family may deal with serious illness in an elderly person by stating, "He has led a good life" or "She had so much pain the past years." In this way, the young prepare themselves for that person's death. This same reasoning is rarely applied to a child or younger adult who is ill.

When an elderly person is ill, adult sons and daughters may face conflicting responsibilities. A daughter who lives some distance away needs to maintain her job and look after her own family, but at the same time her parents need her in another city. How often should she visit? How should she fulfill her responsibilities? These questions pose problems for many families today who live far apart.

The financial problems of the sick elderly can be a major problem for a family as well as a community. Because illness in this age group tends to be chronic, the costs of illness are often considerable. The greatest change in life-style is that the family must now allot time for hospital visits to the elderly relative.

Sick Parents

When the sick person is a parent, the degree to which the family experiences change is related to the responsibilities the individual has and the number and age of dependents in the person's care. For example, when a father is ill for a long time, his roles are usually taken over by other members of the family, frequently the mother. Such tasks as doing chores in the house or attending a child's basketball games, for example, are either reassigned or not performed at all. Anxiety of family members about the outcome of a parent's illness is usually high, especially if the parent is a wage earner. The implications to the family of prolonged illness or death are great in almost all areas of living because of the needs of the dependents.

Prolonged illness of the mother can have equally serious consequences. Often the children do not understand why their mother is in the hospital, and they may feel lonely and unwanted. Sometimes the mother's functions are taken over by grandparents or by aunts and uncles as well as by the father. When a young mother has a serious illness of unknown outcome, the father and family face worrisome problems of how to manage over a long period of time. Most arrangements have financial implications and involve role changes for the father and children. In this situation, the father must become both father and mother and give up many of his normal social activities. The children may also need to assume more housekeeping functions.

Sick Children

Because a child is dependent on parents for so many daily needs, both sick children and their families may need to make fewer role adjustments than sick adults and their families. Task reassignments are also generally minimal. Sometimes a younger sibling takes over a paper route for a sick brother or sister, and other members of the family share the sick child's chores.

However, all members of the family experience anxiety if the outcome of the child's illness is in doubt. A permanent disability has implications for schooling, earning a living, and future needs. Financial responsibility for chronic illness or a disability often can be a serious problem for young parents. Other children may feel neglected if an unusual amount of attention is given to the ill child. Husband and wife may also expend most of their energies visiting the hospital and have little time for each other. If extended, this situation can place great stress on a marriage.

When a child is admitted to the hospital, parents and siblings may experience some sense of loss; however, children usually continue with their daily activities, and there frequently is minimal disruption in the home.

CURRENT HEALTH TRENDS

The health of North Americans is steadily improving. Probable reasons for this improvement include the following:

- Earlier preventive efforts based on new knowledge obtained through research.
- Improvements in sanitation, housing, nutrition, and immunization essential to disease prevention.
- Individual measures to promote health and prevent disease. For example, increasing attention is being paid to exercise, nutrition, environmental health, and occupational health.

Trends

Evidence of current health status and changes in the last few decades are measured in various ways. Measurements are made of the type of health behavior people practice; longevity (life expectancy); mortality rates and causes; morbidity rates and causes; and the amount and kind of health services used.

The following facts and statistics are derived from *Statistical Abstract of the United States,* 109th ed. (U.S. Bureau of the Census 1989) unless otherwise indicated.

Health Behaviors The number of cigarette smokers in America has declined since 1964, when the Surgeon General's first *Report on Smoking and Health* was released. The sharp rise in smoking among teenage females that occurred in the 1970s has been curbed. However, the ratio of male to female smokers was about equal in 1983, whereas in 1965 male smokers outnumbered female smokers by 150%. In addition, among people who smoke, the percent who smoke 25 or more cigarettes per day has been increasing (U.S. DHHS 1985, p. 17).

Dietary practices, especially those related to the consumption of saturated fats, have had notable effects on the health of people. Over the past 20 years, the mean serum cholesterol level of adults aged 20 to 74 years has declined for every age group for both men and women. High serum cholesterol levels are associated with heart attacks and strokes. Another indicator of positive health behavior relates to hypertension control. The proportion of people with hypertension who kept their blood pressure below the level of 160/95 mm Hg nearly doubled from 1960–1962 to 1976–1980. This is thought to be due in part to adherence to prescribed medication regimens (U.S. DHHS 1985, p. 18). See also Tables 13–3 and 13–4.

TABLE 13-3 *Health Behaviors of People Over 18 Years (1985)*

Behavior	Percentage of Population
Current smokers	30.1
Have 5 or more alcoholic drinks per day	37.5
Obese (30% or more above desirable weight)	13.0
Less physically active than contemporaries	16.4
Never eat breakfast	24.3
Snack every day	39.0
Sleep 6 hours or less	22.0

Source: U.S. National Center for Health Statistics, U.S. Bureau of the Census, *Health promotion and disease prevention,* United States 1985 series 10, no. 163, In *Statistical abstract of the United States,* 109th ed. (Washington D.C.: U.S. Government Printing Office, 1989), p. 118, Table 190.

TABLE 13-4 *Percentage of Women Who Performed or Obtained Breast Self-Exam and Pap Smear in 1985*

Knew how to do it	87.0
Did at least 12 times per year	37.3
Had breast exam within past year	50.3
Had Pap smear within past year	45.6

Source: U.S. Bureau of the Census, *Statistical Abstract of the United States,* 109th ed. (Washington D.C.:U.S. Government Printing Office, 1989), p. 117, Table 189.

Longevity In 1950, life expectancy at birth for males was 65.6 years and for females 71.1 years. By 1987, it had reached 71.5 years for males and 78.3 years for females, an increase of 5 to 7 years. Differences, however, exist between white and black people; the life expectancy for blacks is 4 to 6 years less. In 1987, life expectancy for black males was only 65.4 years and for black females 73.8 years.

Mortality The infant mortality rate has declined by over 50% since 1960. In 1986, the rate fell to 10.4 per 1000 live births from 26.0 per 1000 in 1960. This decline is attributed largely to advances in medical science related to newborn treatment, improved socioeconomic conditions, and increased availability of maternal and infant care services. Infant mortality rates, however, are still relatively high for certain groups; rates are higher for black babies and babies of unmarried mothers, teenage mothers, and mothers over 35 years of age.

The major causes of death in infants during the first 6 days of life are immaturity (low birth weights) and birth-associated events, such as lack of oxygen. Among infants 1 year and younger, the three most important causes of death are congenital malformations, sudden infant death syndrome, and respiratory distress syndrome. Major causes of death in the general population were shown earlier in Table 13–2.

Morbidity Morbidity means illness; the morbidity rate is the ratio of sick to well people in a population. Morbidity statistics are more difficult to obtain than mortality statistics. Two ways to measure the illness of children is to determine (a) absenteeism from school and (b) changes in average heights and weights, since growth is characteristic of healthy, well-fed children.

The health of adults can be measured by considering the days of work lost, bed-disability days, and restricted-activity days. Many people may be limiting their activities at the onset of illness to prevent more serious health consequences (U.S. DHHS 1985, p. 7).

Implications for Nursing

As nurses assume an increasingly more visible role in providing health care services, it is helpful to consider the trends and behaviors noted above and to structure nursing services to ensure:

- Increased prenatal maternal and infant care services to reduce factors contributing to low birth weight, such as inadequate nutrition, smoking, and alcohol consumption. Services are especially required for black mothers, teenage mothers, mothers over 35 years of age, and the babies of these mothers.
- Early identification of problems that deprive the fetus of oxygen during labor and delivery, or prompt management of such problems when they do occur.
- Instruction in accident prevention to people of all ages.
- Maintenance of immunization programs to prevent infectious diseases.
- Promotion of measures to ensure optimal childhood development.
- Increased emphasis on supportive emotional care for children of divorced parents.
- Instruction to young adults about motor vehicle safety.
- Improved screening programs to assist in the early identification of disease.
- Improvement in life-styles to help individuals avoid major risk factors responsible for disease.
- Improvement in the health of adolescents and young adults; their physical, psychologic, and social attitudes; and their health habits to prevent later susceptibility to chronic diseases.
- Education to help youths acquire skills and information to prevent pregnancy, alcohol and drug abuse, and sexually transmitted diseases.
- Concerted efforts to reduce respiratory cancer rates by assisting people, especially women between 54 and 64 years of age and teenagers, to stop smoking.
- Increased assistance to help the elderly population with self-care and home management.
- Guidance to help all people acquire early treatment for illness and comply with therapy.
- Attention to occupational and environmental hazards.

CHAPTER HIGHLIGHTS

▶ The perspective from which health is viewed has changed; instead of absence of disease, health has come to mean a high level of wellness or the fulfill-ment of one's maximum potential for physical, psychosocial, and spiritual functioning.

- Models developed to explain health include the clinical, ecologic, role performance, adaptive, and eudaemonistic models.

- Because notions of health are highly individual, the nurse must determine each client's perception of health in order to provide meaningful assistance. Nurses too should be aware of their own personal definitions of health.

- Each person's concept of health is molded by social and cultural influences, previous experiences, expectations of self, and perceptions of self.

- Illness, sickness, and disease all have different meanings. Illness and sickness are usually associated with disease but may occur independently of it.

- The single-causation theory of disease is being replaced by a multiple-causation theory. For many diseases, the cause is still unknown.

- Five categories of risk factors that predispose individuals to illness and disease are genetic, age, physiologic, life-style, and environment.

- Marc Lalonde's *health field concept* views all causes of death and disease as having four contributing elements: human biologic factors, unhealthy lifestyles, environmental hazards, and inadequacies in the health care system.

- Wellness is an active, six-dimensional process of becoming aware of and making choices toward a higher level of well-being.

- The health status of a person is affected by many internal and external variables over which the person has varying degrees of control.

- Whether or not people choose to implement health behaviors depends on such factors as the importance of health to the person, perceived control, a perceived threat of a particular disease, perceived familial susceptibility, perceived seriousness of an illness, perceived benefits of preventive actions, and perceived value of early detection.

- Whether or not people take action to improve their health often depends on the cost, inconvenience, and unpleasantness involved and on the degree of life-style change necessary.

- People realize they are ill when certain symptoms indicate that something is wrong; they accept that they are ill when significant others or a health care professional verifies the illness.

- Increasingly, persons are being held responsible for some illnesses but are excused from certain roles and tasks during the illness; they are obliged, however, to get well as quickly as possible and to seek competent help.

- Nurses need to be aware that the illness of one member of a family affects all other members.

- Nurses need to be aware of a hospitalized client's life-style, roles, economic situation, and need for privacy and autonomy, and must provide care accordingly.

- People have the right and ability to make judgements about complying with health regimens after obtaining complete information.

- Health trends indicate that nurses need to assume a major role in helping people make life-style and environmental changes that will prevent accidents, disease, and occupational hazards.

LEARNING ACTIVITIES

- Using the questions in the box on page 231, develop your own definition of health.
- Select a disease process common in your area of clinical nursing practice. What is the etiology of the disease? What are the risk factors? What illness behaviors are seen with this problem? What are the current morbidity and mortality data relative to this disease? How can the nurse intervene to reduce the morbidity and mortality associated with this disease?

READINGS AND REFERENCES

SUGGESTED READINGS

Collins, H. L. May 1989. How well do nurses nurture themselves? *RN* 52:39–41.

This author reports the results of a poll about whether nurses take their own health as seriously as they take their clients'. Diet, exercise, rest and relaxation, and preventive medicine practices are surveyed.

Hogsteal, M. O., and Kashka, M. January/February 1989. Staying healthy after 85. *Geriatric Nursing* 10: 16–18.

These researchers interviewed 302 individuals 85 years or older about longevity patterns in their families, their life-long health practices, and their major health care problems and needs. Eleven factors they believed contributed most to their long life are provided. Included are exercise, religion, and a positive attitude.

RELATED RESEARCH

Allen, J. D. 1987. Identification of health risks in a young adult population. *Journal of Community Health Nursing* 4:223–33.

Lichtenstein, R. L., and Thomas, J. W. Winter 1987. A comparison of self-reported measures of perceived health and functional health in an elderly population. *Journal of Community Health* 12:213–30.

Williams, R. O. September/October 1988. Factors affecting the practice of breast self-exam in older women. *Oncology Nursing Forum* 15:611–16.

Woods, N. F. October 1988. Being healthy: Women's images. *Advances in Nursing Science* 11:36–46.

SELECTED REFERENCES

Abdellah, F. G. et al. 1960. *Patient-centered approaches to nursing.* New York: Macmillan.

Bauman, B. 1965. Diversities in conceptions of health and physical fitness. In Skipper, J. K., Jr. and Leonard, R. C., editors. *Social interaction and patient care.* Philadelphia: J. B. Lippincott Co.

Becker, M. H., editor. 1974. *The health belief model and personal health behavior.* Thorofare, N. J.: Charles B. Slack.

Canadian Department of National Health and Welfare. 1974. *A new perspective on the health of Canadians: A working document.* Ottawa: Department of National Health and Welfare.

Clark. C. C. 1986. *Wellness nursing.* New York: Springer Publishing Co.

Colantonio, A. September/October 1988. Lay concepts of health. *Health Values* 12:3–7.

Dubos, R. 1978. Health and creative adaptation. *Human Nature* 74(1):entire issue.

Dunn, H. L. November 1959. What high-level wellness means. *Canadian Journal of Public Health* 50:447.

————. 1973. *High-level wellness.* Arlington, Va.: R. W. Beatty Co.

Grasser, C., and Craft, B. J. G. June 1984. The patient's approach to wellness. *Nursing Clinics of North America* 19:207–18.

Hall, L. E. 1969. The Loeb Center for Nursing and Rehabilitation. *International Journal of Nursing Studies* 6:81–95.

Henderson, V. 1966. *The nature of nursing: A definition and its implications for practice, research, and education.* New York: Macmillan.

Henderson, V., and Nite, G. A. 1978. *The principles and practice of nursing.* New York: Macmillan.

Hettler, B. 1979. *Six dimensions of wellness.* Stevens Point, Wis.: National Wellness Institute, Inc.

Horgan, P. A. December 1987. Health status perceptions affect health-related behavior. *Journal of Gerontological Nursing* 13:30–33, 34–35.

Igun, U. A. 1979. Stages in health-seeking: A descriptive model. *Social Science and Medicine* 13A:445—56.

Jahoda, M. 1958. *Current concepts of positive mental health.* New York: Basic Books.

Johnson, D. E. 1980. The behavioral system model for nursing. In Riehl, J. P., and Roy, C. *Conceptual models for nursing practice. 2d ed.* New York: Appleton-Century-Crofts.

King, I. M. 1981. *A theory for nursing: Systems, concepts, process.* New York: John Wiley and Sons.

Kneisl, C. R., and Ames, S. W. 1986. *Adult health nursing: A biopsychosocial approach.* Menlo Park, Calif.: Addison-Wesley Publishing Co.

Leddy, S., and Pepper, J. M. 1989. *Conceptual bases of professional nursing.* 2d ed. Philadelphia: J. B. Lippincott Co.

Levine, M. E. 1973. *Introduction to clinical nursing.* 2d ed. Philadelphia: F. A. Davis.

MacElveen-Hoehn, P. 1983. The cooperation model for care in health and illness. pp. 515–39. In Chaska, N.L., editor. *The nursing profession: A time to speak.* New York: McGraw-Hill.

McCann/Flynn, J. B., and Heffron, P. B. 1988. *Nursing: From concept to practice.* 2d ed. East Norwalk, CT: Appleton & Lange.

Mitchell, P. H., and Loustau, A. 1981. *Concepts basic to nursing.* 3d ed. New York: McGraw-Hill.

Muhlenkamp, A. F., and Broerman, N. A. May 1988. Health beliefs, health value, and positive health behaviors. *Western Journal of Nursing Research* 10:637–46.

Murray, R. B., and Zentner, J. P. 1985. *Nursing concepts for health promotion.* 3d ed. Englewood Cliffs, N.J.: Prentice-Hall.

Newman, B. 1982. *The Newman systems model: Application to nursing education and practice.* Norwalk, Conn.: Appleton-Century-Crofts.

Newman, M. A. 1986. *Health as expanding consciousness*. St. Louis: C. V. Mosby Co.

Nightingale, F. 1969. *Notes on nursing: What it is and what it is not*. New York: Dover Books.

Nightingale, F. 1954. *Selected writings*. Compiled by Lucy R. Seymer. New York: Macmillan.

Orem, D. E. 1971. *Nursing: Concepts of practice*. New York: McGraw-Hill.

———. 1980. *Nursing: Concepts of practice*. 2d ed. New York: McGraw-Hill.

———. 1985. *Nursing: Concepts of practice*. 3d ed. New York: McGraw-Hill.

Overfield, T. 1985. *Biologic variation in health and illness: Race, age, and sex differences*. Menlo Park, Calif.: Addison-Wesley Publishing Co.

Parse, R. R. 1981. *Man-Living-Health: A theory of nursing*. New York: John Wiley and Sons.

Parsons, T. 1972. Definitions of health and illness in the light of American values and social structure. In Jaco, E. G., editor. *Patients, physicians and illness*. 2d ed. New York: Free Press.

Payne, L. September 1983. Health: A basic concept in nursing theory. *Journal of Advanced Nursing* 8:393–95.

Pender, N. J. June 1975. A conceptual model for preventive health behavior. *Nursing Outlook* 23:385–90.

———. 1987. *Health promotion in nursing practice*. 2d ed. East Norwalk, Conn.: Appleton & Lange.

President's Commission on Health Needs of the Nation. 1953. *Building American's health*. Vol. 2 Washington, D.C.: U.S. Government Printing Office.

Redeker, N. S. Spring 1988. Health beliefs and adherence in chronic illness. *Image: Journal of Nursing Scholarship* 20:31–35.

Reynolds, C. L. July 1988. The measurement of health in nursing. *Advances in Nursing Science* 10:23–31.

Rogers, M. E. 1970. *An introduction to the theoretical basis of nursing*. Philadelphia: F. A. Davis.

Rosenstock, I. M. 1974. Historical origins of the health belief model. In Becker, M. H., editor. *The health belief model and personal health behavior*. Thorofare, N.J.: Charles B. Slack

Roy, Sr. C. March 1970. Adaptation: A conceptual framework in nursing. *Nursing Outlook* 18:42–45.

———. 1976. *Introduction to nursing: An adaptation model*. Englewood Cliffs, N.J.: Prentice-Hall.

———. 1984. *Introduction to nursing. An adaptation model*. Englewood Cliffs, N.J.: Prentice-Hall.

Ryan, R. S., and Travis, J. W. 1981. *Wellness workbook for health professionals*. Berkeley, Calif.: Ten Speed Press.

Schuster, E. A. October 1976. Privacy: The patient and hospitalization. *Social Science Medicine* 10:245.

Smith, J. A. April 1981. The idea of health: A philosophical inquiry. *Advanced Nursing Science* 3:43–50.

Suchman, E. A. 1972. Stages of illness and medical care. In Jaco, E. G., editor. *Patients, physicians and illness*. 2d ed. New York: Free Press.

Twaddle, A. C. 1977. *A sociology of health*. St. Louis: C. V. Mosby Co.

U.S. Bureau of the Census. 1989. *Statistical abstract of the United States*. 109th ed. Washington, D.C.: U.S. Government Printing Office.

U.S. Department of Health, Education, and Welfare. 1979. *Healthy people: The surgeon general's report on health promotion and disease prevention*. Pub. no. 79-55071. Washington D.C.: U.S. Government Printing Office.

U.S. Department of Health and Human Services. December 1985. *Health United States 1985*. Pub. no. (PHS) 86-1232. Hyattsville, Md.: Public Health Service.

World Health Organization. 1947. *Constitution of the World Health Organization: Chronicle of the World Health Organization 1*. Geneva: WHO.

Yoos, L. September/October 1981. Compliance: Philosophical and ethical considerations. *Nurse Practitioner* 6:27, 29–30, 34.

Contemporary Health Care Delivery Systems

HEALTH CARE SYSTEM

A *health care system* is the totality of services offered by all health disciplines. Traditionally, the health care delivery system in North America provides two general types of services: illness care services (restorative) and health care services (preventive). Illness care services help the ill or injured. Health care services promote better health and help prevent disease and accidents. Although most facilities within the system—for example, hospitals,

clinics, and physicians' offices—provide both types of services, illness care services predominate. In recent years, however, there has been increased awareness of the need to promote health and to prevent disease. Considerable emphasis has been placed on the role of the nurse in these areas.

In the past, health care facilities have been influenced largely by the needs of the people providing the service. For example, hospitals have developed in relation to medical and technologic advances and generally reflect the needs of physicians. Also, the public viewed health care facilities as sources of help primarily for the ill or injured. As a result, preventive health care facilities have been slower to develop. This delay can be attributed in great part to three factors:

1. Physicians are largely oriented to illness in their practice.
2. Consumers have been more aware of treatment of illness than of prevention and health promotion.
3. The nurse's role as the chief provider of preventive health care and health promotion has been slow to evolve, and frequently the treatment of illness takes precedence over preventive health care activities.

In recent years, however, many people have become more conscious of their health, and comprehensive health care, including health promotion and disease prevention services, are receiving increased attention. In the future, increased efforts by nurses, all health professionals, and governments can be instrumental in helping people gain a greater awareness of health as a way of life. Greater emphasis must be given to the ill effects of smoking, excessive consumption of alcohol, taking illicit drugs, and overuse of prescribed and over-the-counter medications, rather than treatment of the consequences of these activities. Measures to prevent disease or reduce risks must also be emphasized. Examples are immunizing children; reducing the incidence of road accidents, particularly among adolescents; and preventing accidents in the home, especially among children and older people.

FACTORS INFLUENCING HEALTH CARE SERVICES

People in this society generally believe that health care is a right of everyone. This does not mean that health itself is a right; people can work toward being healthy, but the health care system may not provide health for all people. However, society can strive to provide health care for all people. The question is not whether all people should have health care but how it can be provided.

Change within the health care system has accelerated during the past decade. This change and future changes are a result of many influences in society.

Health Care Consumer
Comprehensive, holistic, and humanistic health care is being emphasized today. People want comprehensive care. They want to have their health care needs met at one time at one agency rather than to seek help for an abdominal pain at one place, for a tooth problem at another place, and for an emotional problem at yet another. Holistic health practitioners emphasize the effects of one problem on the person as a biopsychosocial whole. Consumers, therefore, expect health care that reflects this view of the total person and the person's roles and functions.

In the past few decades, many North Americans have come to expect more of the health care system than disease prevention or cure. Consumers today are more aware and knowledgeable about the effects of life-style on health. As a result, they desire more information and services related to health promotion and illness prevention. Although the diagnosis and treatment of illness are still a necessity, the focus of health care has changed. Traditionally, health care was viewed as synonymous with professional and medical care. Now health care professionals are increasingly viewed as a supplementary resource for individuals carrying out their own health maintenance and health promotion activities. As a result, a wide range of health promotion programs have arisen. Some are provided through the traditional health care agencies, but many are developing in community facilities along with physical fitness centers. The media, too, reflect this change. It is not rare for characters in movies, for instance, to exhibit positive health behaviors, such as exercising and not smoking. In Canada, alcohol and tobacco advertisements have been restricted.

Mutual Support and Self-Help Groups
In North America today, there are more than 500 mutual support or *self-help groups* that focus on nearly every major health problem or life crisis people experience. Such groups arose largely because people felt their needs were not being met by the existing health care system. Alcoholics Anonymous, which formed in 1935, served as the model for many of these groups. The National Self-Help Clearinghouse provides information on current support groups and guidelines about how to start a self-help group. Groups vary in effectiveness, but most provide education to encourage self-care as well as social and emotional support. Before referring clients to specific groups, the nurse needs to assess the group's effectiveness and availability to the client.

Feminist Movement
The feminist movement has been instrumental in changing health care practices. Examples are the provision of childbirth services in more relaxed hospital settings or the home, the provision of overnight facilities for parents in children's hos-

pitals and the development of women's health care centers. The literature on the health concerns of women and research into women's unique health experiences are growing. Recently concern has been expressed about the amount of research and funding related to women's health issues, causing the federal government to review its policies.

Family Characteristics

The characteristics of the North American family have changed considerably in the last few decades. There is a marked increase in single-parent families because of divorce and increased acceptance of children born out of wedlock. Most single-parent families are headed by women. Serious illness or hospitalization can create major financial and home management difficulties for single-parent families. See Chapter 16 for additional information on family health.

Increasing Population

Statistics reflect an increase in the total population and indicate the need for increased health services. See Figure 14–1. In both the United States and Canada, there has been tremendous population growth. The impact of the growing elderly population on the health care system is a major social issue. About 30 cents of each health care dollar in the United States are allocated to this group, which now exceeds 28 million and constitutes almost 12% of the population (U.S. Department of Commerce 1984).

By the year 2000, it is estimated that the elderly will number approximately 35 million, constituting 13.1% of the population (U.S. Bureau of the Census 1989, p. 25). In Canada, a similar increase in the number of older people is anticipated: from 1.9 million in 1976 (Statistics Canada 1980, p. 10) to 3.2 million by the year 2000. By the year 2031, 21% of the population will be over age 65 (Statistics Canada 1981). Since only 5% of older people are institutionalized because of health problems, substantial home management and nursing support services are required to assist those in their homes and communities.

The frail aged population over age 85 is the second fastest growing population in North America, exceeded only by the baby boom generation now between 40 and 55. More research into the health and economic conditions of this population is needed. See also Special Needs of the Elderly later in this chapter.

Environmental Change

Air and water pollution from industrial waste is a notable change in this century. Many cities publish a daily air quality index so that persons with respiratory disease will know whether the

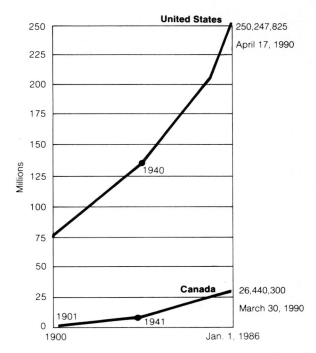

Figure 14-1 Increases in population in the United States, 1900–1987, and in Canada, 1901–1986. *Source:* U.S. Department of Commerce, Bureau of the Census, *Population profile of the United States,* April 17, 1990, 1980 Series P, no. 363 (Washington, D.C.: U.S. Government Printing Office, June 1981), p. 9; Statistics Canada, *The Daily: Quarterly Demographic Statistics for Canada, Provinces and Territories,* March 30, 1990; and Statistics Canada, *Census of Canada* Ottawa: Minister of Supplies and Services, 1981), p. 6.

outside air is safe to breathe. Tragic industrial and nuclear leaks are also of concern.

Many work environments also pose health hazards for employees. Coal miners and textile workers are prone to lung disease. Increasingly, the public is demanding smokeless air in work settings. Many corporations and cities have already banned smoking in certain work areas.

Cultural Diversity

The health care system of North America reflects largely Western, white values and does not adequately accommodate the values of the many different cultural groups living in this country. Language barriers and inequities in income and education hinder access of minority ethnic groups to health care. The more sophisticated and impersonal health services become, the less accessible they are to ethnic groups, who often have a strong family tradition, and prefer personalized care from someone who understands them and their families. Many such people look on the modern health care system with distrust. See Chapter 24 for more information about cultural diversity.

Economic Influences

The health care delivery system is very much affected by a country's total economic status. Inflation and the economic recession of the early 1980s brought increasing concern about escalating health care costs. The United States spends $1 billion a day on health care, and costs are still rising. Medical care costs have increased more than 400% since 1965. They increased an average of 12.6% annually between 1970 and 1984 and about 7.5% in 1986 (Dougherty 1988, p. 16). In Canada, health care expenditures have increased at a similar rate. Some reasons for this sizable increase are advanced techniques and technology, inflation, increased utilization of health services, and the system of payment for hospitals and physicians.

Prospective payment system (PPS)

Efforts to curtail health care costs in the United States were made in 1983, when Congress passed legislation putting the *prospective payment system* into effect. This legislation limits the amount paid to hospitals that are reimbursed by Medicare. Reimbursement is made according to a classification system known as *diagnostic related groups (DRGs)*. The system has categories that establish pretreatment diagnosis billing categories.

Under this system, the hospital is paid a predetermined amount for clients with a specific diagnosis. For example, a hospital that admits a client with a diagnosis of uncomplicated asthma is reimbursed a specified amount, such as $1300, regardless of the cost of services, the length of the stay, or the acuity or complexity of the client's illness. In the past, Medicare reimbursed hospitals according to the reasonable cost of services provided to its clients. The hospital billed retrospectively, after the services were rendered. In contrast, prospective payment or billing is formulated before the client is even admitted to the hospital; thus, the record of admission, rather than the record of treatment, now governs payment. DRG rates are set in advance of the prospective year during which they apply and are considered fixed except for major, uncontrollable occurrences. The prospective rates are paid by clients and/or third parties.

This legislation has had a tremendous impact on health care delivery in the United States, since the providers of care, rather than Medicare or other third-party payers, run the risk of monetary losses. If a hospital's cost per case exceeds the defined limit, it incurs a loss; if the cost is less than the defined limit, it receives a sur-

plus. Thus, PPS offers financial incentives for withholding unnecessary tests or procedures and avoiding prolonged hospital stays.

Notable effects of the DRG system to date are earlier discharge of clients, a decline in admissions, and a reduction of services and staff, especially nurse's aides and LPN/LVN staff. With the decline in admissions, most clients now admitted are seriously ill and have multiple health problems. Many hospitals are now employing only registered nurses (RNs), believing that RNs can provide the broadest range of nursing care. The earlier discharge of clients has given rise to home care agencies that provide needed home nursing care.

To protect clients from DRG abuses, Medicare introduced state peer review organizations (PROs). Made up of physicians and other health care professionals, PROs are intended to monitor the hospitals and ensure high-quality care under DRGs. PROs have developed screening guidelines that govern whether admissions or procedures should occur and are used to review records, render payment decisions, and handle difficulties.

The implication of DRGs for nursing education, practice, and research are many. The Health Care Financing Administration (HCFA) funds research to study alternative systems for classifying severity of illness through nursing diagnosis (Caterinicchio 1984, p. 130) and to shed light on the relationship between DRGs, nursing resource utilization, and nursing costs (ANA 1985).

Unemployment and poverty

Unemployment and poverty, whether the result of recessions, new microchip technology, or inadequate education and technical skills, affect which health services are offered and used. Because the unemployed do not receive employment-based health insurance, they do not use health care services to the same extent as the general population. Even though some government aid is available, eligibility for government insurance programs and benefits varies considerably from state to state. Canada's economic problems are similar to those of the United States; however, the overall effects are not always as apparent because Canada has a smaller population. The National Health Care program in Canada ensures medical care and hospitalization for the poor and unemployed.

Political Influences

Health care is affected by political decisions. For example, political decisions affect health insurance programs, health care funding, allocation of resources (people, money, and equipment), and laws governing the duties of health care workers and the rights of clients, e.g., of women to have abortions. The attitude of people in government health ministries largely determines whether the focus of health care delivery is primary care, secondary care, or tertiary care. *Political activity by nurses* (see Chapter 12) *is essential.*

FINANCING HEALTH CARE SERVICES

Funding for personal health care can come from a variety of sources: Governments (social insurance), the client, and health insurance are the major sources.

Social Insurance

Federal funding is largely through the social insurance programs Medicare and Medicaid in the United States, and the National Medical Care Insurance program in Canada. A nationally funded program to cover the health costs of all United States citizens has been discussed for the past 20 years.

United States   In the United States, the 1965 Medicare amendments (Title 18) to the Social Security Act provided a national and state health insurance program for the aged. By the mid 1970s, virtually everyone over 65 years was protected by hospital insurance under Part A, which also includes posthospital extended care and home health benefits. Medicare Part B is a voluntary medical insurance that supplements Part A. It is jointly paid for by general tax dollars and subscriber fees. Part B provides up to 80% of "reasonable" charges for doctors' services, outpatient treatment, and home health care. Medicaid was established the same year under Title 19 of the Social Security Act. It is funded jointly by the federal and state governments and is administered at the state level to provide financial assistance for medical care to people of any age who cannot afford care.

In 1972, Congress directed the Department of Health, Education, and Welfare to create professional standards review organizations (PSROs) to monitor the appropriateness of hospital use under the Medicare and Medicaid programs. In 1974, the National Health Planning and Resources Development Act established health systems agencies (HSAs) throughout the United States for comprehensive health planning. In 1978, the Rural Health Clinics Act provided for the development of health care in medically underserved rural areas. This act opened the door for nurse practitioners to provide primary care.

In addition, disabled or blind persons may be eligible for special payments called Supplemental Security Income (SSI) benefits. These benefits are also available to people not eligible for Social Security, and payments are not restricted to health care costs. Clients often use this money to purchase medicines or to cover costs of extended health care.

Canada   The Canadian National Hospital Insurance program was started in 1958, and the National Medical Care Insurance Program (Medicare) began in 1968. Through these programs, every Canadian can obtain health insurance. Not all hospital and medical services are covered by provincial hospital insurance or Medicare plans; there are slight differences between provinces. The Canada Health Act was passed in 1984 by Parliament to provide federal government reimbursement to provincial governments for health services they provide. This act replaced two acts: the Hospital Insurance and Diagnostic Services Act and the Medical Care Act. The new act penalizes provinces that permit extra billing of clients by physicians by a levy of a dollar-for-dollar assessment. The act also creates incentives for home care, community health clinics, and health promotion.

Voluntary Insurance

Health care costs are also covered by private insurance plans. The costs of these insurance plans, such as Blue Shield and Blue Cross, are borne by the individual or shared by the employer and the employee. One type of voluntary health insurance is the prepaid group plan offered by HMOs. Prepaid group plans provide for services required by the participants 24 hours a day. By advance payment, the individual takes out insurance against any health requirements in the future. These plans place heavy emphasis on promotion of health and prevention of disease and injury among participants.

Workmen's Compensation

Workers who are injured on the job may collect workmen's compensation payments during their recovery. In some instances, all health care costs are paid by workmen's compensation. Employer companies contribute to a workmen's compensation fund to make money available when accidents occur.

Charitable Resources

Charitable resources for medical payments are supported by donations from individuals or groups and by bequests. Charitable donations are still made by some philanthropic organizations to assist the poor and to support innovations. On the whole, however, charitable donations as a means of paying for health care are declining in importance.

HEALTH CARE AGENCIES

Official Agencies

Government (official) agencies are established at the local, state (provincial), and federal levels. Health agencies at the state, county, or city level vary according to the need of the area. Their funds, generally from taxes, are administered by elected or appointed officials. Local health departments (county, bicounty, or tricounty) traditionally have responsibility for developing programs to meet the health needs of the people, providing the necessary staff and facilities to carry out these programs, continually evaluating the effectiveness of the programs, and monitoring changing needs. State health organizations are responsible for assisting the local health departments. In some remote areas, state departments also provide direct services to people.

The Public Health Service (PHS) of the United States Department of Health and Human Services is an official agency at the federal level. Its functions include conducting research and providing training in the health field, providing assistance to communities in planning and developing health facilities, and assisting states and local communities through financing and provision of trained personnel. Also at the national level in the United States are research institutions such as the National Institutes of Health (NIH). The National Institute on Drug Abuse, the National Institute on Alcohol Abuse and Alcoholism, and the National Institute of Mental Health work with federal, regional, and state agencies. The Centers for Disease Control (CDC) in Atlanta, Georgia, administer a broad program related to surveillance of diseases. By means of laboratory and epidemiologic investigations, data are made available to appropriate authorities. The CDC also publishes recommendations about the prevention and control of infections and administers a national health program. The federal government also administers a number of Veterans Administration (VA) hospitals in the United States.

The Canadian Department of Health and Welfare (CDHW) administers such federal programs as native health in the north and health care in the territories. However, provincial governments generally have responsibility for administering health services to the people of each province.

Agencies Providing Health Care

Health care agencies can be viewed as giving primary, secondary, and tertiary care.

Primary Care Primary care agencies are the point of entry into the health care system, i.e., the point at which initial health care is given. Primary care includes health maintenance, health promotion, and disease prevention activities. Aydelotte writes, "The major purposes of primary care centers will be to provide: (1) entry into the system; (2) emergency care; (3) health maintenance; (4) long-term and chronic care; (5) treatment of temporary malfunctioning that does not require hospitalization" (Aydelotte 1983, p. 812). It is in this area that increased services are expected to reduce health care costs and improve health. Settings for primary care are various health centers in the community, homes, schools, physicians' offices, and industry and business. Primary care is frequently inadequate in rural and economically depressed areas, due to lack of physicians. Emergency departments of hospitals are often crowded and overtaxed, in many instances with nonemergency health problems.

Ambulatory care centers are being used more frequently in many communities. They usually have diagnostic and treatment facilities and may or may not be attached to or associated with an acute care hospital. They provide medical, nursing, laboratory, and radiologic services. Some ambulatory care centers provide services to people who require minor surgical procedures that can be performed outside the hospital. After surgery, the client returns home the same day. These centers have two advantages: They permit the client to live at home while obtaining needed health care, and they free costly hospital beds for seriously ill clients. Nurses in ambulatory care centers frequently function as nurse practitioners or clinical nurse specialists, e.g., in gastroenterology or urology.

The term *ambulatory care center* has replaced the term *clinic* in many places. The term *clinic* can refer to a department in a hospital or a group practice of physicians. Traditionally, a hospital clinic was called an outpatient clinic, serving only outpatients, as opposed to those admitted to the hospital (inpatients). The role of the nurse in a clinic may be similar to that of a nurse practitioner or a nurse in a physician's office.

The *physician's office* is a traditional primary care setting in North America. Nurses employed in physicians' offices have a variety of roles. Some nurses carry out the traditional functions of registering the client, preparing the client for an examination or treatment, and providing information. Other nurses function as nurse practitioners and have the responsibility of providing primary care to clients in stable health.

The *industrial clinic* is gaining importance as a setting for primary care. Employee health has long been recognized as important to productivity. Today, an increasing number of companies are recognizing the value of healthy employees and encouraging healthy life-styles. Some companies provide exercise facilities, while others provide healthy snacks, such as fruit, instead of coffee. More businesses are prohibiting smoking in the work setting.

Community health nurses in the occupational setting have a variety of roles. Worker safety has been a traditional concern of occupational nurses. Today, nursing functions include health education, screening for such health problems as hypertension and obesity, counseling, and initial care after accidents.

A *health maintenance organization (HMO)* is a group health care agency that provides basic and supplemental health maintenance and treatment services to voluntary enrollees. The enrollees prepay a fixed periodic fee that is set without regard to the amount or kind of services received. The basic idea of the HMO arose in the 1930s, when prepaid health care experiments were sponsored by unions, cooperatives, corporations, municipalities, and other organized groups. HMOs did not become popular, however, until after the passage, in 1973, of the Health Maintenance Organization Act. In 1984, 11 million people were served by HMOs (Curtin and Zurlage 1984, p. 34).

To be federally qualified, an HMO company must meet certain requirements. It must offer physicians' services, hospital and outpatient services, emergency services, short-term mental health services, treatment and referral for drug and alcohol problems, laboratory and radiologic services, preventive dental services for children under 12, and preventive health services. By encouraging preventive health care and by offering ambulatory services, HMOs have reduced the cost of health insurance to the consumer.

A client of an HMO signs a contract to pay a specified amount to the HMO for unlimited care. The plan stresses wellness; the better the health of the person, the less the client needs HMO services and the greater the agency's profit. Because of the emphasis on health promotion and prevention of illness, nurses who work in HMOs focus on these aspects of care, frequently as nurse practitioners, client educators, and consultants.

Although not in every community, HMOs have been established across the United States. The largest HMO, the Kaiser-Permanente Medical Care Program, serves clients in California, Oregon, Hawaii, Ohio, and Colorado. A person with private health insurance can obtain services in most hospitals, but the clients of an HMO must use its facilities.

The *preferred provider organization (PPO)* has emerged as another alternative health delivery system. It consists of a group of physicians or a hospital that provides companies with health services at a discounted rate. Hospitals, physicians, and insurance companies are the major sponsors of PPOs. PPOs were first established in 1980 in the United States. Physicians can belong to one or several PPOs, and the client can choose among the physicians belonging to that PPO.

Individual practice associations (IPA) are somewhat like HMOs and PPOs. The IPA provides practice in offices, just as the providers belonging to a PPO do. The difference is that clients pay a fixed prospective payment to the IPA, and the IPA pays the provider. In some instances, the health care provider bills the IPA for services; in others, the provider receives a fixed fee for services given. At the end of the fiscal year, any surplus money is divided among the providers; any loss is assumed by the IPA.

Crisis centers provide emergency services. The clients are often people experiencing life crises. These centers may operate out of a hospital or in the community and usually provide 24-hour telephone service. Some also provide direct counseling to people at the center or in their homes. The primary purpose of a crisis center is to help people cope with an immediate crisis and then provide guidance and support for long-term therapy.

Nurses working in crisis centers need well-developed communication and counseling skills. The nurse must immediately identify the person's problem, offer assistance to help the person cope, and perhaps later provide guidance about resources for long-term support.

Secondary Care Secondary care focuses on preventing complications of disease conditions. It has traditionally been the province of hospitals; however, other agencies now increasingly provide this level of service. Secondary care centers of the future will focus on the treatment of temporary dysfunctions that require hospitalization but not highly skilled services and high-risk interventions, the evaluation of long-term illness that requires hospitalization to determine any needed change in treatment, and the provision of counseling and therapy that cannot be provided in a primary care center (Aydelotte 1983, p. 813). Agencies that provide secondary care include hospitals, home health agencies, and ambulatory care centers.

Hospitals traditionally have provided restorative care to the ill and injured. They vary in size from the 12-bed rural hospital to the 1500-bed metropolitan hospital with a 50-bed day surgery center. Hospitals can be classified according to their ownership or control as governmental (public) and nongovernmental (private). Governmental hospitals are either federal, state, city, or county hospitals in the United States and federal or provincial hospitals in Canada. In both countries, governments have traditionally provided hospital facilities for veterans, merchant mariners, and individuals with long-term illness.

Although hospitals are chiefly viewed as institutions that provide care, they have other functions, such as providing resources for health-related research and teaching.

Hospitals also are classified by the services they provide. General hospitals admit clients requiring a variety of services, such as medical, surgical, obstetric, pediatric, and psychiatric services. Other hospitals offer only specialty services, such as psychiatric or pediatric care.

Hospitals can be further described as acute or chronic. An acute hospital provides assistance to clients who are acutely ill or whose illness and need for hospitalization are relatively short-term, for example, 2 days. Long-term hospitals provide health services for longer periods, sometimes for years or the remainder of the client's life.

Hospitals in the United States are undergoing massive change. In the past, hospitals were virtually the sole providers of secondary care; however, ambulatory care centers and HMOs have forced hospitals to reorganize and adopt different practices. Some hospitals have merged or sold out to large multihospital for-profit corporations, e.g., Humana, Inc., and Hospital Corporation of America. Other hospitals are providing innovative services, such as fitness classes, day care for elderly people, and nutrition classes. Some hospitals have even established alternative birth centers (ABCs) to attract new families.

In the United States today, all but the most seriously ill are treated outside of a hospital. Because so many of these are elderly, some general hospitals are becoming acute care hospitals solely for the elderly. Because of the increasing acuity of illness among clients, general hospitals are becoming intensive care centers.

Tertiary Care

Tertiary care is also called rehabilitation or long-term care. It is largely provided through home health care, long-term care facilities, rehabilitation centers, and hospices. *Home health care agencies* are rapidly becoming major tertiary care providers. Their purposes include promoting, maintaining, and restoring health, specifically maximizing independent functioning and minimizing the disabling effects of illness, including terminal illness. Services appropriate to the needs of clients and their families are planned, coordinated, and delivered by providers organized for the delivery of home health care through the use of contractual arrangements, employed staff, or a combination of the two.

Home care may or may not be associated with a hospitalization. It may precede or follow institutional care in a hospital or long-term care facility, or it may be provided along with ambulatory care (Lundberg 1984). Self-care and care given by health professionals and allied health personnel in the home account for the majority of health care provided in this country today. The time a person spends in a hospital receiving care for acute conditions is generally a very small percentage of the person's life. The need for home care services is increasing as the population of the United States ages and the incidence of chronic illness increases correspondingly (Lundberg 1984).

The nature of home care services has broadened to include both acute, short-term care as well as long-term monitoring of problems associated with chronic illness. Comprehensive home care includes both direct and indirect services.

Direct services involve direct contact between a caregiver and a client for the purposes of administering treatment or nursing care measures, assessment, teaching, counseling, or planning care. Direct services provided may be complex technical procedures, such as intravenous chemotherapy for cancer and respiratory therapy. Such services are becoming more widely available at home. Symptom management, teaching for self-care, monitoring adaptation to long-term illness, family counseling, physical and occupational therapy, and nutritional counseling are direct services provided by a variety of home care agencies. Such basic nursing care measures as bathing, skin care, assistance with ambulation, toileting, feeding, dressing changes, catheter care, and administration of medications have long been and continue to be direct service components of home care. Home care nursing also includes such direct services as providing ongoing assessment, anticipation and planning for problems or crises before they occur, helping clients think through problems and their options for dealing with them, managing symptoms, teaching, counseling, and assisting individuals and families to meet their health care goals.

Indirect services in home care include those measures taken to provide or facilitate direct services in nursing practice (McCorkle and Germino 1984). Consulting with other professionals and allied health personnel about client problems and needs, coordinating care within the home care agency, coordinating community resources and referrals outside the agency, supervising allied health workers providing services, and evaluating the effectiveness of care provided are all examples of indirect services currently provided by home care nurses. In addition, nurses involved in home care may be liaisons with acute care facilities and serve as facilitators and contact persons for clients and families who need access to special health care resources.

Long-Term Care Facilities

There are a wide variety of long-term care facilities. Traditionally, they were all called nursing homes. Long-term care facilities now include skilled nursing facilities for extended care, intermediate care, and personal care for those who are chronically ill or are no longer able to care for themselves without assistance.

Because long term illness occurs most often in the elderly, many long-term care facilities have programs that are oriented to the needs of this age group. Nursing homes are intended for people who require not only personal services (such as assistance in bathing and dressing, and meal preparation) but also some regular nursing care and occasional medical attention. However, the type of care provided varies considerably. Some admit and retain only residents who can dress themselves and are ambulatory. Other long-term care facilities provide bed care for clients who are more incapacitated. Nursing homes can, in effect, become the clients' home, and consequently the people who live there are frequently referred to as residents rather than patients or clients.

In 1987, the Congress of the United States passed the Omnibus Budget Reconciliation Act (OBRA) to bring a measure of quality assurance to the nursing home industry. There was growing concern whether minimal essential standards were being met in many nursing home facilities. One of the provisions of OBRA that concerns nursing is the requirement for nurse's aide training. Specific requirements include the following:

- A training program of 75 hours in length for nurse's aides
- Competency evaluation of newly trained nurse's aides
- Competency evaluation of nurse's aides already providing care
- A registry for nurse's aides

For nursing, implications of this OBRA 1987 provision include the following (Kelly 1989, p. 792):

1. Concern about which state agency is to be responsible for implementing the requirements. If the state agency is other than a board of nursing, the nursing community could have less than the desired control over nursing functions to be delegated by licensed nurses to nurse's aides. Legally, a licensed registered or practical nurse is accountable for acts delegated.

2. The 75-hour training requirement may not be sufficient to prepare aides to carry out routine care for nursing home clients who have complex problems.

3. The evaluation requirement necessitates job analysis and the development of standard criteria at the state level.

4. The establishment of a registry system for nurse's aides implies the establishment of a discipline function and a process to identify those at risk to the public. Licensed nurses, therefore, will need to be alerted to their responsibilities in monitoring for the three problems cited by OBRA as calling for the investigation of care provided by aides: (a) neglect of residents, (b) abuse of residents, and (c) misappropriation of resident property.

Rehabilitation Centers

Rehabilitation centers usually are independent community centers or special units in hospitals. However, rehabilitation ideally starts the moment a client enters the health care system. Thus, nurses are involved in rehabilitation whether they are employed on pediatric, psychiatric, or surgical units of hospitals or in the community. Today, the concept of rehabilitation is applied to all illness (physical and mental), to injury, and to chemical addiction. Rehabilitation affects every age group and segment of society. *Rehabilitation* is a process of restoring people to useful function in physical, mental, social, economic, and vocational areas of their lives. Rehabilitation, then, is a process of restoring people to their previous level of health (i.e., to their previous capabilities) or to the level that is possible for them. Rehabilitation, as distinct from maintenance, is an active concept and can be considered largely an educational function.

Hospice Services

Traditionally, a *hospice* was a place where travelers could rest. Recently, the term has come to mean a health care facility for the dying. The hospice movement subsumes a variety of services given to the terminally ill, their families, and support persons. The movement sprang initially from dissatisfaction with the preoccupation of health personnel with technologic care and insufficient emphasis on caring and psychologic support. In the 1970s, the movement gained momentum. It derived impetus from new attitudes toward death and from the work of such people as Elisabeth Kübler-Ross, whose books challenged prevailing attitudes, and Cicely Saunders, founder of St. Christopher's Hospice in London, England. Saunders believed that the physical and social environments of dying people are as important as medical interventions on their behalf.

In recent years, hospices have provided a variety of services to terminally ill clients and their families; indeed, hospices have inspired a social movement. Basic to the movement is a humanistic belief in the individuality of people and their needs. Hospice programs are institution and community based. Some supply services in the home, either directly or through community resources. Reimbursement for these services is variable, often voluntary.

Hospices are a haven for the dying because they emphasize the needs of the individual and help clients and their families plan for death. The central concept of the hospice movement, as distinct from the acute care model, is not saving life but improving or maintaining the quality of life until death. Important in this care are *palliative measures* for relief rather than cure. Comfort and relief from pain are frequently the most important needs of the dying. Hospice care addresses the needs of the mind and the spirit as well: It is truly holistic.

RIGHTS TO HEALTH CARE

The movement for clients' rights in health care arose in the late 1960s. At that time, the broad goals of the movement were to improve the quality of health care and to make the health care system more responsive to clients' needs. Today, clients are also seeking more self-determination and control over their own bodies when they are ill. Informed consent, confidentiality, and the right of the client to refuse treatment are all aspects of this self-determination. The need for clients' rights is largely the result of two circumstances: the vulnerability of the client because of illness and the complexity of the relationships in the health care setting.

When people are ill, they are frequently unable to assert their rights as they would if they were healthy. Asserting rights requires energy and an underlying awareness of one's rights in the situation.

The complexity and variety of health care relationships also increase the need for clients' rights. In this day of specialization, a client is often helped by a variety of health professionals. The client becomes one person among many health professionals. Thus, the client's needs or priorities, for example, can become lost in the communications among health professionals.

A new pattern of health care relationships is emerging as a result of several forces in society, including a more knowledgeable consumer and recognition of the role of life-style in disease. Today, the goals of health include the return of autonomy and independence to the client and the acceptance of good health as a responsibility of the care provider, the client, and society. These goals cannot be met unless clients accept active responsibility for their health and health care and unless clients and care providers have mutual respect.

Annas and Healey (1974, p. 26) list four rights that are assertable in a health care facility: (a) the right to the whole truth, (b) the right to privacy and personal dignity, (c) the right to retain self-determination by participating in decisions regarding one's health, and (d) the right of complete access to medical records, both during and after the hospital stay.

A Patient's Bill of Rights

In 1973, the American Hospital Association published "A Patient's Bill of Rights" in an effort to promote the rights of hospitalized clients. See Table 14–1. Frequently clients do not know their rights, although many hospitals today give clients upon admission a statement of their rights while in hospital.

The nursing implications of the Patient's Bill of Rights are:

1. *The patient has a right to considerate and respectful care.* The client has a right to an explanation about what will happen, why, and when. Clients also have the right to participate in planning their care. Considerate and respectful care also includes respect for the dignity of each person. Nurses can convey respect by listening carefully to clients and their support persons and reporting their concerns to the appropriate people.

2. *The patient has the right to obtain from his physician complete current information concerning his diagnosis, treatment, and prognosis, in terms the patient can be reasonably expected to understand.* The responsibility for divulging this information belongs to the physician. If a client asks a nurse for this information, the nurse should relay the questions to the physician and document the client's questions and the nurse's actions on the client's record.

   Many people believe that even when ill, clients still have a right to the whole truth, i.e., complete information about their health care. Nurses should

TABLE 14-1 *A Patient's Bill of Rights*

1. The patient has the right to considerate and respectful care.

2. The patient has the right to obtain from his physician complete current information concerning his diagnosis, treatment, and prognosis, in terms the patient can be reasonably expected to understand. When it is not medically advisable to give such information to the patient, the information should be made available to an appropriate person in his behalf. He has the right to know by name the physician responsible for coordinating his care.

3. The patient has the right to receive from his physician information necessary to give informed consent prior to the start of any procedure and/or treatment. Except in emergencies, such information for informed consent should include but not necessarily be limited to the specific procedure and/or treatment, the medically significant risks involved, and the probable duration of incapacitation. Where medically significant alternatives for care or treatment exist, or when the patient requests information concerning medical alternatives, the patient has the right to such information. The patient also has the right to know the name of the person responsible for the procedures and/or treatment.

4. The patient has the right to refuse treatment to the extent permitted by law and to be informed of the medical consequences of his action.

5. The patient has the right to every consideration of his privacy concerning his own medical care program. Case discussion, consultation, examination, and treatment are confidential and should be conducted discreetly. Those not directly involved in this care must have the permission of the patient to be present.

6. The patient has the right to expect that all communications and records pertaining to his care should be treated as confidential.

7. The patient has the right to expect that within its capacity a hospital must make reasonable response to the request of a patient for services. The hospital must provide evaluation, service, and/or referral as indicated by the urgency of the case. When medically permissible, a patient may be transferred to another facility only after he has received complete information and explanation concerning the needs for and alternatives to such a transfer. The institution to which the patient is transferred must first have accepted the patient for transfer.

8. The patient has the right to obtain information as to any relationship of his hospital to other health care and educational institutions insofar as his care is concerned. The patient has the right to obtain information as to the existence of any professional relationships among individuals, by name, who are treating him.

9. The patient has the right to be advised if the hospital proposes to engage in or perform human experimentation affecting his care or treatment. The patient has the right to refuse to participate in such research projects.

10. The patient has the right to expect reasonable continuity of care. He has the right to know in advance what appointment times and physicians are available and where. The patient has the right to expect that the hospital will provide a mechanism whereby he is informed by his physician or a delegate of the physician of the patient's continuing health.

11. The patient has the right to examine and receive an explanation of his bill regardless of source of payment.

12. The patient has the right to know what hospital rules and regulations apply to his conduct as a patient.

Source: American Hospital Association. 1973. A patient's bill of rights, *Nursing Outlook,* February 1973, 21:82, and January 1976, 24:29. Reprinted with the permission of the American Hospital Association.

explain independent nursing actions truthfully and completely. Because these activities are solely in the nurse's domain, the nurse has sole responsibility for explaining them. However, dependent nursing functions, i.e., those nursing activities ordered by the physician, should be explained only after the nurse completely understands the physician's and client's positions. See Chapter 8 for information about independent and dependent nursing actions. Usually, a physician has no objection to a client understanding the ordered treatments; however, occasionally a physician does not wish a client to be fully informed, e.g., about a medication for a malignancy before the client has been informed of the diagnosis. Although the client has a right to be fully informed, not all jurisdictions accept the Patient's Bill of Rights as law. Therefore nurses should inform the physician about the client's questions, discuss the matter thoroughly, and document the client's questions.

3. *The patient has the right to receive from his physician information necessary to give informed consent prior to the start of any procedures and/or treatment.* The client has the right to give or withhold informed consent. Obtaining informed consent is primarily the physician's responsibility. The nurse's role in obtaining informed consent is discussed in Chapter 10.

An important nursing strategy is to "coordinate the medical, technical, and nursing activities on behalf of the patient's well-being into a meaningful process that the patient and family can utilize in the shared decision process" (Bandman and Bandman 1990, p. 95). It has been found that in many instances treatments are refused because of conflicting information. Therefore, when nurses and other health professionals collaborate and encourage the client's participation, the client feels more secure and more comfortable about making decisions regarding care.

4. *The patient has the right to refuse treatment to the extent permitted by law and to be informed of the medical consequences of his action.* Clients have the right to self-determination. Just as they have the right to informed consent, they also have the right to refuse a treatment. An adult client who is conscious and medically competent has the right to refuse any medical or surgical procedure (Annas 1975, p. 79). When the client refuses treatment, no person has the right to impose the treatment. The clients still have the right to the best possible care within the limitations they impose. In regard to a parent's refusal to allow treatment of a child, Annas states: "It is only in extreme cases involving the potential of death or permanent disability to the child that courts are likely to overrule a parent's refusal of treatment for a child" (Annas 1975, p. 87).

5. *The patient has the right to every consideration of his privacy concerning his own medical care program.* People vary in what they consider an invasion of privacy and a threat to dignity. Therefore only the client can decide whether to permit any invasion of privacy. Although a client who signs a consent form for an examination or treatment may be giving up certain aspects of privacy in the course of the examination or treatment, the invasion of the client's privacy must be kept to the minimum. For example, a client who consents to a physical examination is expected to disrobe; however, the nurse can provide some degree of privacy by supplying an appropriate gown, drapes, and a room or enclosed

area. Also, by consenting to the examination, the client does not also agree to the presence of people other than those directly involved in the examination.

The right to privacy is closely linked to the individual's personal dignity. Individuals "on exhibit" can feel demeaned and embarrassed. The experience of being viewed by a group of health professionals, e.g., nursing students, can live in a person's memory for many years as a distasteful incident. Nurses must ensure that the client fully understands and consents to the presence of health personnel not directly involved in treatment. The right to privacy is the second item in the ANA Code (ANA 1976, p. 2).

Clients have a right to privacy even after death. Privacy also means not intruding into the client's private life and disclosing confidential information. Nurses can be held legally liable for taking any action without consent that would offend a reasonable person's sensibilities (Good Intentions Gone Awry 1986, p. 55). Ways of intruding into a client's private life include eavesdropping on a conversation, searching a client's clothes or handbag, taking photographs of an unconscious client, or asking questions that have no relation to the client's health. See Chapter 10 for additional information regarding the invasion of privacy.

6. *The patient has the right to expect that all communications and records pertaining to his care should be treated as confidential.* Privacy is closely related to confidentiality. Only clients have the power to let people not directly involved in their care view their medical records. Only the client has the right to provide information to support persons or others. Confidentiality is also included in the ANA ethical code. See Chapter 11.

Another aspect of confidentiality is related to computers. Although computers have facilitated health care in a number of ways, any person who knows an access code can view confidential client information. Therefore, nurses and all health professionals must guard the confidentiality of client records and not give computer codes to unauthorized people.

7. *The patient has the right to expect that within its capacity a hospital must make a reasonable response to the request of a patient for services.*

8. *The patient has a right to obtain information as to any relationship of his hospital to other health care and educational institutions insofar as his care is*

concerned. Rights 8 and 9 are largely related to hospital administration. However, nurses are becoming increasingly involved in such matters as budget as it relates to client care. Clients who believe their care is inadequate should communicate this fact to the appropriate person in the hospital. Every health agency should have a procedure for handling client grievances. One trend in health care is client advocacy, a function assumed by nurses in some settings.

9. *The patient has the right to be advised if the hospital proposes to engage in or perform human experimentation affecting his care or treatment.* Clients also have a right to consent or refuse to participate in any research or experimentation. Both the ANA and the CNA have published guidelines for nurses who participate in research.

10. *The patient has the right to expect reasonable continuity of care.* Clients have a right to know what health care they will need after they are discharged from a hospital. It is often the nurse's responsibility to teach follow-up care and to make appropriate referrals to other health agencies. Discharge planning is discussed in Chapter 8.

11. *The patient has the right to examine and receive an explanation of his bill regardless of the source of payment.* Nurses often record billable items such as dressings, medications, and the like. In some settings, it may be the nurse's responsibility to explain a bill to a client, although this task is often carried out by someone in the hospital's business office.

12. *The patient has the right to know what hospital rules and regulations apply to his conduct as a patient.* Some agencies provide pamphlets that list rules, such as those governing visiting hours, and explain services, such as cafeteria and telephone service. Often nurses clarify information and answer a client's questions about hospital rules. Nurses also explain rules associated with special procedures, such as those that apply when oxygen is in use or when a client has an infection.

Another right not mentioned specifically in the AHA Patient's Bill of Rights is the *right of access to medical records.* Although in some jurisdictions clients have the right of access to their health records, agency practices vary widely in this regard. Some hospitals, e.g., military hospitals, permit clients to keep records at the bedside. At the other extreme, some agencies release records to clients only if they have a subpeona. A number of state legislatures have passed laws requiring health agencies to establish reasonable policies by which clients are permitted access to their records. Laws about access to records have changed in recent years, and it is generally recognized that only clients can grant others access to their records or permit the release or transfer of their records.

PROBLEMS IN THE HEALTH CARE SYSTEM

Although the health care system is changing, problems still exist. Many of the problems stem, at least partially, from the enormous changes in health care during the past 30 years. Major advances in medicine and technology have meant better care for many. With this improved care, however, have come such problems as fragmentation of care and high costs.

Other problems have always existed with health care delivery systems and are present today. Some of these are unmet needs of low-income people and the special needs of the homeless and the elderly. Another problem is uneven national distribution of health care services; limited resources are available in rural and inner-city areas, whereas more services are available in more prosperous urban and suburban areas. The consumer is becoming more aware of these problems and is exerting increasing pressure to have them corrected, but corrections are gradual and must accommodate to economic and political realities.

Fragmentation of Care

Highly specialized techniques and new knowledge emerging during the past 30 years of research mean that an increasing number of health care personnel provide specialized services. They may be highly specialized technicians or technologists who have relatively narrow but exacting jobs, such as respiratory technologists, biomedical electronic technologists, and nuclear medicine technologists. Increased specialization is evident also among physicians. In 1982, about 83% of all physicians classified themselves as being in a specialty (Jonas 1986, p. 128). All this specialization means fragmentation of care and, often, increased cost of care. To clients, it may mean receiving care from 5 to 30 people during their hospital experience. This seemingly endless stream of personnel is often confusing and frightening. The individual feels like a cog in the wheel and asks, "Who really cares about me?" and "Who is really responsible?" The increasing number of health workers creates problems with the smooth flow of information and plans to help the client. Again, the person wonders, "Will someone forget to order my medication?" The concept of total care is more difficult to implement when so many people are involved.

Increased Cost of Services

The problem of financing health-illness services is increasingly severe. There are six major reasons for increased costs:

1. Existing equipment and facilities are continually becoming obsolete as research uncovers new and better methods in health-illness care.
2. Additional space and sophisticated equipment are required to provide the newest diagnostic and treatment methods.
3. Inflation increases all costs.
4. The total population has grown, and the demand for services has increased.
5. People increasingly recognize that health is a right of *all* people, hence larger numbers of people are seeking assistance in health matters.
6. The relative number of people who provide health-illness services has increased.

Health Care for the Homeless

The number of homeless people in towns and cities continues to grow. Estimates vary widely, but advocates of the homeless estimate this number at 2 million to 3 million in the United States. Reasons for this increase include the following (Lindsay 1989, p. 78):

- Rising cost of housing
- Reduction in federal subsidies for low-income housing
- Economic recessions of the late 1970s and early 1980s resulting in continued low or minimum wages, plant closures, and unemployment
- Alcohol and drug abuse
- Deinstitutionalization of mental health facilities and a change in the laws governing commitment of the mentally ill. About 30 to 40% of the homeless are mentally ill.

The homeless differ from those who are poor; they are alone, lack some type of permanent residence, and are disaffiliated from family and friends. Because of the con-

ditions in which homeless people live (in shelters, on the streets, in parks, in tents, under scrap material covers, under viaducts, in all-night movie theaters, in transportation terminals, or in cars), their health problems are often exacerbated and sometimes become chronic. Major health problems of the homeless include the following (Lindsay 1989, p. 79):

- Chronic health problems such as diabetes, hypertension, and drug and alcohol abuse
- Risk of communicable diseases such as tuberculosis, scabies, lice, and AIDS
- Hypothermia in the winter
- Malnutrition
- Dental problems
- Peripheral vascular problems
- Traumatic injuries and risk of assault
- Children at risk of abuse, neglect, and missing immunizations, making them vulnerable to disease

The 1987 Report of the Panel on Health Goals for Ontario has suggested several basics to good health (Spasoff 1987): "peace; an adequate income; adequate housing and food; a valued role to play in family, work, and community; a safe environment; and a healthy lifestyle." These basics, however, are beyond the reach of the homeless population, many of whom are multiply handicapped by physical, mental, social, and emotional problems. Several factors contribute to poor health among the homeless (see the accompanying box).

Factors Contributing to Poor Health of the Homeless

- Poor physical environment resulting in increased susceptibility to infections
- Inadequate rest and privacy
- Improper nutrition
- Poor access to facilities for personal hygiene
- Exposure to the elements
- Lack of social support
- Few personal resources
- Questionable personal safety (physical assault is a constant threat)
- Inadequate health care
- Poor compliance with treatment plans

One of the most critical contributors to poor health of the homeless is the lack of access to health care services, even though most of the homeless live in the cities that have an abundance of health services. In the United States, the majority of homeless people have no benefits such as Medicare, Aid for Families with Dependent Children, veteran's benefits, and private health insurance. In Canada—even with its national health insurance system—many homeless have lost their hospital insurance number and other forms of identification and lack other resources such as money and a home address to obtain new identification. Homeless people without proper identification find it humiliating to be turned away when they seek health care.

Because the life-style of the homeless is usually outside the experience of health care providers, it is difficult for them to understand and appreciate the health care needs of this group. In addition, many health care providers find it distasteful to deal with the homeless because of their poor hygiene, unkempt appearance, body odors, and sometimes offensive remarks and behavior. Those who have had experience with the homeless have learned that traditional approaches and routine health care instructions are not appropriate for this group of people. For example, Judd and Forgues (1989, p. 19) state that simple treatment instructions such as "get plenty of rest," "drink clear fluids," and "soak your wound in salt and water three times a day" may be impossible for homeless persons to carry out, given their meager resources (e.g., no bed, no money, and no hygienic facilities). Experienced health professionals have learned, too, that the homeless want to be healthy and that they will, with support, benefit from health care services.

Health care workers can help in providing health care to the homeless in these ways (Judd and Forgues 1989, p. 19):

■ Valuing the right of the homeless to receive the same health care as others in the society

■ Establishing nursing care services in shelters and on the streets

In 1983, the Robert Wood Johnson Foundation (RWJ) and the Pew Memorial Trust announced the Health Care for the Homeless Program (The RWJ/Pew homeless program initiative), in which they would provide funds for four-year demonstration projects providing health care to the homeless. Several cities in the United States have successfully applied for funding and have demonstrated that the homeless can be reached and that health care can be provided to them. In Canada, one approach to helping the homeless was started in Toronto in 1985 by Dilin Baker, who originated a service called Street Health. Street Health is owned and operated by street people who are members of the board of directors and who work in the clinics. This type of service enables nurses to establish contact, gain trust, act as resource persons, attend to minor wounds and conditions, listen to and act on their concerns, teach illness management to shelter workers, help the homeless secure identification, and through the office provide an address for these people to receive mail. The ultimate goal of Street Health is to lead the homeless to existing health services.

Special Needs of the Elderly

Because people over 65 are becoming an increasingly large part of the population, their health needs deserve special concern. Long-term illnesses are most prevalent in this group, making special housing, treatment services, and financial support necessary. By the year 2030, the world population over the age of 65 years is expected to increase from 10% in 1975 to 18–20% (Bezold 1982, p. 14).

In addition, at any given time about 10 million adults over the age of 25 years are providing care to elderly relatives. These people often require respite from the care-giving role, as well as reassurance and support. About 5% of adults over 65 years reside in nursing homes or other long-term care facilities, and more than twice that number of frail elderly are cared for in the home. (Baldwin 1990, pp. 172–73). By the year 2050, it is expected that the number of elderly requiring nursing home care will have quadrupled (Andreoli and Musser 1985, p. 47).

Among the health services required by the elderly, screening and assessment programs are important in order to detect disease early and thereby prevent subsequent problems from developing. Tertiary prevention programs for the elderly are needed to promote independent functioning and prevention of further deterioration due to disease.

The elderly also need to know about home care agencies in their community. Nurses can help hospitalized clients make a smooth transition home by providing discharge planning and referrals to appropriate community agencies. Adult day care programs offer the elderly person a change of environment and stimulation while providing the care-giver with some respite.

Developing a healthy life-style is as important for the elderly as it is for other people. Many diseases that affect the elderly can be modified or prevented through life-style changes. Factors such as diet, exercise, and cigarette smoking, for example, can affect the incidence of cancer, heart disease, and stroke.

Uneven Distribution of Health Services

Serious problems in the distribution in health services exist in both the United States and Canada. Two facets of this problem are (a) uneven distribution and (b) increased specialization. Uneven distribution is evidenced by the relatively higher number of nurses per population in the New England states and the lowest number in Louisiana and Oklahoma. Physicians are also unevenly distributed: Mississippi has the lowest number of physicians per 100,000 (120), whereas Massachusetts has the highest (306) (Jonas 1986, pp. 61, 103).

CHALLENGES FOR THE FUTURE

Health for All

In 1977, the World Health Organization launched the movement known as Achieving Health for All. The goal of this movement was—and still is today—for all persons to obtain a level of health by the year 2000 that will permit them to lead socially and economically productive lives.

Achieving the goal of equal access to appropriate health care for all people in the future requires the efforts of all people and a focus on the following (O'Neill 1983, pp. 117–18):

1. Establishment of community-based health systems in which primary health care is the major function. Such systems would need to be backed up by hospital services and other specialty services. Health and welfare centers of the future need to be planned together and cover all aspects of health. Such centers should be places that the local people can approach whatever their health requirement.

2. Redistribution of health and specialty services to overcome regional inequities. Currently, health care services and professionals are concentrated in the more prosperous urban areas. In rural and low-income areas, such as declining inner city areas, there is a notable lack of services.

3. Emphasis on self-reliance and participation by the individual and community members in health matters. This will require a changed emphasis by health work-

ers on home and community care rather than institutional care. More research will be needed about the cost-effectiveness of home and community services, self-care, and self-help approaches.

4. Increased emphasis on provision of services to specific target groups, such as children and adolescents, the elderly, the disabled, the dying, single mothers, the mentally ill, and working mothers. A whole array of services that now exist need expansion. Examples are health education for children, home help, and child care for working women.

5. Increased involvement of existing health organizations and groups. Many existing health and social groups, e.g., AA, groups for the elderly, and paraplegic associations, can use their specialized talents to bring about change.

6. Expanded education of health professionals—medical practitioners, nurses, nurse-midwives—in community and health care as well as traditional hospital and acute care. Graduating physicians and nurses will need to think and practice in terms of health rather than disease, apply techniques of prevention and health promotion in addition to those of cure and rehabilitation, focus practice on the family and community and not the individual sick person, and work as members of a health team that invites the active participation of the consumer. Clients are now beginning to play a critical, active role rather than their traditional, uncritical role of passively accepting everything the health professional says and does.

7. Expansion of traditional roles and change in the current hierarchical health profession. As O'Neill (1983, p. 72) says: "Health professionals have before them a dramatic new role in addition to the exercise of their clinical skills: that of health leaders, educators, guides, and generators of simpler and more socially acceptable technologies. To fulfill this role they will require a combination of sagacity, scientific and technical knowledge, social understanding, managerial acumen and, above all, political persuasiveness."

8. New focus by government on health rather than cure and on the roles that transportation, housing, and industry can play in bringing about a healthy society.

Future Health Care Environment

O'Malley, Loveridge, and Cummings (1989) state that the changing health care environment challenges nurses to redesign nursing care delivery systems. Several future changes in the health care environment are outlined in the accompanying box.

Aydelotte (1987, p. 118) predicts a health care system divided into four branches:

1. Health promotion, health education, self-help, and health evaluation
2. Chronic disease management
3. Trauma and severe illnesses
4. Care of the frail elderly, the physically limited elderly, and the dying

Within each of these branches at least four classes of nursing roles are needed (Aydelotte 1987, p. 119):

1. Provider of direct services
2. Researcher and developer, who will develop new knowledge, educational programs, technology, media, *telematics* (new information technologies), and the like
3. Case manager in the health promotion and maintenance branch, who will emphasize prevention rather than remedy
4. Executives to administer groups of nurses in the units, who will secure resources; allocate resources; develop policy; and distribute, evaluate, and revise services

Nurses will provide these services through four different arrangements (Aydelotte 1987, p. 119):

1. Professional corporations headed by nurses, which will contract with specific groups or other organizations to provide nursing services such as school nursing, home health care, or intensive care
2. Nurse specialty practice groups, which will provide special services such as counseling, health maintenance, and certain technological services on a contractual basis with individuals or groups
3. Practice on an individual basis, which will provide highly specialized nursing service on a one-to-one basis or consultation with other health care professionals (this service will also be arranged by contracts).
4. Employment in profit and nonprofit health care systems primarily oriented toward acute care

Implications for Nursing

The changes and future trends in the health care system have many implications for nursing practice. Aydelotte

---

Future Changes in the Health Care Environment

- The elderly will be the fastest growing segment of the population, because the baby boomers are entering middle age; therefore, the number who are young and who provide services to this group will be relatively small.

- Hospitals will restructure their organizations and redirect their goals toward a health-maintenance versus illness-based culture.

- Health promotion services, child-rearing services, and weight reduction programs will increasingly be provided by the same organizations that offer long-term care and physical rehabilitation.

- The organizational design of the health care service will be decentralized and information-based rather than centralized and bureaucratic.

- The service focus will become consumer focused and information-based rather than treatment focused and highly technologic.

Source: J. O'Malley, C. E. Loveridge, and S. H. Cummings, The new nursing organization, *Nursing Management,* February 1989, 20:29–32.

(1987, pp. 118–20; 1983, pp. 814–15) describes the following strategies:

- The nature of the profession needs to be clarified and understood. The knowledge of nursing should be exclusive, and the education of nurses should be on a professional level. The title "nurse" should be more highly restricted to only one class, i.e., the *professional,* and not include support personnel.

- Individuals entering nursing must meet high standards of intelligence and motivation, especially motivation to public service. The nursing profession must be concerned with building a nucleus of true professionals.

- The nursing education system needs to be remodeled, so that it will be much more extensive and sound. Such a remodeling should include more depth in the sciences, an understanding of economics, emphasis on legal and ethical issues, an introduction to management and business, an increased understanding of information technology, and greater clinical application.

- Preparation in self-governance and self-management is needed for the professional of the future. Ways to develop clinical nursing judgment need to be explored and made available to students.

- Nursing's relationship with the public and the power elite must change. Political action should extend beyond the legislative arena into every aspect of community affairs. Nursing leaders need to make a concerted effort to become college and university presidents and vice presidents, leaders in business and community affairs, heads of corporations, and chairpersons of boards. Increased leadership skills for functioning in corporate structures will be needed.

- The costs of nursing services will need to be established. Currently, nursing costs are often disguised as hospital room costs or payments to nonnurse supervisors. Thus, a system of reimbursement that pays directly to nursing services obtained by contracts needs to be developed. To develop such a system, nurses will need to learn the management of contracts and business, attach a value to services, and, at the same time, ensure the maintenance or quality of care provided.

- Nursing strategies need to be designed to meet the health promotion and health maintenance needs of people, especially the elderly, low-income persons, rural residents, the chronically ill, the unemployed, pregnant women, working women, children, and adolescents. The nurse's role in primary care needs to be expanded in hospitals, homes, and industry, and the public and government need to be convinced that such services would coordinate care, decrease fragmentation, and be cost-efficient. Nurses will need to develop the following:
  a. Improved assessment and evaluation skills
  b. Increased skills in communication, e.g., a second language or computer skills
  c. Increased knowledge and acceptance of cultural diversity
  d. Increased acceptance of change
  e. Increased use of technology in teaching clients

- Nurses need to understand and appreciate their own worth and actively participate in meeting the challenges of providing quality health care for all. Nurses must educate the public about nursing's unique capabilities in meeting health care needs. Nursing care can be an alternative as well as an adjunct to medical care.

Humanizing Health Care

Although the goal of any health care delivery system is intrinsically human, the system is perceived as increasingly dehumanizing. Dehumanization is associated with vulnerability, powerlessness, and loss of identity in large, faceless institutions. The blame usually falls on society in general, technologic change, the rat race, or bureaucratic red tape.

Howard and Strauss (1975, p. 73) discuss four ways nurses and other health care professionals can humanize care:

1. Value the concept of inherent worth, which reflects notions of equality among people. Health systems now recognize the inherent worth of persons by trying to prolong life, reduce pain, and restore social functioning. Clients themselves emphasize that they should be treated with dignity and respect even if discriminated against in the larger society. The concept of inherent worth needs to apply to *all* professional/ client interactions and must be reflected in institutional policy.

2. Recognize that each person is a unique individual, even though all humans have some commonalities, and avoid stereotyping or treating clients in a routine, uniform way. Remember that at any given moment, the sum of a person's past and present experience influences the person's feelings, attitudes, and actions.

3. Recognize that although humans do not have infinite freedom of action, most people have considerable control and choice over their destinies and need to be given the freedom to consider all options available to them. Clients are restricted by such factors as illness, ignorance, and financial constraints. Practitioners are restricted by institutional commitments, colleague pressures, scarce resources for therapy, and cost considerations. Sharing decision making and responsibility (a) reflects the ideology that all clients, regardless of education, have a right to participate as much as possible in decisions about their care and (b) makes the client and provider partners and therefore, in a way, equals. To share in decision making, the client must be informed about prognoses, alternative therapies, and the rationales behind them.

   The client's level of education will influence the client's desire and capacity to accept shared responsibility for care. In addition, some clients may be too sick, anxious, or irrational to analyze facts and to make appropriate decisions.

4. Convey empathy and positive affect. *Empathy* is the ability to identify and sympathize with others. Clients

expect health care professionals to show sympathy and concern. Otherwise, clients feel depersonalized and dehumanized. For example, in the words of one client, "He should know how much my leg hurts and what it means to me." The dilemma of the practitioner is that too much empathy can be emotionally draining. In some instances, it may also be impossible to put oneself in the client's shoes. For example, an able-bodied nurse who cares for paraplegics knows that these clients are well aware the nurse has two legs and cannot possibly identify with them as well as another paraplegic. Thus, a balance between too little and too much empathy is necessary. The means of achieving this balance needs research.

Positive affect is the conveying of genuine feelings of warmth to the client. Positive feelings appear to be necessary for continued human-to-human contact.

CHAPTER HIGHLIGHTS

▶ Consumer attitudes—their view of health care as a right and their demand for comprehensive, holistic, and humanistic health care—are noticeably influencing health care delivery.

▶ Consumers are demanding greater emphasis on health promotion and illness prevention rather than on treatment of disease.

▶ The idea that health is the responsibility of each individual in society is gaining greater acceptance.

▶ Social changes, such as the feminist movement, the rise in single-parent families and in women working outside the home, cultural diversity, and the growing elderly population, are influencing the type and quantity of health care services needed.

▶ Health care services are currently financed through social insurance, such as Medicaid and Medicare in the United States and the National Medical and Hospital Insurance programs in Canada; direct client payments; voluntary insurance plans, such as Blue Cross and Blue Shield; and charitable donations.

▶ The prospective payment system (PPS) was introduced in the United States to curtail the escalating costs of health care.

▶ Because of fewer hospital admissions, earlier discharges, and staff reductions—the results of PPS—the need for home health care has increased.

▶ Government health care agencies, established at the local, state (provincial), and federal levels, are supported by revenues obtained through taxes.

▶ Agencies providing health care can be viewed as giving primary, secondary, and tertiary care.

▶ *Primary care* agencies focus on health maintenance, health promotion, and disease prevention.

Secondary care agencies, such as hospitals and ambulatory care clinics, focus on the treatment of illness and the prevention of complications of disease conditions.

Tertiary care agencies provide long-term care and rehabilitation services and focus on restoring the client to optimum functioning after physical or mental illness.

▶ Several alternative health care delivery systems, such as health maintenance organizations, preferred provider organizations, and individual practice associations, have arisen in the past decade to encourage preventive health care and to reduce the cost of health care to the consumer.

▶ A variety of hospice services meets the special needs of the terminally ill in settings other than acute care agencies; caring and psychologic support are emphasized.

▶ Health care services are provided by a variety of health care personnel in a variety of settings.

▶ Problems in the health care system include fragmentation of care, increased costs, and health care for the homeless, elderly, and low-income groups.

▶ The unemployed and poverty-stricken have unique health care needs that require increasing attention. ▶

CHAPTER HIGHLIGHTS *(continued)*

▸ Future challenges in health care delivery are to promote health as a way of life, to prevent ill health, and to provide community care for all.

▸ In the future, nurses will need to be prepared to practice in primary care settings and to develop the skills to work in these settings. They will also need to learn the management of contracts and business.

LEARNING ACTIVITIES

■ Review the "Health for All" foci listed on page 266. How can you and other nurses in your community help achieve the goal of equal access to health care for all by the year 2000? What specific actions are required? What systems need to be changed or created?

■ Review the demographic changes in your community. Contact your local government or health department. What are the specific health concerns in your community? List the identified health concerns in order of priority. Share your list with other nurses. Do they agree with the identified health concerns? Do they agree with the prioritization? How can nursing as a force in your community address the identified health concern?

READINGS AND REFERENCES

SUGGESTED READINGS

Davis, G. C. November/December 1988. Nursing values and health care policy. *Nursing Outlook* 36:289–92.
   Davis describes the relationship between society's and nursing's values and how these relate to public policy. Five nursing beliefs are described, and some suggestions for influencing health policy conclude the article.

Dimond, M. March/April 1989. Health care and the aging population. *Nursing Outlook* 37:76–77.
   Dimond relates the increasing number of aging people in the population to the problems in the present health care delivery system. Dimond then explains some of the challenges facing health care providers given the limited financial resources. Long-term care as a health care deficiency and the problem of aging as a women's problem are described.

Grassi, L. C. 1989. Nurses' assessment of DRGs on quality patient care. *Nursing Forum* 24:32–34.
   Grassi describes a survey of how several nurses perceive the impact of DRGs on client care. The survey revealed that the nurses had specific concerns about the quality of health care for their clients.

RELATED RESEARCH

Beachy, W. November 1988. Multicompetent health professionals: Needs, combinations, and curriculum development. *Journal of Allied Health* 17:319–29.

Bremer, A. 1989. A description of community health nursing practice with the community-based elderly. *Journal of Community Health Nursing* 6:173–84.

Cameron, E.; Badger, F.; and Evers, H. May 1989. District nursing, the disabled and the elderly: Who are the black patients? *Journal of Advanced Nursing* 14:376–82.

Wilson, S. L.; Rudman, S. V.; and Snyder, J. R. May/June 1989. Health educators in HMOs: A study of utilization and effectiveness. *Health Values* 13:9–14.

SELECTED REFERENCES

American Nurses' Association. 1976, 1985. *Code for nurses with interpretative statements*. Kansas City, Mo.: ANA.

American Nurses' Association. Center for Research. June 1985. *DRGs and nursing care*. Kansas City, Mo.: ANA.

American Hospital Association. January 1976. A patient's bill of rights. *Nursing Outlook* 24:29 (also February 1973, *Nursing Outlook* 21:82).

Andreoli, K. G., and Musser, L. A. January 1985. Trends that may affect nursing's future. *Nursing Health Care* 1:46–51.

Annas, G. J. 1975. *The rights of hospital patients: The basic ACLU guide to a hospital patients' rights.* New York: Avon Books.

Annas, G. J., and Healey, J. May/June 1974. The patient rights advocate. *Journal of Nursing Administration* 4:25–31.

Aydelotte, M. K. 1983. The future health care delivery system in the United States. In Chaska, N. L. *The nursing profession: A time to speak.* New York: McGraw-Hill.

———. May/June 1987. Nursing's preferred future. *Nursing Outlook* 35:114–20.

Baldwin, B. A. July/August 1990. Family caregiving: Trends and forecasts. *Geriatric Nursing* 11:172–74.

Bandman, E. L., and Bandman, B. 1990. *Nursing ethics in the lifespan.* 2d ed. Norwalk, CT.: Appleton and Lange.

Bezold, C. August 1982. Health care in the U.S.: Four alternative futures. *Futurist* 1:14–18.

Brecht, M. C. January/February 1990. Nursing's role in assuring access to care. *Nursing Outlook* 38:6–7.

Caterinicchio, R. P., editor. 1984. *DRGs: What they are and how to survive them—A sourcebook for professional nursing.* Thorofare, N.J.: Charles B. Slack.

Curtin, L. L., and Zurlage, C. 1984. *DRGs: The reorganization of health.* Chicago: S-N Publications.

Deines, E. October 1985. Coping with PPS and DRGs: The levels of care approach. *Nursing Management* 16:43–44, 46–48, 52.

Dimond, M. March/April 1989. Health care and the aging population. *Nursing Outlook* 37:76–77.

Dougherty, C. J. 1988. *American health care: Realities, rights, and reforms.* New York: Oxford University Press.

Edelman, C. L., and Mandle, C. L. 1990. *Health promotion throughout the lifespan.* 2d ed. St. Louis: C. V. Mosby Co.

Good intentions gone awry. March/April 1986. *Nursing Life* 6:55–56.

Hamilton, C. L., and Wilson, C. N. January 1989. The new Medicare Catastrophic Coverage Act: Will it affect nursing? *Nursing and Health Care* 10:30–34.

Hamilton, J. January/February 1986. Consumer alert: DRGs—Are hospitals saving money at your expense? *American Health* 41–45.

Howard, J., and Strauss, A., editors. 1975. *Humanizing health care.* New York: John Wiley and Sons.

Jonas, S. 1986. *Health care delivery in the United States.* 3d ed. New York: Springer Publishing Co.

Judd, V., and Forgues, C. November 1989. Canada's homeless: Breaking down the barriers to health care. *Canadian Nurse* 85:18–19.

Kelly, M. September 1989. The Omnibus Budget Reconciliation Act of 1987: A policy analysis. *Nursing Clinics of North America* 24:791–94.

Lindsay, A. M. March/April 1989. Health care for the homeless. *Nursing Outlook* 37:78–81.

Lundberg, C. J. 1984. Home health care: A logical extension of hospital services. *Topics in Health Care Financing* 11:22–33.

McCorkle, R., and Germino, B. 1984. What nurses need to know about home care. *Oncology Nursing Forum* 11:63–69.

Micheletti, J. A., and Shlala, T. J. October 1985. PROs and PPS: Nursing's role in utilization management. *Nursing Management* 16:37–42.

Nornhold, P. January 1990. 90 predictions for the '90's. *Nursing 90.* 34–41.

Omachonu, V. K., and Nanda, R. April 1989. Measuring productivity: Outcome vs. output. *Nursing Management* 20:35–38, 40.

O'Malley, J.; Loveridge, C. E.; and Cummings, S. H. February 1989. The new nursing organization. *Nursing Management* 20:29–32.

O'Neill, P. 1983. *Health crisis 2000.* London: William Heinemann.

Porter-O'Grady, T. October 1985. Strategic planning: Nursing practice in the PPS. *Nursing Management* 16:53–56.

RNABC News. January/February 1990. Health in the 1990's. *RNABC News* 22:11–13.

Smith, C. E. January 1985. DRGs: Making them work for you. *Nursing 85* 15:34–41.

Spasoff, R. 1987. *Health for all: Report of the Panel on Health Goals for Ontario.* Toronto: Ontario Ministry of Health.

Statistics Canada. 1980. *Perspectives Canada III.* Ottawa: Minister of Supply and Services.

———. 1981. *Canada year book 1980–81.* Ottawa: Statistics Canada.

Thatcher, R. M. September 1989. Community support: Promoting health and self-care. *Nursing Clinics of North America* 24:725–31.

U.S. Bureau of the Census. 1989. *Statistical abstract of the United States.* 109th ed. Washington, D.C.: U.S. Government Printing Office.

U.S. Department of Commerce. July 1, 1984. *Statistics on elderly population.* Washington, D.C.: Bureau of the Census.

Walker, A. 1987. Demand and supply of health care services. In Economics Council of Canada, *Aging with limited health resources: Proceedings of a colloquium on health care, May 1986.* Ottawa: Minister of Supplies and Services.

Zarle, N. C. September 1989. Continuity of care: Balancing care of elders between health care settings. *Nursing Clinics of North America* 24:697–705.

Health Promotion

CONTENTS

CONCEPT AND SCOPE OF HEALTH PROMOTION

Considerable differences appear in the literature regarding the use of the terms *health; wellness; health promotion; primary, secondary, and tertiary prevention; health protection;* and *illness prevention.* These differences are confusing to both health professionals and the consumers of health care services. Authors in nursing and the health care fields present different definitions of

health promotion and primary prevention and offer different ideas about their application. See Table 15–1.

Leavell and Clark (1965, p. 21) define three levels of prevention: primary, secondary, and tertiary. There are five steps that describe these levels: (1) health promotion and (2) specific protection are *primary preventions;* (3) early diagnosis and (4) prompt treatment to limit disability are *secondary preventions;* and (5) restoration and rehabilitation are *tertiary preventions.*

In the model used by Leavell and Clark, primary pre-

TABLE 15-1 *Definitions of Health Promotion*

Author	Definition
Pender (1987)	Activities directed toward increasing the level of well being and actualizing the potential of individuals, families, and groups; a category separate from primary prevention
Leavell and Clark (1965)	Maintaining or improving the general level of health of individuals, families, and groups; part of primary prevention
Julius Richmond, U.S. Surgeon General (1979)	Individual and community activities to promote healthful lifestyles
Amelia Mangay Maglacas, Chief Nurse WHO (1988)	*Positive* health promotion is the process of enabling people to increase control over and improve their own health; aimed primarily at improving health potential and maintaining health balance

Sources: N. J. Pender, *Health promotion in nursing practice,* 2d ed. (Norwalk, Conn.: Appleton & Lange, 1987), p. 4; H. R. Leavell and E. G. Clark, *Preventive medicine for the doctor in the community,* 3d ed. (New York: McGraw-Hill, 1965), p. 21; *Healthy people: The Surgeon General's report on health promotion and disease prevention* (Washington, D.C.: U.S. Department of Health, Education, and Welfare, 1979), p. 119; A. M. Maglacas, Health for all: Nursing's role, *Nursing Outlook,* November 1988, 88:67.

vention precedes any disease symptoms. The purpose of primary prevention is to encourage optimal health and to increase the person's resistance to illness (Edelman and Mandle 1986, p. 9). Examples of primary prevention include health education concerning the hazards of smoking and specific protection against a particular disease, such as the vaccine against poliomyelitis.

The second level, secondary prevention, presumes the presence of a disease or illness. Screening procedures, such as a blood sugar test for a client with diabetes mellitus, and the Denver Developmental Screening Tests to assess developmental delays, are facets of secondary prevention. Screening procedures facilitate early discovery and allow treatment to begin before the illness progresses. Disability limitation, another step in secondary prevention, is also more effective in the early stages of a disease.

Tertiary prevention relates to situations where a disability is already present. The goal of tertiary prevention is to restore individuals to their optimal level of functioning within the limitations imposed by their condition.

Pender (1987, p. 4) considers health promotion separate from primary prevention. She defines health promotion as "activities directed toward increasing the level of well being," and primary prevention as "activities directed toward decreasing the probability of specific illnesses." In this instance, health promotion is considered to be an approach behavior, whereas primary prevention is considered avoidance behavior. Health promotion is not disease oriented; that is, no specific problem is being avoided. By contrast, primary prevention activities are geared toward avoiding specific problems (Pender 1987, p. 5). Having analyzed the terms used in the health promotion literature, Brubaker (1983, p. 4) agrees with Pender's definition and further argues that even dictionary definitions support differences between the terms health promotion and primary or illness prevention. Brubaker notes that promotion is geared to "helping and encouraging to flourish," whereas to prevent is defined as "to keep from occurring." For example, a 40-year-old male may begin a program of walking 3 miles each day. If the goal of his program is to "decrease the risk of heart disease," then the activity would be considered prevention. By contrast, if his walking regime is instituted to "increase his overall health and feeling of well being," then the activity would be considered health promotion behavior. Most authors do not take health promotion to mean simply the avoidance of risk factors or the maintenance of stability. Rather, health promotion is seen as being directed toward self-development, growth, and a high level of wellness (Brubaker 1983, pp. 4–5).

In a 1979 document called *Healthy People,* the Surgeon General of the United States differentiates health promotion, health protection, and preventive health services. He outlines specific activities for each category:

- *Health promotion*—individual and community activities to promote healthful life-styles. Examples of health promotion activities include improving nutrition, preventing alcohol and drug misuse, maintaining fitness, and exercising.

- *Health protection*—actions by government and industry to minimize environmental health threats. Health protection relates to activities such as maintaining occupational safety, controlling radiation and toxic agents, and preventing infectious diseases and accidents.

- *Preventive health services*—actions of health care providers to prevent health problems. These services include control of high blood pressure, control of sexually transmitted diseases, immunization, family planning, and health care during pregnancy and infancy.

The chief scientist for nursing from the World Health Organization (WHO), Amelia Mangay Maglacas, uses the terms *positive health* and *positive health promotion* and presents them in a broader context. According to Maglacas, *positive* health for all does not mean the eradication of every disease or the healing of every body part. Rather, health should be considered in the context of its contribution to social and economic development, so that all people have the necessary social and economic support to lead satisfying lives (1988, p. 67). *Positive* health promotion is the process of enabling people to improve and to increase their control over their own health. The aim of positive health promotion is the improvement of health potential and the maintenance of health balance. This goal of positive health is attained by caring for ourselves and for others, by controlling life's circumstances with careful and conscientious decision making, and by ensuring that conditions in society allow people to attain health.

Health promotion organizations, wellness centers, and traditional health care centers all offer a different approach to client care. Table 15–2 demonstrates these differences. Health promotion activities take place before any disease occurs and can be considered a part of primary prevention. Health promotion strategies are geared toward raising the level of the health and well-being of the individual, family, or community. These activities can be carried out on a governmental level (e.g., a national program to improve knowledge of nutrition) or on a personal level (e.g., an individual exercise program).

Health promotion programs on an individual level can be active or passive. With *passive* strategies, the client is a recipient of the health promotion effort. Many health professionals participate in national programs to define and institute these passive strategies. Examples of passive government strategies are maintaining the cleanliness of water and promoting a healthy environment by enforcing sewage regulations to decrease the spread of disease. *Active* strategies depend on individuals' commitment to and involvement in adopting a program directed toward their health promotion. Active strategies are more important in that they encourage individuals to take control of their lives and assume the responsibility for their health. Examples of active strategies that involve changes in life-style are (1) a diet management program to improve nutrition, (2) a self-help program to reduce stress related to parenting, (3) an exercise program to improve muscle strength and endurance, or

TABLE 15–2 *Focus of Traditional Health Care Contrasted with Health Promotion and Wellness*

	Traditional	Health Promotion	Wellness
Primary goal	Identify and correct problem	Disease prevention and risk reduction	Increased health
Dominant message	"Health care professionals will take care of you."	"You will live longer if you avoid illness."	"You are responsible, and your efforts to be well will be supported."
Change agent	Treatment	Information and behavior change	Positive experience and cultural influences
Target	The problem	Individuals, families, and communities	Clients within cultures
Duration of intervention	Ends when the problems clear up	Length of class or program	Ongoing

Source: Adapted from J. P. Opatz, *A primer of health promotion: Creating healthy organizational cultures* (Washington, D.C.: Oryn Publications, 1985), p. 101.

(4) a combination diet and exercise regime for weight reduction or control. For optimal health and well-being, a combination of both active and passive strategies is suggested (Edelman and Mandle 1986, p. 10).

Types of Health Promotion Programs

A variety of programs can be used for the promotion of health, including (1) information dissemination, (2) health appraisal and wellness assessment, (3) life-style and behavior change, (4) worksite wellness programs, and (5) environmental control programs.

Information dissemination is the most basic type of health promotion program. This method makes use of a variety of media to offer information to the public about the risk of particular life-style choices and personal behavior, as well as the benefits of changing that behavior and improving the quality of life. Billboards, posters, brochures, newspaper features, books, and health fairs all offer opportunities for the dissemination of health promotion information. Alcohol and drug abuse, driving under the influence of alcohol, good nutrition, and hypertension are some of the topics frequently discussed. Recently, information about AIDS, including how it is transmitted, techniques for prevention, and the issue of sexual responsibility, has been distributed. The intent is to reduce unjustified fear, correct misinformation, and educate the public about this disease. Information dissemination is a useful strategy for raising the level of knowledge and awareness of individuals and groups about health habits.

Health appraisal/wellness assessment programs are used to apprise individuals of the risk factors that are inherent in their lives in order to motivate them to reduce specific risks and develop positive health habits. Wellness assessment programs are focused on more positive methods of enhancement, in contrast to the risk factor approach used in the health appraisal. A variety of tools are available to facilitate these assessments. Some of these tools are computer based and can therefore be offered to educational institutions and industries at a reasonable cost.

Life-style and behavior change programs require the participation of the individual and are geared toward enhancing the quality of life and extending the life span. Individuals generally consider life-style changes after they have been informed of the need to change their health behavior and become aware of the potential benefits of the process. Many programs are available to the public, both on a group and individual basis, some of which address stress management, nutrition awareness, weight control, smoking cessation, and exercise.

Worksite wellness programs are found in a variety of settings and are generally developed to serve the needs of individuals spending a great deal of time in the work environment. These include programs that address air quality standards for the office, classroom, or plant; programs aimed at specific populations, such as accident prevention for the machine worker or back-saver programs for the individual involved in heavy lifting; programs to screen for high blood pressure; or health enhancement programs, such as fitness information and relaxation techniques.

Environmental control programs have been developed in response to the recent growth in the number of contaminants of human origin that have been introduced into our environment (Logan and Dawkins 1986, p. 313). The amount of contaminants that are already present in the air, food, and water will affect the health of our descendants for several generations. The most common concerns of community groups are toxic and nuclear wastes, nuclear power plants, air and water pollution, and herbicide and pesticide spraying.

Sites for Health Promotion Activities

Health promotion programs are found in many settings. Programs and activities may be offered to individuals and families in the home or in the community setting, at schools, hospitals, or worksites. Some individuals may feel more comfortable having the nurse, diet counselor, or fitness expert come to their home for teaching and following up individual needs. This type of program, however, is not cost-effective for most individuals. Many people prefer the group approach, find it more motivating, and enjoy the socializing and group support. Most programs offered in the community are group oriented.

Community programs are frequently offered by cities and towns. The type of program depends on the current concerns and the expertise of the sponsoring department or group. Program offerings may include health promotion, specific protection, and screening for early detection of disease. The local health department may offer a townwide immunization program or blood pressure screening. The fire department may disseminate fire prevention information; the police may offer a bicycle safety program for children or a safe-driving campaign for young adults.

Hospitals began the emphasis on health promotion

and prevention by focusing on the health of their employees. Because of the stress involved in caring for the sick and the various shifts that nurses and other health care workers must work, the life-styles and health habits of health care employees was seen as a priority.

Programs offered by health care organizations initially began with the specific focus of prevention, i.e., infection control, fire prevention and fire drills, limiting exposure to x rays, and the prevention of back injuries. Gradually, issues related to the health and life-style of the employee were addressed with programs such as smoking cessation, exercise and fitness, stress reduction, and time management. Increasingly, hospitals have offered a variety of these programs and others (e.g., women's health) to the community as well as to their employees. This community activity of the health care institution enhances the public image of the hospital, increases the health of the surrounding population, and generates some additional income.

School health promotion programs may serve as a foundation for children of all ages to learn basic knowledge about personal hygiene and issues in the health sciences. Because school is the focus of a child's life for so many years, the school provides a cost-effective and convenient setting for health-focused programs. The school nurse may teach programs about basic nutrition, dental care, activity and play, drug and alcohol abuse, domestic violence, child abuse, and issues related to sexuality and pregnancy. Classroom teachers may include health-related topics in their lesson plans, e.g., the way the normal heart functions or the need for clean air and water in the environment.

Worksite programs for health promotion have developed out of the need for businesses to control the rising cost of health care and employee absenteeism (Greiner 1987, p. 53). Many industries feel that both employers and employees can benefit from healthy life-style behavior. The convenience of the worksite setting makes these programs particularly attractive to many adults who would otherwise not be aware of them or motivated to attend them. Health promotion programs may be held in the company cafeteria so that employees can watch a film or have a discussion group during their lunch break. Program offerings include diet, relaxation techniques, or physical fitness. Benefits to the worker may include an increased feeling of well-being, fitness, weight control, and decreased stress. Benefits to the employer may include an increase in employee motivation and productivity, an increase in employee morale, a decrease in absenteeism, and a lower rate of employee turnover, all of which may decrease business and health care costs.

The Nurse's Role in Health Promotion

Changes in the health care system, the demands of society, environmental and social issues, and the increased use of modern technology have all affected the role of the nurse. Clients are spending less time in acute care facilities. The focus is shifting to community and preventive nursing services. Nurses, as the largest group of health care workers, must prepare for the shift in emphasis and anticipate the nursing services that consumers will require. The nurse may act as advocate, consultant, teacher, or coordinator of services. For examples of the nurse's role in health promotion, see the accompanying box. In this role, the nurse may work with all age groups or be limited to a specific population, e.g., new parents, school-age children, or senior citizens. In any case, the nursing process is a basic tool for the nurse in a health promotion role. Although the process is the same, the emphasis is on teaching the client self-care responsibility. The clients decide the goals, determine the health promotion plans, and take the responsibility for the success of the plans. The steps of the nursing process in health promotion are health assessment, formu-

---

The Nurse's Role in Health Promotion

- Model healthy life-style behaviors and attitudes.
- Facilitate client involvement in the assessment, implementation, and evaluation of health goals.
- Teach clients self-care strategies to enhance fitness, improve nutrition, manage stress, and enhance relationships.
- Assist individuals, families, and communities to increase their levels of health.
- Educate clients to be effective health care consumers.
- Assist clients, families, and communities to develop and choose health-promoting options.
- Guide clients' development in effective problem solving and decision making.
- Reinforce clients' personal and family health-promoting behaviors.
- Advocate in the community for changes that promote a healthy environment.

lation of a nursing diagnosis, development of a health promotion/protection plan, implementation of the plan, and evaluation.

ASSESSING

A thorough assessment of the client's health status is basic to health promotion. Components of this assessment are the health history and physical examination, physical-fitness assessment, nutrition assessment, health risk appraisal, life-style assessment, health beliefs review, and life-stress review (Pender 1987, p. 103). As nurses move toward greater autonomy in providing client care, expanded assessment skills are essential to provide the meaningful data needed for health planning.

Health History and Physical Examination

The health history and physical examination provide a means for detecting any existing problems.

Physical-Fitness Assessment

During an evaluation of physical fitness, the nurse takes girth and skinfold measurements, administers the step test, and assesses strength and endurance of muscles and flexibility of joints.

Girth measurements The nurse measures the girth of the chest, waist, hips, upper arm (biceps), thigh, calf, and ankle. Guidelines for appropriate body proportions are shown in Table 15–3.

Skinfold measurements Skinfold measurements indicate the amount of body fat. To take skinfold measurements, the nurse grasps the skinfold (skin layers and subcutaneous fat) between the thumb and forefinger and measures the skinfold with special calipers.

The step test For this test, the client steps up and down a 17-inch step for 3 minutes. The following movements constitute one step: left foot up, right foot up, left foot down, right foot down. The rate should be 24 steps per minute for women and 30 steps for men (Getchell 1979, pp. 72–73). After the test, the client sits in a chair while the nurse assesses the pulse rate for 30 seconds at prescribed intervals:

TABLE 15–3 *Guidelines for Appropriate Girth Measurements*

	Males	Females
Chest or bust	Same size as hips	Same size as hips
Waist	About 13 to 18 cm less than chest	About 25 cm less than bust
Upper arm	Twice the wrist size	Twice the wrist size
Thigh	20 to 25 cm less than abdomen	15 cm less than abdomen
Calf	18 to 20 cm less than thigh	15 to 18 cm less than thigh
Ankle	15 to 18 cm less than calf	13 to 15 cm less than calf

Source: N. J. Pender, *Health promotion in nursing practice,* 2d ed. (Norwalk, Conn.: Appleton & Lange, 1987), p. 112. Used by permission.

1. 1 to 1½ minutes after the test
2. 2 to 2½ minutes after the test
3. 3 to 3½ minutes after the test

The sum of these three 30-second pulse rates is referred to as the *recovery index*. Normal values for women are 154–170; for men, 149–165 (Getchell 1979, pp. 72–73).

Muscle strength and endurance There are several tests of muscle strength and endurance. One is performing sit-ups with knees bent (bent-knee sit-ups). Women are asked to do these for 1 minute; men, for 2 minutes. The average rate for women is about 20 to 25 sit-ups per minute; for men, 50 to 60 per 2 minutes (Getchell 1979, p. 56).

Joint flexibility Range of motion in joints can be assessed quickly by asking the person to touch the toes several times. The average touch point is 1 to 3 inches in front of the toes.

Nutritional Assessment

To assess nutritional status, the nurse compares the client's weight to body build and height, measures mid-upper arm circumference to determine muscle mass, observes for signs of malnutrition, and takes a dietary history.

Health Risk Appraisal

A *health risk appraisal* (HRA) or health hazard appraisal (HHA) is an assessment and educational tool that indicates a client's risk of disease or injury over the next 10 years by comparing the client's risk with the mortality risk of the corresponding age, sex, and racial group. The client's health behavior and demographic data are compared to behaviors of and data about a large national sample. The principle behind risk appraisal is that each person, as a member of a specific group, faces certain quantifiable health hazards and that average risks are applicable to a client if the health professional knows the client's characteristics and the mortality of a large group of cohorts with similar characteristics (Pender 1987, p. 119).

Many HRA instruments are available today. In 1970, Drs. Lewis Robbins and Jack Hall used the medical health model to develop an HRA called Health Hazard Appraisal. Since that time, other health care groups have adapted this tool and marketed it under several names. More recently HRAs have begun to reflect a broader approach to health. The new focus is on the assessment of life-style factors and health behaviors. The objectives of most HRAs are twofold:

1. To assess risk factors that may lead to health problems. A *risk factor* is a phenomenon (e.g., age or lifestyle behavior) that increases a person's chance of acquiring a specific disease. The concept of at-risk aggregate is increasingly being used in community nursing practice. An *at-risk aggregate* is a subgroup within the community or population that is at greater risk of illness or poor recovery (Logan and Dawkins 1986, p. 18).

2. To change health behaviors that place the client at risk of developing an illness.

An HRA may have from 25 to 300 or more questions. Clients either score their responses themselves or send them to an organization for computer printouts. Scores are often tabulated according to an overall life-style profile, levels of health risk, and life expectancy.

Risk factors may be categorized according to (a) age, (b) genetic factors, (c) biologic characteristics, (d) personal health habits, (e) life-style, and (f) environment. Clients cannot control some of the risk factors appraised, such as age, sex, and family history; others, such as blood pressure, stress, and cigarette smoking, can be partially or totally controlled.

Pender (1987, pp. 123–130) developed a comprehensive risk factor assessment tool. She classifies risk factors into five categories: (a) risk of cardiovascular disease, (b) risk of malignant disease, (c) risk of automobile accidents, (d) risk of suicide, and (e) risk of diabetes. Contributing factors, such as family and personal medical history, habits, sex, age, environment, and life-style patterns, are included. See Figure 15–1 for Pender's risk appraisal form.

A client is usually appraised as being at high risk of developing a specific disease when two or three of the risk factors are at the highest level or four of the risk factors are at the two highest levels.

Life-Style Assessment

Life-style assessment focuses on the personal life-style and habits of the client as they affect health. Categories of life-style generally assessed are physical activity, nutritional practices, stress management, and such habits as smoking, alcohol consumption, and drug use. Other categories may be included.

Several tools are available to assess life-style. Pender (1987, pp. 138–143) outlines a comprehensive 10-category, 100-item tool that includes the following:

1. Competence in self-care, including dental hygiene, breast self-examination, knowledge about the danger signs of cancer, blood pressure, and other health care practices

2. Nutritional practices

3. Physical or recreational activity

4. Sleep patterns

5. Stress management

6. Self-actualization, including outlook on life and feelings about self, work, and accomplishments

7. Sense of purpose in life and knowledge of what is important in one's life

8. Relationships with others

9. Environmental control to make living areas free of hazards

10. Use of the health care system

The number of statements in each category ranges from 4 to 16. The reader is referred to Pender 1987 (see Selected References) for detailed information.

Walker, Sechrist, and Pender (1987) have developed the Health-Promoting Lifestyle Profile (HPLP), a 48-item tool that measures six dimensions of a healthy life-style: nutrition, exercise, health responsibility, stress management, interpersonal support, and self actualization. This

Risk Factor		⟶ Increasing Risk ⟶					

Risk for cardiovascular disease

Sex and age		Female under 40	Female 40-50	Male 25-40	Female after menopause	Male 40-60	Male 61 or over
Family history (parents, siblings)	High blood pressure	No relatives with condition	One relative		Two relatives		Three relatives
	Heart attack	No relatives with condition	One relative with condition after 60	Two relatives with condition after 60	One relative with condition before 60	Two relatives with condition before 60	
	Diabetes	No relatives with condition	One or more relatives with maturity onset		One or more relatives with pre-adolescent or adolescent onset		
Blood pressure*	Systolic	120 or below	121-140	141-160	161-180	181-200	Above 200
	Diastolic	70 or below	71-80	81-90	91-100	101-110	Above 110
Diabetes*		No diagnosis	Maturity onset, controlled	Maturity onset, uncontrolled	Adolescent onset, controlled	Adolescent onset, uncontrolled	
Weight*		At or slightly below recommended weight	10% overweight	20% overweight	30% overweight	40% overweight	50% overweight
Cholesterol*† level (mg/100 ml)		Below 180	181-200	201-220	221-240	241-260	261-280	Above 280
Serum triglycerides* (mg/dl) fasting		150 or below	151-400		401-1000		Above 1000
Percentage of fat in diet*		20%-30%	31%-40%		41%-50%		Above 50%
Frequency of exercise*	Recreational	Intensive recreational exertion (35-45 minutes at least 4 times a week)	Moderate recreational exertion		Minimal recreational exertion	No recreational exertion	
	Occupational	Intensive occupational exertion	Moderate occupational exertion		Minimal occupational exertion	Sedentary occupation	
Sleep patterns* (hours per night)		7-8	More than 8				4-6
Cigarette smoking*	No. per day	Nonsmoker	1-10	11-20	21-30	31-40	Over 40
	No. years smoked	Nonsmoker	Less than 10	11-15	16-20	21-30	31 or more

*Indicates risk factors that can be fully or partially controlled.

†Serum lipid analysis is also recommended to determine low-density (beta) and high-density (alpha) lipoprotein levels. Evidence suggests that high-density lipoprotein (HDL) carries cholesterol from tissues for metabolism and excretion. An inverse correlation appears to exist between HDL and coronary artery disease.

‡Chemicals such as asbestos, nickel, chromates, arsenic, chlormethyl ethers, radioactive dust, petroleum or coal products, and iron oxide.

Figure 15-1 Pender's risk appraisal assessment tool. *Source:* N. J. Pender, *Health promotion in nursing practice,* 2d ed. (Norwalk, Conn.: Appleton & Lange, 1987), pp. 123–129. Used by permission.

Risk for cardiovascular disease—cont'd

Stress*	Domestic	Minimal	Moderate	High	Very high
	Occupational	Minimal	Moderate	High	Very high

Behavior pattern* (particularly males)	*Type B* Relaxed, appropriately assertive, not time dependent, moderate to slow speech	*Type A* Excessively competitive, aggressive, striving, hyperalert, time dependent, loud and explosive speech

Air pollution*	Low	Moderate	High
Use of oral contraceptives* (females)	Do not use oral contraceptives	Under age 40 and use oral contraceptives	Over age 40 and use oral contraceptives

Risk for malignant disease

Breast cancer (women)

Age	20-29	30-39		40-49		50 or over
Race	Oriental		Black			White
Family history (grandmother, mother, sister)	None	Mother, sister, or grandmother		Mother and grandmother		Mother and sister
Onset of menstruation	Over age 12					Under age 12

Pregnancy*

Time	First pregnancy before age 25	First pregnancy after age 25	No pregnancies
No.	Three or more	One or two	None
Weight*	0% to 40% overweight		More than 40% overweight
Personal history	No evidence of dysplasia or previous breast cancer	Breast dysplasia	Previous breast cancer

Lung cancer
Cigarette smoking*

No. per day	Nonsmoker	1-10	11-20	21-30	31-40	Over 40
No. years smoked	Nonsmoker	Less than 10	11-15	16-20	21-30	31 or more

Occupational exposure to toxic chemicals‡

Years of exposure	Less than 1	1-5	6-10	11-15	Over 15
Frequency and intensity of exposure	Low frequency and low intensity	Low frequency, moderate intensity (or vice versa)	Moderate frequency, moderate intensity	Moderate frequency, high intensity (or vice versa)	High frequency, high intensity

▶

Risk Factor	→ Increasing Risk →			

Risk for malignant disease—cont'd

Cervical cancer

Onset of sexual activity*	After age 28	Age 22-27	Age 16-21	Before age 16
Number of sexual partners*	Two	Three		Four or more
Marital status*	Single			Married
Sexual partner*	Circumcised			Uncircumcised

Colorectal cancer

Age	Under 45			Over 45
Personal history	No history of ulcerative colitis	Ulcerative colitis less than 10 years	Ulcerative colitis more than 10 years	
Fiber content of diet*	High	Moderate		Low
Weight* (men)	Less than 40% overweight		More than 40% overweight	
Rectal bleeding or black bowel movement	Never	Occasionally		Frequently

Uterine and ovarian cancer

Age	Under 45			Over 45
Weight*	Less than 40% overweight		More than 40% overweight	
Vaginal bleeding other than during menstrual period	Never	Occasionally		Frequently

Skin cancer

Complexion	Dark	Medium		Fair
Sun exposure (without protection)	Never or seldom	Occasionally		Frequently

Risk for auto accidents

Alcohol consumption*	Nondrinker	Occasionally small to moderate consumption	Frequently small to moderate consumption	Occasionally heavy consumption	Frequently heavy consumption
Miles driven per year*	Under 5000	5001-10,000	10,001-20,000		Over 20,000
Use of seat belt*	Always	Usually	Occasionally		Never
Use of shoulder harness*	Always	Usually	Occasionally		Never

Figure 15-1 Pender's risk appraisal assessment tool. *(continued)*

Risk Factor	Increasing Risk →			
Risk for auto accidents—cont'd				
Use of drugs or medication that decrease alertness*	No use	Occasional use	Moderate use	Frequent use
Risk of suicide				
Family history	No history	One family member		Two or more family members
Personal history*	Seldom experience depression	Periodically experience mild depression	Frequently experience mild depression	Periodically experience deep depression	Frequently experience deep depression
Access to hypnotic medication*	No access	Access to small or limited dosages		Unlimited access to large dosages
Risk for diabetes Weight*	Desired weight	15% over-weight	30% over-weight	45% over-weight	More than 45% overweight
Family history (parent or sibling)	None	Either parent or sibling		Both parent and sibling

tool allows researchers to investigate patterns of a healthy life-style and measure the effects of health promoting interventions.

Ryan and Travis (1981) have developed a shorter, 16-item life-style assessment form entitled the Wellness Index. This tool may be used for initial assessments when client time is limited. See Figure 15–2.

The goals of life-style assessment tools are

1. To provide an opportunity for clients to assess the impact of their present life-style on their health
2. To provide a basis for decisions related to desired behavior and life-style change.

Health Care Beliefs

Clients' health care beliefs need to be clarified, particularly those beliefs that determine how they perceive control of their own health care status.

Locus of control is a concept from social learning theory. It is also relevant when determining who is most likely to take action regarding health, i.e., whether clients believe that their health status is under their own or others' control. People who believe that they have a major influence on their own health status, i.e., who believe health is largely self-determined, are called *internals*. Persons who are internally controlled are more likely than others to take the initiative in their own health care, be more knowledgeable about their health, and adhere to prescribed health care regimens. By contrast, people who believe their health is largely controlled by outside forces (e.g., chance, luck, or powerful others) and is beyond their control are referred to as *externals*. Edelman and Mandle (1986, p. 53) suggest that externally controlled people may need assistance to become more internally controlled if behavior changes are to be successful.

Locus of control is a measurable concept that can be used to predict which people are most likely to change their behavior. Wallston, Wallston, and DeVellis (1978) have developed two Multidimensional Health Locus of Control (MHLC) instruments to assess perceptions of health control. See Figure 15–3 (page 285) for one such instrument. Assessment of clients' health care beliefs provides the nurse with an indication of how much the clients believe they can influence or control health through personal behaviors.

The results of a study by Lewis suggest that greater personal control over one's life is associated with higher

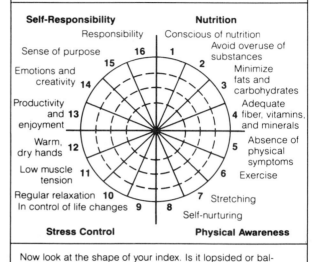

Circle the category that most closely answers the question.

1. I am conscious of the ingredients of the food I eat and their effect on me.   Rarely, Sometimes, Very Often (R, S, VO)

2. I avoid overeating and abusing alcohol, caffeine, nicotine, and other drugs.   R, S, VO

3. I minimize my intake of refined carbohydrates and fats.   R, S, VO

4. My diet contains adequate amounts of vitamins, minerals, and fiber.   R, S, VO

5. I am free from physical symptoms.   R, S, VO

6. I get aerobic cardiovascular exercise.   R, S, VO   (Very Often is at least 12–20 minutes 5 times per week vigorously running, swimming, or bike riding)

7. I practice yoga or some other form of limbering/stretching exercise.   R, S, VO

8. I nurture myself.   R, S, VO   (Nurturing means pleasuring and taking care of oneself, for example, massages, long walks, buying presents for self, "doing nothing," sleeping late without feeling guilty, etc.)

9. I pay attention to changes occurring in my life and am aware of them as stress factors.   R, S, VO   (See Life-Change Index—a score of over 300 is considered very stressful!)

10. I practice regular relaxation.   R, S, VO   (Suggested: 20 minutes a day "centering" or "letting go" of thoughts, worries, etc.)

11. I am without excess muscle tension.   R, S, VO

12. My hands are warm and dry.   R, S, VO

13. I am both productive and happy.   R, S, VO

14. I constructively express my emotions and creativity.   R, S, VO

15. I feel a sense of purpose in life and my life has meaning and direction.   R, S, VO

16. I believe I am fully responsible for my wellness or illness.   R, S, VO

Using your answers at the left to guide you, you can synthesize a graphic picture of your wellness. Each numbered pie-shaped segment of the circle below corresponds to the same numbered question on the preceding page. (They are divided into quarters representing four major dimensions of wellness.) Color in an amount of each segment corresponding to your answer to the question with the same number. The inner broken circle corresponds to "rarely," the next one to "sometimes," and third to "very often." You don't need to restrict yourself to these categories, however, and can fill in any amount in between. You may use different colors for each section if you like.

Now look at the shape of your index. Is it lopsided or balanced? This should provide beginning suggestions for improving your lifestyle and health habits.

Figure 15-2   Wellness index. Reprinted from *Wellness Workbook* © 1981, 1988 by John W. Travis, M.D. and Regina Sara Ryan with permission of Ten Speed Press, Berkeley, CA.

levels of self-esteem, greater purpose in life, and decreased self-report of anxiety (Lewis 1982, p. 113). Nurses can use this information about a client's locus of control to plan internal reinforcement training if necessary in order to improve client compliance. However, according to Shillinger (1983, p. 63):

Greater emphasis should be placed on assisting the client to make his own informed decisions, helping to identify and find solutions to problems that may interfere with compliance, and giving support and guidance as needed. In essence, this means building a partnership, an alliance, with the client rather than having compliance as the major goal.

The Health Belief Model (HBM) discussed in Chapter 13 suggests that the motivation to engage in a behavior is based on the person's belief that (a) one is vulnerable to the health problem, (b) the illness or problem is a threat, (c) the recommended health action will reduce the threat without substantial inconvenience, and (d) people should be generally concerned about health matters and be willing to accept medical advice (Becker et al. 1972, p. 852). The HBM is focused on susceptibility to disease and is therefore considered appropriate to explain health-protecting or preventive behaviors. It is not considered an appropriate model for health promoting behaviors.

Researchers have not been able to validate a significant association between a person's health beliefs and behaviors (Muhlencamp et al. 1985, p. 327). Cox (1985, p. 178) therefore has developed a new measure of motivation called the Health Self-Determination Index

Figure 15-3 Multidimensional health locus of control scale (Form B). *Source:* K. A. Wallston, B. S. Wallston, and R. DeVellis, Development of multidimensional health locus of control (MHLC) scales, *Health Education Monographs,* Spring 1978, 6:164–65. Reprinted by permission of John Wiley & Sons, Inc.

(HSDI). She believes that motivation is multidimensional, i.e., based on many factors. The process of choosing between behaviors is a primary factor.

Cox's HSDI includes a 20-item scale that has four interrelated subscales or factors:

1. *Self-determined health judgments.* Self-determinism in health judgments is assessed by the client's responses to statements such as:

   "Whatever the doctor suggests is OK with me."

2. *Self-determined health behavior.* Self-determinism in health behavior is assessed by the client's responses to statements such as:

   "I know without a doctor's telling me so that I'm doing the right things for my health."

3. *Perceived competency in health matters.* Perceived competency is determined by the client's responses to statements such as:

   "I feel good about how I take care of my health."

4. *Responsiveness to internal and external cues.* Responsiveness is measured by response to statements such as:

   "Some people think the doctor should decide about their health, but I think I should."

Although this tool has not been tested sufficiently to be used as a diagnostic aid, the data obtained in Cox's study strongly support the multidimensionality of motivation and the contributing roles of judgment, behavior, sense of competency, and responsiveness to internal or external cues. With further refinement and research, the HSDI will enable nurses to (Cox 1985, p. 182)

- Identify people at risk for decreased health and well-being owing to specific motivational responses
- Examine the motivational responses of clients throughout the life span for trends and changes
- Evaluate the differential effects of chronic versus acute illness on a person's motivational response
- Examine the effectiveness of interventions on specific health outcomes

This questionnaire is designed to determine the way in which different people view certain important health-related issues. Each item is a belief statement with which you may agree or disagree. Beside each statement is a scale that ranges from strongly disagree (1) to strongly agree (6). For each item we would like you to circle the number that represents the extent to which you disagree or agree with the statement. The more strongly you agree with a statement, the higher will be the number you circle. The more strongly you disagree with a statement, the lower will be the number you circle. Please make sure that you answer every item and that you circle *only one* number per item. This is a measure of your personal beliefs; obviously, there are no right or wrong answers.

Please answer these items carefully, but do not spend too much time on any one item. As much as you can, try to respond to each item independently. When making your choice, do not be influenced by your previous choices. It is important that you respond according to your actual beliefs and not according to how you feel you should believe or how you think we want you to believe.

1 = Strongly Disagree; 2 = Moderately Disagree; 3 = Slightly Disagree; 4 = Slightly Agree; 5 = Moderately Agree; 6 = Strongly Agree.

1. If I become sick, I have the power to make myself well again. 1 2 3 4 5 6
2. Often I feel that no matter what I do, if I am going to get sick, I will get sick. 1 2 3 4 5 6
3. If I see an excellent doctor regularly, I am less likely to have health problems. 1 2 3 4 5 6
4. It seems that my health is greatly influenced by accidental happenings. 1 2 3 4 5 6
5. I can only maintain my health by consulting health professionals. 1 2 3 4 5 6
6. I am directly responsible for my health. 1 2 3 4 5 6
7. Other people play a big part in whether I stay healthy or become sick. 1 2 3 4 5 6
8. Whatever goes wrong with my health is my own fault. 1 2 3 4 5 6
9. When I am sick, I just have to let nature run its course. 1 2 3 4 5 6
10. Health professionals keep me healthy. 1 2 3 4 5 6
11. When I stay healthy, I'm just plain lucky. 1 2 3 4 5 6
12. My physical well-being depends on how well I take care of myself. 1 2 3 4 5 6
13. When I feel ill, I know it is because I have not been taking care of myself properly. 1 2 3 4 5 6
14. The type of care I receive from other people is what is responsible for how well I recover from an illness. 1 2 3 4 5 6
15. Even when I take care of myself, it's easy to get sick. 1 2 3 4 5 6
16. When I become ill, it's a matter of fate. 1 2 3 4 5 6
17. I can pretty much stay healthy by taking good care of myself. 1 2 3 4 5 6
18. Following doctor's orders to the letter is the best way for me to stay healthy. 1 2 3 4 5 6

Life-Stress Review

There is abundant literature about the impact of stress on mental and physical well-being. Assessment of stressors, signs of anxiety, and stress is discussed in Chapter 23.

Validation of Assessment Data

Following the collection of assessment data, the nurse and client need to review, validate, and summarize the information. This step is carried out jointly by the nurse and the client. During this process, the nurse verbally reviews the current practices and attitudes of the client. This allows validation of the information by the client and may increase awareness of the need to change behavior. The following information should be considered (Pender 1987, p. 214):

- Any existing health problems
- The client's perceived degree of control over health status
- Level of physical fitness and nutritional status
- Illnesses for which the client is at risk
- Current positive health practices
- Ability to handle stress
- Information needed to enhance health care practices

DIAGNOSING

Following assessment, validation, and summarizing of data, nursing diagnoses are identified. The nurse and client may agree on potential nursing diagnoses that will assist the client in decreasing the risk of developing specific diseases. Diagnoses such as **High risk for altered nutrition: More than body requirements** are meaningful to a client who is interested in decreasing the risk factors related to cardiac disease.

Nursing diagnoses accepted by NANDA (North American Nursing Diagnosis Association) have generally focused on altered health patterns. Nurses caring for basically healthy individuals would find it necessary to use statements such as **High risk for altered nutrition** to describe a healthy client on a moderate weight-loss program, or **High risk for altered parenting** to describe new parents wanting information about child care. Houldin, Saltstein, and Ganley find the use of problem-oriented diagnoses somewhat inappropriate for a healthy population and suggest using a wellness-oriented classification system. Nursing diagnosis statements that describe motivational and wellness behaviors will identify client strengths, recognize self-care potential, reinforce healthy life-styles, assist the nurse in providing comprehensive, meaningful nursing care, and achieve the goals of health promotion and the prevention of illness (1987, pp. 16–17).

Wellness- or strength-oriented diagnoses can be applied at all levels of prevention but are particularly useful in primary care settings such as schools, industries, clinics, and community health facilities. When the nurse and client conclude that the client has positive function

---

Wellness Nursing Diagnoses

- Appropriate health maintenance related to balanced pattern of activity and rest
- Potential for adequate health maintenance related to good parenting skills
- Potential for adequate safety precautions related to knowledge of unsafe and unhealthy practices
- Adequate nutrition for body requirements related to support of spouse and awareness of balance between nutrition and exercise
- Satisfactory bowel elimination related to effective intestinal function and adequate fluids
- Optimal physical fitness related to regular exercise routine and motivation
- Potential for adequate physical fitness related to motivation
- Effective sleep pattern related to ability to fall asleep and adjust to interruptions in sleep
- Potential for successful coping of diminished sensory abilities related to willingness to change and ability to develop new coping skills
- Productive family processes related to adequate physical health of family members and ability to accept family responsibilities
- Positive social functioning related to personal maturity and respect for others
- Satisfactory sexual functioning related to healthy relationship with spouse
- Adequate personal coping related to appropriate emotional control and balance of work and recreational activities

in a certain pattern area, such as adequate nutrition or effective coping, the nurse can use this information to help the client reach a higher level of functioning. Some examples of wellness nursing diagnoses adapted from Houdin, Saltstein, and Ganley (1987) are listed in the box on page 286 in the right column. NANDA nursing diagnoses written as *high risk* diagnostic statements can also direct activities related to health promotion. See the examples of NANDA diagnoses in the accompanying box.

PLANNING

During the diagnosis phase of the health promotion process, the client has determined areas of potential problems and risks as well as areas of strength or positive health. The client then determines a health promotion plan. Health promotion plans need to be developed according to the needs, desires, and priorities of the client. The client decides on health promotion goals, the activities or interventions to achieve those goals, the frequency and duration of the activities, and the method of evaluation. During the planning process the nurse acts as a resource person rather than as an adviser or counselor. The nurse provides information when asked, emphasizes the importance of small steps to behavioral change, and reviews the client's goals and plans to make sure they are realistic, measurable, and acceptable to the client.

Steps in Planning

Pender (1987, p. 214) outlines several steps in the process of health promotion planning, which are carried out jointly by the nurse and the client:

1. *Identify health care goals.* The client selects two or three top priority goals or areas for improvement. Common goals are:
   a. To reduce the risk of cardiovascular disease
   b. To achieve or maintain a desired weight
   c. To improve or increase physical fitness
   d. To initiate and maintain relationships with a peer group
   e. To adjust to life-style changes effectively
   f. To decrease the amount of tobacco use
   g. To maintain an optimal balance between activity and rest
   h. To increase knowledge of safety practices in the home
   i. To improve relationships with family members

NANDA Nursing Diagnoses Related to Health Promotion

- Health-seeking behaviors related to new role as parent
- Health-seeking behaviors related to optimal nutrition for age and body size
- Altered nutrition: More than body requirements related to young-adult eating habits and adjustment to college life
- Altered nutrition: Less than body requirements related to lack of scheduled meals
- High risk for altered health maintenance related to tobacco use
- High risk for altered health maintenance related to insufficient finances
- High risk for altered growth and development related to school-related stressors
- High risk for diversional activity deficit related to postretirement status
- High risk for ineffective individual coping related to new parenting role
- High risk for decisional conflict related to college and career choices
- High risk for altered sexuality patterns related to job stress
- High risk for injury related to knowledge deficit of environmental hazards
- High risk for impaired adjustment related to divorce and inadequate support from family members
- High risk for activity intolerance related to lack of motivation

---

2. *Identify possible behavior changes.* For each of the selected goals or areas in step 1, determine what specific behavioral changes are needed to bring about the desired outcome. For example, to reduce the risk of cardiovascular disease, the client may need to change these specific behaviors:
   a. Stop smoking
   b. Lose weight
   c. Increase activity level
   d. Learn to relax
   e. Decrease animal fat in diet

f. Discontinue use of oral contraceptives

g. Sleep 7 to 8 hours per night

3. *Assign priorities to behavior changes.* Behavior must be acceptable to the client if it is to be adopted and integrated. From the list of behavior options in step 2, the clients select and assign priorities to those changes they are most willing to try. For example, the client may select increasing activity level, losing weight, and stopping smoking, in that order. It is helpful if the client first selects a behavior change area in which change is most readily perceived as positive. A successful beginning experience is important.

4. *Make a commitment to change behavior.* In the past, commitments to change behavior have usually been verbal. Increasingly, a formal, written behavioral contract is being used to motivate the client to follow through with selected actions. Motivation to follow through is provided by a positive reinforcement or reward stated in the contract. Contracting is based on the belief that all persons have the potential for growth and the right of self-determination, even though their choices may be different from the norm. Contracts are of two types: nurse-client contracts or self-contracts. Here is a sample of a self-contract:

I, Amy Martin will exercise strenuously for 20 minutes three times per week for a period of 2 weeks and will then buy myself six yellow roses.

> Amy Martin
> July 30, 1992

To ensure that a contract is explicit and meaningful, Kort (1984, p. 25) recommends that the client review it against the SMART checklist:

Specific: Do I know how, when, where, with whom, and how long I will do this?

Measurable: Will I know when it's done?

Acceptable: Will I feel good about doing this?

Realistic: Am I able to do this?

Truthful: Do I really want to?

Before a contract can be made, the client needs to identify actions that will bring about the desired behavior change. If, for example, the behavior change is to increase activity level, the client needs to consider and adopt specific actions. The client may consider swimming for 30 minutes three times a week, walking briskly for 1 hour daily, or some similar activity.

5. *Identify effective reinforcements and rewards.* Rewards tend to provide an incentive for behavior change, more so than individual willpower, provided the reward is meaningful to and selected by the client. Rewards can be objects, experiences, family activities, or praise. Examples of objects used as rewards are books, educational pamphlets, and personal care items. Examples of experiences used as rewards are having a 15-minute talk with a consultant, renting a cassette about a specific health matter, or going to a concert or health spa. Family trips, sports, or picnics are strong reinforcement for some people.

6. *Determine barriers to change.* Some specific barriers to change are
   a. Lack of support from family members
   b. Lack of space to carry out a certain activity
   c. Inappropriate weather
   d. Lack of motivation
   e. Fatigue or boredom
   f. Strong anxiety
   g. Cost of change
   h. Inconvenience
   i. Lack of time
   j. Culture or peer pressure

7. *Develop a schedule for implementing the behavior change.* Clients need to set up a time frame to make the behavior changes required to meet each goal. Time frames may be several weeks or months. Scheduling short-term goals and rewards can offer encouragement to achieve long-term objectives. Clients may need help to be realistic and to deal with one behavior at a time.

Exploring Available Resources

Another essential aspect of planning is identifying support resources available to the client. These may be community resources, such as a fitness program at a local gymnasium, or educational programs, such as stress management, breast self-examination, nutrition, smoking cessation, and health lectures. The nurse, too, may meet some of the client's educational needs. A major nursing role is to support the client. The nurse can contact the client or be available at specified intervals to review the contract and to assist with problem solving.

IMPLEMENTING

Implementing is the "doing" part of behavior change. Self-responsibility is emphasized for implementing the plan. The client, therefore, is the primary decision maker, seeking out the expertise of the nurse where it will assist in goal achievement. The strategies to be used, their frequency, and the priorities have all been determined in the plan. To increase the likelihood of a successful implementation, the nurse ascertains that the assessment has been accurate and complete and that the goals are individualized and attainable. Depending on the clients' needs, the nursing strategies may include supporting, teaching, consulting, coordinating, facilitating, counseling, and enhancing the behavior change.

Providing and Facilitating Support

A vital component of life-style change is ongoing support that focuses on the desired behavior change and is provided in a nonjudgmental manner. Support can be offered by the nurse on an individual basis or in a group setting. The nurse can also facilitate the development of support networks for the client, such as family members and friends.

Individual counseling sessions   Counseling sessions may be routinely scheduled as part of the plan or may be provided if the client encounters difficulty in carrying out interventions or meets insurmountable barriers to change. In a counseling relationship, the nurse and client share ideas. In this sharing relationship, the nurse acts as a facilitator, promoting the client's decision making regarding the health promotion plan.

Telephone counseling   Regular telephone sessions may be provided to the client to help in answering ques-

---

RESEARCH NOTE

What Are the Health Promotion Practices of Nursing Students?

Nursing students have the power to act as role models for classmates, family, friends, and clients. How well do they play this role? The purpose of this study was to identify the health practices of nursing students and to find out their overall opinion toward primary preventive practices. The sample for this study consisted of 1081 female nursing students from ten schools in the Buffalo, New York area. The ten schools included diploma, associate degree, and baccalaureate programs. The ages of the students ranged from 17 to 55 years, with a mean age of 24.

The results showed considerable variation in the extent to which students practiced health promotion and prevention. On the positive side, the majority of students obtained 6–8 hours of sleep per night, did not or had never smoked, brushed their teeth regularly, exercised regularly, had routine dental care, and had a yearly physical examination. However, less than half of the students ate breakfast daily, three-fourths of those surveyed ate between meals, and less than half limited fats, salt, and sugar in their diets. Breast self-examination was done by only one-third of the group; most did not wear seat belts; and 90% consumed alcoholic beverages.

The preventive health orientation (PHO) of the sample was measured by a 14-item index. The scores ranged from 1 to 13, with a mean of 7.1. Thus, the typical nursing student practiced about half the desired behaviors.

Both age and type of educational program were significant factors with respect to preventive health practices. Scores on the PHO index were significantly higher for older students versus younger ones, and for associate degree and baccalaureate students versus diploma students.

These findings indicate that although nursing students, as future health care professionals, are expected to act as role models, their own health practices need improvement.

Implications: The authors suggest that faculty take a more active role in promoting positive health promotion behaviors by (a) increasing students' awareness regarding the information and resources that are available for facilitating behavior change, (b) increasing content related to health promotion and prevention within the core curriculum and in courses relating to health and life-styles, and (c) instituting no-smoking policies in classrooms and school buildings. In addition, nursing faculty members should be aware of their role in setting the appropriate example by practicing health promotion and prevention.

S. Dittmar, B. Hoyghey, R. O'Shea, and J. Brasure. Health practices of nursing students. *Health Values,* March/April 1989, 13:24–31.

tions, reviewing goals and strategies, and reinforcing progress. The client may find that scheduling a weekly telephone session is helpful or may wish to initiate a call if a problem occurs. The client is asked, "Is your plan working?" If the plan is not working, the nurse asks, "What would you like to do?" The client may wish to continue or may wish to change the plan to a more realistic one. Telephone support is efficient for the busy client who may not have the time for regular, in-person sessions.

Group support   Group sessions provide an opportunity for participants to learn the experiences of others in changing behavior. Group contact gives individuals a renewed commitment to their goals. Groups can be scheduled at monthly or less frequent intervals for over a year.

Facilitating social support   Social networks, such as families and friends, can facilitate or impede the efforts directed toward health promotion and prevention. The nurse's role is to assist the client to assess, modify, and develop the social support necessary to achieve the desired change (Pender 1987, p. 393). In order to provide the necessary support, families must communicate effectively, be aware of and support each other's needs and goals, and provide help and assistance to one another to achieve those goals. The client may wish the nurse to meet with the family or significant others and help in enlisting their understanding and support.

Providing Health Education

Health education programs on a variety of topics can be provided to groups, individuals, or communities. Group programs need to be planned carefully before they are implemented. The decision to establish a health promotion program must be based on the assessed health needs of the people; also, specific health promotion goals must be set. After the program is implemented, program outcomes must be evaluated.

In the evaluation of health promotion programs, the client's understanding must be ascertained. Simply asking clients if they understand may be inappropriate (Byham and Vickery 1988, p. 10). In some cases, the client may understand the information but may not be able to apply it or may have anxiety about doing a particular task. For instance, a new parent may understand all the principles of giving an infant a bed bath but have considerable anxiety about safely managing the procedure. Giving clients ample opportunity to demonstrate or practice routines and procedures, asking them to repeat

important steps or information, and clarifying any unclear statements allows the nurse to evaluate the clients' knowledge and competence more fully.

Nurses may offer an abundance of information less formally. To do so, however, nurses need up-to-date knowledge, the ability to assess learning needs, and effective teaching skills. See Chapter 19 for detailed information. For example, nurses often disseminate information about parenting, breast and testicular self-examination, prevention of sexually transmitted disease, nutritional needs, and monitoring blood pressure and pulse rates.

Health fairs are a recent method being used to disseminate information to the public about health promotion and disease prevention and early detection. Nurses are often the initiators of health fairs and may provide participants of all age groups with information, teaching, counseling, or screening. Health fairs are usually offered in convenient locations such as shopping malls, schools, hospitals, and business settings in order to encourage maximum participation.

Enhancing Behavior Change

Whether people will make and maintain changes to improve health or prevent disease depends on many interrelated factors. See the section on assessing health care beliefs, earlier in this chapter. Murphy (1982, p. 427) says that the distances between wanting to change, attempting to change, and being able to change can be enormous. She emphasizes this statement by pointing out the difficulty many people have in acquiring regular dental flossing habits. When a client succeeds in making healthy behavior changes because of information the nurse has provided, the nurse feels satisfied and pleased. When, however, the client does not succeed in planned behavioral changes, the nurse tends to feel frustrated and often describes the person as "resistant," "uninterested," "unmotivated," or "noncompliant."

Murphy (1982) says the nurses are erroneously inclined to believe (a) that change will occur simply by bringing unhealthy behavior to the client's attention and (b) that when the client does not change, the desire to change is absent.

To help clients succeed in implementing behavior changes, the nurse needs to understand the process of change and the nature of the client's motivation or the client's current situation. An application of Lewin's stages of change (Lewin 1951) can help the nurse recognize the client's needs (Murphy 1982, p. 428). See Chapter 12 for additional information on Lewin's stages.

In *Stage 1 (unfreezing),* the client's motivation to

change emerges. The client recognizes the need to change and becomes uneasy about the present way of doing things. At this stage, the nurse must help the client feel safe enough to explore and consider alternatives. Murphy says, " 'Unfreezing' or 'unlearning' old habits is probably the most important stage of change but it is also the most difficult and challenging for the health promoter" (1982, p. 428). The nurse can best help the client by emphasizing what that person values. Loss of an unhealthy behavior may then become tolerable. For example, a client may start to "unfreeze" a habit of eating excessive carbohydrates if emphasis is placed on maximizing energy potential through a balanced food intake rather than just on the components of a healthy diet. In *Stage 2 (moving),* the client is ready to change and develop new responses. Many health promoters tend to focus their efforts on this stage of eliciting new desired responses (Murphy 1982). In *Stage 3 (refreezing),* the client internalizes behavior changes and stabilizes a new level of functioning.

The response of the nurse to lack of change in the client is generally to provide more information or to withdraw from the interaction after concluding that there is no point wasting time on people who do not want to change. Both responses deny such clients the opportunity to improve their health. By providing more information to the client, the nurse assumes that the client lacks knowledge. If, however, the client has understood the information, repeating or amplifying the information more than likely will annoy the client. The nurse has failed to identify the problem clearly. Withdrawal from clients who have difficulty changing implies that the nurse's health promotion efforts will be directed toward persons who readily and willingly comply. Such people, however, are probably the ones who least need the nurse's help. Additional guidelines for assisting the client toward behavior change are offered in the accompanying box.

Modeling

Modeling consists of observing the behavior of other people who have successfully achieved the goal that clients have set for themselves (Pender 1987, p. 265). Modeling is not imitating. Through observing a model, the client acquires ideas for behavior and coping strategies for specific problems. The client is not expected to mimic the sequence of actions or behavior patterns of the model.

The nurse and client should mutually select models with whom the client can identify, since the cultural and ethnic backgrounds of the nurse and client often differ.

CLINICAL GUIDELINES
Enhancing Behavior Change

■ Recognize that motivation is the basis of all behavior whether it is healthy or unhealthy, good or bad.

■ Recognize that people are motivated by their needs.

■ Avoid labeling people as unmotivated. The label simply means that the person does not comply with the wishes of the nurse who applies the label.

■ Focus on the sources or factors that motivate the person's behavior rather than on the presence or absence of motivation.

■ Remember that resistance is a normal part of change and a healthy response to a threat.

■ Understand that a client may choose to keep unhealthy habits for many reasons.
  a. The habit may be a culturally learned response such as cigarette smoking and alcohol consumption. In North America, these habits were once associated with a glamorous or sophisticated lifestyle and a certain kind of satisfaction.
  b. The client may be directing all available energies to meet other needs. A person who is grieving the loss of a loved one, or a recently divorced person, for example, may not have the energy to follow a weight-loss diet.
  c. The conditions required to change may be absent. For example, clients need help first to "unlearn" or "unfreeze" old habits and recognize the benefits of new habits before they can consider or undertake action.

■ Cast aside the idea that the client *must* change. This attitude is not conducive to a helping relationship with the client and does not convey respect for the client. The client who does not change is entitled to the nurse's interest and nonjudgmental response.

■ Measure your competence in terms of how well you understand clients' needs and implement clients' care rather than by the extent to which clients change their behavior.

(Murphy 1982, p. 429)

Models should be frequently available during the early learning and change stages of unfreezing and moving. Models should also be people the client respects.

Nurses should serve as models of wellness. In order to model effectively, nurses need to have a philosophy and life-style that demonstrate good health habits. Pender (1987, p. 463) believes that undergraduate nursing students should work with faculty and college health services to develop a wellness program. Through such a plan, students can assess their own life-styles, develop a health promotion plan, and actually carry out the implementation strategies. The college years offer access to facilities and health services that may not be available when students begin their working life. Once students have had a firsthand experience with creating a health promotion plan and with the difficulties involved with behavior change, they will be able to work more effectively with peers and clients. Clients are more likely to respect and trust the nurse who can tell them what worked in the nurse's personal situation.

EVALUATING

Evaluation takes place on an ongoing basis, both during the attainment of short-term goals and after the completion of long-term goals. During evaluation, the client may decide to continue with the plan, reorder priorities, change strategies, or revise the health promotion contract. Evaluation of the plan is a collaborative effort between the nurse and the client. Goals are written during the planning phase and a date determined for attaining the specific results or behaviors that are desired to promote health or prevent illness. The following is an example of a nursing diagnosis, goal statements, planned interventions, and evaluative statements.

- *Nursing Diagnosis*
  Health-seeking behaviors related to desire for information on breast self-examination

- *Long-Term Goal*
  The client performs breast self-examination regularly by 10/15/19xx.

- *Short-Term Goals*
  #1. The client passes a test on the basic facts about breast cancer by 2/2/19xx.
  #2. The client performs breast self-examination accurately by 3/4/19xx.

- *Interventions*
  The client attends two educational sessions to learn basic information on breast cancer and breast self-examination.
  The client practices and demonstrates procedures on models.
  The client demonstrates procedure on self.

- *Evaluation*
  Goal #1 attained. By the date specified, the client was able to pass a test on basic knowledge of the subject. Because this is an objective measure of cognitive knowledge, the nurse can clearly evaluate whether the client has learned the material and met this short-term goal.

  Goal #2 attained. By the date specified, the client was able to perform the breast self-examination accurately. This is a psychomotor objective that the nurse can evaluate by having the client demonstrate breast self-examination using the appropriate techniques.

- *Evaluation of the Long-Term Goal*
  In this example, the long-term goal may be evaluated during a meeting or planned telephone conversation with the client. Achievement of the long-term goal is ascertained by asking the client if she performed accurate breast self-examination each month. The client states, "Yes, I have done the procedure every month for the past five months." In this example, goal achievement is measured solely on the basis of information the client gives the nurse. There is no objective measure to ascertain that this was done. It is up to the client to be honest in her self-assessment and commitment to the health promotion goal.

Using the nursing process for promotion of health and prevention of illness assumes that the client is a motivated, self-directed, responsible consumer. The nurse's role is to assist clients in achieving their goals. The nurse is available to lend expertise in the assessment of health, the implementation of a health promotion plan, and the evaluation of the goals. The nurse also enhances the potential for client success in goal achievement by using strategies such as teaching, counseling, support, and the modeling of good health behaviors.

CHAPTER HIGHLIGHTS

▶ Health promotion activities are directed toward developing client resources that maintain or enhance well-being.

▶ The goal of health promotion is to raise the client's level of health.

CHAPTER HIGHLIGHTS (continued)

▶ Health protection activities are geared toward the prevention of specific diseases, such as obtaining immunizations to prevent poliomyelitis.

▶ Health promotion programs can be categorized as information dissemination, health appraisal and wellness assessment, life-style and behavioral change, worksite wellness, and environmental control programs.

▶ Wellness-oriented nursing diagnoses identify client strengths, recognize self-care abilities, and enhance health promotion goals.

▶ A thorough assessment of the client's health status is basic to health promotion.

▶ Health risk or hazard appraisals provide the data that often spur the client to adopt a healthier life-style.

▶ Life-style assessment tools give clients the opportunity to assess the impact of their present life-styles on their health and to make decisions about life-style changes.

▶ Clients' health care beliefs provide the nurse with an indication of how much clients believe they can influence or control health through personal behaviors.

▶ To help clients change their life-styles or health behaviors, the nurse provides ongoing support, supplies additional information and education, and explores the motivating sources of the client's behavior.

▶ During planning the client may wish to make a behavioral contract. A contract usually includes the client goal, activities needed to achieve the goal and the methods of evaluation to measure goal achievement.

▶ Nurses, in order to be role models for their clients, should develop attitudes and behaviors that reflect healthy life-styles.

▶ During the evaluation phase of the health promotion process, the nurse assists clients in determining whether they will continue with the plan, reorder priorities, or revise the plan.

LEARNING ACTIVITIES

■ Identify health promotion goals for your community. You may need to consult with public health or civil officials.

■ Identify health promotion or wellness programs in your community. Where are they (schools, hospitals, industry, private enterprise, civic groups, and so on)? What service do they provide? What are the criteria to participate? What fees are required?

■ 1. Using Pender's Health Risk Appraisal instrument on pages 280–283, conduct your own personal assessment of health risk. What are your health risk factors? Which are changeable? Which are not changeable?
2. Conduct your own Wellness Index as described on page 284. What is your Wellness Index?
3. What areas could you improve? Develop a written plan to decrease your health risks and increase your Wellness Index. How will you go about implementing your plan?

READINGS AND REFERENCES

SUGGESTED READINGS

Ireland, D. November 1988. Reading, writing and reasons for health. *American Journal of Nursing* 88:1506.

Ireland describes the development, philosophy, staffing, and types of services offered at an adolescent health center located on the grounds of a high school. Each visit to the clinic is seen as an opportunity for health teaching. The staff also reaches out to the classroom and community centers with career days, tutoring, film festivals, walking programs, and other such "sideline sessions."

McMahon, A., and Maibush, R. M. November 1988. How to send quit-smoking signals: Timing is everything when encouraging a patient to decide to quit smoking. *American Journal of Nursing* 88:1498–99.

McMahon and Maibush outline a three-step process nurses can use to assist clients to quit smoking. The authors suggest using quit-smoking messages that are brief, direct, and informative. A chart with examples of "the do's and don'ts of quit-smoking messages" is provided.

Maglacas, A. M. March/April 1988. Health for all: Nursing's role. *Nursing Outlook* 36:66–71.

This author shares her vision of health for all in the 21st century and describes the role and responsibility of the nurse if the vision is to become reality. The future role of the nurse will emphasize not interventions related to disease but support of the total person to meet all the individual's needs. To prepare for this new role, the nurse must develop new skills that enable people to accept responsibility for self-care, self-help, environmental improvement, and positive health promotion.

RELATED RESEARCH

Boyd, A. September/October 1988. Level of wellness of nursing students. *Health Values* 12:14–20.

Byham, L. D., and Vickery, C. E. July/August 1988. Compliance and health promotion. *Health Values* 12:5–13.

Campion, V. Summer 1989. Effect of knowledge, teaching method, confidence and social influence on breast self-examination. *Image: Journal of Nursing Scholarship* 21:76–80.

SELECTED REFERENCES

Becker, M.; Drachman, R; and Kirscht, J. 1972. Motivation as predictors of health behavior. *Health Services Reports* 87:852–62.

Brubaker, B. H. April 1983. Health promotion: A linguistic analysis. *Advances in Nursing Science* 5:1–14.

Byham, L. D., and Vickery, C. E. July/August 1988. Compliance and health promotion. *Health Values* 12:5–12.

Clark, C. C. 1986. *Wellness Nursing*. New York: Springer Publishing Co.

Cox, C. L. May/June 1985. The health self-determinism index. *Nursing Research* 34:177–83.

Donoghue, J.; Duffield, C.; Pelletier, D. et al. 1990. Health promotion as a nursing function: Perceptions held by university students of nursing. *International Journal of Nursing Studies* 27:51–60.

Edelman, C., and Mandle, C. L. 1986. *Health promotion throughout the life span*. St. Louis: C. V. Mosby Co.

Getchell, B. 1979. *Physical fitness: A way of life*. 2d ed. New York: John Wiley and Sons.

Greiner, P. A. November 1987. Nursing and worksite wellness. *Holistic Nursing Practice* 2:53–60.

Hales, D. 1989. *An invitation to health*. 4th ed. Redwood City, Calif.: Benjamin/Cummings Publishing Co.

Healthy People: The Surgeon General's Report on Health Promotion and Disease Prevention. 1979. Washington, D.C.: U.S. Department of Health, Education and Welfare.

Houldin, A.; Saltstein, S.; and Ganley, K. 1987. *Nursing Diagnosis for Wellness*. Philadelphia: J. B. Lippincott Co.

Ireland, D. F. November 1988. Reading, writing and reasons for health. *American Journal of Nursing* 88:1506.

Kort, M. April 1984. Support: An important component of health promotion. *Canadian Nurse* 80:24–26.

Leavell, H. R., and Clark, E. G. 1965. *Preventive medicine for the doctor in the community*. 3d ed. New York: McGraw-Hill.

Lewin, K. 1951. *Field theory in social science*. New York: Harper and Row.

Lewis, F. M. March/April 1982. Experienced personal control and quality of life in late-stage cancer patients. *Nursing Research*. 31:113–18.

Logan, B. B., and Dawkins, C. E. 1986. *Family-centered nursing in the community*. Menlo Park, Calif.: Addison-Wesley.

Maglacas, A. M. March/April 1988. Health for all: Nursing's role. *Nursing Outlook* 36:266–71.

Montoye, H. J.; Christian, J. L.; Nagle, F. J.; and Levin, S. M. 1988. *Living Fit*. Menlo Park, Calif.: Benjamin/Cummings Publishing Co.

Muhlenkamp, A. F.; Brown, N. J.; and Sands, D. November/December 1985. Determinants of health promotion activities in nursing clinic clients. *Nursing Research* 34:327–32.

Murphy, M. M. November/December 1982. Why won't they shape up? Resistance to the promotion of health. *Canadian Journal of Public Health* 73:427–30.

Murray, R. B., and Zentner, J. P. 1989. *Nursing assessment and health promotion strategies through the life span*. 4th ed. Norwalk, Conn.: Appleton & Lange.

Pender, N. J. 1987. *Health promotion in nursing practice*. 2d ed. Norwalk, Conn.: Appleton & Lange.

Ryan, R. S., and Travis, J. W. 1981. *Wellness workbook for health professionals*. Berkeley, Calif.: Ten Speed Press.

Walker, S. N.; Sechrist, K. R.; and Pender, N. J. March/April 1987. The health-promoting lifestyle profile: Development and psychometric characteristics. *Nursing Research* 36:76–81.

Wallston, K. A.; Wallston, B. S.; and DeVellis, R. Spring 1978. Development of the multidimensional health locus of control (MHLC) scales. *Health Education Monographs* 6:164–65.

Family Health

Janice Denehy, RN, PhD

ROLES AND FUNCTIONS OF THE FAMILY

Considerable evidence underscores the importance of the family. Definitions of *family* are as numerous and different as the many forms of family seen in today's society. There has been a resurgence of interest in the family unit and its impact on the health, values, and productivity of individual family members. In the nursing profession, this interest in the family as a unit has been expressed by the emergence of *family-centered nursing:* nursing that considers the health of the family as a

unit in addition to the health of individual family members.

Membership in a family has a tremendous influence on the individual through genetic endowment, ethnicity, and the development of personal, social, moral, and cultural values. Nurses must consider the family's influence on the individual as they assess, diagnose, plan, implement, and evaluate nursing care.

When one envisions a family, usually the first image

that comes to mind is a mother and father—the husband and wife—and their children, usually a boy and a girl. A family of parents and their offspring is known as the *nuclear family*. The relatives of nuclear families, such as grandparents or aunts and uncles, comprise the *extended family*. In some families, members of the extended family live with the nuclear family. Such multigenerational families were more common during the last century but are still seen today in many cultures as well as in many North American homes. Although members of the extended family may live in different areas, they are a frequent source of support and companionship for the family.

The family is frequently defined as two or more persons who are related through marriage, blood, birth, or adoption (Duvall 1977). Although this definition characterizes a large number of families, it does not adequately describe the membership of many families today. In many family groups, there are no legal or blood relationships among members. As the structure of the family has become more diverse, it has been necessary to define the family more broadly to encompass the wide variety of family forms seen in today's society. To provide flexibility in the study of families, Friedman (1981, p. 8) defines the family as follows: "A family is composed of people (two or more) who are emotionally involved with each other and live in close geographical proximity." Emotional involvement is demonstrated through caring and a commitment to a common purpose.

The family is the basic unit of society. Its major roles are to protect and socialize its members. Among the many functions it serves, of prime importance is the role the family plays in providing emotional support and security to its members through love, acceptance, concern, and nurturing. This affective (emotional) component holds families together, gives family members a sense of belonging, and develops a sense of kinship.

In addition to providing an emotionally safe environment for members to thrive and grow, the family is also a basic unit of physical protection and safety. This is accomplished by meeting the basic needs of its members: food, clothing, and shelter. Provision of a physically safe environment requires knowledge, skills, and economic resources.

In modern society, the economic resources needed by the family are secured by adult members through employment or government programs. The family also protects the physical health of its members by providing adequate nutrition and health care services. Nutritional and life-style practices of the family not only influence the health of family members but also directly affect the developing health attitudes and life-style practices of children.

In addition to providing an environment conducive to physical growth and health, the family creates an atmosphere that influences the cognitive and psychosocial growth of its members. Children and adults in healthy, functional families receive support, understanding, and encouragement as they progress through predictable developmental stages, as they move in or out of the family unit, and as they establish new family units. In families where members are physically and emotionally nurtured, individuals are challenged to achieve their potential in the family unit. As individual needs are met, family members are able to reach out to others in the family and the community, and to society.

The family is a major educator of its members. Parents are often called a child's first teachers. This early learning plays an influential part in the development of a child's attitudes about family, education, health, work, and recreation. These attitudes persist throughout their lives. In addition, families play a major role in the transmission of religious, cultural, and societal values. As the family socializes its new members to the expectations of home, community, and society, it provides a place of warmth, acceptance, and nurturing that insulates its members from the demands of society.

The family is a place of roots, refuge, and rejuvenation. It is a small network where members communicate and work together, delegating roles and responsibilities with a shared purpose: the protection and growth of its members. Through the experiences of family life, the individual learns to participate in and contribute productively to society.

FRAMEWORKS FOR STUDYING THE FAMILY

According to *systems theory,* a system is a unit composed of parts that are interdependent. (See Chapter 4 for systems theory.) The family unit can be viewed as a system. Its members are interdependent, working toward specific purposes and goals. Many families are described as *open systems,* for they are continually interacting and influenced by other systems in the community. Boundaries regulate the input from other systems that interact with the family system; they also regulate output from the family system to the community or to society. Boundaries protect the family from the demands and influences of other systems. Open families are likely to welcome input from without, encouraging individual members to adapt beliefs and practices to meet the changing demands of society. Such families are more likely to seek out health care information and use community resources. These families are adaptable and therefore better prepared to cope with changes in lifestyle needed to restore, maintain, or promote health.

Family systems also can be described as *closed systems*. Closed families are self-contained units resistant to outside interaction or influence. Such families may be suspicious of others and are content with the status quo. They are less likely to change values and practices; they tend to exert more control over the lives of their members and distrust recommendations made by nonfamily members. It is more difficult for closed family systems to use community resources that may be helpful in dealing with a family health crisis or to incorporate new behaviors that may promote a healthier family. The boundaries of most families, however, are permeable and flexible, regulating input and output according to family needs, values, and developmental stage.

The *structural-functional theory*, as the name implies, focuses on family structure and function. The structural component of the theory addresses the membership of the family and the relationships among family members. Intrafamily relationships are complex because of the numerous relationships that exist within the family structure—mother-daughter, brother-sister, husband-wife, and so on. These relationships are constantly evolving as children mature and leave the family nest and adults age and become more dependent on others to meet their daily needs.

The functional aspect of the theory examines the effects of intrafamily relationships on the family system, as well as their effects on other systems. Some of the main functions of the family include developing a sense of family purpose and affiliation, adding and socializing new members, and providing and distributing care and services to members. A healthy family organizes its members and resources in meeting family goals; it functions in harmony, working toward shared goals.

Developmental theory views families as ever-changing and growing. Crucial, yet predictable, tasks occur at each level or stage of development. Achievement of tasks appropriate at one level is a prerequisite for successfully achieving the tasks expected at the next level. A major task of the family, from a developmental perspective, is to create an environment where the family can master critical developmental tasks. This ensures orderly progression through the stages of the family life cycle.

THE FAMILY IN TODAY'S SOCIETY

It is difficult to describe the family of today except as uniquely diverse. Improvements in health care have led to healthier people living longer and more productive lives. The development of reliable contraceptives and the legalization of abortion have resulted in greater control in the planning of families. Today's economic realities, coupled with liberation ideology, have moved many women out of the home and into the workplace, changing traditional family roles. Higher divorce rates and the acceptance of children born to unmarried mothers have led to a dramatic increase in the number of single-parent families. Individuals are also grouping together to form new family units based on sexual preference or economic need.

Traditional Families

The *traditional family* is often viewed as an autonomous unit in which both parents reside in the home with their children, the mother assuming the nurturing role and the father providing the necessary economic resources. The traditional family is still very much a part of North American culture, but it is no longer the predominant family form. Although members of the extended family are not likely to live with traditional nuclear families, they remain an important source of information, support, and security. Contact with members of the extended family is vital to mobile families in times of stress or crisis because contact gives a sense of stability in a complex, impersonal society.

In the modern family, changes are occurring in traditional role patterns. Today's fathers are more involved with their children and family life. Many attend prenatal classes and witness the birth of their infants. In addition, fathers are more involved with household chores as role stereotypes are challenged, even though wives continue to perform a large portion of the housework. Likewise, females are less bound by traditional role patterns in today's society.

Two-Career Families

In *two-career*, or *dual-career, families*, both the husband and wife are employed. Such families have been steadily increasing since the 1960s. The reasons for this trend are many, including the increased educational and career opportunities available to women, a desired increase in standard of living, and economic necessity. Many two-career families are young couples without children who desire to complete and use their education. Other working couples postpone childbearing until they are financially secure, have paid debts, and have purchased some of life's extras. Two-career families may also be parents who have launched their children and find they have many healthy, productive years to spend in the marketplace prior to retirement.

It is estimated that 60% to 70% of working women have children in the home, many of whom are preschoolers. When both parents work, the roles each partner plays are variable. Many husbands become more involved in the care of children and the management of household chores. Time and personal energy constraints also may lead to reevaluation of family activities and goals. Attention must be given to maintaining the husband-wife relationship and individual interests amidst the pressures of juggling family and career commitments.

The increased number of working parents has created a need for quality, affordable child care. Finding such child care is one of the greatest stresses faced by today's working parents. Many children spend part of each working day in daycare homes or child-care centers that may expose them at a young age to a host of people with a wide range of ideas and values.

Once children reach school age, parents find that few resources for after-school child care are available. Many school-age children come home to empty houses or apartments to care for themselves. These latchkey children, as they are called because they carry their own house key, may become bored or frightened as they wait for the parents to return from work (McClelland 1984). Parents and professionals are realizing the importance of preparing these children with information about safety and household management to reduce their anxiety and help them make the most of these hours alone. Children of working parents are growing up with new family role models, which will no doubt have an effect on the families of tomorrow.

Single-Parent Families

Today it is estimated that over 50% of North American children live in a *single-parent family*—a home headed by one parent—sometime during their childhood. There are many reasons for single parenthood, including death of a spouse, separation, divorce, birth of a child to an unmarried woman, or adoption of a child by a single man or woman. Single parents frequently express concern about child care, adequate financial resources, social isolation, and lack of adult companionship. Single parents who work outside the home experience fatigue and role overload in managing growing children, household tasks, and a job. At times, these concerns seem to occupy their entire lives, leaving little time for personal or recreational activities.

Nearly 90% of single-parent families are headed by a female. Because these women are often young and poorly prepared for the job market, many single-parent families live with financial strain or poverty. In homes where a divorce has occurred, there is frequently a drop in the standard of living. Child support payments may dwindle after the first year and in many cases are never received. When families live with inadequate financial resources, the health of the family is likely to suffer from substandard living conditions, poor nutrition, stress, and inadequate health care services. The self-esteem of the family is impaired because members, particularly the head of the household, find it difficult to raise their standard of living due to stigma or lack of skills, time, and energy. Depression and despair are common among women struggling to raise a family (Duffy 1982); these feelings not only affect the woman but also influence the outlook of growing family members, who learn to view society as hostile, not as a place full of challenges and hope for the future.

Single-parent families need to identify a support system. Members of the extended family or friends who are supportive provide an opportunity for mutual caring and sharing of concerns. Such support networks reduce social isolation and provide opportunities for relaxation and recreation. A support system helps the single parent cope with and reduce stress; in addition, it gives the individual a chance to have fun and regain self-esteem. Referral to appropriate community resources helps the single parent locate child care, take advantage of financial or social programs, and develop job skills through education or job-training programs.

Blended Families

Existing family units who join together to form new family units are known as *blended* or *reconstituted families*. Families with children living with a birth parent and a nonbirth parent are commonly called step families. The blending of two families presents a unique set of challenges to the individuals involved. The joining of two families is often met with hope and anticipation. Each family brings its own history and expectations to the new family constellation. Often expectations for instantaneous adaptation and affection are too high. Children, depending on their ages and past experiences, usually adjust slowly to new patterns of communication and family authority. Family reintegration requires time and effort. Stress occurs as blended families get to know each other, respect differences, and establish new patterns of behavior (Reutter and Strang 1986).

The greatest success in blending families comes when each family member enters the new relationship with realistic expectations and plans to take the time to make the new family unit succeed. Successful parents get along with and enjoy each other, enjoy life, and bring a sense of humor to the challenge of blending the lifestyles and values of two families into one.

Adolescent Parents

A disturbing trend is the growing proportion of infants born each year to adolescent parents. These young parents, who are still mastering the developmental tasks of childhood, are physically, emotionally, and financially ill prepared to undertake the responsibilities of parenthood. Over 600,000 infants in America are born each year to adolescent mothers (*The Adolescent Family* 1984, p.1). An increasing number of these mothers are 15 years and younger. A disproportionate number of adolescent births are to members of minority racial or ethnic groups.

Pregnant adolescents are at greater risk for health problems during pregnancy because of poor nutritional status, physiologic immaturity, and lack of prenatal care. They are more likely to deliver premature infants who are, in turn, at greater risk for subsequent health and developmental problems. In addition, adolescent mothers are more likely to give birth to another infant while still in their teens. Today there is a greater acceptance of unmarried parenthood, and fewer pregnant teens feel pressured to marry the father of the infant or to relinquish the infant for adoption.

Adolescent pregnancy frequently interrupts education and may necessitate changes in life goals of many young women. The newly formed family unit is often dependent upon others for physical, emotional, and financial assistance. Support systems are crucial to its success. Parenting skills need to be developed, and the completion of at least a high school education should be encouraged. While helping the new mother understand the needs of her growing infant is an important intervention for nurses, so is assisting the young mother progress through the developmental tasks of adolescence into adulthood.

The children of adolescent parents are at greater risk for health and social problems as they grow up. These children experience more accidents during their preschool years than their peers, are frequently behind in receiving their childhood immunizations, and are more prone to exhibit learning and behavior problems when they enter school. Often raised in poverty, children of adolescent mothers may have few role models to help them break out of the cycle of poverty and subsequent adolescent parenthood.

Cohabiting Families

A current and growing trend in alternate family forms is unrelated individuals or families cohabiting or living under one roof, forming new family units called *cohabiting* or *communal families*. Some individuals join together out of a need for companionship; for example, two widowed adults who share common interests found that living together eliminated previously lonely hours during the evening. Others cohabit to achieve a sense of family or belonging. Many unmarried couples choose to cohabit; some have no desire for a long-term commitment, others wish to test a relationship prior to marriage.

Financial need often leads to the formation of cohabiting families. In these situations, individuals or families share living expenses as well as the responsibilities of household management. Others may cohabit to share services. For example, a single mother moved in with an elderly man who desired to remain in his home but needed help with cooking and cleaning. The single mother was able to provide these services, and she benefited because she and her daughter were now regularly sitting down to nutritious meals, something they rarely experienced previously. An added bonus was the close friendship the elderly man established with her 6-year-old daughter. The formation of cohabiting families illustrates the flexibility and creativity of the family unit in adapting to meet individual challenges and responding to changing societal demands.

Gay and Lesbian Families

Of recent interest is the awareness of the number of homosexual adults in today's society who have formed *gay* and *lesbian families* based on the same goals of caring and commitment seen in heterosexual relationships. While homosexual relationships have been stereotyped as short term and casual, many gay and lesbian relationships are based on long-term mutuality. As the society becomes more educated about homosexuality, it will better understand the complex emotional attachments and affiliation of many homosexual couples and will provide a more accepting atmosphere for these relationships.

Although homosexual marriages are not legally recognized, many homosexual relationships are the basis of new family units. Lesbian women are more likely to live together or cohabit than gay men. Lesbians have fewer sexual partners, are more likely to spend time with their partner, and place a higher value on sexual fidelity than their male counterparts (Williamson 1986). Lesbian women are also more likely to bring children from previous marriages into their partnerships than gay men are. Although many are concerned about the effects of parental homosexuality on the growing child, studies have shown that these children develop sex-role orientations and behaviors similar to children in the general population (Hoeffer 1981). The greatest danger to children reared in gay and lesbian families is the prejudice and ridicule expressed by others in society. For this reason, many homosexual parents keep their sexual preference private to spare their children pain during early childhood, choosing to explain their sexual preference when the children are able to understand homosexuality and emotionally ready to deal with its implications.

Families from Different Cultures

Families from different cultures are an integral part of North America's rich heritage. Each family has values and beliefs *(cultural heritage)* that are unique to their culture of origin and that shape the family's structure, methods of interaction, health care practices, and coping mechanisms. These factors interact to influence the health of families. Families from different cultures may cluster to form mutual support systems and to preserve their heritage; however, this practice may isolate them from the larger society.

Children in cultural clusters often have greater contact with the world around them than adults; through school, children become more proficient in language and more comfortable with new customs and behaviors. Sometimes children create conflict in the family when they bring home new ideas and values. They want to become part of the culture in which they live and incorporate new practices into existing family customs. In the process, they may reject previously cherished cultural traditions.

Becoming acculturated is a slow, stressful process of learning the language and customs of a new country. Chapter 24 presents information that helps the nurse understand the family traditions, beliefs, and practices of different cultures. This information helps the nurse pro-

vide nursing care that is sensitive to the unique needs of families from different cultural heritages.

Single Adults Living Alone

Although individuals living alone, by definition, are not considered a family unit, in today's society many individuals live by themselves. When society is studied from a family perspective, these individuals are frequently overlooked, yet they represent a significant proportion of the population. Singles may include young, newly emancipated adults who have left the nuclear family and achieved independence. These young adults may have completed their education and entered the job market, becoming self-sufficient and self-supporting. As young adults postpone marriage or choose singleness, living alone is becoming a more prevalent life-style.

On the other end of the age spectrum is the older adult living alone. Having launched their families, many older adults find themselves single through divorce, separation, or death of a spouse. Some older adults remain in their homes, while others find an apartment more suitable to their changing needs. As they age, and depending on their health status and financial resources, some single adults relocate into retirement homes or extended care facilities. Although many older adults live alone, they may have frequent contacts with other family members, especially adult children and grandchildren. As they enter the golden years, their sense of family becomes stronger, and they seek to communicate the history and values of the family to the new generation.

ASSESSING THE HEALTH OF FAMILIES

The importance of family assessment cannot be overemphasized. The information gathered during assessment is the basis for planning and delivering nursing care to family members or to the family as a whole. Numerous family assessment tools are available. The nurse must consider a number of factors in selecting a family assessment tool or in developing a tool that meets the demands of the families served in a particular practice setting. The home care nurse, for instance, may develop a tool to assess the unique needs and problems of a family who has a member with diabetes.

A family assessment tool should be holistic, eliciting information about a wide variety of family characteristics, beliefs, and behaviors. The tool should be understandable and acceptable to both the family and the nurse (Speer and Sachs 1985). In other words, the nurse must use terminology comprehensible to a wide range of clients, and the tool should be quickly and easily administered. The instrument should also yield clinically relevant data about the family—information useful in formulating nursing diagnoses and planning nursing interventions that promote the health of families.

Overall Family Assessment

The purpose of family assessment is to determine the level of family functioning, to clarify family interaction patterns, to identify family strengths and weaknesses, and to describe the health status of the family and its individual members (Logan & Dawkins, 1986, p. 185).

An overall assessment of the family includes:

- Identification of family members
- Description of the living environment
- Health status of family members
- Financial status, including health insurance and patterns of health care utilization
- Health beliefs and goals of the family
- Occupation of family members
- Education level and aspirations of the family
- Social and community agencies utilized by the family
- Social patterns of the family

Also important are family living patterns, including communication, child rearing, coping strategies, and health practices. An overall family assessment gives an overview of the family process and helps the nurse identify areas that need further assessment. Nurses carry out a more detailed assessment in specific target areas as they become more acquainted with the family and begin to understand family needs and strengths more fully. In planning interventions, nurses need to focus not only on problems but also on family strengths and resources as part of the nursing care plan.

The family APGAR is a screening tool that reveals how family members perceive the level of functioning of the family unit as a whole (Smilkstein 1978) (see Figure 16–1). Open-ended questions assess family functioning in the areas of adaptation, partnership, growth, affection, and resolve. The nurse then elicits information on family satisfaction with each of the functional components of family functioning. The information gained provides basic data about the level of family functioning and gives the nurse an idea about which areas need more detailed assessment and intervention and about

family strengths that can be mobilized in solving other family problems.

Health Appraisal

The *health appraisal* begins with a complete health history. The nurse focuses first on the family unit and then on the individuals in that family. The health history is one of the most effective ways of identifying existing or potential health problems. The history is followed by physical assessment of family members. If further evaluation is indicated, referral is made to the appropriate health care professional. Frequently the physical examination focuses on identifying disease conditions or the potential for them rather than on appraisal of health. When the focus is on health, the appraisal includes information on life-style behaviors and health beliefs. The nurse uses data from the health appraisal to formulate a health profile. The health profile provides the data necessary to establish a nursing diagnosis and to plan appropriate nursing interventions to promote optimal health through life-style modification.

Health Beliefs

To promote health, the nurse must understand the health beliefs of individuals and families and use this information in planning and delivering nursing care. Health beliefs may reflect a lack of information or misinformation about health or disease. They may also include folklore and practices from different cultures. Because of the many advances in medicine and health care during the last few decades, many clients have out-dated information about health, illness, treatment, and prevention. The nurse is frequently in a position to give information or correct misconceptions about health. This function is an important component of the nursing care plan. For additional information on health beliefs, see Chapter 15.

Family Communication Patterns

The effectiveness of family communication determines its ability to function as a cooperative, growth-producing unit. Messages are constantly being communicated among family members, both verbally and nonverbally. The information transmitted influences how members work together, fulfill their assigned roles in the family, incorporate family values, and develop skills to function in society. *Intrafamily communication* plays a significant role in the development of self-esteem, which is necessary for the growth of personality.

Family APGAR Questionnaire

	Almost always	Some of the time	Hardly ever
I am satisfied that I can turn to my family* for help when something is troubling me.	_____	_____	_____
I am satisfied with the way my family talks over things with me and shares problems with me.	_____	_____	_____
I am satisfied that my family accepts and supports my wishes to take on new activities or directions.	_____	_____	_____
I am satisfied with the way my family expresses affection and responds to my emotions, such as anger, sorrow, and love.	_____	_____	_____
I am satisfied with the way my family and I share time together.	_____	_____	_____

Scoring: The patient checks one of three choices, which are scored as follows: "Almost always" (2 points). "Some of the time" (1 point), or "Hardly ever" (0). The scores for each of the five questions are then totaled. A score of 7 to 10 suggests a highly functional family. A score of 4 to 6 suggests a moderately dysfunctional family. A score of 0 to 3 suggests a severely dysfunctional family.

*Family is defined as the individual(s) with whom you usually live. If you live alone, your "family" consists of persons with whom you now have the strongest emotional ties.

Figure 16-1 Family APGAR questionnaire. *Source:* G. Smilkstein, M.D. and W.R. Moore, Professor, The APGAR Questionnaires. Screening for social support: family, friends, and work associates. Department of Family Practice, University of Louisville, Louisville, KY, May 1988, p. 33.

Families who communicate effectively transmit messages clearly. Members are free to express their feelings without fear of jeopardizing their standing in the family. Family members support one another and have the ability to listen, empathize, and reach out to one another in times of crisis. When the needs of family members are met, they are more able to reach out to meet the needs of others in society.

When patterns of communication among family members are dysfunctional, messages are often communicated unclearly. Verbal communication may be incongruent with nonverbal messages. Power struggles may be evidenced by hostility, anger, or silence. Members may be cautious in expressing their feelings because they cannot predict how others in the family will respond. Many things remain unsaid to preserve family unity and tranquility. When family communication is im-

paired, the growth of individual members is stunted. Members often turn to other systems to seek personal validation and gratification.

The nurse needs to observe intrafamily communication patterns closely. Nurses should pay special attention to who does the talking for the family, which members are silent, how disagreements are handled, and how well the members listen to one another and encourage the participation of others. Nonverbal communication is important because it gives valuable clues about what people are feeling.

Family Coping Mechanisms

Family coping mechanisms are the behaviors families use to deal with stress or changes. Coping mechanisms can be viewed as an active method of problem solving developed to meet life's challenges. The coping mechanisms families and individuals develop reflect their individual resourcefulness. Friedman (1981, p. 249) states that families may use the same coping patterns rather consistently over time or may change their coping strategies when new demands are made on the family. Coping is a basic function that helps the family meet demands imposed both from within and without. The success of a family depends on how well it copes with the stresses it experiences.

Nurses working with families realize the importance of assessing coping mechanisms as a way of determining how families relate to stress. Also important are the resources available to the family. Internal resources, such as knowledge, skills, effective communication patterns, and a sense of mutuality and purpose within the family, assist in the problem-solving process. In addition, external support systems promote coping and adaptation. These external systems may be extended family, friends, religious affiliations, health care professionals, or social services. The development of social support systems is particularly valuable today, when many families, due to stress, mobility, or poverty, are isolated from resources that would help them cope.

Identifying Families at Risk for Health Problems

Risk assessment helps the nurse identify individuals and groups at higher risk than the general population of developing specific health problems, such as stroke, diabetes, and lung cancer. Risk may be related to genetic factors; for example, persons who have a family history of diabetes are at greater risk of developing diabetes than persons with no family history of diabetes. Certain practices also increase the risk of health problems; for instance, cigarette smokers are at greater risk of developing lung cancer than nonsmokers. Environmental factors, such as air pollution or exposure to toxic chemicals, increase the risk of certain health problems.

Risk reduction among individuals and groups identified as at risk poses a special challenge to health care professionals. Once the individuals or groups are identified, the nurse's role is to plan and implement interventions to reduce health risks when possible or to optimize the current health status of those individuals or groups when risks cannot be reduced. The vulnerability of family units to health problems may be based on family developmental level, age of family members, heredity or genetic factors, sociologic factors, and life-style practices. The goal of the nurse is to promote optimal family health and functioning.

Developmental Factors Families at both ends of the age continuum are at risk of developing health problems. Newly formed families entering the childbearing and childrearing phases of development experience many changes in roles, responsibilities, and expectations. These changes occur when adult family members are attempting to establish financial security. The many, often-conflicting demands on the young family cause stress and fatigue, which may impede growth of family members and the functioning of the group as a unit.

Adolescent mothers, because of their developmental level and lack of knowledge about parenthood, and single-parent families, because of role overload experienced by the head of the household, are more likely to develop health problems. Moreover, the elderly are at risk of developing degenerative and chronic health problems. Because of the emphasis on youth in today's society, many elderly persons feel a lack of purpose and decreased self-esteem. These feelings in turn reduce their motivation to engage in health-promoting behaviors, such as exercise or community and family involvement.

Hereditary Factors Persons born into families with a history of certain diseases, such as diabetes or cardiovascular disease, are at greater risk of developing these conditions. A detailed family health history, including genetically transmitted disorders, is crucial to the identification of persons and families at risk. These data are used not only to monitor the health of individual family members but also to recommend modifications in health practices that potentially reduce the risk, minimize the consequences, or postpone the development of genetically related conditions.

Other family units or family members may be at risk of developing a disease by reason of sex or race. Males, for example, are at greater risk of having cardiovascular disease at an earlier age than females, and females are at greater risk of developing osteoporosis, particularly after menopause. While at times it is difficult to separate genetic factors from cultural factors, certain risk factors seem to be related to race. Some diseases are more prevalent among whites than blacks, and vice versa. Sickle-cell anemia, for example, is a hereditary disease limited to blacks of African descent (McFarlane 1977). Native Americans and Asians seem more susceptible to certain diseases and less susceptible to others than the general population.

Life-Style Factors

As the understanding of health and illness increases, it has become clear that many diseases are preventable, the effects of some diseases can be minimized, or the onset of disease can be delayed through life-style modification. Cancer, cardiovascular disease, adult-onset diabetes, and tooth decay are among the life-style diseases. The incidence of lung cancer, for example, would be greatly reduced if people stopped smoking. Proper nutrition, good dental hygiene, and use of fluoride—in the water supply, in toothpaste, as a topical application, or as supplements—have been shown to reduce dental decay or caries, one of America's most prevalent health problems. Automobile accidents, the leading cause of death among adolescents and young adults, are frequently associated with alcohol consumption and increased risk taking.

In addition to health practices and nutrition, other important life-style considerations are exercise, stress management, and rest. Today, health professionals have the knowledge to prevent or minimize the effects of some of the main causes of disease, disability, and death. Too often, there is little consideration of health until sickness occurs. The challenge is to disseminate information about prevention and to motivate families to make life-style changes prior to the onset of illness. Many demands are made on today's family. An important question is: Will people take the time to be responsible for their own health?

Sociologic Factors

Poverty is a major problem that affects not only the family but also the community and society. Over 35 million people, or nearly one out of every six Americans, live in poverty (Moccia and Mason 1986, p. 20). A disproportionate number of today's poor belong to ethnic or racial minority groups. Poverty is a real concern among the rising number of one-parent families headed by a female, and, as the number of these families increases, poverty will affect a large number of growing children.

Because many poor families do not possess the skills or support systems necessary to break out of the cycle of poverty, it is likely that poverty will continue to escalate rapidly in the future. When ill, the poor are likely to put off seeking services until the illness reaches an advanced state and requires longer or more complex treatment. Even though the Surgeon General has reported that the health of the American people has never been better (U.S. DHEW 1979), it is clear that this progress has not benefited all segments of society, particularly the poor.

DIAGNOSING AND PLANNING

Data gathered during a family assessment may lead to the nursing diagnoses: **Altered family processes,** the state in which a normally supportive family experiences a stressor that affects its functioning; **Family coping: potential for growth,** the state in which a family member exhibits a desire and readiness for enhanced health and growth; **Ineffective family coping: disabling,** the state in which a family demonstrates destructive behavior or adapts detrimentally to a stressor; **Ineffective family coping: compromised,** a state similar to *altered family processes;* **Altered parenting,** the state in which one or more caregivers is unable to create an environment that promotes the optimal growth and development of a child or children; and **Impaired home maintenance management,** the state in which an individual or family is unable to independently maintain a safe, growth-promoting immediate environment. Examples of contributing factors for these diagnoses follow.

Altered family processes related to:

- Illness of family member
- Loss of family member
- Gain of new family member
- Economic crises (e.g., unemployment)
- Change in family role (e.g., working mother)
- Retirement
- Divorce

Family coping: potential for growth related to:

- Role changes (e.g., marriage, parenthood)

See also contributing factors for *Health seeking behaviors*

Ineffective family coping: disabling related to:

- Alcoholic parent
- Drug-addicted family member
- Dependent elderly parent
- Emotionally disturbed parent or child
- Terminally ill parent or child

Ineffective family coping: compromised related to:

See *Altered family processes*

Altered parenting related to:

- Impaired parental infant attachment
- Mental or physical illness

Impaired home maintenance management related to:

- Chronic debilitating disease
- Injury to family member
- Parent with cognitive, motor, or sensory deficit

Planned nursing interventions need to focus on assisting the family to plan realistic strategies that enhance family functioning, such as improving communication skills, identifying and utilizing support systems, developing and rehearsing parenting skills, and becoming involved in community activities. For families who are functioning well, anticipatory guidance may assist families in preparing for predictable developmental transitions that occur in the life of families (Denehy 1990).

Examples of outcome criteria to evaluate the achievement of client goals and the effectiveness of nursing interventions follow.

The client or family:

- Expresses feelings freely and appropriately
- Participates in problem-solving processes directed at appropriate solutions for the crisis
- Participates in care of the ill family member
- Encourages ill family member to handle situation in own way, progressing toward independence
- Seeks appropriate external resources as needed
- States an intent to use positive coping mechanisms and constructive stress management
- Expresses more realistic understanding and acceptance of the family member demonstrating destructive or maladaptive behavior
- Seeks assistance for abusive behavior
- Verbalizes realistic expectations of parenting role
- Demonstrates appropriate parenting behaviors, e.g., attachment
- Identifies own needs as well as strengths and resources to meet needs
- Begins to verbalize positive feelings about infant
- Identifies factors that restrict self-care and home management
- Demonstrates ability to perform skills necessary for individual or home care

HEALTH PROMOTION IN THE FAMILY

Today's families are concerned about living healthy, productive, fulfilling lives. The media regularly inform the public that many personal behaviors endanger life

RESEARCH NOTE

Health Promotion in the Family

Duffy reviewed current research in health promotion for the family and suggests directives for future research. Four nursing journals—*Nursing Research, Research in Nursing and Health, Western Journal of Nursing Research,* and *International Journal of Nursing Studies*—were reviewed to identify the number of studies related to health promotion in the family published between January 1980 and June 1986. The review revealed a dearth of nursing research in family health promotion. Of the 105 issues reviewed, only five articles (4.8%) addressed health promotion activities in the family.

Duffy used the findings from these studies, as well as other research literature, to develop future directives, or areas for study. These directives address both the internal and external environment of the family. Areas related to the *internal environment* of the family include (a) family definitions of health and health promotion, (b) descriptions of current family health promotion behaviors and those practiced over time, (c) decision-making, (d) influence of parenting, (e) influence of fathering, and (f) methods of intervention most effective in encouraging health promotion in the family. Research of the *external* environment includes (a) the societal norms that facilitate or impede health promotion behaviors, (b) societal interventions, such as those that decrease the impact of poverty in families, and (c) the effects of social institutions on the practice of health.

Implications: Without further nursing research on health promotion in the family, nurses will not have a sufficient body of knowledge to influence public and health policies and to work with individuals and families in the promotion of their health.

Duffy, M. E. January 1988. Health promotion in the family: Current findings and directives for nursing research. *Journal of Advanced Nursing* 13:109–17.

and health, yet at the same time they accept advertising revenues from products that do not promote health. Much has been learned about the effects of diet, stress, and exercise on health, but changing long-established preferences and practices is difficult. Substance abuse, particularly of tobacco and alcohol, as well as personal and environmental safety hazards have needlessly decreased the productivity and shortened the lives of many persons.

To make changes that improve its own well-being, the family must be aware of potential health problems and their relationship to life-style practices. Information on how to reduce risks within the context of the family's value system is crucial. Support and encouragement of life-style changes help ensure that these changes are not temporary but become an important health value that influences lifelong health practices. The role of health education is to inform, motivate, and facilitate adoption of healthful life-style practices—activities that promote the well-being of individuals and families.

One of the major goals of health promotion is to help families take responsibility for their own health through self-care. *Self-care* is defined as activities individuals perform in their own behalf to maintain health and well-being (Orem 1980). Effective self-care requires knowledge and skills relating to health and illness. It includes knowing how to solve health problems of the family, as well as knowing when to seek outside guidance in meeting health problems. Self-care also encompasses health promotion for the family. Through health promotion, families can realize higher levels of wellness, productivity, self-awareness, and personal growth. For a more comprehensive discussion of health promotion, see Chapter 15.

THE FAMILY EXPERIENCING A HEALTH CRISIS

Illness of a Family Member

Illness of a family member is a crisis that affects the entire family system. The family is disrupted as members abandon their usual activities and focus their energy on restoring family equilibrium. Roles and responsibilities previously assumed by the ill person are delegated to other family members, or those functions may remain undone during the duration of the illness. The family experiences anxiety because members are concerned about the sick person and the resolution of the illness. This anxiety is compounded by additional responsibili-

ties when there is less time or motivation to complete the normal tasks of daily living.

Many factors determine the impact of illness on the family unit. Among these are:

- The nature of the illness, which can range from minor to life-threatening.
- The duration of the illness, which ranges from short term to long term.
- The residual effects of the illness, including none to permanent disability.
- The meaning of the illness to the family and its significance to family systems.
- The financial impact of the illness, which is influenced by factors such as insurance and ability of the ill member to return to work.
- The effect of the illness on future family functioning. For instance, previous patterns may be restored or new patterns may be established.

The family's ability to deal with the stress of illness depends on the members' coping skills. Families with good communication skills are better able to discuss how they feel about the illness and how it affects family functioning. They can plan for the future and are flexible in adapting these plans as the situation changes. An established *social support network* provides strength, encouragement, and services to the family during the illness. During health crises, families need to realize that it is a strength, not a sign of weakness, to turn to others for support. Nurses can be part of the support system for families, or they can identify other sources of support in the community.

During a crisis, families are often drawn together by a common purpose. In this time of closeness, family members have the opportunity to reaffirm personal and family values and their commitment to one another. Indeed, illness may provide a unique opportunity for family growth.

Intervening in Families Experiencing Illness

Nurses committed to family-centered care involve both the ailing individual and the family in the nursing process. Through their interaction with families, nurses can give support and information. Nurses make sure that not only the individual but also each family member understands the disease, its management, and the effect of these two factors on family functioning. The nurse also assesses the family's readiness and ability to provide continued care and supervision at home when warranted. After carefully planned instruction and practice, families are given an opportunity to demonstrate their ability to provide care under the supportive guidance of the nurse. When the care indicated is beyond the capability of the family, nurses work with families to identify available resources that are socially and financially acceptable (McClelland et al. 1985).

In helping families to reintegrate the ill person into the home, nurses use data gathered during family assessment to identify family resources and deficits. By formulating mutually acceptable goals for reintegration, nurses help families cope with the realities of the illness and the changes it may have brought about, which may include new roles and functions of family members or the need to provide continued medical care to the ill or recovering person. Working together, nurses and families can create environments that restore or reorganize family functioning during illness and throughout the recovery process.

Death of a Family Member

The death of a family member has a profound effect on the family. The structure of the family is altered, and this change may in turn affect how it functions as a unit. Individual members experience a sense of loss. They grieve for the lost person, and they grieve for the family that once was. (See Chapter 27 for a discussion of loss and grieving.) Some of the early stages of grief accompany family disorganization. However, as the family begins to recover, a new sense of normalcy develops, the family reintegrates its roles and functions, and it comes to grips with the reality of the situation. This painful blow takes time to heal. After the death of a member, families may need counseling to deal with their feelings and to talk about the person who died. They may also want to talk about their fears about and hopes for the future. At this time, families often derive comfort from their religious beliefs and their spiritual adviser. Support groups are also available for families experiencing the pain of death. It is often difficult for nurses to deal with grieving families because the nurses also feel the loss and feel inadequate in knowing what to say or do. By understanding the effect death has on families, nurses can help families resolve their grief and move ahead with life.

CHAPTER HIGHLIGHTS

▶ The family is the basic unit of society.

▶ The family plays an important role in forming the health beliefs and practices of its members.

▶ Family-centered nursing addresses the health of the family as a unit, as well as the health of family members.

▶ Through family assessment, the nurse identifies health beliefs and practices that influence the wellness of the family.

▶ In working with the wide variety of family forms in today's society, the nurse must be aware of many factors that affect the health of families.

▶ Nurses must examine their own values about family, health, illness, and death to be effective in supporting families in crisis.

▶ Nurses can help families realize their potential and their dreams for health and happiness by promoting healthy family functioning.

LEARNING ACTIVITIES

■ Select a cooperative client family in your area of clinical nursing practice. Assess the family functioning using the assessment criteria on page 301.

■ Ask the client family members to complete the Family APGAR Questionnaire. What are the results of your assessment. What interventions would you plan to promote family functioning?

READINGS AND REFERENCES

SUGGESTED READINGS

Johnson, S. H. 1986. *Nursing assessment and strategies for the family at high risk: High risk parenting.* 2d ed. Philadelphia: J. B. Lippincott Co.

Identification of and intervention in families at risk are essential to reduce the potential health care problems of these groups.

Logan, B. B., and Dawkins, C. E. 1986. *Family-centered nursing in the community.* Menlo Park, Calif.: Addison-Wesley.

The authors integrate the areas of family and community health into a family-focused community-health nursing text, reflecting contemporary trends and changes in the family, communities, and health policies, and demonstrating the impact of these changes on community health nursing. Contemporary issues discussed include adolescent pregnancy, substance abuse, chronic mental illness, and family violence.

Wright, L. M., and Leahey, M. 1984. *Nurses and families: A guide to family assessment and intervention.* Philadelphia: F. A. Davis.

This book illustrates how family theory can be applied to clinical practice and emphasizes the development of interviewing skills with families.

RELATED RESEARCH

Lasky, P., Buckwalter, K. C.; Whall, A., Lederman, R.; Speer, J.; McLane, A.; King, J. M.; and White, M. A. February 1985. Developing an instrument in the assessment of family dynamics. *Western Journal of Nursing Research* 7:40–57.

Sund, K., and Oswald, S. K. November/December 1985. Dual-earner families' stress levels and personal and life-style-related variables. *Nursing Research* 34:357–61.

SELECTED REFERENCES

The adolescent family. 1984. Columbus Ohio: Ross Laboratories.

Bradley, R., and Caldwell, B. M. 1977. Home environment, social status, and mental test performance. *Journal of Educational Psychology* 69:697–701.

Clemen-Stone, S., Eigsti, D., and McGuire, S. 1987. *Comprehensive family and community health nursing.* 2d ed. New York: McGraw-Hill.

Denehy, J. A. 1990. Anticipatory guidance. In Craft, M. J., and Denehy, J. A., editors. pp. 53–67. *Nursing Interventions for Infants and Children.* Philadelphia: W. B. Saunders Co.

Duffy, M. A. September/October 1982. When a woman heads a household. *Nursing Outlook* 30:468–73.

Duvall, E. M. 1977. *Marriage and family development.* 5th ed. Philadelphia: J. B. Lippincott Co.

Feetham, S. L., and Humenick, S. S. 1982. The Feetham family functioning survey. In Humenick, S. S. pp. 259–68. *Analysis of current assessment strategies in the health care of young children and childbearing families.* Norwalk, Conn.: Appleton-Century-Crofts.

Friedman, M. 1981. *Family nursing: Theory and assessment.* Norwalk, Conn.: Appleton-Century-Crofts.

Hoeffer, B. 1981. Children's acquisition of sex-role behavior in lesbian-mother families. *American Journal of Orthopsychiatry* 51: 536.

Logan, B. B., and Dawkins, C. E. 1986. *Family-centered nursing in the community.* Menlo Park, Calif.: Addison-Wesley Publishing Co.

McClelland, M. A. May/June 1984. On their own: Latchkey children. *Pediatric Nursing* 10:198–204.

McFarlane, J. December 1977. Sickle cell disorders. *American Journal of Nursing* 77:1948–54.

Moccia, P. and Mason, D. J. January/February 1986. Poverty Trends: Implications for nursing. *Nursing Outlook* 34:20–24.

Mott, S. R., James, S. R., and Sperhac, A. M. 1990. *Nursing care of children and families.* 2d ed. Redwood City, Calif.: Addison-Wesley Nursing.

Orem, D. E. 1980. *Nursing concepts of practice.* 2d ed. New York: McGraw-Hill Book Company.

Pender, N. J. 1987. *Health promotion in nursing practice.* 2d ed. Norwalk, Conn.: Appleton & Lange.

Reutter, L. and Strang, V. July/August 1986. Yours, mine and ours: Stepparents and their children. *The American Journal of Maternal/Child Nursing* 2:264–66.

Smilkstein, G. 1978. The family APGAR: A proposal for a family function test and its use by physicians. *The Journal of Family Practice* 6:1231–39.

Speer, J. J., and Sachs, B. September/October 1985. Selecting the appropriate family assessment tool. *Pediatric Nursing* 11:349–55.

U. S. Department of Health, Education, and Welfare. 1979. *Healthy people: The Surgeon General's report on health promotion and disease prevention.* DHEW Pub. no. 79–555071. Washington, D. C.: U. S. Department of Health, Education, and Welfare.

Williamson, M. 1986. Lesbians. In Griffith-Kinney, J., Editor. pp. 278–96. *Contemporary women's health: A nursing advocacy approach.* Menlo Park, Calif.: Addison-Wesley Publishing Co.

Wright, L. M., Leahey, M. February 1990. Trends in nursing of families. *Journal of Advanced Nursing* 15:148–54.

Community Health

CONTENTS

DEFINITIONS OF A COMMUNITY

A *community* is a collection of people who share some attribute of their lives. It may be that they live in the same locale, attend a particular church, or even share a particular interest, such as skiing. When the community is identified as a *place* or locale, an epidemiologic approach is often used to assess such demographic data as morbidity and mortality. Groups that constitute a community because of common member interests are often referred to as a *community of interest* (e.g., religious and ethnic groups). A community can also be defined as a *social system* in which the members interact formally or informally and form networks that operate for the benefit of all people in the community.

Although there are many types of communities, for purposes of health care a community may be described as having a particular location, a common interest, and a health problem (Spradley 1985). Neuman (1989) states that the community may be viewed in terms of three components: a practice setting, a target of service, or a small group within a larger community. For example, a nurse who collects data about adolescent mortality using local records is focusing on the practice setting. A nurse who collects data about the number of upper respiratory infections of preschoolers at a day-care center is focusing on a small group within the larger community. A nurse who collects data about the reduction in childhood injuries in the home after an intensive childhood safety education program for families is focusing on a target of service.

THE FUNCTIONS OF A COMMUNITY

According to Warren (1978), a community has five functions: (1) production, distribution, and consumption of goods and services, (2) socialization, (3) social control, (4) social interparticipation, and (5) mutual support.

Production, distribution, and consumption of goods and services provides for the economic needs of the members of the community. It includes not only the supplying of food and clothing but also the provision of water, electricity, and police and fire protection and the disposal of refuse. In this function a community is usually interdependent with other communities and with businesses and organizations outside its boundaries.

Socialization is the process of transmitting values, knowledge, culture, and skills to others. Communities usually contain a number of established institutions for socialization: families, churches, schools, media, voluntary and social organizations, and so on. See Chapter 3 for further information regarding socialization.

Social control refers to the way in which order is maintained in a community. Laws are enforced by the police; public health regulations are implemented to protect people from certain diseases. Social control is also exerted through the family, church, and schools.

Social interparticipation refers to community activities that are designed to meet people's needs for companionship. Families and churches have traditionally met this need; however, many public and private organizations also serve this function.

Mutual support, the fifth function of a community, is its ability to provide resources at a time of illness or disaster. Although the family is usually relied on to fulfill this function, health and social services may be necessary to augment the family's assistance if help is required over an extended period.

COMMUNITY HEALTH NURSING

Community health nursing is a specialized area of nursing practice. The community health nurse specialist is prepared in graduate nurse programs at universities and colleges. These programs usually prepare the nurse for leadership and coordinating functions in the community. Staff nurses (community health nurse generalists) are prepared at the baccalaureate level. The client of the community health nurse may be an individual, a family, a group in the community, or a specific population. Hegyvary (1990, p. 7) states that community health nurses "care for individuals and families who are parts of aggregates. The focus on populations is a basis for program planning, not for individual care . . ." The many roles of the community health nurse can include client advocate, consultant, coordinator, manager, educator, and collaborator. See Chapter 3 for additional information about the roles of the professional nurse.

Community health nursing is an area of nursing practice that applies knowledge and skills from both nursing and public health. According to the American Nurses' Association (1980), *community health nursing* is a synthesis of nursing practice and public health practice applied to promoting and preserving the health of populations. The practice is general and comprehensive. It is not limited to a particular age group or diagnosis and is continuing, not episodic. The dominant responsibility is to the population as a whole; nursing directed to individuals, families, or groups contributes to the health of the total population. Health promotion, health maintenance, health education, and continuity of care are utilized in a holistic approach to the management and coordination of the health care of individuals, families, and groups in a community.

How do community health and public health differ? In theory there is no difference. However, the term *public* is usually associated with "efforts of government agencies that are governed by law and financed by taxes." (Spradley 1985, p. 15). In contrast, many community health agencies are private agencies funded through private sources. Community health practices encompass the efforts of both in an organized, cooperative manner. The aim is to promote the physical, emotional, and social health of all individuals in a specific community.

An essential aspect of community health nursing is its interdisciplinary nature. Community health nurses usually work closely with other health professionals and with people in the community. In many situations they meet on a regular basis with other members of a community team, including social workers, psychiatrists, physicians, speech therapists, and so on. Collaboration with other health professionals is one of the major roles of many community nurses. Even in rural areas of the country, where community nurses often function with a great deal of autonomy, they must have occasional direct interaction with other health professionals.

ELEMENTS OF COMMUNITY HEALTH PRACTICE

There are six basic elements of community health practice: (1) promotion of healthful living, (2) prevention of health problems, (3) remedial care for health problems, (4) rehabilitation, (5) evaluation, and (6) research. (Spradley 1985, p. 15)

Promotion of Healthful Living
The promotion of the health of individuals and groups has long been recognized as an important aspect of community health nursing. Health promotion programs are provided to raise the levels of wellness of individuals, families, groups, and the entire community. At the individual level, programs may include smoking cessation, reduction of alcohol and drug abuse, exercise and fitness, and stress management. At the family level, preventive health services such as family planning, pregnancy and infant care, immunizations, and information about sexually transmitted diseases may be offered. At the group level, occupational safety and health, and accidental injury may be considered. At the community level, toxic agent control, fluoridation of water supplies, and infectious agent control are of significance. See Chapter 15 for additional information on health promotion.

Prevention of Health Problems
Health protection activities are highly varied. They may include the prevention of nutritional deficiency, accidents at work and at home, communicable diseases, cardiovascular disease, lung cancer, child abuse, poisoning, pollution, and so on. Levels of prevention were first discussed by Leavell and Clark in the 1950s. Their concept was based on public health concepts. Shamansky and Clausen (1980, p. 106) clarified the concept of prevention levels in a nursing context:

> *Primary prevention* is prevention in the true sense of the word; it precedes disease or dysfunction and is applied to a generally healthy population. The targets are those individuals considered physically or emotionally healthy, exhibiting normal or maximum functioning. Primary prevention is not therapeutic; it does not consist of symptom identification and use of therapeutic skills. Primary prevention includes generalized health promotion as well as specific protection against disease.
>
> *Secondary prevention* emphasizes early diagnosis and prompt intervention to halt the pathological process, thereby shortening its duration and severity and enabling the individual to regain normal func-

tion at the earliest possible point. Early diagnosis is illustrated by the use of a comprehensive nursing assessment, which may reveal the need for further medical evaluation.

> Screening procedures of any type, whether they be breast self-examination; screening for hypertension, PKU, or sickle cell anemia; the use of the Denver Developmental Screening Test (DDST); or any multiphasic screening procedure, are by definition secondary prevention. In all of these examples, screening is done in order to detect problems at an early stage.
>
> *Tertiary prevention* comes into play when a defect or disability is fixed, stabilized, or irreversible. Rehabilitation, the goal of tertiary prevention, is more than halting the disease process itself; it is restoring the individual to an optimum level of functioning within the constraints of the disability.

Remedial Care for Health Problems
Community health care nurses provide direct and indirect services to individuals with chronic health problems. A variety of health care services provide *direct* services, such as home visits for the assessment and monitoring of health problems, dietary planning, administration of injections, personal care, homemaking services, and information about equipment resources (e.g., bath seats, wheelchairs, canes, walkers, syringes, dressing materials, and so on). *Indirect* services focus on assisting people with health problems to obtain treatment. For example, a community health nurse may assist a person to get a physician's appointment after eliciting data about an elevated blood pressure, a persistent cough, or vaginal bleeding. In other instances, the nurse may refer an individual or family to other agencies that provide information and/or therapy such as (a) a family therapy and counselling program, (b) a self-help group or association, or (c) a chemical dependency counselling and treatment center.

On a community level, individual community members and health workers may lobby for the development of programs to remedy unhealthy situations or to initiate services that are lacking. Examples of unhealthy situations are an inadequate school lunch program, inhumane conditions in a nursing home, and excessive pollution of water supplies from industrial wastes. Examples of new initiatives are increased shelters for abused women, low-cost housing for the elderly, the establishment of nursing services on the streets, and provision of health care to the homeless.

Rehabilitation
Rehabilitative services that focus on reducing disability and/or restoring function are pro-

vided at the individual, family, and community level. At the individual level, a community health nurse in conjunction with other allied health workers (e.g., physical and occupational therapists) may assist physically handicapped persons (e.g., those with cerebrovascular accidents, heart conditions, amputations, or paralysis) regain some degree of lost function, prevent further disability, and develop new skills that enable them to assume an appropriate vocation or degree of independence. Many rehabilitative community groups are available to assist families and individuals with chronic health problems. Examples are colostomy clubs, postmastectomy groups, halfway houses for the discharged mentally ill, and Alcoholics Anonymous. The community health nurse can be instrumental in informing clients of available services.

Evaluation   Ongoing evaluation of health and health care services at the individual, national, and international levels is an essential component of community health practices. Its aim is to (a) determine the effectiveness of current activities, (b) determine needs, and (c) develop improved services. For example, evaluation of services available for rape victims may reveal a need for more comprehensive counselling programs.

Research   Research, a critical component of community health care practice, provides the means to identify problems and examine improved methods of providing health services. Research occurs at all levels—from federal agencies such as the U.S. Public Health Service to state and municipal groups. Researchers may investigate (a) patterns of illness and health, (b) possible causes and means of preventing specific problems such as child abuse, suicide, homicide, trauma, and substance abuse, (c) deficiencies in services such as day care centers or services for the elderly, (d) the effectiveness of treatment programs such as weight reduction, stress management, or substance abuse programs, (e) the effect of societal and environmental changes on existing services, and (f) utilization of existing health services.

EPIDEMIOLOGY

Epidemiology is the study of the distribution and determinants of health and illness status in population groups (Spradley 1985). Epidemiologic studies provide health professionals with information about the health and illness patterns of a specified population, the people involved, and any causal factors. Most health problems are currently thought to be the result of multiple causes. That is, a multiplicity of factors interact to result in coronary heart disease or teenage pregnancy, for example.

Types of Studies

Epidemiologists use three types of studies: analytic, descriptive, and experimental. In *analytic studies* the epidemiologist uses prospective (forward looking) and retrospective (backward looking) and/or experimental studies to test hypotheses about health and illness. (Prospective and retrospective studies are further described in the next paragraph.) *Descriptive studies* rely primarily on existing data. The epidemiologist describes the people most likely to be affected by a disease, the geographic region in which it will occur, when it will occur, and its overall effect. *Experimental studies* are often conducted to determine the effectiveness of a particular therapeutic modality. Subjects are assigned to one of two groups: the experimental group or the control group. People in the experimental group are, for example, exposed to a condition thought to improve health, to prevent disease, or to influence a person's health status in some manner, such as walking for a half hour each day. The members of the matched control group are not exposed to the experimental condition. Any subsequent differences in the health patterns between the two groups are then attributed to the manipulated factor.

In a *prospective study,* the epidemiologist determines the variables and the investigation method and establishes possible hypotheses. Data are then collected to see whether the hypothesis is supported. For example, a nurse may establish a hypothesis about the relation of dietary habits to weight, then follow a group of people, collecting data regarding their diet. In a *retrospective study* the investigator goes back over existing records to collect data that may or may not support a hypothesis. For example, when studying weight loss patterns among a group of people, a nurse might refer to records about the activity and diet of these people.

Population, in the context of epidemiology, is the universe of people in the study (Spradley 1985). Two types of rates are commonly used when describing health patterns in a population: the incidence rate and the prevalence rate. The *incidence rate* reflects the number of people with a particular health problem or characteristic over a given unit of time, such as a year:

$$\text{Incidence rate} = \frac{\text{Number of people developing the condition}}{\text{Total number of people at risk}}$$

The *prevalence rate* describes a situation at a given point in time. For example, if 63 students in a school have chickenpox, the number of students who have the disease is divided by the number of students in the school:

$$\text{Prevalence rate} = \frac{\text{Total people with disease or condition}}{\text{Number in the population}}$$

For information about other frequently used rates see Table 17–1.

Mapping Community Health Problems

Commercial computerized systems are available to analyze, integrate, and display locational data. These packages, referred to as Geographic Information Systems (GISs), place dots on a map electronically. Varying dot densities display data such as clusters of specific health problems. Because commercial GIS packages are costly, alternative methods using a personal computer may be used. For example, community nurses may decide to map health problems such as childhood accidents or accidents to elderly people. This mapping process involves (a) the collection of data by community nurses in a specific area, such as an electoral district, (b) provision of reports to the community projects office, (c) input into the office computer, and (d) dissemination of information to interested nurses on a regular basis. The information recorded may include the number of accidents by age, sex, type of injury, residential data, cause of the injury and so on. Such a system can be beneficial in providing the information community nurses need to predict work loads, by identifying high-risk areas in which people need the most help.

APPLICATION OF THE NURSING PROCESS

The nursing process is the basic framework for the practice of nursing in a community. Regardless of whether the client is a person, a family, a group of people, or the entire community, the nursing process provides a systematic means of collecting data, establishing nursing diagnoses, planning nursing strategies, implementing nursing activities, and evaluating the effectiveness of these nursing actions. Viewing the nursing process in the context of the individual and family was discussed in Chapters 6 through 9 and Chapter 16. Viewing the client

as a community requires a different perspective. If a problem relates to air pollution, for example, it can involve a number of states or even countries.

The manner in which a health care system approaches a community depends on a number of variables, including the size of the community, the health problems, the expertise required to deal with the problems, the time permitted to deal with the problems, and the technology available. It is important for nurses to have some concept of a healthy community before initiating any assessment. The question "What is a healthy community?" is not simply answered. There is probably no such thing as a completely healthy community. Spradley (1985, p. 391) suggests ten characteristics of a healthy community:

1. A healthy community is one in which members have a high degree of awareness that "we are a community."

2. A healthy community uses its natural resources while taking steps to conserve them for future generations.

3. A healthy community openly recognizes the existence of subgroups and welcomes their participation in community affairs.

4. A healthy community is prepared to meet crises.

5. A healthy community is a problem-solving community; it identifies, analyzes, and organizes to meet its own needs.

6. A healthy community has open channels of communication that allow information to flow among all subgroups of citizens in all directions.

7. A healthy community seeks to make each of its systems' resources available to all members.

8. A healthy community has legitimate and effective ways to settle disputes that arise within the community.

9. A healthy community encourages maximum citizen participation in decision making.

10. A healthy community promotes a high level of wellness among all its members.

Assessing

A Systems Approach Several community assessment frameworks have been devised. Stewart (1985) proposes a general systems theory as a framework for community assessment. She identifies nine subsystems of the community for analysis: health, communication,

TABLE 17-1   *Frequently Used Rates*

Natality

Crude birth rate	$\dfrac{\text{Total number of live births}}{\text{Total population}}$	$\times\,1,000$
Fertility rate	$\dfrac{\text{Total number of live births}}{\text{Number of women 15–44 years of age}}$	$\times\,1,000$

Morbidity

Incidence rate	$\dfrac{\text{Number of new cases of a specified disease reported during a given time interval}}{\text{Estimated mid-interval population at risk}}$	$\times\,1,000^{*}$
Attack rate	$\dfrac{\text{Number of new cases of a specified disease reported during a limited time interval}}{\text{Population at risk during same time interval}}$	$\times\,100$
Prevalence rate	$\dfrac{\text{Number of cases (new and old) of specified disease existing at a given point in time}}{\text{Estimated population at the same point in time}}$	$\times\,1,000$

Mortality

Crude death rate	$\dfrac{\text{Total number of deaths}}{\text{Estimated mid-interval population}}$	$\times\,1,000$
Crude cause-specific death rate	$\dfrac{\text{Total number of deaths from a specific cause}}{\text{Estimated mid-interval population}}$	$\times\,1,000$
Case fatality rate	$\dfrac{\text{Number of deaths from specified disease}}{\text{Number of cases of the disease}}$	$\times\,100$
Fetal death rate	$\dfrac{\text{Number of fetal deaths of 28 weeks or more gestation}}{\text{Number of live births}}$	$\times\,1,000$
Neonatal mortality rate	$\dfrac{\text{Number of deaths under 28 days of age}}{\text{Number of live births}}$	$\times\,1,000$
Post-neonatal mortality rate	$\dfrac{\text{Number of deaths from 28 days to 1 year}}{\text{Number of live births}}$	$\times\,1,000$
Infant mortality rate	$\dfrac{\text{Number of deaths under 1 year}}{\text{Number of live births}}$	$\times\,1,000$
Maternal mortality rate	$\dfrac{\text{Number of deaths assigned to causes related to pregnancy}}{\text{Number of live births}}$	$\times\,10,000^{\dagger}$

* May be expressed per 10,000 or 100,000 when the number of cases is small.
† May be expressed per 100,000 when the number of cases is small.

Source: Dawkins, C. E. and Logan, B. B. *Family-centered nursing in the community* (Menlo Park, Calif.: Addison-Wesley Publishing Co., 1986), pp. 138–39. Used with permission.

economy, education, law, politics, recreation, religion, and social life. See Table 17–2 for details about assessment data for these subsystems.

Assessment of the *health subsystem* of a community includes collecting data about population size, rate of growth, density, and composition; life expectancy; overall health status of individuals; health care facilities and services and accessibility to the facilities; and quantity and types of caseloads of health professionals. The *communication subsystem* is an important part of the health of a community since a community relies on the abilities of individuals and groups to exchange ideas and feelings and work toward common goals. The *economic subsystem* or economic status of the community significantly affects the physical and emotional health of its citizens. Successful industries and high income and employment levels provide financial support for health, education, and recreational services. The *education subsystem* promotes intellectual development and socialization of the community's youth. Communities that expend a great deal of energy on educational, social, and cultural activities achieve a higher level of development than those whose energies are directed toward law enforcement and economic concerns (Hanchett 1979). The *law subsystem* ensures social order and the safety of a community and thus preserves the emotional and physical security of its members. In regard to the *political subsystem,* "political jurisdictions identify the formal boundaries of many of a community's subsystems such as school, health, and police districts" (Stewart 1985, p. 371). Local and other governments carry specific responsibilities for all community subsystem services that directly and indirectly affect the health of a community. The *recreational subsystem* provides facilities and activities that are essential for the physical, emotional, and social health of individuals and families. The *subsystem of religion* functions to promote the spiritual health of citizens. It is often a pervading force in providing support to individuals and families in times of crisis. *Social life* as a subsystem consists of all the social, economic, and ethnic classes of people in the community and the social clubs and organizations that function to promote cohesiveness of all members of the community.

When viewing a community as a system it is important to identify five elements: the boundaries, the focal unit, the proximity of members, the similarity of members, and resistance of members to intrusion and internal communications (Logan and Dawkins 1986).

The *boundary* of the system is the first aspect of the system that needs to be determined. Does the community have geographic boundaries? Or are the boundaries of a different sort, such as the boundaries of a workplace or the boundaries of a group of people who have a particular occupation?

When considering the second aspect, the *focal unit,* Braden and Herban (1976) suggest three levels: micro, mezzo, and macro. A person in a family is an example of a focal unit on the microlevel. A larger and more complex focal unit, such as a factory or a school, is at the mezzolevel. The most extensive and complex units, such as a state health organization, are at the macrolevel.

The *proximity of the members* of a community allows determination of where interactions take place. For example, are the members in a house, an apartment, or a school? The *similarity of the members* refers to shared membership in the same family or the same organization or to some other set of shared characteristics.

The last aspect of the community viewed as a system is the degree of *resistance of the members to external influence.* How resistant is a family to outside help? How readily will a school accept new students into its activities? Also, how effective are the communication channels within the system? Do members of a family communicate regularly? Do all members of an organization obtain information they require on a regular basis?

Sources of Data   Sources of data for a community assessment are abundant. Some sources, with examples of information obtainable, include:

1. City maps to locate community boundaries, roads, churches, schools, parks, hospitals, and so on.

2. State or provincial census data for population composition and characteristics.

3. Chamber of Commerce for employment statistics, major industries, and primary occupations.

4. State or provincial and municipal health departments for location of health facilities, occupational health programs, numbers of health professionals, numbers of welfare recipients, and so on.

5. City health planning boards for health needs and practices.

6. Telephone book for location of social, recreational, and health organizations, committees, and facilities.

7. Public and university libraries for district social and cultural research reports.

8. Health facility administrators or supervisors for information about employee caseloads, prevalent types of problems, and dominant needs.

9. Recreational directors for programs provided and participation levels.

(text continues on p. 319)

TABLE 17-2 *Systems Framework for Community Assessment*

System	Assessment Data	Rationale
Health	Size	Size influences the number and size of health care agencies.
	Rate of growth or decline	Rapid growth may place excessive demands on health care services.
	Density	Density affects the availability of health care services.
	Composition	Composition may identify the types of health care needs.
	Life expectancy	Life expectancy indicates the need for services for the aged or the physically and mentally incapacitated.
	Health status, including nutritional status	This reflects the overall physical, emotional, and social health of the members of the community.
	Health care facilities and services, including resource allocation and utilization, health programs, and age groups served	These indicate the degree to which the health needs of the community are being met.
	Geographic, economic, and cultural accessibility to health care services	Accessibility to health care services is considered a basic right by many people regardless of economic status, ethnic origin, or geographical location.
	Consumer participation in health care programs	Consumer participation reflects people's interest in and values about health maintenance and promotion.
	Number, type, and routine caseloads of health professionals (e.g., community health nurses, nutritionists, dental hygienists, family physicians and specialists, public health inspectors)	Caseload numbers and types indicate physical and emotional health problems prevalent in the community.
	Sources of health knowledge	This identifies information about agencies and available services for consumers.
	Levels of immunization among children	This information reflects the citizens' knowledge and values about disease prevention.
	Ambulance services	The availability of emergency services indicates the ability of the community to respond to life-threatening situations.
	Sanitation services	Quality sanitation services prevent disease.
	Opinions about community health services	Satisfaction with current services and proposed improvements can be determined.
	Environmental conditions of air, water, and soil	The state of the environment can affect physical and emotional health.
Communication	Existence and frequency of public forums	Public forums enable inputs or feedback to the system, thus enhancing satisfaction with and survival of the system.
	Telephone services	Telephones promote communication among members and ability to contact health services.
	Newspapers and television	Newspapers and television provide an ongoing flow of information about community activities and health care.

▶

TABLE 17–2   *(continued)*

System	Assessment Data	Rationale
	Transportation and road networks	Transportation influences access to health care facilities and programs, as well as to recreational and educational facilities that indirectly affect health.
Economy	Industries and occupations	A strong industrial base in a community provides financial support for health, education, and recreational facilities.
	Number or percentage of population employed or attending school	Social health problems such as stress, depression, drug abuse, and crime are frequently widespread where there are economic problems such as high unemployment.
	Income levels and quality and types of housing (private dwellings, apartments, mobile homes, etc.)	Overcrowded and poor-quality dwellings may affect the health of residents.
	Occupational health programs	The presence of occupational health programs can help workers maintain health and prevent accidents.
Education/schools	School health facilities, services, and personnel	Quality health facilities and services can provide information and assistance to maintain and promote health.
	Existence of nutritious lunch programs, extracurricular sports activities, libraries, and counseling services	These services contribute to children's physical, emotional, and social health.
	Number and types of health problems handled by the school nurse	The number and types of problems reflect individual and family health problems in the community.
	Adjunctive services for the physically and mentally handicapped (e.g., resource teachers, community volunteers)	Available services and resources for the handicapped indicate the attitudes of the community toward these citizens.
	Type of continuing education or evening extension classes provided	Continuing education programs can affect the development of a community, the literacy of its adults, and its overall health values.
	Parent-teacher associations and the extent of parental involvement in the schools	Maximum parental involvement in the schools can indicate minimal individual and family health problems such as school dropouts, teenage pregnancies, drug abuse, vandalism, etc.
Law	Caseloads of police force and lawyers	These caseloads identify the social problems of a community (e.g., child abuse, vandalism, drug addiction, alcoholism, juvenile crime, etc.). Such problems reflect the social order of the community, the safety of the citizens, and the need for special programs such as youth recreation, arts and crafts for older adults, and child abuse programs.

▶

TABLE 17-2 *Systems Framework for Community Assessment*

System	Assessment Data	Rationale
Politics	Responsibilities of local and other governments and community councils for all community subsystem services (e.g., health and welfare councils, housing authorities, transportation authorities, sanitation authorities	Formal political channels and authority to direct use of the health care dollar are reflected in government responsibilities.
	Political leaders or other influential people in community affairs	This helps the nurse determine and recognize the power framework and perhaps leaders' issues of concern.
	Election issues and average election turnout	Election turnouts can indicate the degree of citizen involvement, community cohesiveness, and desire to influence change.
Recreation	Location of *inexpensive* recreational services for all age groups, including use made of schools and other vacant buildings	Recreational activities provide physical and emotional outlets and intellectual stimulation that promote and maintain health.
	Number of playgrounds, pools, sports fields, and parks and utilization of them	Existence and use of recreational facilities indicates the community system's goals and values about them.
	Participation levels in fitness programs	Low participation levels may indicate the need to provide inexpensive programs for certain age groups, such as senior citizens.
	Number of family-centered programs	Family-centered programs assist in the maintenance of family health and cohesiveness.
	Persons responsible for developing and maintaining playgrounds and parks	Knowledge of those responsible for playgrounds and parks helps the citizens provide direct input about any problems.
Religion	Number and types of churches and religious programs	Church members provide support to individuals and families, particularly in times of crisis.
	Level of participation in various church programs	Church programs help people grow spiritually and morally, both of which are important influencing factors in the development and maintenance of a healthy self-concept.
Social life	Predominant social classes, racial and ethnic makeup, language, values, and childrearing practices	The community's classes, cultures, and values affect its health and its ability to make use of input from the environment.
	Number and type of social committees, organizations, and clubs, and kinds of services offered	These groups promote cohesiveness of the system's citizens. Such groups, whether formal government agencies or informal friendship groups, often provide financial assistance, emotional support, counseling, and rehabilitation services to the handicapped and to senior citizens.
	Number of persons who belong to social groups and participate in volunteer activities	The level of participation and numbers of volunteers are indicators of community health.

Source: Modified from M. Stewart, Community and aggregates: Systematic community health assessment. In Stewart, M., Innes, J., Searl, S., and Smillie, C. *Community health nursing in Canada* (Toronto, Ontario: Gage Educational Publishing Co., 1984), pp. 363–77.

10. Police department for incidence of crime, vandalism, and drug addiction.

11. Teachers and school nurses for incidence of children's health problems and information on facilities and services to maintain and promote health.

12. Local newspapers for community activities (lectures, adult courses, and so on).

Diagnosing

Freeman and Heinrich (1981, p. 316) state that an ecologic approach is essential to a community health diagnosis. Ecology is concerned with the interactions of humans with their environment. Nursing diagnoses are based on three interacting and changing conditions:

1. The health status of the community, including the population's level of vulnerability.

2. Community health capability, or the ability of the community to deal with its health problems.

3. Community action potentials, or the ways and directions in which the community is likely to work on its health problems.

NANDA diagnoses have largely focused on individual and family responses. The diagnosis **Knowledge deficit** or some wellness diagnoses, such as **Enhanced potential for nutrition** or **Enhanced activity tolerance,** may be used for larger groups (see Chapters 7 and 15). Specific nursing diagnoses for the community have yet to be developed. In a survey of community health nurses, educators, and administrators, it was noted that the diagnosis of population groups was the responsibility of community-nurse administrators (Anderson 1983, p. 40).

Porter (1986, p. 308) developed the following five nursing diagnoses for population groups after conducting an inductive study to isolate the fundamental concepts of the diagnostic reasoning process of 34 community-nurse administrators.

- **Vulnerable population group** Used in situations where the population group had characteristics that increased the possibility of specific health problems. Characteristics may include age, developmental status, racial/cultural heritage, life-style, family medical history, personal medical history, social history.

- **Population-at-risk** Used in situations where an environmental hazard threatened the health of a population group. Properties may include unsafe environment (e.g., air, water, noise pollution), environmental deficiency (e.g., lack of fluoridated water), endemic or epidemic communicable disease, unsanitary environment, threats to safety, and crowded living conditions.

- **Vulnerable population group-at-risk** Used in situations where the personal characteristics of group members and the environmental conditions listed above are combined, i.e., the group is innately vulnerable and faces an environmental hazard.

- **Need-service-mismatch** Used when a change in service is proposed where (a) there is no existing program to meet need; (b) the need for the service no longer exists; (c) there is duplication of services by agencies; (d) there is lack of coordination among agencies who provide a service cooperatively; (e) the service format is ineffective in meeting the need; or (f) the service format is inefficient.

- **Need-service-match** Used in situations when an existing community service could meet or was meeting the need (e.g., after confirming the need of elderly for cardiovascular screening, a nurse finds that the required services are being provided by physician's office nurses).

These diagnoses were based on decisions (1) to confirm the health needs of a population group and (2) to initiate or discontinue a related community health service. Two nursing diagnoses were made before a service change was considered. The first diagnosis involved the group's health status (see the first three diagnoses above); the second involved the degree of match between the group's need and the existing services that might meet the need (see the last two diagnoses above). These diagnoses differ from NANDA diagnoses in another aspect: They relate to a health *need* rather than a probable *cause*. Porter (1986, p. 313) suggests that (a) the group's health need may provide a more precise direction for nursing intervention than would an etiology of its health state and (b) the diagnoses of need-service match and mismatch may have a broader application than the realm of community nursing administration.

Planning

Planning community health may be oriented toward improved crisis management, disease prevention, health maintenance, or health promotion (Logan and Dawkins 1986). One or many of these factors may serve to guide the establishment of nursing strategies. Ruybal (1978) listed three factors that are essential for community health planning:

1. a community or social structure
2. a cultural belief system
3. a process or rational action

The responsibility for planning at the community level is usually broadly based. The exact resources and skills of members of the community will often be dependent on the size of the community. A broadly based planning group is most likely to create a plan that is acceptable to members of the community. Also, people who are involved in planning become educated about the problems, the resources, and the interrelationships within the system relative to health and problems.

Planning involves setting priorities, establishing goals and outcome criteria, planning nursing strategies, and developing a plan (see Chapter 8).

Priorities

At this stage health planners must work with consumers, interest groups, or other involved persons to prioritize health problems. It is important to take into consideration the values and interests of community members, the severity of the problems, and the resources available in order to identify and act on the problems. Because any plan will probably result in change, members of the planning group should be cognizant of and employ planned change theory. See Chapter 12.

Establishing Goals and Outcome Criteria

Establishing goals also requires consumer participation. The goals should reflect a desirable state—for example, to reduce infant mortality 15%. National statistics may be helpful in keeping goals realistic. Among the many other factors that must be considered are the traditions of people in the community, vested interests, current organizations, and resources, all of which may be barriers to change. An example of a goal of a community would be to reduce the incidence of infectious diseases in a school.

Outcome criteria or objectives are specific, measurable targets, such as increasing immunization levels by 20% by September 1992.

Planning Nursing Strategies

Part of planning nursing strategies is selecting from available alternatives. It is important to consider the consequences of all alternatives. Bower (1972) gives three guidelines to assist nurses:

1. Choose the alternative that leads to as many desirable consequences as possible.

2. Select the alternative that best meets the desired intent but that minimizes risk to all involved.

3. Choose the alternative that is of least risk to the client and secondly to the agency.

Planners should evaluate each alternative in terms of the planned results and the possible consequences. At the same time, the values and interests of the people and the resources of the planners must be considered. Resources such as money, professional practitioners, literature, and transportation, for example, can often affect the viability of plans.

Developing a Plan

The last aspect of the planning phase is the development of a plan. After the most desirable strategy has been determined, the phases of the plan and the resources required should be written down. What staff is needed? What buildings? What rooms? What supplies? Each aspect of the plan should have a target date for completion, and a mechanism should be devised for a periodic review of progress. At this time responsibilities for various aspects for implementing the plan can be determined. Each person involved should understand her or his responsibilities and how to carry out the plan.

Implementing

Implementing nursing strategies in community health is generally a collaborative action. According to Spradley (1985), nurses are also frequently catalysts and facilitators in implementation of plans. The primary goal in community health nursing is to help people help themselves.

Freeman and Heinrich (1981) identify three approaches to obtaining goal-directed action: motivating, mobilizing, and delegating. To *motivate* others is to induce them to accept a certain viewpoint or to take a specific action. A community health nurse may need to motivate a client to change his diet or a group to take certain actions in order to get rid of rats living in a neighborhood. To *mobilize* is to involve and organize people so that they effectively deal with specific health problems. For example, various members of a family may need to be mobilized to care for a sick elderly parent. To *delegate* is to deputize or designate another person to carry out certain actions. A nurse may delegate a committee with the task of gathering data about a specific nutrition problem among school children in a community.

Because an interdisciplinary approach is frequently used, another mechanism commonly employed by the community health nurse is referral. The object of referral, according to Freeman and Heinrich (1981), is to introduce the client and the resource, to clarify their respective expectations regarding the client's health problems, and to facilitate coordination of the services being provided.

Freeman and Heinrich (1981, p. 79) suggest that the referral process should meet the following criteria:

1. Provide *specific* information, i.e., time, place, person, travel instructions, documents.
2. Interpret the coping level of significant people and explain the purpose of the referral. The agency's expectations, procedures, and constraints should also be outlined.
3. Inform the agency to which the referral is being sent as to concurrent care being provided by other health professionals.

4. Provide for the return of information through reports and records.

Evaluating

Evaluation determines whether the nursing actions have led to the established goals (standards). For example, was the incidence of child abuse reduced? Evaluation should be continuous throughout the nursing process. As a consequence of evaluation, community health needs—such as organized recreational activities for senior citizens or a volunteer network to assist the disabled—may become evident.

CHAPTER HIGHLIGHTS

▶ A community is a collection of people who share some attribute of their lives.

▶ According to Warren, a community has five functions: production, distribution, and consumption of goods and services; socialization; social control; social interparticipation; and mutual support.

▶ In community health nursing the client can be a person, a group, a family, or the entire community.

▶ Collaboration with other health professionals and people in the community is a major role of the community health nurse.

▶ Six elements of community nursing practice are (1) promotion of healthful living, (2) prevention of health problems, (3) remedial care for health problems, (4) rehabilitation, (5) evaluation, and (6) research.

▶ Epidemiology is the study of the distribution and determinants of health and illness status in population groups, and is one of the bases of community health.

▶ Three types of epidemiological studies are analytic, descriptive, and experimental.

▶ A number of statistical rates are used to describe the incidence of significant health data in the community.

▶ The nursing process provides a comprehensive approach to community nursing practice.

▶ A systems theory can provide a comprehensive framework for community assessment.

▶ When using systems theory to view a community, the focal unit can be at a microlevel, mezzolevel, or macrolevel.

LEARNING ACTIVITIES

■ Identify one health problem in your community. Analyze the problem, identifying incidence (how many people have the problem), population group at risk (e.g., age, sex, occupation, socioeconomic status), location in the community where the problem is most prevalent. What specific interventions might nurses in your community implement to prevent and/or resolve the problem?

■ Community resources may be public or private. They may provide service, education, or psychosocial support. What health related resources are available in your community to meet the needs of the public? Is there a directory available listing community resources? If one is not available, consider developing such a directory.

READINGS AND REFERENCES

SUGGESTED READINGS

Anderson, E., McFarlane, J., and Helton, A. September/October 1986. Community-as-client: A model for practice. *Nursing Outlook* 34:220–24.

The four central concepts for this model are person, health, environment, and nursing. According to this model, the community has eight major subsystems: recreation, safety and transportation, communication, education, health and social services, economics, politics and government, and the physical environment. This model is intended to operationalize the definition of public health nursing as a synthesis of public health and nursing. A table describes the three levels of prevention as applied to battering during pregnancy.

Begg, E. October 1989. Planning a health fair. *Community Outlook* 19–22.

Begg describes the steps involved in planning a health fair to promote healthier life-styles. The steps include (a) preliminary planning that focuses on the desired goals and how best to achieve them, (b) selecting contributors, (c) gaining local interest to obtain financial support, (d) planning and coordination, (e) publicizing the event, (f) obtaining necessary equipment, such as display boards, wooden boxes for fitness tests, a computer to assess risks of health/disease, video recorders, and so on, and (g) evaluating the event in terms of quality of information content and presentation, popular topics, and further actions participants might take as a result of the day.

Laffrey, S. C., and Page, G. December 1989. Primary health care in public health nursing. *Journal of Advanced Nursing* 14:1044–50.

Despite similarities in primary health care and public health nursing, Laffrey and Page point out that several obstacles impede public health nursing's ability to perform its role in achieving the World Health Organization's (WHO) goal of health for all by the year 2000. This article includes information about (a) the essential components of primary health care and public health nursing, (b) obstacles to fulfillment of public health nursing's primary health care role, and (c) possible solutions at the levels of education, practice, and research to overcome these obstacles.

RELATED RESEARCH

Porter, E. J. 1986. The nursing diagnosis of population groups. *Classification of nursing diagnoses. Proceedings of the seventh conference. North American Nursing Diagnosis Association.* St. Louis: C. V. Mosby Co. pp. 306–14.

Wong, J., Wong, S. and Nolde, T. et al. 1990. Effects of an experimental program on post-hospital adjustment of early discharged patients. *International Journal of Nursing Studies* 27(1):7–20.

SELECTED REFERENCES

American Nurses' Association, Division on Community Health Nursing. 1980. *A conceptual model of community health nursing.* Kansas City, Mo.: ANA.

Anderson, E. January/February 1983. Community focus in public health nursing: Whose responsibility? *Nursing Outlook* 31:44–48.

Anderson, E. T., and McFarlane, J. M. 1988. *Community as client. Application of the nursing process.* Philadelphia: J. B. Lippincott Co.

Bower, F. L. 1972. *The process of planning nursing care: A theoretical model.* St. Louis: C. V. Mosby.

Braden, C. J. 1984. *The focus and limits of community health nursing.* Norwalk, Conn.: Appleton-Century-Crofts.

Braden, C. J., and Herban, N. L. 1976. *Community health: A systems approach.* New York: Appleton-Century-Crofts.

Cookfair, J. M. 1991. *Nursing process and practice in the community.* St. Louis: Mosby-Year Book Inc.

Freeman, R. B., and Heinrich, J. 1981. *Community health nursing practice.* 2d ed. Philadelphia: W. B. Saunders Co.

Hanchett, E. 1979. *Community health assessment: A conceptual tool kit.* New York: John Wiley and Sons.

Hegyvary, S. T. January–February 1990. Education: redefining community. *Journal of Professional Nursing* 6:7.

Leavell, H. R. et al. 1965. *Preventive medicine for the doctor in the community.* 3d ed. New York: McGraw-Hill Book Co.

Logan, B. B., and Dawkins, C. E. 1986. *Family-centered nursing in the community.* Menlo Park, Calif.: Addison-Wesley Publishing Co.

Neuman, B. 1989. *The Neuman systems model.* 2d ed. Norwalk, Conn.: Appleton and Lange.

Porter, E. J. 1986. The nursing diagnosis of population groups. *Classification of nursing diagnoses. Proceedings of the seventh conference. North American Nursing Diagnosis Association.* St. Louis: C. V. Mosby Co.

Ruybal, S. E. April 1978. Community health planning. *Family and Community Health* 1:9–18.

Shamansky, S. L., and Clausen, C. E. February 1980. Levels of prevention: Examination of the concept. *Nursing Outlook* 28:104–8.

Spradley, B. W. 1985. *Community health nursing concepts and practice.* 2d ed. Boston: Little, Brown and Co.

Stewart, M. 1985. Community and aggregates: Systematic community health assessment. In Stewart, M., Innes, J., Searl, S., and Smillie, C., editors. *Community health nursing in Canada.* Toronto, Ontario: Gage Educational Publishing Co.

Thomas, E. February 1990. Mapping community health. *Community Outlook* 6:8.

Warren, R. L. 1978. *The community in America.* 3d ed. Chicago: Rand McNally.

INTERACTIVE PROCESSES

Helping and Communicating

CONTENTS

THE HELPING RELATIONSHIP

Nurse-client relationships are referred to by some as *interpersonal relationships,* by others as *therapeutic relationships* and by still others as *helping relationships*. Helping is a growth-facilitating process in which one person assists another to solve problems and to face crises in the direction the assisted person chooses (Brammer 1988, p. 5). Several terms are used to describe the persons involved in a helping relationship: *helper* and *helpee; giver* and *receiver;* and *counselor* and *client*. For purposes of consistency, in this text the term *nurse* or *helper* will refer to the person who gives the help, and the term *client* will denote the person receiving the help. However, we recognize that various people in all walks of life act as helpers and receivers of help.

Imogene King (1981) uses the terms *nurse/client interaction* rather than *interpersonal relationship*. According to King (1981, p. 60), "The process of *interactions* between two or more individuals represents a sequence of verbal and nonverbal behaviors that are goal directed." In King's theory, *interpersonal relationships* are a subconcept of the *interaction*. She points out that in many nurse practice settings, such as critical care, where the nurse only has time to attend to physiologic variables that are life-threatening, interpersonal relationships cannot be established. In the interactive process, two individuals mutually identify goals and the means to achieve them. When they agree on the means to implement the goals, they move toward transactions. *Transaction* is defined as goal attainment (King 1981, p. 61).

Phases of the Helping Relationship

This relationship process can be described in terms of four sequential phases, each of which is characterized by identifiable tasks and skills. Progression through the stages must occur in succession, as each builds on the one before. Nurses can identify the progress of a relationship by understanding these phases: preinteraction phase, introductory phase, working (maintaining) phase, and termination phase. Table 18–1 summarizes the tasks and skills required for each phase.

Preinteraction Phase The *preinteraction phase* is similar to the planning stage before an interview. In most situations, the nurse has information about the client before the first face-to-face meeting. Such information may include the client's name, address, age, medical history, and/or social history. Planning for the initial visit may generate some anxious feelings in the nurse. By recognizing these feelings and identifying specific information to be discussed, positive outcomes will evolve.

Introductory Phase The *introductory phase* is also referred to as the *orientation phase* or the *prehelping phase*. This phase is important, since the tone for the rest of the relationship phases is set during this phase. Three stages of this introductory phase are (a) opening the relationship, (b) clarifying the problem, and (c) structuring and formulating the contract (Brammer 1988, p. 51). Other important tasks of the introductory phase include getting to know each other and developing a degree of trust.

During the initial parts of the introductory phase, the client may display some resistive behaviors and some testing behaviors. *Resistive behaviors* are those that inhibit involvement, cooperation, or change. Three major reasons for their occurrence are (a) difficulty in acknowledging the need for help and thus a dependent role, (b) fear of exposing and facing feelings, and (c)

anxiety about the discomfort involved in changing problem-causing behavior patterns. *Testing behaviors* are those that examine the nurse's interest and sincerity.

By the end of the introductory phase, the client begins to develop trust in the nurse. Both participants also begin to view each other as unique individuals. Characteristics of trusting individuals include (a) a feeling of comfort with growth in self-awareness, (b) an ability to share this awareness with others, (c) acceptance of others as they are without needing to change them, (d) openness to new experiences, (e) consistency between words and actions, (f) openness and honesty about motives, (g) willingness to confide, offer information and opinions, and (h) ability to delay gratification (Thomas 1970, p. 118; and Kaul and Schmidt 1971, p. 542).

Working Phase During the *working phase* the nurse and the client begin to view each other as unique individuals. They begin to appreciate this uniqueness and care about each other. *Caring* is sharing deep and genuine concern about the welfare of another person. Once caring develops, the potential for empathy increases. The working phase has three successive stages: (a) responding and exploring, (b) integrative understanding and dynamic self-understanding, and (c) facilitating and taking action (Egan 1975, pp. 34–40).

Stage 1: Responding and exploring In addition to listening and attending skills, the nurse requires four skills for this first stage.

1. *First-level empathy*. Nurses must communicate (respond) in ways that indicate they have listened to what was said and understand how the client feels. The nurse responds to content or feelings or both, as appropriate. The nurse's nonverbal behaviors are also important. In a study of five nurses and five clients, Hardin and Halaris (1983, p. 15) found that nonverbal communication and specific nonverbal behaviors may be linked to empathy. They observed the engaging and defensive nonverbal behaviors of clients and nurses and compared nurses whom the clients rated as either highly empathetic or not empathetic. Nonverbal engaging behaviors included direct gaze, slight smile, laugh, forward torso, gestures, head nods, and leg position. Defensive behaviors included crossed arms and crossed legs. Their findings indicated that *high-empathy nurses* employed moderate head nodding, a steady gaze, moderate gesturing, and little activity or body movement. The *low-empathy nurse* used frequent head nodding and gesturing, laughed more than the high-empathy nurse,

TABLE 18-1 · *Tasks and Skills for Each Phase of the Helping Relationship*

Phase	Tasks	Skills
Preinteraction phase	The nurse reviews pertinent knowledge, considers potential areas of concern, and develops plans for interaction.	Recognizing limitations and seeking assistance as required.
Introductory phase 1. Opening the relationship	Both client and nurse identify each other by name. When the nurse initiates the relationship, it is important to explain the nurse's role to give the client an idea of what to expect. When the client initiates the relationship, the nurse needs to help the client express concerns and reasons for seeking help. Vague, open-ended questions, such as "What's on your mind today?" are helpful at this stage.	A relaxed attending attitude to put the client at ease. It is not easy for all clients to receive help.
2. Clarifying the problem	Because the client initially may not see the problem clearly, the nurse's major task is to help clarify the problem.	Attentive listening, paraphrasing, clarifying, and other effective communication techniques discussed in this chapter. A common error at this stage is to ask too many questions of the client.
3. Structuring and formulating the contract (obligations to be met by both the nurse and client)	Nurse and client develop a degree of trust and verbally agree about: (a) location, frequency, and length of meetings, (b) overall purpose of the relationship, (c) how confidential material will be handled, (d) tasks to be accomplished, and (e) duration and indications for termination of the relationship.	Communication skills listed above and ability to overcome resistive and/or testing behaviors if they occur.
Working phase	Nurse and client accomplish the tasks outlined in the introductory phase, enhance trust and rapport, and develop caring.	
1. Responding and exploring	The nurse assists the client to explore thoughts, feelings, and actions. The client explores feelings and actions associated with problems (self-exploration or self-disclosure).	Listening and attending skills and four responding skills: first-level empathy, respect, genuineness, and concreteness.
2. Integrative understanding and dynamic self-understanding	The nurse acquires integrative understanding about the client. The client develops the skill of listening and gains insight into personal behavior.	In addition to those of the first stage, skills required by the nurse are advanced-level empathy, self-disclosure, and confrontation. Skills required by the client are nondefensive listening and dynamic self-understanding.
3. Facilitating and taking action	The nurse plans programs within the client's capabilities and considers long- and short-term goals. The client needs to learn to take risks (i.e., accept that either failure or success may be the outcome). The nurse needs to reinforce successes and help the client recognize failures realistically.	Decision-making and goal-setting skills. In addition: For the client: risk-taking. For the nurse: reinforcement skills.
Termination phase	Nurse and client accept feelings of loss. The client accepts the end of the relationship without feelings of anxiety or dependence.	For the nurse: summarizing skills. For the client: ability to handle problems independently.

and displayed more eye movement, leg movement, and torso movement.

2. *Respect.* The nurse must show respect for the clients, willingness to be available, and desire to work with the client.

3. *Genuineness.* Personal statements can be helpful in solidifying the rapport between the nurse and the client. The nurse might offer such comments as "I recall when I was in (a similar situation), and I felt angry about being put down." Egan (1982, p. 128) states that the helper "must be spontaneous, open. He can't hide behind the role of counselor. He must be a human being to the human being before him." Egan refers to this quality as *genuineness* and outlines five behaviors that are components of it. See the accompanying box. Nurses need to exercise caution when making references about themselves. These statements must be used with discretion. The extreme of matching each of the client's problems with a better story of the nurse's own is of little value to the client.

4. *Concreteness.* The nurse must assist the client to be concrete and specific rather than to speak in generalities.

During this first stage of the working phase, the intensity of interaction increases, and feelings such as anger, shame, or self-consciousness may be expressed. If the nurse is skilled in this stage and if the client is willing to pursue self-exploration, the outcome is a beginning understanding on the part of the client about behavior and feelings.

Stage 2: Integrative understanding and dynamic self-understanding   In this second stage, clients achieve an objective understanding of themselves and their world (dynamic self-understanding). This ultimately enables clients to change and to take action. More self-exploration occurs, and more information is produced. As a result of this process, isolated pieces of information can now be integrated into larger contexts that reveal behavior patterns or themes.

For this stage, the nurse needs the following three skills in addition to those of the first stage:

1. *Advanced-level empathy.* The nurse responds in ways that indicate an understanding not only of what is said but also of what is hinted at or implied nonverbally. Isolated statements become connected.

2. *Self-disclosure.* The nurse willingly but discreetly shares personal experiences.

3. *Confrontation.* The nurse points out discrepancies between thoughts, feelings, and actions that inhibit the client's self-understanding or exploration of specific areas. This is done empathetically, not judgmentally.

Stage 3: Facilitating and taking action   Ultimately the client must make decisions and take action to become more effective. The responsibility for action belongs to the client. The nurse, however, collaborates in these decisions, provides support, and may offer options or information.

Termination Phase   This phase of the relationship is often expected to be difficult and filled with ambivalence. However, if the previous phases have evolved effectively, the client generally has a positive outlook and feels able to handle problems independently. However, because caring attitudes have developed, it is natural to expect some feelings of loss, and each person needs to develop a way of saying good-bye.

Many methods can be used to terminate relationships. Summarizing or reviewing the process can produce a sense of accomplishment. This may include sharing reminiscences of how things were at the beginning of the relationship, compared to now. It is also helpful for both the nurse and the client to express their feelings about termination openly and honestly. Thus termination discussions need to start in advance of the termination interview. This allows time for the client to adjust to independence. In some situations referrals are necessary, or it is appropriate to offer an occasional standby meeting to give support as needed.

Developing Helping Relationships

Whatever the practice setting, the nurse establishes some sort of helping relationship in which mutual goals are set with the client, or with support persons if the client is unable to participate. Although *special* training in counseling techniques is advantageous, there are many ways of helping clients that do not require special training. Shanken and Shanken (1976, pp. 24–27) have outlined 11 of these:

1. *Listen actively.* (See the discussion of attentive listening, later in this chapter.)

2. *Help to identify what the person is feeling.* Often clients who are troubled are unable to identify or to label their feelings and consequently have difficulty working them out or talking about them. Responses by the nurse such as "You seem angry about taking orders from your boss" or "You sound as if you've been lonely since your wife died" can help clients recognize what they are feeling and talk about it.

3. *Put yourself in the other person's shoes.* The ability to do this is referred to as *empathy*. According to Egan (1975, p. 76), empathy involves the ability to discriminate what the other's world is like and to communicate to the other this understanding in a way that shows the other that the helper has picked up both the client's *feelings* and the *behavior* and *experience* underlying these feelings.

4. *Be honest.* In effective relationships nurses honestly recognize any lack of knowledge by saying, "I don't know the answer to that right now"; openly discuss their own discomfort by saying, for example, "I feel uncomfortable about this discussion"; and admit tactfully that problems do exist, for instance, when a client says "I'm a mess, aren't I?"

5. *Do not tell a person not to feel.* Feelings expressed by clients often make nurses uncomfortable. Common examples are a client's expressions of anger or worry or a client's crying. When a nurse feels this discomfort, common responses are "Don't worry about it, everything will be fine" or "Please don't cry." Such responses inhibit the client's expression of feelings. Unless feelings are extremely inappropriate, it is best to encourage the client to ventilate (voice) them. Ventilation allows the client to express feelings in words and examine them objectively. Indirectly, such an attitude conveys this message: "Your feelings are not that awful, since I am not bothered by them."

6. *Do not tell a person what to feel.* Statements that indicate to clients how they should feel, rather than how they actually do feel, in essence deny clients' true feelings and suggest that they are inappropriate.

7. *Do not make excuses for the other person.* When a person reacts with an intense feeling such as anger or grief and seems to have lost control of behavior to the astonishment or discomfort of others, a common error is to explain the behavior by offering excuses. Responses such as "I guess you've had a tough session in physical therapy" discourage and divert the person from discussing feelings of anger or inadequacy. The nurse has made assumptions about the reasons for the client's behavior and therefore inhibits exploration of what the client is really experiencing and feeling.

8. *Be genuine.* See the discussion of this topic earlier in this chapter.

9. *Use your ingenuity.* There are always many courses of action to consider in handling problems. Whatever course is chosen needs to further achievement of the client's goals, be compatible with the client's value system, and offer the probability of success. The client needs to choose the ways to achieve goals; however, the nurse can assist in identifying options.

10. *Know your role and your limitations.* Every person has unique strengths and limitations. When the nurse feels unable to handle some problems, the client should be informed and referred to the appropriate health professional.

COMMUNICATION IN NURSING

The term *communication* has various meanings, depending on the context in which it is used. To some, communication is the interchange of information between two or more people; in other words, the exchange of ideas or thoughts. This kind of communication uses methods such as talking and listening or writing and reading. However, painting, dancing, and story telling are also methods of communication. Thoughts are conveyed to others not only by spoken or written words but also by gestures or body actions.

Communication may have a more personal connotation than the interchange of ideas or thoughts. It can be a transmission of feelings, or a more personal and social interaction between people. In this context, communication often is synonymous with relating. Frequently one member of a couple comments that the other is not communicating. Some teenagers complain about a generation gap—being unable to communicate with understanding or feeling to a parent or authority figure. Sometimes a nurse is said to be efficient but lacking in something called *bedside manner*. For the purpose of this text, *communication* is any means of exchanging information or feelings between two or more people. It is a basic component of human relationships.

The intent of any communication is to elicit a response. Thus, communication is a process. It includes all the techniques by which an individual affects another. It has two main purposes: to influence others and to obtain information. Communication can be described as helpful or unhelpful. The former encourages a sharing of information, thoughts, or feelings between two or more people. The latter hinders or blocks the transfer of information and feelings.

Communication is a significant aspect of nursing practice. Nurses who communicate effectively are better able to initiate change that promotes health, establish a trusting relationship with a client and support persons, and prevent legal problems associated with nursing practice. Effective communication is essential for the establishment of the nurse-client relationship.

Nursing practice involves three kinds of communication: social, structured, and therapeutic. *Social communication* is unplanned communication, often carried out in an informal setting and usually at a leisurely pace. It is usually satisfying to all parties participating. *Structured communication* refers to definite planned content (Sundeen, Stuart, Rankin, and Cohen 1989, p. 129). An example of structured communication is teaching a client to give an injection or discussing postoperative care with a person anticipating surgery. *Therapeutic communication* is also used by nurses. It is defined by Ruesch as a process that helps "overcome temporary stress, to get along with other people, to adjust to the unalterable, and to overcome psychological blocks which stand in the way of self-realization" (1961, p. 7). Therapeutic communication is used by nurses in many settings and in many circumstances, for example, to support the anxious preoperative client or to help the person who has cancer accept and cope with this diagnosis. Structured communication is discussed in Chapter 19.

MODES OF COMMUNICATION

Communication is generally carried out in two different modes: verbal and nonverbal. *Verbal communication* uses the spoken or written word; *nonverbal communication* uses other forms, such as gestures or facial expressions. Although both kinds of communication occur concurrently, the majority of communication (some say 80 to 90%) is nonverbal. This may be surprising to those who associate communication with only verbal expression. Learning about nonverbal communication is thus an important consideration for nurses in developing effective communication patterns and relationships with clients.

Verbal Communication

Verbal communication is largely conscious, because people choose the words they use. The words used vary among individuals according to culture, socioeconomic background, age, and education. As a result, countless possibilities exist in the way ideas are exchanged. An abundance of words can be used to form messages. In addition, a wide variety of feelings can be conveyed when talking. The intonation of the voice can express animation, enthusiasm, sadness, annoyance, or amusement. The number of different intonations heard when people say "hello" or "good morning" illustrates the variety that is possible. The pacing or rhythm of a person's communication is another variable. Monotonous rhythms or very rapid rhythms can be products of lack of energy or interest, anxiety, or fear.

When choosing words to say or to write, nurses need to consider several criteria of effective communication. These include (a) simplicity, (b) clarity, (c) timing and relevance, (d) adaptability, and (e) credibility.

Simplicity The best teachers can state complex ideas in simple words. The same holds true for persons communicating everyday concerns. Simplicity includes the use of commonly understood words, brevity, and completeness. Many people have a tendency to overcommunicate. Their messages are wordy, contain too many extraneous explanations, or use words that are highly academic, technical, or slangy. In the world of nursing, many complex technical terms become natural to nurses. However, these terms can often be misunderstood even by informed laypeople. Words such as *vasoconstriction* or *cholecystectomy* are meaningful to the speaker and easy to use but are ill-advised when communicating with clients. Nurses need to learn to select simple words intentionally even though effort is required to do so. For example, instead of saying to a client, "The nurse will be catheterizing you tomorrow for a urine specimen," it is better to say "Tomorrow we need a sample of urine and we will collect it by putting a tube into your bladder." The latter statement is likely to produce a response from the client about why it is needed and whether it will hurt or be uncomfortable. The former statement may simply make the client wonder what the nurse means.

Another aspect of simplicity is brevity. Most people have heard others give lengthy explanations of events, to which they respond, "Get to the point." By using short sentences and avoiding unnecessary material, the speaker or writer can achieve brevity. Brevity is of particular importance in writing, e.g., nurse's notes. Reports or memos need to be concise and should be condensed into a single paragraph or page, if possible.

The opposite of overcommunicating is undercommunicating. Shortcuts for the sake of simplicity can lead to incomplete or unclear communication. For example, initials or abbreviations such as b.i.d. (twice a day) or ICU (intensive care unit) should be avoided unless the nurse is certain that the client will understand them. Because clarification is required, abbreviations can waste the listener's or reader's time. At the first use, names should be expressed in full; later they can be shortened when the nurse is sure that the client or reader knows the meanings.

Clarity

Clarity means saying exactly what is meant. It also is aligned with meaning what is said. The latter involves a blending of the speaker's behavior (nonverbal communication) with the words that are spoken. When the words and the behavior blend together or are unified, the communication is regarded as consistent or congruent.

The goal of clarity is to communicate so that people know the what, how, why (if necessary), when, who, and where of any specific event. Without knowing these facts, people are left to make assumptions. To ensure clarity in communication, the nurse also needs to speak slowly and enunciate words well. It may be helpful to repeat the message and to reduce distractions such as surrounding noises.

Some common pitfalls that can produce unclear communications are ambiguous statements, generalizations, and opinions. For example, "Men are stronger than

---

RESEARCH NOTE

The Words Clients Don't Understand

Some nurses think that today's clients are better informed than clients of years ago because they receive better health education and watch more television. However, in a research study of 100 randomly selected clients, Aina Apse found that many are bewildered by 41 commonly used clinical terms: Not one of the research subjects could correctly define all of the terms. The results ranged from one client who understood only 4% of the terms to another who understood 97%. Most of the clients understood between 51% and 75% of the terms.

The least understood terms included *N.P.O., ambulate,* and *impaction.* Surprisingly, 63% didn't understand the term *blood pressure;* and 29% didn't understand *malignant.* Some clients thought *dilate* means "smaller," *orally* means "every hour," *P.O.* means "afternoon."

Implications: This research demonstrates how important it is for the nurse to find out which terms a particular client understands and then to avoid using potentially confusing terms.

A. Apse, Avoiding terms of bewilderment, *Nursing 85,* December 1985, 15:42–43.

---

women" is both a generalization and an opinion, and the term *stronger* is open to several interpretations. Another example is a nurse's statement to a client, "Mrs. Smith, you need to keep busy today." The specific actions Mrs. Smith is expected to carry out and the reasons for them are open to many interpretations.

Timing and Relevance

No matter how clearly or simply words are stated or written, the timing needs to be appropriate to ensure that words are heard. Moreover, the messages need to relate to the person or to the person's interests and concerns. Consider the woman whose children are crying and whose doorbell is ringing while she is on the telephone with a salesperson. This is not the best time to make a sale, even if the woman is interested.

Nurses need to be aware of both relevance and timing when communicating with clients. This involves being sensitive to the client's needs and concerns. For example, if a female client is enmeshed in fear of cancer, she may not hear the nurse's explanations about the expected procedures before and after her gallbladder surgery. In this situation it is better for the nurse first to encourage her to express her concerns, and to then deal with those concerns. The necessary explanations can be provided at another time.

Another pitfall is to ask several questions at once. For example, a nurse enters a client's room and says in one breath, "Good morning, Mrs. Brody. How are you this morning? Did you sleep well last night? Your husband is coming to see you before your surgery, isn't he?" The client no doubt would feel bombarded and confused and wonder which question to answer first, if any. A related pattern of poor timing is to ask a question and then not wait for an answer before making another comment.

Adaptability Spoken messages need to be altered in accordance with behavioral cues from the receiver. This adjustment is referred to as *adaptability*. Moods and behavior may change minute by minute, hour by hour, or from day to day. In this sense the nurse needs to avoid routine or automatic speech. What the nurse says and how it is said must be individualized and carefully considered. This requires astute assessment and sensitivity on the part of the nurse.

Credibility *Credibility* means worthiness of belief, trustworthiness, reliability. Credibility may be the most important criterion of effective communication. A nurse's credibility to clients depends in part on the opinion of others. If other health professionals and clients regard the nurse as trustworthy, then the client also is likely to.

To become credible, the nurse needs to be knowledgeable about the subject matter being discussed and to have accurate information. Nurses also need to convey confidence and certainty in what they are saying. This is often referred to as *positivism*. People tend to perceive confidence, which is dynamic and emphatic, as more credible than hesitance or uncertainty, which is less forceful and less active. However, the nurse should not sound overconfident or authoritarian. To avoid this perception by the client, the nurse states messages in a constructive way and focuses on being helpful to clients.

Reliability is developed by being consistent, dependable, and honest. People value the nurse who acknowledges limitations and can say, "I don't know the answer to that, but I'll find someone who does."

Nonverbal Communication

Nonverbal communication is sometimes called *body language*. It includes gestures, body movements, and physical appearance, including adornment. The majority of communication is nonverbal. Nonverbal communication often tells others more about what a person is feeling than what is actually said, because nonverbal behavior is controlled less consciously than verbal behavior. Nonverbal communication either reinforces or contradicts what is said verbally. For example, a nurse may say to a client, "I'd be happy to sit here and talk to you for a while," yet if she glances nervously at her watch every few seconds, the actions contradict the verbal message. The client is more likely to believe the nonverbal behavior, which conveys "I am very busy."

Observers cannot always be sure of the correct interpretation of the feelings expressed nonverbally. On the one hand, the same feeling can be expressed nonverbally in more than one way. For example, anger may be communicated by aggressive or excessive body motion, or it may be communicated by a frozen stillness. On the other hand, a variety of feelings, such as embarrassment, pleasure, or anger, can be expressed by a single nonverbal cue, such as blushing.

Observing and interpreting the client's nonverbal behavior are essential skills for nurses. Interpreting the observations requires validation with the client. The nurse's own nonverbal behavior is under constant scrutiny by clients. It is therefore necessary for nurses to gain awareness of their actions and to learn to convey understanding, respect, and acceptance to clients.

To observe nonverbal behavior efficiently requires a systematic approach. As part of an initial assessment, the nurse should observe the person's overall physical appearance, including adornments, posture, and gait, and then assesses specific parts of the body, such as the face and the hands for nonverbal cues. The person's overall appearance includes physical characteristics and manner of dress. Physical characteristics can denote the person's state of health. Skin color and texture, length of fingernails, weight, and deformities causing physical limitations are a few examples. The skin may appear dry, mottled, or pale. Weight may indicate malnourishment. Nails may be well manicured or extremely short. Whatever is observed, the nurse needs to exercise caution in interpretation. For example, pale skin may be normal for that person. Nails may be short because they were bitten nervously or because they were broken by hard manual labor.

Clothing and adornments are sometimes rich sources

of information about a person. Choice of apparel is highly personal. Clothing may convey social and financial status, culture, religion, group association, and self-concept. Adornments such as jewelry, perfume, and cosmetics reveal additional information.

How a person dresses is often an indicator of how the person feels. People who are tired or ill may not have the energy or the desire to maintain their normal grooming. The nurse also needs to be alert to sudden changes in a person's dress. When a person known for immaculate grooming becomes lax about appearance, the nurse may suspect a loss of self-esteem or a physical illness. For clients in acute general hospital settings, a change in grooming habits or personal adornment often signals that the client is feeling better. A male client may request a shave, or a female client may request a mirror and her lipstick.

Posture and Gait   The ways people walk and carry themselves are often reliable indicators of self-concept, current mood, and health. Erect posture and an active, purposeful stride suggest a feeling of well-being. Slouched posture and a slow, shuffling gait suggest dejection or physical discomfort. Tense posture and a rapid, determined gait suggest anxiety or anger. Likewise, the sitting or lying postures of clients can communicate feelings.

Facial Expression   No part of the body is as expressive as the face. Feelings of joy, sadness, fear, surprise, anger, and disgust can be conveyed by facial expressions. The muscles around the eyes and the mouth are particularly expressive. Although actors learn to control these muscles to convey emotions to audiences, facial expressions generally are not consciously controlled.

Clients are quick to notice the nurse's facial expression, particularly when they feel unsure or uncomfortable. The client who questions the nurse about a feared diagnostic result will watch the nurse to see whether the nurse maintains eye contact or looks away when answering. The client who has had disfiguring surgery will examine the nurse's face for signs of disgust. Nurses, like actors, need to be aware of their facial expressions and what they are communicating to others. Although it is impossible to control all facial expressions, the nurse must learn to control feelings such as fear and disgust in certain situations.

Many facial expressions convey a universal meaning. The smile conveys happiness. Contempt is conveyed by the mouth turned down, the head tilted back, and the eyes directed down the nose. No single expression can be interpreted accurately, however, without considering (a) other reinforcing physical cues, (b) the setting in which it occurs, and (c) the expression of others in the same setting.

Eye contact is another essential element of facial communication. Traditionally in Western society mutual eye contact acknowledges recognition of the other person and a willingness to maintain communication. Often a person initiates contact with another person with a glance, capturing the person's attention prior to communicating. A person who feels weak or defenseless often averts the eyes or avoids eye contact. The communication received may be too embarrassing or too dominating. Animals are known to succumb to dominance by averting first their eyes and then their presence.

Hand Movements and Gestures   Like faces, hands are expressive. They can communicate feelings at any given moment. An anxious person, for instance a man awaiting word about his daughter in surgery, may wring his hands or pick his nails; relaxed persons may interlock their fingers over their laps or allow their hands to fall over the ends of armrests. Hands also communicate by touch: slapping someone's face or caressing another's head communicates obvious feelings.

Hands are frequently involved in gestures. The handshake, the victory sign, the wave good-bye, the hand motion to ask a visitor to sit down are gestures that have relatively universal meanings. Some gestures, however, are culture-specific. European women walk together holding hands as a sign of friendship; in North American society, this gesture may be regarded as unacceptable. Even the same gesture can have different meanings in different cultures. The North American gesture meaning "shoo away" or "go away" means "come here" or "come back" in some Asian cultures.

Hands are also very expressive in illustrating or stylizing verbal communication. The French and Italians are noted for using their hands in this manner. When describing the shape and size of an object, a French person uses the hands to reinforce the verbal message.

For people with special communication problems, such as the deaf, the hands are invaluable in communication. Many deaf people learn sign language. Ill persons who are unable to reply verbally can similarly devise a unique communication system using the hands. The client may be able to raise an index finger once for "yes" and twice for "no." Other signals can often be devised by the client and the nurse to denote other meanings.

THE COMMUNICATION PROCESS

There are two major models of nurses' communication in nurse-client interaction: the therapeutic model and "interpersonally competent" model. The *therapeutic model* originated as part of the patient-centered approach to nursing that emphasized the nurse's responsibility to the total well-being of the client. This model focuses on the learning and practicing of a now well-accepted set of skills and abilities such as listening, responding empathetically, using non-evaluative language and nonverbal cues, and demonstrating behaviors that stress confirmation and acknowledgment. See the discussion of therapeutic responses, later in this chapter.

The *interpersonally competent model* was introduced by Kasch in 1984. This model assumes that communication is related to health outcomes. It defines effective communication as that which is interpersonally competent rather than that which is psychologically therapeutic. It is based upon two types of abilities. The first is *social cognitive competence*: the ability to interpret the message content in interactions from many perspectives and to make judgments about the effectiveness and appropriateness of potential responses. The second is *strategic message competence*: the ability to control and strategically use language and other behavioral capabilities to achieve objectives of the nursing process (Harrison et al 1989, p. 77).

Both models emphasize the necessity to learn and perform certain basic communication skills, but the interpersonally competent model stresses these skills as part of the strategic message competence. It adds to these basic skills analytic and interpretational skills in communicating (Harrison et al. 1989, p. 77). Interpretation involves perception, symbolization, memory, and thinking.

The purpose of a model is to break down the process of communication into its essential components so that it can be better understood. A communication model has two main parts: people and messages. In face-to-face communication there is a sender, a message, a receiver, and a response (feedback). See Figure 18–1. In its simplest form, communication is a two-way process involving the sending and the receiving of a message. Since the intent of communication is to elicit a response, the process is ongoing; the receiver of the message then becomes the sender of a response, and the original sender then becomes the receiver.

Sender

The sender, a person or group who wishes to convey a message to another, is sometimes called the *source-encoder*. This term suggests that the person or group sending the message must have an idea or reason for communicating (source) and must put the idea or feeling into a form that can be transmitted. *Encoding* involves the selection of specific signs or symbols (codes) to transmit the message, such as which language and words to use, how to arrange the words, and what tone of voice and gestures to use. For example, if the receiver speaks English, English words will usually be selected. If the message is "No, Johnny, you may not have any more cookies before dinner!" the tone of voice selected will be one of firmness, and a shake of the head or a pointing index finger can reinforce it. The nurse must not only deal with dialects and foreign languages but also must cope with two language levels—the layperson's and the health professional's.

Message

The second component of the communication process is the message itself—what is actually said or written, the body language that accompanies the words, and how the message is transmitted. Various channels can be used to convey messages, and frequently combinations are used. It is important that the channel be appropriate for the message and make the intent of the message clear.

Talking face-to-face with a person may be more effective in some instances than telephoning or writing a message. Recording messages on tape or communicat-

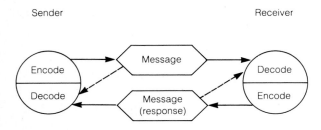

Figure 18-1 The communication process. The dashed arrows indicate internal feedback from the sender of the message (or response).

ing by radio or television may be more appropriate for larger audiences. Written communication is often appropriate for long explanations or for a communication that needs to be preserved. The nonverbal channel of touch is often highly effective.

Receiver

The receiver, the third component of the communication process, is the listener, who must listen, observe, and attend. This person, sometimes called the *decoder,* must perceive what the sender intended (sensation) and then analyze the information received (interpretation). Perception involves use of all the senses to receive all verbal and nonverbal messages. To *decode* means to relate the message perceived to the receiver's storehouse of knowledge and experience and to sort out the meaning of the message. Whether the message is decoded accurately by the receiver, according to the sender's intent, depends largely on their similarities in knowledge and experience.

Response

The fourth component of the communication process, the response, is the message that the receiver returns to the sender. It is also called *feedback.* Feedback can be either positive or negative. Nonverbal examples are a nod of the head or a yawn. Either way, feedback allows the sender to correct or reword a message. The sender then knows the message was interpreted accurately. However, now the original sender becomes the receiver, who is required to decode and respond.

The receiver is not the sole source of feedback. Communicators constantly receive *internal feedback* from themselves. Internal feedback is often used for written messages. For example, after composing a letter, a person will read it silently or out loud to see how it sounds; or a person who makes a social blunder (*faux pas*) may instantly realize the mistake and say, "That isn't what I really meant" or "I didn't mean it that way."

Factors Influencing the Communication Process

In addition to factors such as a person's sociocultural background, language, age, and education, and the limitations and attributes of nonverbal communication, the following factors affect the communication process: ability of the communicator; perceptions; personal space; territoriality; roles and relationships; time; environment; attitudes; and emotions and self-esteem.

Ability of the Communicator   The person's abilities to speak, hear, see, and comprehend stimuli influence the communication process. People who are hard of hearing may require messages that are short, loud, and clear. Those who are unable to read will be unable to comprehend written information. Some, because of disease processes, are unable to see or to speak, and individual methods for communication need to be devised with them.

The receiver of a message also needs to be able to interpret the message. Mental faculties can be impaired for such reasons as brain damage or use of sedative drugs or alcohol. Even if a client is free of physical impairments, the nurse needs to determine how many stimuli the client is capable of receiving in a given time frame. Frequently the receiver is expected to assimilate too much information. The nurse may be talking too quickly or presenting too many ideas at once. This is of particular importance when offering health instruction.

Perceptions   Because each person has unique personality traits, values, and life experiences, each will perceive and interpret messages differently. It is important in many situations to validate or correct the perceptions of the receiver.

Personal Space   *Personal space* is the distance people prefer in interactions with others. *Proxemics* is the study of distance between people in their interactions. Middle-class North Americans use definite distances in various interpersonal relationships, along with specific voice tones and body language. Communication thus alters in accordance with four distances, each with a close and a far phase, that have been described by Hall (1969, p. 45):

1. Intimate: Physical contact to 1½ feet
2. Personal: 1½–4 feet
3. Social: 4–12 feet
4. Public: 12 feet and beyond

Intimate distance communication is characterized by body contact, heightened sensations of body heat and smell, and vocalizations that are low. Vision is intense, restricted to a small body part, and may be distorted. Intimate distance is frequently used by nurses. Examples occur in cuddling a baby, touching the sightless client, positioning clients, observing an incision, and restraining a toddler for an injection. It is a natural protective instinct for people to maintain a certain amount of space immediately around them, and the amount varies with individuals. When someone who wants to communicate steps too close, the receiver automatically steps back a pace or two. In their therapeutic roles, nurses often are required to violate this intimate space. However, it is important for them to be aware when this will occur and to forewarn the client. In many instances, the nurse can respect (not come as close as) a person's intimate distance. In other instances, the nurse may come within intimate distance to communicate warmth and caring.

Personal distance is less overwhelming than intimate distance. Voice tones are moderate, and body heat and smell are noticed less. Physical contact such as a handshake or touching a shoulder is possible. More of the person is perceived at a personal distance, so that nonverbal behaviors such as body stance or full facial expressions are seen with less distortion. Much communication between nurses and clients occurs at this distance. Examples occur when nurses are sitting with a client, giving medications, or establishing an intravenous infusion. Communication at a close personal distance can convey involvement by facilitating the sharing of thoughts and feelings. At the outer extreme of 4 ft, however, less involvement is conveyed. Bantering and some social conversations are usual at this distance.

Social distance is characterized by a clear visual perception of the whole person. Body heat and odor are imperceptible, eye contact is increased, and vocalizations are loud enough to be overheard by others. Communication is therefore more formal and is limited to seeing and hearing. The person is protected and out of reach for touch or personal sharing of thoughts or feelings. Social distance allows more activity and movement back and forth. It is expedient in communicating with several people at the same time or within a short time. Social distance is important in accomplishing the business of the day. However, it is frequently misused. For example, the nurse who stands in the doorway and asks a client "How are you today?" will receive a more noncommittal reply than the nurse who moves to personal distance to inquire.

Public distance requires loud, clear vocalizations with careful enunciation. Although the faces and forms of people are seen at public distance, individuality is lost. Instead, a general notion is perceived about a group of people or a community.

Territoriality   *Territoriality* is a concept of the space and things that an individual considers as belonging to the self. Territories marked off by people may be visible to others. For example, clients in a hospital often consider their territory as bounded by the curtains around the bed unit or by the walls of a private room.

This human tendency to claim territory must be recognized by all health care workers. Clients often feel the need to defend their territory when it is invaded by others; for example, when a visitor removes a chair to use at another bed, the visitor has inadvertently violated the territoriality of the client whose chair was moved.

Roles and Relationships   The roles and the relationship between sender and receiver affect the communication process. Roles such as nursing student and instructor, client and physician, or parent and child will affect the content and responses in the communication process. Choice of words, sentence structure, and tone of voice vary considerably from role to role. In addition, the specific relationship between the communicators is significant. The nurse who meets with a client for the first time will communicate differently from the nurse who has previously developed a relationship with that client.

Time   The time factor in communication includes the events that precede and follow the interaction. The hospitalized client who is anticipating surgery or who has just received news that a spouse has lost a job will not be very receptive to information. A client who has had to wait for some time to express needs may respond quite differently from one who has endured no waiting period. The setting also influences communication. If the room lacks privacy or is hot, noisy, or crowded, the communication process can break down.

Nurses' use of time can facilitate or inhibit a client's communication. The nurse who tells a client "I'll be back in a moment" while delivering medications is likely to convey "I haven't time now" or "I've got work to do." This inhibits client communications. However, if this nurse says to the client, "Would you tell me now what your concern is about, and then when I've finished delivering medications I'll come back and help you with it," the communication process is facilitated.

Environment   People usually communicate most effectively in a comfortable environment. Temperature extremes, excessive noise, and a poorly ventilated environment can all interfere with communication. Also, lack of privacy may interfere with a client's communication about matters the client considers private. For example, a client who is worried about the ability of his wife to care for him after discharge from hospital may not wish to discuss this concern with a nurse within the hearing of other clients in the room. Environmental distraction can impair and distort communication.

Attitudes   Attitudes convey beliefs, thoughts, and feelings about people and events. They are communicated convincingly and rapidly to others. Attitudes such as caring, warmth, respect, and acceptance facilitate communication, whereas condescension, lack of interest, and coldness inhibit communication.

Caring and *warmth* convey a feeling of emotional closeness, in contrast to impersonal distance. Caring is more enduring and intense than warmth. It conveys deep and genuine concern for the person. Warmth, on the other hand, conveys friendliness and consideration, shown by acts of smiling and attention to physical comforts (Brammer 1988, p. 37). Caring involves giving feelings, thoughts, skill, and knowledge. It requires psychologic energy and poses the risk of gaining little in return, yet by caring, people usually reap the benefits of greater communication and understanding.

Respect is an attitude that emphasizes the other person's worth and individuality. It conveys that the person's hopes and feelings are special and unique even though similar to others in many ways. People have a need to be different from—and at the same time similar to—others. Being too different can be isolating and threatening. Respect is conveyed by listening open-mindedly to what the other person is saying, even if the nurse disagrees. Nurses can learn new ways of approaching situations when they conscientiously listen to another person's perspective.

Acceptance emphasizes neither approval nor disapproval. The nurse willingly receives the client's honest feelings and actions without judgment. An accepting attitude allows clients to express personal feelings freely and to be themselves. The nurse may need to restrict acceptance in situations where clients' actions are harmful to themselves or to others.

In contrast, *condescension* is an attitude that conveys superiority over the other person. Clients who feel helpless often perceive nurses to be in a superior position because of their knowledge and skill. In these instances, the nurse may convey condenscension by an air of superiority and intellectualism. One common condescending act by nurses is to call clients "honey" or "dear." This casts the nurse in the role of the superior mother and the client in the role of the inferior child. Another condescending act is patting an elderly client on the head.

Lack of interest also inhibits communication by saying "I'm not concerned" or "What you say is not important." The nurse conveys lack of interest by forgetting part of the client's conversation or not concentrating on it sufficiently to respond. Being tired near the end of a long day's work or in a hurry to complete tasks may contribute to giving the appearance of not being interested in the client.

Coldness is the opposite of caring and warmth. Nurses convey this attitude to clients by appearing more interested in the technical and procedural aspects of nursing than in the concerns of the person receiving the therapy. For example, the nurse can convey coldness by appearing more concerned about the neatness of the client's bed than about the client's restlessness or more interested in the efficient functioning of a cardiac monitor than in the client's anxiety. A rigid body posture and aloof tone of voice also convey a nurse's lack of genuine concern for the client.

Emotions and Self-Esteem   Most people have experienced overwhelming joy or sorrow that is difficult to express in words. Anger may produce loud, profane vocalizations or controlled speechlessness. Fright may produce screams of terror or paralyzed silence.

Emotions also affect a person's ability to interpret messages. Large parts of a message may not be heard, or the message may be misinterpreted when the receiver is experiencing strong emotion. This situation occurs frequently in nursing. For example, the client feeling great fear may not remember all the preoperative instructions offered by a nurse.

Self-esteem also influences communication patterns. People whose self-esteem is high communicate honestly, with confidence, and with *congruence* (agreement or coinciding) between verbal and nonverbal messages. For example, a nurse explaining the importance of preoperative exercises would present a sincere and serious facial expression. Those with low self-esteem or under high stress tend to give double messages; that is, their verbal and nonverbal messages are incongruent (lack consistency). For example, while explaining about a client's colostomy to the client's family, a nurse laughs.

ASSESSING COMMUNICATION

When nurses assess the communication of clients, they need to include language development, nonverbal behavior, and communication style.

Language Development

The nurse assesses the following aspects of language development:

- The language skills presented by the client, compared to the language skills normally expected
- Adequacy of the language skills in relation to the individual's need
- The chief method of communicating, e.g., words or gestures
- Obstacles to language development, such as deafness or absence of environmental stimuli
- Specific forms of language impairment, e.g., a school-age child's inability to write or lack of abstractions in the language of an adult
- Cultural influences on language development, e.g., the language used in the home or customs about when and how to speak

Nonverbal Behavior

In assessing nonverbal communication, the nurse considers the following:

- Gestures used by the individual.
- Posture and facial expressions employed.
- Use of touch as a means of communication. See the discussion of touch, later in this chapter.
- The interpersonal distance with which the person feels comfortable, e.g., whether the person assumes an intimate distance for most discussions.
- The grooming and appearance of the individual. These may affect the communication process, e.g., when dress is inconsistent with a setting or presents a stereotype that may evoke biases.

Style of Communication

A person's style of communication is often affected by such factors as health, culture, education, stress level, fatigue, and cognitive ability. In assessing communication style, the nurse considers the following:

- The vocabulary of the individual, particularly any changes from the vocabulary normally used. For example, a person who normally never swears may indicate increased stress or illness by an uncharacteristic use of profanity.
- The use of symbols and gestures to communicate. Some uses of symbols and gestures are culturally determined; for example, a Puerto Rican girl may be taught not to look an adult in the eyes, as a sign of

respect and obedience; the gesture should not be interpreted as a sign of guilt.
- The presence of hostility, aggression, assertiveness, reticence, hesitance, anxiety, or loquaciousness (incessant verbalization) in the communication.
- Difficulties with verbal communication, such as slurring, stuttering, inability to pronounce a particular sound, lack of clarity in enunciation, inability to speak in sentences, loose association of ideas, flight of ideas, or the inability to find or name words or identify objects.
- Refusal or inability to speak.

DIAGNOSING COMMUNICATION PROBLEMS

Impaired verbal communication is the nursing diagnosis given to clients with verbal communication problems. Impaired verbal communication is the "state in which an individual experiences, or could experience, a decreased ability to send or receive messages, i.e., has difficulty exchanging thoughts, ideas, or desires" (Carpenito 1989, p. 227). Contributing factors for impaired verbal communication follow.

Impaired verbal communication related to:

- Development or age-related stage(s)
- Anatomic deficit, such as cleft palate
- Cultural difference or inability to speak dominant language
- Physical conditions such as cerebrovascular accident or brain tumor, or surgery such as laryngectomy or tracheostomy.
- Psychologic conditions, such as extreme anger, severe anxiety or panic, moderate and severe depression, fear, shyness, loneliness, and unrealistic or inadequate self-concept
- Pharmacologic therapy, such as central nervous system depressant

Ineffective individual coping, Ineffective family coping, Anxiety, and **Fear** may be appropriate diagnoses for some clients. These definitions, defining characteristics, and contributing factors are discussed in Chapter 23.

PLANNING FOR EFFECTIVE COMMUNICATION

When problems in communication have been identified, the nurse and client set goals and begin planning ways to promote effective communication. The overall client goal for persons with impaired verbal communication is to reduce or resolve the impaired communication. Specific nursing interventions are planned from the stated etiology. Among these interventions are (a) developing listening skills, (b) becoming aware of how people respond and (c) developing a helping relationship. More specific interventions may include the following:

- Anticipate needs until effective communication is established.
- Discuss individual methods of dealing with the impairment.
- Keep communication simple, using visual, auditory, and kinesthetic modes for conveying information.
- Plan for alternate methods of communication, such as a typewriter, slate, or letter/picture board.
- Respond with simple, straightforward, honest statements to provide reality orientation and correct faulty perception.
- Use and assist clients to learn facilitative communication techniques, e.g., active listening skills. See the discussion of therapeutic and nontherapeutic communication skills later in this chapter.
- Help the client look at the effects of nonfacilitative communication techniques.
- Teach and encourage expression of feelings.
- Point out discrepancies in verbal and nonverbal behavior.
- Encourage the client to ask for feedback when communicating with others.
- Refer the client to appropriate resources such as speech therapy, group therapy, or individual or family counseling.

Examples of outcome criteria to evaluate the achievement of client goals and the effectiveness of nursing interventions follow.

The client:

- Attends to appropriate communication input.
- Perceives input accurately.
- Gives clear, concise, understandable messages.

- Uses effective communication techniques, e.g., active listening, silence, reflecting, restating.
- Avoids the use of nonfacilitative techniques such as offering advice.
- Expresses congruent verbal and nonverbal behavior.
- Expresses feelings appropriately.
- Uses resources appropriately.
- Establishes a method of communication in which needs can be expressed.

IMPLEMENTING

Techniques for Therapeutic Communication

Therapeutic communication promotes understanding by both the sender and the receiver. A number of techniques can help establish a constructive relationship between the nurse and the client, although the use of the techniques is no guarantee of effective communication. So many factors are involved in communication that the nurse is ill-advised to rely on any one technique or even several techniques. Not all people feel comfortable with all techniques, and skill in using them appropriately is essential. The nurse must be comfortable with the technique used and convey sincerity to the client. A phony or false response is usually quickly identified by clients and hinders the development of an effective relationship.

Nurses can learn much by examining and becoming aware of their own reactions (feelings) and responses. Although it is difficult for nurses to see their own nonverbal communication other than by videotape feedback, much can be learned by reflecting on what was heard, what the nurse said, and when and how it was said. Methods such as role playing, process recordings, and audiotapes can be useful.

Nurses need to respond not only to the content of a client's verbal message but also to the feelings expressed. It is important to understand how the client views the situation and feels about it before responding. The content of the client's communication is the words or thoughts, as distinct from the feelings. Sometimes people can convey a thought in words while their emotions contradict the words; i.e., words and feelings are incongruent. For example, a client says, "I am glad he has left me; he was very cruel." However, the nurse observes that the client has tears in her eyes as she says this. To respond to the client's *words,* the nurse might simply rephrase, saying "You are pleased that he has left you." To respond to the client's *feelings,* the nurse would need to acknowledge the tears in the client's eyes, saying, for example, "You seem saddened by all this." Such a response helps the client to focus on her feelings. In some instances, the nurse may need to know more about the client and her resources for coping with these feelings.

Sometimes clients need time to deal with their feelings. Strong emotions are often draining. People usually need to deal with feelings before they can cope with other matters, such as learning new skills or planning for the future. This is most evident in hospitals when clients learn that they have a terminal illness. Some require hours, days, or even weeks before they are ready to start other tasks. Some need only time to themselves, others need someone to listen, others need assistance identifying and verbalizing feelings, and others need assistance making decisions about future courses of action.

Attentive Listening   It is essential, in therapeutic communication, that nurses listen and respond to clients purposefully and deliberately. Attentive listening is listening actively, using all the senses, as opposed to listening passively with just the ear. It is probably the most important technique in nursing. Attentive listening is an active process that requires energy and concentration. It involves paying attention to the total message, both verbal messages and nonverbal messages that can modify what is spoken, and noting whether these communications are congruent. Attentive listening means absorbing both the content and the feeling the person is conveying, without selectivity. The listener does not select or listen to solely what the listener wants to hear; the nurse does not focus on the nurse's own needs but rather on the client's needs. Attentive listening conveys an attitude of caring and interest, thereby encouraging the client to talk. In summary, attentive listening is a highly developed skill, but fortunately it can be learned with practice.

A nurse can convey attentiveness in listening to clients in various ways. Common responses are nodding the head, uttering "uh huh" or "mmm," repeating the words that the client has used, or saying "I see what you mean." Each nurse has characteristic ways of responding, and the nurse must take care not to sound insincere or phony.

Egan (1982, pp. 60–61) has outlined five specific ways to convey physical attending. He defines physical attending as the manner of being present to another or being with another. Listening, in his frame of reference, is what a person does while attending. The five actions of physical attending, which convey a "posture of involvement," follow:

1. *Face the other person squarely.* This position says, "I am available to you." Moving to the side lessens the degree of involvement.

2. *Maintain good eye contact.* Mutual eye contact, preferably at the same level, recognizes the other person and denotes a willingness to maintain communication. Eye contact neither glares at nor stares down another but is natural.

3. *Lean toward the other.* People move naturally toward one another when they want to say or hear something—by moving to the front of a class, by moving a chair nearer a friend, or by leaning across a table with arms propped in front. The nurse conveys involvement by leaning forward, closer to the client.

4. *Maintain an open posture.* The nondefensive position is one in which neither arms nor legs are crossed. It conveys that the person wishes to encourage the passage of communication, as the open door of a home or an office does.

5. *Remain relatively relaxed.* Total relaxation is not feasible when the nurse is listening with intensity, but the nurse can show relaxation by taking time in responding, allowing pauses as needed, balancing periods of tension with relaxation, and using gestures that are natural.

These five attending postures need to be adapted to the specific needs of clients in a given situation. For example, leaning forward may not be appropriate at the beginning of an interview. It may be reserved until a closer relationship grows between the nurse and the client. The same applies to eye contact, which is generally uninterrupted when the communicators are very involved in the interaction.

Paraphrasing   Paraphrasing, also called *restating,* involves listening for the client's basic message and then repeating those thoughts and/or feelings in similar words. Usually fewer words are used. Paraphrasing conveys that the nurse has listened and understood the client's basic message. It may also offer clients a clearer idea of what they have said. The client's response to the paraphrase may tell the nurse whether the paraphrase was accurate or helpful. (It may be necessary for the nurse to ask for a response.)

Client: I couldn't manage to eat any of my dinner last night—not even the dessert.

Nurse: You had difficulty eating yesterday.

Client: Yes, I was very upset after my family left.

Clarifying

Clarifying is a method of making the client's message more understandable. It is used when paraphrasing is difficult, when the communication has been rambling or garbled. To clarify the message the nurse can make a guess and restate the basic message or confess confusion and ask the client to repeat or restate the message (Davis 1984, p. 9). In the former situation, if the client says, "I didn't sleep at all last night," the nurse might say, "You didn't sleep at all last night." In the latter instance the nurse might say, "I'm puzzled" or "I'm not sure I understand that" and "Would you please say that again?" or "Would you tell me more?"

Nurses sometimes need to clarify their own messages to clients. The need to do so is generally discovered from the client's nonverbal feedback. Then the nurse might ask a question or say, "It seems to me I didn't make that clear" and repeat or rephrase the message. Sometimes only one word or phrase in a message needs clarifying.

Clarifying also includes *verifying what is implied*. In this instance, the client implies or hints at something without actually saying it. The nurse then tries to clarify the client's statement without interpreting it.

Client: There is no point in asking for a pain pill.

Nurse: Are you saying that no one gives you an analgesic when you have pain?

Another clarifying technique is *perception checking*, or *consensual validation*. This verifies the accuracy of the nurse's listening skills by giving and receiving feedback about what was communicated. It involves paraphrasing what the nurse believes to have heard and asking the client for confirmation. It is important to allow the client to correct inaccurate perceptions. The advantage of frequent perception checking is that inaccurate perceptions are corrected before communications become confused and misunderstandings arise. Examples of perception checking are: "You sound annoyed with me—is that correct?" or "You seem to have some doubts about the decision you made, and I'd like to see if what I'm hearing is accurate."

Sometimes it is important for nurses to clarify reality when a client has misrepresented it. This assists the client to differentiate the real from the unreal.

Client: Someone took my magazine last night.

Nurse: Your magazine is here in your drawer.

It may also be necessary to clarify a sequence of events or a time period.

Client: I feel that I have been asleep for weeks.

Nurse: You had your operation Monday, and today is Tuesday.

Using Open-Ended Questions and Statements

The use of *open-ended questions* is discussed in Chapter 6. Examples of *open-ended statements* are "I'd like to hear more about that" and "Tell me about . . ."

Focusing

Focusing is used when the client's communication is vague, when the client is rambling, or when the client seems to be talking about numerous things. Focusing can be compared to using a telephoto lens, which focuses sharply on a certain aspect of a view; similarly, the nurse assists or leads the client to focus on one specific aspect of a communication. It is important for the nurse to wait until the clients think they have talked about the main concerns before attempting to focus. The focus may be an idea or a feeling; however, a feeling is often emphasized, to help the client recognize an emotion disguised behind words.

Client: My wife says she will look after me, but I don't think she can, what with the children to take care of, and they're always after her about something—clothes, homework, what's for dinner that night.

Nurse: You are worried about how well she can manage.

Being Specific, Tentative, and Informative

When responding to another person's comments, it is helpful to make statements that are (a) specific rather than general, (b) tentative rather than absolute, and (c) informative rather than authoritarian. Examples are: "You scratched my arm" (specific statement); "You're as clumsy as an ox" (general statement); "You seemed unconcerned about Mary" (tentative statement); "You don't give a damn about Mary and you never will" (absolute statement); "I haven't finished yet" (informative statement); "Stop interrupting!" (authoritarian statement).

In being informative, the nurse needs to present facts or specific information simply and directly. If the nurse does not know some fact, this is also stated simply, together with a suggestion about where or how the information can be obtained.

Client: I don't know the visiting hours.

Nurse: The visiting hours are 9 A.M. to 9 P.M. each day.

Another way to be informative is to make an observation. This indicates that the nurse has noticed a change of behavior but is not placing a value judgment on it. For example: "You have washed your hair" (neutral observation); "Your hair looks better now that you have washed it" (value judgment); "You are holding your arm carefully; is it painful?" (observation; verifying implication).

Using Touch   Certain forms of touching indicate affection. For example, cheek patting, hand patting, and putting an arm over the person's shoulder are valued forms of affection in North America. The "laying on of hands" is a common expression indicating curative and comforting actions. This expression is often attributed to individuals in the healing professions such as religion, medicine, and nursing. Tactile contacts vary considerably among individuals, families, and cultures. Some families have a great deal of tactile contact among members. Other families, even within the same culture, have minimal contact. Appropriate forms of touch can be helpful in reinforcing caring feelings by the nurse. The use of touch alone often says much more than words for clients, such as for those who are terminally ill or who are unable to speak for whatever reason. It is important, however, for the nurse to be sensitive to the differences in attitudes and practices related to touch among individuals, including the nurse's own attitudes.

Using Silence   In everyday conversations natural pauses or silences are often accepted without thought. The listener attentively waits until the talker resumes conversation. These natural pauses are generally used to recall a name or event or to put thoughts or feelings into the most accurate words possible. Pauses or silences that extend for several seconds or minutes, however, make some listeners extremely uncomfortable. The listener who interjects thoughts, questions, or explanations to reduce the discomfort in essence "puts words into the other person's mouth." The unfortunate result is that self-expression is blocked for the initial communicator.

When people are ill, communication about how they feel is often difficult for them. Many prefer to remain sto-

ically silent until they are sure that the nurse is interested or trustworthy. Once communication is initiated, it may be expressed awkwardly, with many pauses. The nurse needs to learn to be silent in these situations and to wait patiently until the person is able to put thoughts and feelings into words.

Providing General Leads   By providing a general lead, the nurse encourages the client to verbalize and at the same time choose the topic of conversation.

Client: I am sure glad yesterday is over.

Nurse: Perhaps you would like to talk about it.

Summarizing   Summarizing the main points of a discussion is a useful technique near the end of an interview, after a significant discussion, or to review a health-teaching session. It clarifies for both the nurse and the client the relevant points discussed and often acts as an introduction to future care planning. For example, the nurse might say, "During the past half hour we have talked about. . . . Tomorrow afternoon we may explore this further" or "In a few days, I'll review what you have learned about the actions and effects of your insulin." A word of caution about summarizing: No new material should be added.

Nontherapeutic Responses

Nurses need to recognize nontherapeutic techniques that interfere with effective communication. These include failing to listen; unwarranted reassurance; judgmental responses; defensive responses; and probing, testing or challenging responses.

Failing to Listen   Because listening is the most effective technique to facilitate communication, the opposite, failure to listen, is the primary inhibitor to communication. It says to the client, "I'm not interested" or "I'm bored" or "You are not important." It suggests that nurses need to be entertained, that the nurses' needs require attention, or that nurses prefer to discuss topics that concern themselves.

Unwarranted Reassurance   Statements such as "You'll feel better soon," "I'm sure everything will turn out all right," "Don't worry," and "You're looking better each day" are futuristic and intended to provide hope for the client. However, they disregard the client's feelings of the moment and in many instances are said when there is no hope of improvement. The client who fears death, for example, needs to express these concerns rather than have them dismissed with false reassurance. The nurse who offers reassurance in this manner needs to examine her or his own feelings and recognize that this type of response is of more help to the nurse than to the client.

Judgmental Responses

Passing judgment on the client implies that the client *must* think as the nurse thinks—the client's values must be the same as the nurse's—if the client is to be accepted. Approving or disapproving responses, such as "That's good (bad)," "You shouldn't do that," and "That's not good enough," tell clients they must measure up to the nurse's standards rather than to their own goals. Perhaps what the nurse considers "bad" the client considers "good."

Giving common advice, another nontherapeutic response, removes decision-making control from the client to the nurse. It suggests that the client is inferior and less wise than the nurse. Moreover, it fosters dependence, and often the advice is not followed. Note that *common,* not *expert,* advice is spoken of here. This differentiation is significant, since giving expert advice can be therapeutic. Brammer (1988, p. 92) writes:

> Advice can be helpful if it is given by trusted persons with expert opinions based on solid knowledge of a supporting field such as law, medicine, or child rearing. Sometimes . . . clients need a recommended course of action supported by wide experience and . . . facts.

Common advice, on the other hand, refers to matters dealing with individual choice. For example, a client asks, "Should I move from my home to a nursing home?" or "I'm separated from my wife. Do you think I should have sexual relations with another woman?" Offering advice such as "If I were you . . ." is unwise for the nurse. Clients need support to make their own decisions.

Stereotyping responses are judgmental, since they categorize clients and negate their uniqueness as individuals. *Stereotypes* are generalized and oversimplified beliefs we hold about various groups of people, which are based upon experiences too limited to be valid. The less one knows about a person, the more the tendency to stereotype. Examples of stereotyping statements are: "Two-year-olds are brats," "Women are complainers," and "Men don't cry." Communication between nurse and client can be inhibited, depending on how emotionally charged the stereotype is for the nurse. For example, if the nurse is not deeply committed to the "brat" theory, the communication pattern with a 2-year-old who is cooperative may be only temporarily affected. On the

other hand, the nurse who has marked feelings about men who cry will probably ignore the individualism of a male client who expresses his grief in that manner.

Another common error is to offer meaningless stereotyped responses to clients.

Client: I'm sure having a lot of pain.

Nurse: Really? Most people don't have pain after this type of surgery.

Agreeing and disagreeing imply that the client is either right or wrong and that the nurse is in a position to judge this. They can deter clients from thinking through their position. Disagreement sometimes causes the client to defend a position.

Client: I don't think Dr. Broad is a very good doctor. He doesn't seem interested in his patients.

Nurse: Dr. Broad is head of the Department of Surgery and is an excellent surgeon.

Defensive Responses

Many clients offer opinions or comments about their care, directed toward the nurse, the nurse's colleagues, or the institution. Feeling threatened or attacked, the nurse may become defensive and prevent the client from expressing feelings.

Client: The food here is lousy.

Nurse: It's a lot better here than in the county hospital. You should consider yourself lucky.

These responses prevent the client from expressing true concerns. The nurse is saying, "You have no right to complain." Defensive responses protect the nurse from admitting weaknesses in the health care services, including personal weaknesses.

Probing, Testing, and Challenging Responses

Probing, testing, and challenging are often considered hostile responses. *Probing* is asking for information chiefly out of curiosity rather than with the intent to assist the client. Usually probing is considered prying, and the client feels that privacy is not being respected. Often asking "why" is probing and can place the client in a defensive posture:

Client: I didn't ask the doctor when he was here.

Nurse: Why didn't you?

Testing is questioning by nurses to make clients admit to something. With testing, the nurse usually asks a question that permits the client only limited answers. Testing often meets the nurse's need rather than the client's. Examples of testing questions are: "Who do you think you are?" This question forces clients to admit that their status in the health care agency is that of "only a client." Another testing question is "Do you think I am not busy?" which forces the client to admit that the nurse really *is* busy.

Challenging is giving a response that makes clients prove their statement or point of view. Usually clients' feelings are not considered, and they feel it necessary to defend a position. Challenging a client's perceptions rarely changes them; often it strengthens them, because the client feels forced to find proof to support the position.

Client: I feel as if I am dying.

Nurse: I don't understand, how can you feel that way when your pulse is 60?

EVALUATING COMMUNICATION

Evaluation activities involve an appraisal of both client communication and nurse communication. To evaluate whether client goals have been achieved, the nurse obtains data in relation to the outcome criteria established. This is accomplished by actively listening to the client's style of verbal communication and observing the client's nonverbal communication with the nurse and others. Examples of evaluative statements indicating goal achievement are "The client expressed feelings of anger and fear about diagnosis and inability to speak," or "Using slateboard effectively to indicate needs × 1 week."

For nurses to evaluate the effectiveness of their own communications with clients, process recordings are frequently used. A *process recording* is a verbatim (word-for-word) account of a conversation. It can be taped or written, and it includes all verbal and nonverbal interactions.

One method of writing a process recording is to make three columns on a page. The first column lists what the client said and did, the second what the nurse said and did, and the third contains interpretive comments about the nurse's responses. See Table 18–2.

Once a process recording his been completed, it should be analyzed in terms of (a) the direction and development of the interaction (process), and (b) the content. The nurse's interaction can be analyzed for process according to a number of questions:

1. Was the client's verbal and nonverbal behavior really heard and seen?

2. Were any cues missed?

3. Were the nurse's verbal responses and behavior congruent?

4. Did the client respond to the nurse or independently of the nurse?

5. Did the communication process flow smoothly?

6. Were the nurse's responses consistent with what the nurse observed and heard? Or were they unrelated, exaggerated, or underresponsive?

7. Were the nurse's responses therapeutic or nontherapeutic? See the previous sections on responding therapeutically or nontherapeutically.

Each response can also be analyzed for content in terms of facilitating or inhibiting communication. See Table 18–2 for a sample analysis.

GROUP INTERACTION

People are born into a group (i.e., the family) and interact with others at all stages of their lives in various groups: peer groups, work groups, recreational groups, religious groups, and so on. A *group* is defined as two or more persons who have shared needs and goals, who take each other into account in their actions, and who thus are held together and set apart from others by virtue of their interactions. Groups exist to help people achieve goals that would be unattainable by individual effort alone. For example, groups can often solve problems more effectively than one person by pooling the ideas and expertise of several individuals; in addition, information can be disseminated to groups more quickly than to individuals. Moreover, groups often take greater risks than do individuals. Just as responsibilities for actions are shared by group members, so are the consequences of actions. The overall effectiveness of groups in attaining goals depends on many factors, discussed in this chapter.

Classifications of Groups

Groups are classified as either primary or secondary, according to their structure and type of interaction. A *primary group* is a small, intimate group in which the relationships among members are personal, spontaneous, sentimental, cooperative, and inclusive. Examples are the family, a play group of children, informal work

text continues on p. 347

TABLE 18-2 *Sample Process Recording*

Mary Jane Adams, a nursing aide, reports to Irene Olsen, the staff nurse, that Sandra Barrett, the client in room 815, had finished only her orange juice when Ms. Adams collected the breakfast trays. Mrs. Barrett had been admitted two days earlier for diagnostic studies. Concerned about her client, Miss Olsen walks down the corridor to room 815, knocks, and enters. Mrs. Barrett turns away from the window, tears in her eyes, as Miss Olsen enters.

Client	Nurse	Comments
	Good morning, Mrs. Barrett.	Acknowledging.
Hello.		
	I understand you didn't eat your breakfast.	Making a specific statement, but ignoring the nonverbal.
I wasn't hungry.	Is something wrong?	Asking a closed-ended question that fails to facilitate exploration.
No. (Eyes fill with tears.)	You look sad; as if you're about to cry.	Giving feedback.
(Cries)	I'll sit here a while with you. (Sits down.)	Offering self.
(Continues to cry.)	(After a 30-second pause): Sometimes it's hard to share the things you're concerned about with someone you don't know well. I'd like to be able to help.	Empathizing. Supporting. Offering self.
(Angrily): You can help me by telling me the truth.		
	(Leans forward and maintains eye contact.)	Actively listening and demonstrating interest.
Everyone beats around the bush when I ask them what's wrong with me. The head nurse said, "What do *you* think is wrong?" That kind of put-off drives me up the wall!		
	You're angry because you're not getting any answers. It seems as if the staff knows something about your condition and they're keeping it from you.	Paraphrasing.
They all seem to be in cahoots. Nobody tells me anything. (Pause). (Softly): If the news was good, they wouldn't beat around the bush.		
	I'm wondering if you're worried that because people haven't answered your question it means that you have a serious illness?	Paraphrasing.
Good news is always easy to give.		
	Yes, people do seem to be able to deliver good news easier and faster. I also know that we don't have any news—good or bad—to give you because none of the laboratory or x-ray results are back yet. I know that doesn't help answer your questions, but I hope it relieves you a bit from	Giving information. Supporting.

▶

TABLE 18-2 *Sample Process Recording* (continued)

Client	Nurse	Comments
	worrying that there is some bad news that's being withheld.	
Well, when my father-in-law had surgery for a bleeding ulcer, the x-ray and laboratory results were available immediately.		
	When there's a question of emergency surgery being needed, then tests results are asked for immediately. Usually, though, it's preferable to wait for an accurate reading and a thorough written report.	Giving information.
Are you absolutely sure?		
	You don't sound convinced.	Acknowledging the implied.
Listen, I don't mean to give you a hard time. It's just that . . . it may not seem like an emergency to my doctor or the lab people, but it sure is to me. I can't stand not knowing. I don't know the results of the tests I had yesterday. I don't know how many more tests I have to have. Will I have to have surgery? When can I go home?		
	The problem you need help with now is finding out the answers to four questions: What are the results of yesterday's tests? Is your doctor considering any other tests for you, and if so what are they? Is surgery being planned? And when can you go home? Let's try to figure out how you can get the answers to these questions.	Summarizing. Encouraging problem solving.
Well, I can't call my doctor on the phone. All his receptionist will do is take the message. And, anyway, I'm afraid that he'll be offended if he thinks I'm complaining about him. You won't tell him, will you?		
	No, not unless you and I decide together that it would be the best solution.	Encouraging collaboration.
I suppose I could try to forget about it and be patient, just like everyone tells me to.		
	You've tried that, but you're still worried, fearful, and angry. Let's think of some other possibilities.	Encouraging further exploration.

▶

TABLE 18–2 *Sample Process Recording* (continued)

Client	Nurse	Comments
Maybe you could call his office for me! Since you're a nurse, they'll probably put your call right through.		
	So far there are three possible solutions—calling his office yourself, waiting until he comes to visit you later this afternoon, or having me call his office. Are there any other possible solutions that we haven't considered?	Focusing on solutions.
I can't think of any others.		
	Okay, then, which do you think would be best?	Demonstrating respect for the client.
I guess I'd feel better if you called his office. I just don't want him to think that I'm criticizing him.		
	You're concerned about what he might think of you because of this phone call. Let's discuss how I should handle the call and what I should say.	Paraphrasing. Encouraging collaboration and problem solving.

After a few minutes they develop a plan for calling Mrs. Barrett's physician, and Miss Olsen makes the call. The physician has decided to call both the laboratory and the X-ray department for the results of Mrs. Barrett's tests and promises to phone her as soon as he learns the results. They will discuss further possible tests and treatment plans that afternoon when he makes his hospital rounds. Mrs. Barrett asks Miss Olsen to stay with her while she receives the physician's telephone call about the test.

Courtesy of Carol Ren Kneisl, President and Educational Director, Nursing Transitions, Williamsville, New York.

groups, and friendship groups. Members of a primary group communicate with each other largely in face-to-face interactions and develop a strong sense of unity or "oneness." What belongs to one person is often seen as belonging to the group. For example, a success achieved by one member is shared by all and is seen as a success of the group.

Primary groups set standards of behavior for the members but also support and sustain each member under stresses he or she would otherwise not be able to withstand. Expectations are informally administered and involve primarily internal constraints imposed by the group itself. To its members, the primary group has a value in itself, not merely as a means to some other goal. The group has a sense of "we" and "our" to it, in contrast to "I" and "mine." Affective relationships are stressed.

The role of the primary group, particularly the family, in health care is increasingly recognized. It is to the primary group that people turn for help and support when they have health problems. Treatment and health care of individuals therefore are developing an expanded focus that includes the family.

A *secondary group* is generally larger, more impersonal, and less sentimental than a primary group. Examples are professional associations, task groups, ad hoc committees, political parties, and business groups. Members view these groups simply as means of getting things done. Interactions do not necessarily occur in face-to-face contact and do not require that the members know each other in any inclusive sense. Thus, there is little sentiment attached to such relationships. Expectations of members are formally administered through impersonal controls and external restraints imposed by designated enforcement officials. Once the goals of the group are achieved or change, the interaction is discontinued.

Groups may be also classified as formal, semiformal, or informal. The most common example of the *formal group* is the work organization. People become familiar with many different formal work groups during their lifetimes and spend a major part of their working hours in such groups. Formal groups usually exist to carry out a task or goal rather than to meet the needs of group members. Some examples of *semiformal groups* are churches, lodges, social clubs, PTAs, and some labor unions. Many of a person's social needs and ego needs are satisfied by membership in these groups.

All people, from childhood on, have membership in numerous *informal groups*. These groups provide much of a person's education and develop most cultural values. Five types of groups are representative of the numerous informal groups in existence.

1. *Friendship groups*. The first groups formed in life are friendship groups. They are often formed on the basis of common interests. Many arise out of semiformal group interactions or are formed spontaneously from work organization.

2. *Hobby groups*. Hobby groups bring together a wide variety of people from all walks of life. The differences in members' personalities and backgrounds are largely ignored in the interests of the hobby itself.

3. *Convenience groups*. Many examples of convenience groups are found both in and out of the work setting. Two examples are the car pool and the child-care group organized by mothers.

4. *Work groups*. Informal work groups can make or break an organization. Managers need to be sensitive to such groups and cultivate their cooperation and good will. Friendships often arise out of such groups between a new member and the first person who makes that member feel a welcome addition to the group.

5. *Self-protective groups*. Self-protective groups can be found anywhere but are particularly common in work organizations. They arise spontaneously out of a real or perceived threat. For example, a supervisor may approach a worker too strongly and find a group of workers organizing a united front against the threat. Such groups dissipate as soon as the threat has subsided.

Types of Health Care Groups

Much of a nurse's professional life is spent in a wide variety of groups, ranging from *dyads* (two-person groups) to large professional organizations. As a participant in a group, the nurse may be required to fulfill different roles: member or leader, teacher or learner, adviser or advisee, etc.

Common types of health care groups include task groups, teaching groups, self-help groups, self-awareness/growth groups, therapy groups, and work-related social support groups. There are similarities and differences among the characteristics of these various types of groups and the nurse's role. Task groups and work-related social groups are discussed in Chapter 20.

Teaching Groups   The major purpose of teaching groups is to impart information to the participants. Examples of teaching groups include group continuing education and client health care groups. Numerous subjects are often handled via the group teaching format: childbirth techniques, birth control methods, effective parenting, nutrition, management of chronic illness such as diabetes, exercise for middle-aged and older adults, and instructions to family members about follow-up care for discharged clients. A nurse who leads a group in which the primary purpose is to teach or learn must be skilled in the teaching-learning process discussed in Chapter 19.

Self-Help Groups   A self-help group is a small, voluntary organization composed of individuals who share a similar health, social, or daily living problem (Rollins 1987, p. 403). These groups are based on the helper-therapy principle: those who help are helped most. One of the central beliefs of the self-help movement is that persons who experience a particular social or health problem have an understanding of that condition which those without it do not.

The self-help group process can be classified as either behaviorally or cognitively oriented (Levy 1979). Behaviorally oriented processes include social reinforcement, self-control behaviors, modeling, and promoting change. Cognitively oriented processes include the provision of information and advice, demystifcation of troubling experiences, and discovering alternative perceptions of problems and methods of solutions. There are many self-help groups available for a range of problems (e.g., stillbirth, parenting, pregnant adolescents, divorce, drug abuse, cancer, menopause, mental illness, diabetes, AIDS, women's health, caregivers of elderly people, and grief). Alcoholics Anonymous was the first self-help group established. Positive aspects of self-help groups are outlined in the accompanying box.

There are three major reasons why people join self-help groups. First, individuals want to be self-reliant and as independent as possible from health and/or social

The program of a self-help group has several aspects: First, the members should gain confidence in their abilities to handle their problems. Second, a member's failure to deal with a problem should afford an opportunity for that person to learn how to deal with the failure. Third, peers, in self-help groups need to balance support with critical feedback. Peers in a self-help group are generally judgmental, critical, active, and supportive, whereas a therapist in an orthodox psychotherapy group is usually noncritical, nonjudgmental, and neutral. Fourth, peers in a self-help group serve as role models; therefore they act as reminders to the other members that "it can be done." Fifth, a self-help group helps the members assume a "wellness role" rather than a "sickness role" in which one is dependent and helpless. Finally, the emphasis in these groups is on self-control or will power. The locus of control is within, not external to, the member.

The major functions of the nurse's role in self-help groups include

1. Helping clients form such groups by identifying key people who can act as facilitators.

2. Sharing expertise with clients and helping them gain appropriate knowledge and skills.

3. Informing clients and support persons about existing self-help groups available to them. Some self-help groups are organized nationally, e.g., Alcoholics Anonymous (alcoholism), Weight Watchers (obesity), and United Ostomy Association (any ostomy). Community service organizations and social work agencies can usually provide the name of self-help groups.

4. Participating as a member of a self-help group when this is appropriate. For example, a nurse in a nursing home might participate in a self-help group of elderly clients, or a nurse could be a member of a self-help group in the larger community. The nurse's role is that of a resource person, i.e., being "on tap, but not on top."

5. Helping out in times of crisis. A self-help group may flounder after operating successfully for some time for several reasons. For example, group time may compete with other aspects of a member's social life, or people who are caregivers may not have the time or energy to take part in the activities designed to help them.

Involvement in a self-help group can supplement and complement any health worker's role. They can profit from learning of people's experiences and in turn offer

services. Second, people like to give help as well as receive it—a value is placed on the idea of mutual aid. Third, members feel that they have power through collective action.

According to Katz (1970, p. 58), self-help groups have the following characteristics.

■ They are similar to small autonomous groups and form along the lines of friendship networks.

■ They are problem-centered and organized with reference to a specific problem or problems.

■ Members of the group tend to be peers.

■ The members of the group have common goals, and the group's goals are formed by the group.

■ The action of the group is group action. According to Corbin (1983, p. 12), "this is one of the main reasons for joining a group rather than 'going it alone.' "

■ A norm of the group is helping others. Riessman (1976, p. 42) lists three reasons why people who help others obtain special benefits: (a) the helper is less dependent; (b) in struggling with another's problems that are like one's own, helpers have an opportunity to view their own problems from a distance; and (c) the helper attains a feeling of social usefulness.

■ Power and leadership are on a peer basis. Leaders evolve from the group over a period of time.

more insightful counseling to future clients and their families.

Self-Awareness/Growth Groups

The purpose of self awareness/growth groups is to develop or use interpersonal strengths. The overall aim is to improve the perception of members or to improve the functioning of the group to which they return, whether job, family, or community. From the beginning broad goals are usually apparent, e.g., to study communication patterns, group process, or problem solving. Because the focus of these groups is interpersonal concerns around current situations, the work of the group is oriented to reality testing with a here-and-now emphasis. Members are responsible for correcting inefficient patterns of relating and communicating with each other. They learn group process through participation and involvement.

The leader of self awareness/growth groups is usually referred to as a *trainer* and the members as *trainees*. To maintain effective control of interpersonal tensions, the trainer must have sufficient preparation and skill to understand and facilitate group process and experience. When the trainees learn and implement similar skills, the trainer's superior role diminishes.

Selection criteria are variable. Members may merely express a desire to become more self-aware or to address specific personality characteristics. Members may or may not be interviewed and/or requested to complete a questionnaire regarding personal data and personality characteristics before entry. Effectiveness of these groups is facilitated when an agenda and structure are defined by all members and the leader. A target date for termination is usually set in advance.

Therapy Groups

Therapy groups are clearly defined to do the work of therapy. Members work toward self-understanding, more satisfactory ways of relating or handling stress, and changing patterns of behavior toward health. The focus of the group is member-centered. Depending on the leader's orientation, past experiences may be just as relevant as current concerns.

The leader of the group, referred to as a *therapist,* differs from the members in having superior skills in a specialized area such as group psychotherapy. The therapist never truly becomes a member but may at times take on a member role. The overall role of the therapist is to establish and facilitate group interaction between the therapist and individual members and among group members.

Members of the therapy group are referred to as clients or, in some settings, as patients. They are selected by health professionals after extensive selection interviews that consider the pattern of personalities, behaviors, needs, and identification of group therapy as the treatment of choice. Duration of therapy groups is not usually set. A termination date is usually mutually determined by the therapist and members. Additional information about the nurse's role in leading, managing, and evaluating client-directed therapy groups and staff-directed work groups is presented in Chapter 20.

Characteristics of Effective Groups

To be effective, a group must meet three main criteria:

1. Accomplish its goals
2. Maintain its cohesion (degree of group unity or oneness; sense of members being "we")
3. Develop and modify its structure to improve its effectiveness.

Characteristics of an effectively functioning group are shown in Table 18–3.

Assessing Group Dynamics

During recent years the terms *group dynamics* and *group process* have frequently appeared in literature and discussions among group workers, educators, and professional organizations. *Group dynamics* (or *group process*) are forces in the group situation that determine the behavior of the group and its members. They are a way of looking at groups. Every group has its own unique dynamics and constantly changing patterns of forces, just as each individual has unique forces from within that shape the person's character. To study the dynamics of a group, several factors, in addition to group structure and organization, may be analyzed: (a) commitment, (b) leadership style, (c) decision-making methods, (d) member behaviors, (e) interaction patterns, (f) cohesiveness, and (g) power.

Commitment

The members of effective groups have a *commitment* (agreement, pledge, or obligation to do something) to the goals and output of the group. Because groups demand time and attention, members must relinquish some autonomy and self-interest. Inevitably conflicts arise between the interests of individual members and those of the group. However, many members who are committed to the group feel close to each other and willingly sacrifice their own interests for the group.

TABLE 18-3 *Comparative Features of Effective and Ineffective Groups*

Factor	Effective Groups	Ineffective Groups
Atmosphere	Informal, comfortable, and relaxed. It is a working atmosphere in which people demonstrate their interest and involvement.	Obviously tense. Signs of boredom may appear.
Goal setting	Goals, tasks, and objectives are clarified, understood, and modified so that members of the group can commit themselves to cooperatively structured goals.	Unclear, misunderstood, or imposed goals may be accepted by members. The goals are competitively structured.
Leadership and member participation	Shift from time to time, depending on the circumstances. Different members assume leadership at various times, because of their knowledge or experience.	Delegated and based on authority. The chairperson may dominate the group, or the members may defer unduly. Member participation is unequal, with high-authority members dominating. One or more functions may not be emphasized.
Communication	Open and two-way. Ideas and feelings are encouraged, both about the problem and about the group's operation.	Closed or one-way. Only the production of ideas is encouraged. Feelings are ignored or taboo. Members may be tentative or reluctant to be open and may have "hidden agendas" (personal goals at cross-purposes with group goals).
Decision making	By consensus, although various decision-making procedures appropriate to the situation may be instituted.	By the highest authority in the group, with minimal involvement by members; or an inflexible style is imposed.
Cohesion	Facilitated through high levels of inclusion, trust, liking, and support.	Either ignored or used as a means of controlling members, thus promoting rigid conformity.
Conflict tolerance	High. The reasons for disagreements or conflicts are carefully examined, and the group seeks to resolve them. The group accepts unresolvable basic disagreements and lives with them.	Low. Attempts may be made to ignore, deny, avoid, suppress, or override controversy by premature group action.
Power	Determined by the members' abilities and the information they possess. Power is shared. The issue is how to get the job done.	Determined by position in the group. Obedience to authority is strong. The issue is who controls.
Problem solving	High. Constructive criticism is frequent, frank, relatively comfortable, and oriented toward removing an obstacle to problem solving.	Low. Criticism may be destructive, taking the form of either overt or covert personal attacks. It prevents the group from getting the job done.
Self-evaluation as a group	Frequent. All members participate in evaluation and decisions about how to improve the group's functioning.	Minimal. What little evaluation there is may be done by the highest authority in the group rather than by the membership as a whole.
Creativity	Encouraged. There is room within the group for members to become self-actualized and interpersonally effective.	Discouraged. People are afraid of appearing foolish if they put forth a creative thought.

Source: H. S. Wilson and C. R. Kneisl, *Psychiatric nursing,* 3d ed. (Menlo Park, Calif.: Addison-Wesley Publishing Co., 1988), p. 276. Used by permission.

These are some indications of group commitment:

- Members feel a strong sense of belonging.
- Members enjoy each other.
- Members seek each other for counsel and support.
- Members support each other in times of difficulty.
- Members value the contributions of other members.
- Members are motivated by working in the group and want to do their tasks well.
- Members express good feelings openly and identify positive contributions.
- Members feel that the goals of the group are achievable and important.

Leadership Style   Leadership styles and characteristics of effective leaders are discussed in Chapter 20. To determine which group members carry out leadership functions, the following questions may be asked:

- Who starts the meeting or the work?
- Who contributes additional information to help the group carry out its functions?
- Who represents the group with other groups?
- Who encourages contributions from group members?
- Who provides support to members with difficult situations?
- Who clarifies thoughts expressed in discussions?
- Who keeps the discussions relevant?

Decision-Making Methods   Five methods of decision making have been identified:

1. *Individual or authority-rule decisions.* The designated leader of the group makes the decision, and group members or others involved in the decision are expected to abide by it. Authority-rule decisions may be made without discussion or consultation with the group or may be made after discussing the issue and eliciting the group's ideas and views. Decisions made without discussion are often advantageous for simple, routine matters. Those made after discussion use the resources of the group and gain the benefits of discussion. However, this type of decision making does not develop members' commitment to implement the decision, and it fails to resolve controversies among members.

2. *Minority decision.* A few group members meet to discuss an issue and make a decision that is binding for all. This method of decision making is advantageous when the whole group is unable to meet together because of time pressures. It is useful for routine decisions. Its limitations are similar to those of decision making by authority rule. Often, executive committees of large groups exercise minority control in decision making.

3. *Majority decisions.* More than half of those involved make the decision. This method is commonly used in large groups when complete member commitment is unnecessary. It is an effective method to close a discussion on issues that are not highly important for the group and when sufficient time is lacking for a decision by consensus.

4. *Consensus decisions.* Each group member expresses an opinion, and a decision is made by which members can abide, if not in whole, at least in part. This type of decision making takes a great deal of time and energy and therefore is not effective when time pressures are great or when an emergency is in progress. It is useful, however, when important and complex decisions requiring commitment from all members need to be made. This method has several advantages: (a) it produces creative, high-quality decisions, (b) it elicits commitment by all members and responsibility for implementing action, (c) it uses the resources of all members, and (d) it enhances the future decision-making ability of the group.

5. *Unanimous decisions.* Every group member agrees on the decision and can support the action to be taken. This method is commonly used for issues that are highly important to the group and require complete member commitment. Unanimous decisions are not practical for simple, routine matters or controversial issues, however.

Making sound decisions is essential to effective group functioning. Effective decisions are made when

- The group determines which decision method to adopt.
- The group listens to all members' ideas.
- Members feel satisfied with their participation.
- The expertise of group members is well used.
- The problem-solving ability of the group is facilitated.
- The group atmosphere is positive.
- Time is used well; i.e., the discussion focuses on the decision to be made.
- Members feel committed to the decision and responsible for its implementation.

Group Task Roles   The degree of input by members into goal setting, decision making, problem solving, and group evaluation is due in part to the group structure and leadership style, but members have responsibilities for group behavior and participation. Effective member task roles include the following:

- **Initiator/Contributor** Offers facts, opinions, ideas, suggestions, and relevant information to facilitate group discussion.

- **Information Giver** Offers relevant information based on personal knowledge or experience.

- **Information Receiver** Asks for facts, information, opinions, ideas, and feelings from other members to facilitate group discussion.

- **Opinion Giver** Offers opinions, judgments, or feelings about suggestions.

- **Opinion Receiver** Asks for opinions, judgments, or feelings about suggestions.

- **Summarizer** Restates and summarizes the major points discussed.

- **Energizer** Stimulates a higher quality of work from the group.

- **Elaborator/Evaluator** Examines the practicality and workability of ideas; evaluates alternative solutions and applies them to real situations to see how they will work.

- **Gatekeeper** Encourages everyone to participate, gives recognition for contributions, demonstrates acceptance and openness to the ideas of others.

- **Linker** Enables members to analyze their differences of opinion constructively, searches for common elements in conflicts, and tries to reconcile disagreements.

- **Diagnoser** Identifies sources of difficulties the group has in working effectively and identifies blocks to goal accomplishment progress.

- **Active Listener** Listens and serves as an interested audience for other members.

- **Clarifier** Ensures that each group member understands what other members are saying.

- **Tension Reliever** Eases tensions and increases the enjoyment of group members by joking, suggesting breaks, and proposing fun approaches to group work.

- **Recorder** Keeps notes of ideas, suggestions, or decisions made by the group. May construct sociogram of group interaction.

Other member behaviors may satisfy members' individual needs and can block the effectiveness of the group in achieving its goal. Such behaviors include:

- **Dominator** Attempts to assume group leadership, interrupts others, gives directions, and wants his or her own way.

- **Blocker** Is generally negative, resistant, and disagreeable. Obstructs group progress by reintroducing issues already resolved.

- **Playboy** Does not take the group task seriously; jokes, plays around and makes silly, inappropriate comments.

- **Aggressor** Is overly assertive; attacks and criticizes group members.

- **Monopolizer** Talks continually to the extent that other members do not have an opportunity to speak.

Interaction Patterns   Interaction patterns can be observed and ascertained by a *sociogram,* a diagram of the flow of verbal communication within a group during a specified period, e.g., 5 or 15 minutes. This diagram indicates who speaks to whom and who initiates the remarks. Ideally, the interaction patterns of a small group would indicate verbal interaction from all members of the group to all members of the group. See Figure 18–2. In reality, however, such an interaction pattern does not occur. See Figure 18–3. This second diagram illustrates that not all communication is a two-way process. The lines with arrowheads at each end indicate that the statement made by one person was responded to by the recipient; a short cross-line drawn near one of the arrowheads indicates who initiated the remark. One-way communication is indicated by lines with an arrowhead at only one end. Remarks made to the group as a whole are indicated by arrows drawn to only the middle of the circle. By using a sociogram, nurses can analyze strengths and weaknesses in a group's interaction patterns. Used in conjunction with member behavior tools, this can offer considerable data about the group's dynamics.

Cohesiveness   Cohesive groups (those that cohere or "hang together") possess a certain group spirit, a sense of being "we," and a common purpose. Groups lacking in cohesiveness are unstable and prone to disintegration. Membership attitudes and behaviors and group properties that characterize high-cohesion groups include the following (Kneisl 1988, p. 284):

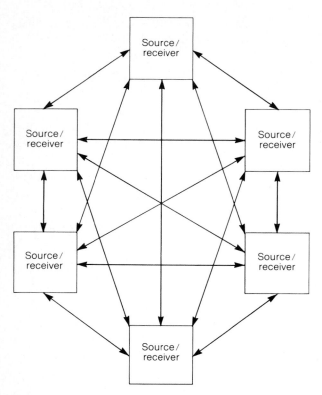

Figure 18-2 An ideal small-group interaction pattern. All members interact with all other members.

- Members like one another, are friendly, and enjoy interacting with one another.
- Members receive support on issues from one another.
- Members praise one another for accomplishments.
- Members share similar opinions and attitudes.
- Members are likely to influence one another and are willing to be influenced by other members.
- Members accept assigned tasks and roles readily and value group goals.
- Members trust one another.
- Members are loyal to group and defend it against external criticism and attack.
- Attendance, risk taking, participation, and communication are high.
- "We" is frequently heard in discussions, and group output and productivity are high.
- Leadership is democratic.
- Satisfaction with members and work of group is high.

Power   Power can be viewed as a vital, positive force that moves people toward the attainment of individual or group goals. It is impossible to interact with others without influencing and being influenced by them; hence, group members are constantly adjusting to one another and modifying their behavior. The various types and sources of power are detailed in Chapter 12.

The unequal distribution of power within a group (i.e., a group in which certain members have much power and others have little) can adversely affect the task and maintenance functions of the group. Members who believe they have little influence in the group are less likely to feel committed to group goals and to participate in decision making. Dissatisfaction with the group decreases its attractiveness and reduces its cohesion.

High-power people often are the most popular or have the most authority. However, neither circumstance is appropriate for high-quality decision making. High-quality decisions are the result of power based on expertise, competence, and relevant information, not on popularity or authority. To ensure rational and humane decision making and to avoid unquestioning obedience

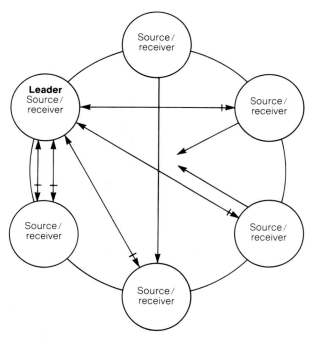

Figure 18-3 A sociogram indicating the flow of verbal communication within a group during a specific period. Note that five questions or comments calling for a response were directed at the leader.

to authority, group members need to assess and critique suggestions from the authority person.

Group Self-Evaluation

Groups need to set up mechanisms for feedback of information to the members about their method of operation. Only when a group acquires information about itself can it make adjustments to improve its efficiency. Several mechanisms can be set up for group feedback and self-evaluation: use of a group-productivity observer, use of a group self-evaluation guide, general open discussion initiated by the group leader prior to the end of the meeting, or combinations of these.

Some groups establish a rotating position for a group-productivity observer, just as positions are established for a recorder; others acquire the assistance of an outsider specially trained in this area. The responsibility of this person is to observe the group during its discussions, rather than participate, and to provide feedback to the group about perceptions of the group's behavior. The observer notes the general atmosphere of the group, leadership techniques, orientation of the group, participation by members, and any factor considered to affect the productivity of the group.

The provision of feedback requires skill by the observer in presenting comments. It is helpful to present objective data first and then phrase comments in the form of tentative hypotheses, alternative solutions, or expressions of the observer's feelings. This allows group members the chance to reject a comment if they are not ready to handle it. The observer can be viewed as "in error." For example, the observer might comment:

Objective data: During the time we were trying to suggest solutions to problems, two of us seemed impatient to tear a new idea apart. Out of five suggestions made, four were immediately criticized. Right after that, suggestions for solutions lagged.

Alternative solution: I was wondering at the time whether more and better ideas might have emerged if we had withheld our critical comments until after most of the ideas about solutions were on the blackboard.

Open discussion needs to follow such comments.

CHAPTER HIGHLIGHTS

▸ The effective nurse-client relationship is a growth-facilitating process.

▸ Four phases of the helping relationship include the preinteraction phase, the introductory phase, the working phase, and the termination phase; each has a specific purpose or goal and requires specific skills of the nurse.

▸ Communication incorporates exchanging information between two or more people and is a basic component of human relationships and nurse-client relationships.

▸ Communication is usually categorized as verbal or nonverbal.

▸ Verbal communication is effective when the criteria of simplicity, clarity, timing, relevance, adaptability, and credibility are met.

▸ Nonverbal communication often reveals more about a person's thoughts and feelings than verbal communication; it includes physical appearance, posture and gait, facial expressions, hand movements, and other gestures.

▸ When assessing nonverbal behaviors, the nurse needs to consider cultural influences and be aware that a variety of feelings can be expressed by a single nonverbal expression.

▸ When communication is effective, verbal and nonverbal expressions are congruent.

▸ Communication is a two-way process involving the sender of the message and the receiver of the message.

▸ Because the sender must encode the message and determine the appropriate channels for conveying it, and because the receiver must perceive the message, decode it, and then respond, the communication process includes four elements: sender, message, receiver, and feedback.

▸ Many factors influence the communication process: the ability of the communicator, perceptions, personal space (intimate, personal, social, and public distance), territoriality, roles and relationships, purposes, time and setting, attitudes, emotions, and self-esteem.

▶ There are three broad areas for assessing communication: language development, nonverbal behavior, and style of communication.

▶ Many techniques facilitate therapeutic communication: attentive listening; paraphrasing; clarifying; using open-ended questions and statements; focusing; being specific; using touch and silence; clarifying reality, time, or sequence; providing general leads; and summarizing.

▶ Techniques that inhibit communication include offering unvalidated reassurance, stating approval or disapproval, giving common (not expert) advice, stereotyping, and being defensive.

▶ Process recordings are frequently made by nurses to evaluate their own communication. With them, nurses can analyze both the process and the content of the communication.

▶ Most people's lives are spent interacting with other human beings in groups. A person's sense of being evolves through membership in groups that help achieve goals they set for themselves.

▶ Groups can be classified as primary or secondary, according to their structure or according to their type of interaction. In small, primary groups, relationships are spontaneous, personal, and sentimental. In larger, secondary groups, relationships are impersonal and less sentimental.

▶ Effective groups produce outstanding results, succeed in spite of difficulties, and have members who feel responsible for the output of the group. They accomplish their goals, maintain cohesion, and develop and modify their structure in ways that improve effectiveness.

▶ Regardless of setting or composition, several forces shape and modify the structure and functioning of groups. They include member commitment, leadership styles and roles, methods of decision making, member behaviors, interaction patterns, cohesiveness, and power and influence.

▶ Sound decision making that leads to well-conceived, well-understood, and well-accepted realistic actions toward the goals agreed on by the group is the hallmark of a group that functions effectively.

▶ Groups make decisions by consensus, selection of a group of experts, averaging members' opinions, majority vote, minority control, authority rule after discussion, and authority rule without discussion. Each method is appropriate at certain times.

▶ Power and influence in groups operate constantly and force members to adjust to one another and modify their behavior.

▶ Group self-evaluation is essential to improving the efficiency of a group.

▶ Nurses interact with groups of clients and colleagues in a wide variety of settings. To use groups rationally and effectively, nurses must understand the forces that underlie small group interactional processes and recognize their own patterns of participation.

LEARNING ACTIVITIES

■ With permission from your client, conduct a process recording on a nurse/client interaction. Using the criteria listed on page 344, analyze the interaction. How would you rate the effectiveness of the interaction?

■ With permission from a nursing colleague, conduct a process recording on a nurse/nurse interaction. Modifying the 7 criteria on page 344 to analyze a nurse/nurse interaction, evaluate the interaction with your nursing colleague. How would you rate the effectiveness of the interaction?

■ Using the following group self-evaluation guide, evaluate a nursing group activity; e.g., a change of shift report or a staff meeting. What are your findings? How effective is your group interaction?

A. Group direction and orientation
    1. How much was achieved?
    2. How clear are goals and purposes?
    3. How clear is procedure to achieve goals?
    4. Was sufficient relevant information available?
B. Group motivation and unity
    5. What degree of interest is there in task?
    6. Was interest maintained throughout?
    7. Is group united in purpose?
C. Group atmosphere
    8. Formal?
    9. Informal?
   10. Permissive?
   11. Inhibited?
   12. Cooperative?
   13. Competitive?
   14. Friendly?
   15. Hostile?

D. Member contributions
   16. What is degree of participation by members?
   17. Were contributions relevant, factual, and problem-centered?
   18. Were members listening to what others said?
   19. How did special members serve group?
     a. Leader
     b. Recorder
     c. Resource person
     d. Others
   20. How did majority of members feel about meeting?
     a. Poor
     b. Mediocre
     c. Okay
     d. Good
     e. Excellent

READINGS AND REFERENCES

SUGGESTED READINGS

Peplau, H. E. July 1960. Talking with patients. *American Journal of Nursing* 60:964–66.
    This classic article differentiates nursing communication with a client from that of a layperson. In this article, Peplau offers the beginning nursing student helpful suggestions for meaningful communication with clients.

Scott, A. L. August 1988. Human interaction and personal boundaries. *Journal of Psychosocial Nursing and Mental Health Services* 26:23–27.
    Scott discusses the different meanings of *boundaries* and their major characteristics. The behaviors of people with open and closed boundaries are listed in a table. The development of an individual's boundaries is reviewed and the assessment of a client's boundaries discussed.

RELATED RESEARCH

Appleby, F. M. March 1987. Professional support and the role of support groups. *Health Visitor* 60:77–78.

Banning, M. R. August 1987. The effects of activity-elicited humor and group structure on group cohesion and affective responses. *American Journal of Occupational Therapy* 41:510–14.

Chapman, G. E. March 1988. Reporting therapeutic discourse in a therapeutic community. *Journal of Advanced Nursing* 13:255–64.

Edwards, E. M. J. September 1988. Group dynamics in psychotherapy. *Canadian Nurse* 84:59.

Trojan, A. 1989. Benefits of self-help groups: A survey of 232 members from 65 disease-related groups. *Social Science and Medicine* 29(2):225–32.

SELECTED REFERENCES

Brammer, L. M. 1988. *The helping relationship: Process and skills.* 4th ed. Englewood Cliffs, N.J.: Prentice-Hall.

Carpenito, L. J. 1989. *Nursing diagnosis. Application to clinical practice.* 3d ed. Philadelphia: J. B. Lippincott Co.

Consider this . . . Social support groups. February 1988. *Journal of Nursing Administration* 18:3.

Corbin, D. E. May/June 1983. Self-help groups: What the health educator should know. *Health Values* 7:10–14.

Davis, A. J. 1984. *Listening and responding.* St. Louis: C. V. Mosby Co.

Dreher, B. B. 1987. *Communication skills for working with elders.* New York: Springer Publishing Co.

Egan, G. 1975. *The skilled helper: A model for systematic helping and interpersonal relating.* Monterey, Calif.: Brooks/Cole Publishing. Co.

———. 1982. *The skilled helper: Model, skills, and methods for effective helping.* 2d ed. Monterey, Calif.: Brooks/Cole Publishing Co.

Gilbey, V. J. April 1987. Self-help. *Canadian Nurse* 83:23, 25.

Hall, E. T. 1969. *The hidden dimension*. Garden City, N.Y.: Doubleday and Co.

Hardin, S. B., and Halaris, A. L. January 1983. Nonverbal communication of patients and high- and low-empathy nurses. *Journal of Psychosocial Nursing and Mental Health Services* 21:15–20.

Harrison, T. M., Pistolessi, T. V., Stephen, T. M. February 1989. Assessing nurses' communication: A cross-sectional study. *Western Journal of Nursing Research* 11:75–91.

Kasch, C. R. 1984. Interpersonal competence and communication in the delivery of nursing care. *Advances in Nursing Science* 6(2):71–88.

Katz, A. H. January 1970. Self-help organizations and volunteer participation in social welfare. *Social Work* 15:57–60.

Kaul, T., and Schmidt, L. 1971. Dimensions of interviewer trustworthiness. *Journal of Counselling Psychology* 34:134–39.

King, I. M. 1981. *A theory for nursing. Systems, concepts, process.* New York: John Wiley and Sons.

Kneisl, C. R. 1988. Group process. In Wilson, H. S. and Kneisl, C. R. pp. 270–289. *Psychiatric nursing*. 3d ed. Menlo Park, Calif: Addison-Wesley Publishing Co.

Levy, L. 1979. Processes and activities in groups. In Lieberman, M. A., and Borman, L. D., and Associates, editors. pp. 244–257. *Self-help groups for coping with crisis: Origins, members, process, and impact.* San Francisco: Jossey-Bass.

Morgan, B. S., and Barden, M. E. September 1985. Nurse-patient interaction in the home setting. *Public Health Nursing* 2:159–67.

Northhouse, P. G., and Northhouse, L. L. 1985. *Health education. A handbook for health professionals.* Englewood Cliffs, N.J.: Prentice-Hall.

Orr, J. August 1987. In our own hands . . . self-help groups are a growing concern. *Nursing Times* 83:26–28.

Raudsepp, E. April 1990. Seven ways to cure communication breakdowns. *Nursing 90* 20:132, 134, 137–38.

Richman, J. M. February 1988. Social support groups. *Journal of Nursing Administration* 18:3, 19.

Riessman, F. 1976. How does self-help work? *Social Policy* 7:41–45.

Rollins, J. A. November/December 1987. Self-help groups for parents. *Pediatric Nursing* 13:403–9.

Ruesch, J. 1961. Therapeutic Communication. New York: W. W. Norton and Co.

Shanken, J., and Shanken, P. February 1976. How to be a helping person. *Journal of Psychiatric Nursing and Mental Health Services* 14:24–28.

Stewart, C. J., and Cash, W. B. 1988. *Interviewing principles and practices.* 5th ed. Dubuque, Iowa: Wm. C. Brown Publishers.

Sundeen, S. J.; Stuart, G. W.; Rankin, E. A. D.; and Cohen, S. A. 1989. *Nurse-client interaction.* 4th ed. St. Louis: C. V. Mosby Co.

Thomas, M. 1970. Trust in the nurse-patient relationship. In Carlson, Carolyn E. editor. *Behavioral concepts and nursing intervention.* Philadelphia: J. B. Lippincott Co.

Wilkinson, R. April 1986. Communication: Learning from the market. *Nursing Management* 17:42J, 42L.

Wilson, M. 1985. *Group theory/process for nursing practice.* Bowie, Md.: Brady Communications Co.

Teaching and Learning

CONTENTS

FACILITATING LEARNING

Education incorporates two processes: teaching and learning. However, these processes are not interdependent. Teaching can occur without any learning taking place, and learning can occur in the absence of teaching. Client education is a major aspect of nursing practice and an important independent nursing function. In 1972, the American Hospital Association passed the Patients' Bill of Rights mandating client education as a right of all clients. In addition, legislation relating to nursing frequently has included client teaching as a function of nursing, thereby making teaching a legal and professional responsibility (Phillips and Heckelman 1983, pp. 42–46).

Client education is multifaceted, involving promoting, protecting, and maintaining health. It involves teaching about reducing health risk factors, increasing a person's level of wellness, and providing information about specific protective health measures.

Clients have a variety of learning needs. A *learning need* is a need to change behavior or "a gap between the information an individual knows and the information necessary to perform a function or care for self" (Gessner 1989, p. 593). *Learning* is a change in human disposition or capability that persists over a period of time and that cannot be solely accounted for by growth. Learning is represented by a change in behavior. An important aspect of learning is the individual's desire to learn and to act on the learning. This is referred to as *compliance*. Compliance is best illustrated when the person recognizes and accepts the need to learn, willingly expends the energy required to learn, and then follows through with the appropriate behaviors that reflect the learning. For example, a man diagnosed as having diabetes willingly learns about the special diet he needs, and then plans and follows the learned diet. Implicit in the definition of learning is *change*. See Chapter 12.

Theories of Learning

Theories of learning have been developed to explain how and why people learn. Three main theoretical areas are behaviorism, cognitivism, and humanism.

Behaviorism was originally advanced by Edward Thorndike, who believed that transfer of knowledge could occur if the new situation closely resembled the old situation. To Thorndike, the term *understanding* was used in the context of building connections. One of his major contributions applicable to client teaching is that learning should be based on the learner's behavior.

Cognitivism depicts learning as a complex cognitive activity. Kurt Lewin's field theory, i.e., theories of motivation and perception, were considered precursors of the more recent cognitive theories. Lewin believed that learning involved four different types of changes: change in cognitive structure, change in motivation, change in one's sense of belonging to the group, and gain in voluntary muscle control.

Humanism or humanistic theories of learning assume that there is a natural tendency for people to learn and that learning flourishes in an encouraging environment. Implementing humanistic theory involves providing options for the client and the resources and equipment for learning.

More recently, in the 1970s and 1980s, theories of adult learning have been increasingly applied in client teaching. Malcolm Knowles coined the term *andragogy*.

Andragogy is "the art and science of helping adults learn" (Knowles 1980, p. 43) in contrast to *pedagogy,* the discipline concerned with helping children learn. Nurses can use the following andragogic concepts about learners as a guide for client teaching (Knowles 1984):

- As people mature, they move from dependence to independence.
- An adult's previous experiences can be used as a resource for learning.

- An adult's readiness to learn is often related to a developmental task or social role.
- An adult is more oriented to learning when the material is immediately useful, not useful sometime in the future.

PRINCIPLES OF LEARNING

Learning involves the entire person and can affect the person's life-style, methods of handling problems, attitudes, and knowledge. Learning requires energy and the ability to concentrate. To be effective client teachers, nurses must understand those factors that facilitate learning and those that inhibit it.

Factors Facilitating Learning

Motivation to learn is the desire to learn. It is a term that describes forces acting on or from within the person to initiate, direct, and maintain behavior and to explain differences in the intensity and direction of behavior (Redman 1988, p. 21). Such motivation is generally greatest when a person recognizes a need and believes the need will be met through learning. It is not enough for the need to be identified and verbalized by the nurse; it must be experienced by the client. Often the nurse's task is to help the client personally work through the problem and identify the need. Sometimes clients or families need help identifying relevant situational elements before they can see a need. For instance, clients with heart disease may need to know the effects of smoking and being overweight before they recognize the need to stop smoking or adopt a weight-reduction diet. Or adolescents may need to know the consequences of an untreated sexually transmitted disease before they see the need for treatment.

Readiness to learn is the behavior that reflects motivation at a specific time. Readiness sometimes comes with time, and the nurse's role is often to encourage its development (Redman 1988, p. 36).

Active involvement in the learning process makes learning more meaningful. For example, if the learner actively participates in planning and discussion, learning is faster and retention is better. Passive learning, such as listening to a lecture or watching a film, does not foster optimal learning.

Once learners have succeeded in accomplishing a task or understanding a concept, they gain self-confidence in their ability to learn. This reduces their anxiety about failure and can motivate greater learning. Successful learners have increased confidence with which to accept failure. People learn best when they believe they are accepted and will not be judged. The person who expects to be judged as a "poor" or "good" client will not learn as well as the person who feels no such threat.

Feedback is information relating a person's performance to a desired goal. It has to be meaningful to the learner. Feedback that accompanies practice of psychomotor skills helps the person to learn those skills. Support or desired behavior through praise, positively worded corrections, and suggestions of alternative methods are ways of providing positive feedback. Negative feedback such as ridicule, anger, or sarcasm can lead people to withdraw from learning. Such feedback, viewed as a type of punishment, may cause the client to avoid the teacher in order to avoid punishment.

Learning is facilitated by material that is logically organized and proceeds from the *simple to the complex*. Such organization enables the learner to comprehend new information, assimilate it with previous learning, and form new understandings. Of course, simple and complex are relative terms, depending on the level at which the person is learning. What is simple for one person may be complex for another.

Repetition of key concepts and facts facilitates retention of newly learned material. Practice of psychomotor skills improves performance of those skills and facilitates their transfer to another setting. When a person appreciates the relevance of specific material, learning is facilitated. For example, the man who understands the relevance to his health of a special diet is often better able to learn about the diet than a person who sees no such connection.

People retain information and psychomotor skills best when the *time between learning and use is short*; the longer the time interval, the more is forgotten. For example, a woman who is taught how to administer her own insulin but is not permitted to do so until discharge from hospital is unlikely to remember much of what she learned. However, if she is encouraged to give her own injections while in hospital, her learning will be enhanced.

An *optimal learning environment* has adequate lighting that is free from glare, a comfortable room temperature, and good ventilation. A hot, stuffy room can cause drowsiness that interferes with concentration. Noise is distracting and may interfere with listening and thinking. For the best learning in a hospital setting, nurses should choose a time when there are no visitors present and interruptions are unlikely. Privacy is essential for some learning. For example; when a client is learning to irrigate a colostomy, the presence of others can be embarrassing and thus interfere with learning.

Factors Inhibiting Learning   A greatly *elevated anxiety* level can impede learning. Clients or families who are very worried may not hear spoken words or may retain only part of the communication. Extreme anxiety might be reduced by medications or by information that relieves uncertainty. By contrast, clients who appear disinterested and unconcerned may need to be told about potential problems, to increase their anxiety slightly and enhance their motivation to learn.

Learning can be inhibited by *physiologic events* such as a critical illness, pain, or impaired hearing. Because the client cannot concentrate and apply energy to learning, the learning itself is impaired. There are also *cultural barriers* to learning, such as language or values. Obviously the client who does not understand the nurse's language will learn little. Another impediment to learning is differing values held by the client and the health team. For example, a client who does not value being thin may have difficulty learning about a reducing diet.

Domains of Learning   Bloom (1956) has identified three domains, or areas of learning: cognitive, affective, and psychomotor. The *cognitive domain* includes intellectual skills such as thinking, knowing, and understanding. The *affective domain* includes feelings, emotions, interests, attitudes, and appreciations. The *psychomotor domain* includes motor skills such as giving an injection. Nurses should include each of these three domains in client teaching plans. For example, teaching a client how to irrigate a colostomy is the psychomotor domain. An important part of such a teaching plan is to teach the client why a specific amount of fluid is used and when the irrigation should be carried out; this is the cognitive domain. Helping the client accept the colostomy and maintain self-esteem is in the affective domain.

TEACHING

Teaching is a system of activities intended to produce learning. The teaching process is intentionally designed to produce specific learning. Teaching is considered one of the functions of nursing. In some states in the United States teaching is included in the legal definition of nursing, making it a required function under the law.

The teaching/learning process involves dynamic interaction between teacher and learner. Each participant

TABLE 19-1 *Comparison of the Teaching Process and the Nursing Process*

Step	Teaching Process	Nursing Process
1	Collect data; analyze client's learning strengths and deficits.	Collect data; analyze client's strengths and deficits.
2	Make educational diagnoses.	Making nursing diagnoses.
3	Prepare teaching plan.	Plan nursing intervention.
4	Implement teaching plan.	Implement nursing strategies.
5	Evaluate client learning (effectiveness of teaching plan)	Evaluate effectiveness of nursing interventions.

in the process communicates information, emotions, perceptions, and attitudes to the other. The teaching process and the nursing process are very much alike. See Table 19–1.

Teaching also involves a type of communication for which there are specific goals. For example, clients who need to administer their own eye drops or to change an incision dressing share these goals with the nurse. Another aspect of teaching is the relationship between the teacher and the learner. It is essentially one of trust and respect. The learner trusts that the teacher has the knowledge and skill to teach, and the teacher respects the learner's ability to attain the recognized goals. Once a nurse starts to instruct a client and/or support persons, it is important that the teaching process continue until the participants reach the goals, change the goals, or decide that the goals will not help meet the learning objectives.

The following five *principles of teaching* may be helpful to nursing students:

1. Teaching activities should help the learner meet individual learning objectives. These objectives should be mutually determined. If certain activities do not assist the learner, these need to be reassessed; perhaps other activities can replace them.

2. Rapport between teacher and learner is essential. A relationship that is both accepting and constructive will best assist learning.

3. The teacher who can use the client's previous learning in the present situation encourages the client and facilitates the learning of new skills.

4. A teacher must be able to communicate clearly and concisely. The words the teacher uses need to have the same meaning to the learner as to the teacher.

5. The teaching activities need to be oriented around the learning objectives. Thus information and skills not related to the learner's objectives need to be eliminated from the teaching process. If they remain, they may confuse the learner or be a distraction from effective learning.

ASSESSING

Assessing for teaching essentially has two foci: the identification of the client's learning needs and the assessment of relevant data about the client.

Identifying Client Learning Needs

Smitherman (1981, pp. 125–28) describes three sources for identifying learning needs.

1. *The client.* Clients' learning needs may be identified by the clients themselves. A client aware of a learning need may ask pertinent questions or seek out the needed information in some other way.

2. *The client's behavior.* Learning needs are not always easily detected; frequently, consultation with the client is necessary to confirm or deny the existence of these needs. For example, a client who appears angry may be insecure or worried because the client does not understand what is happening; only after the discussion with the client can the nurse be sure that the client has a need for information.

3. *Health care professionals.* Anticipatory learning needs related to the client's health problem often are known by health professionals. For example, a client anticipating surgery will probably need to learn about deep breathing and leg exercises. Or a client receiving oxygen who is being discharged from hospital will need to know how to operate the oxygen equipment and the appropriate safety measures to employ while at home.

Relevant Client Data

Particular client data that need to be collected and examined include client readiness, client motivation, and personal characteristics such as socioeconomic factors, age, and health beliefs and practices.

Readiness   Clients who are ready to learn often behave differently from those who are not. A client who is ready may search out information, for instance, by asking questions, reading books or articles, talking to others, and generally showing interest. The person unready to learn is more likely to avoid the subject or situation and hope or believe that someone else will take care of the problem (Smitherman 1981, pp. 126–27). In addition, the unready client may change the subject when it is brought up by the nurse. For example, the nurse might say, "I was wondering about a good time to show you how to change your dressing," and the client responds, "What did you think of the ball game last night?" Furthermore, somatic symptoms (such as headaches, upset stomach, or gas pains experienced by clients having surgery) may make it difficult for clients to pay attention (Laird 1975, p. 1340).

Tyson (1984) points out that in assessing readiness there are two major factors: emotional and experiential. Emotional factors affecting readiness include anxiety. If the anxiety level of the client is high, perceptions are narrowed and thus interfere with learning. Experiential factors include occupational status, client capabilities, and educational level. In health, physical readiness is also important to consider. Clients may be too ill or weak to attend to learning.

Nurses can sometimes facilitate a client's readiness by tactfully calling attention to a learning need (for example, "Have you thought about learning to change your dressing?"). Two other ways to facilitate readiness are by giving the client information to read and by pointing out an opportunity to learn (for instance, "There is a baby bath demonstration at 3 P.M. today in the next room").

Motivation   As discussed earlier, motivation relates to whether the client wants to learn and is usually greatest when the client is ready, the learning need is recognized, and the content is meaningful to the client (Smitherman 1981, p. 127).

Assessment of motivation to learn is often part of a general health assessment or of a more specific problem assessment. A nurse assessing motivation and a client's present abilities must have a full understanding of the subject to be learned. For example, a man who has had

RESEARCH NOTE

Can Clients Understand Our Instructions?

Streiff conducted a study to determine whether or not clients in an ambulatory care setting read at a level that allowed them to comprehend the materials available for client education. This descriptive study consisted of two parts. First, 106 adults waiting for appointments were interviewed and their reported and actual reading levels were compared. Reported levels of reading skill indicated by the last grade completed in school were significantly higher than their actual reading levels, indicated by scores achieved on the Wide Range Achievement Test (WRAT). Second, the readability levels of 28 written materials available for client education were evaluated.

Findings indicated (a) that the mean readability level for the instructional texts examined was 11.2 grades and (b) that the majority of study participants (54.7%) read at levels that did not allow them to comprehend any of the client education materials available at their site of primary care. In addition, 25 percent of the texts examined were beyond the comprehension of *all* participants.

Implications: The significant differences between actual and reported reading levels indicates that reported reading levels cannot be accepted as valid and that the WRAT could be used more widely in health care settings to assess the level at which clients read. In addition, health care providers can encourage those who prepare and distribute client education materials to write them at lower readability levels so that they are usable by a greater number of clients.

L. D. Streiff. Can clients understand our instructions? *Image: Journal of Nursing Scholarship* Summer 1986. 18:48–52.

diabetes for several years may already understand how to test his urine for sugar, but he may not know how to administer insulin hypodermically because he has always taken a medication by mouth.

Increasingly, tools are being developed to measure motivation to learn; for example, focus groups may be formed to help identify trends and knowledge held by a selected group of consumers. Another example is a questionnaire given to clients to elicit information about perceptions and expectations related to their illness.

Nurses can positively influence a client's motivation in three ways:

1. By relating the learning to something the client values and helping the client see the relevance of the learning
2. By helping the client to make the learning situation pleasant
3. By encouraging self-direction

To influence the externally motivated learner a nurse can use *positive reinforcement,* which involves rewarding the learner for achievements, e.g., giving praise, or reading a bedtime story to a child. Reinforcement is most effective when given immediately after the desired response. *Negative reinforcement,* or punishment for undesirable responses, is considered less motivating than positive reinforcement. However, negative reinforcement can be motivating if it is accompanied by encouragement and an explanation of how to correct the response (for instance: "I agree that looks right, but if you place the tube like this the urine should flow more readily").

Socioeconomic Factors   Many cultural groups have their own beliefs and practices, a number of them related to diet, health, illness, and life-style. It is therefore important to know how the practices and values held by client's impinge on their learning needs. Although a nurse may be inclined to assume that because a client belongs to a specific ethnic or cultural group the client will follow the norms of the group, this is not always the case. Thus, nurses should avoid stereotyping and should determine the relevant beliefs and values of each client. For example, although the diet of some Jews excludes pork, other Jews have no objection to eating pork.

Folk beliefs of certain groups in North America, e.g., low-income Hispanics, may also affect learning. Although the client may readily understand the health care information being taught, this learning may not be implemented in the home, where folk medical practices prevail. See Chapter 24 for additional information.

Economic factors can also affect a client's learning. For example, a client who cannot afford to obtain a new sterile syringe for each injection of insulin may find it difficult to learn to administer the insulin when the nurse teaches that a new syringe should be used each time.

Learning Style   Considerable research has been done on people's learning styles. It has been suggested

that in terms of perception, people can be classified as either sensing types or intuitive types. Sensing people use their senses to perceive data, whereas intuitive people use their perception of meanings, relationships, and possibilities by way of insight to perceive data (Lawrence 1982, p. 7). For example, a sensing person will likely gather data by using sight or hearing when meeting another person, whereas an intuitive person will more likely be aware of meanings and relationships in the same situation.

In terms of judgement processes, people may be classified as thinking or feeling persons. A thinking person uses logical decision making to arrive at a conclusion, whereas a feeling person is more likely to arrive at conclusions using subjective personal values. Attitudes in the latter group tend to result from a preference for feeling; these people find interpersonal skills more interesting than technical skills (Lawrence 1982, p. 8). A nurse will best stress logic and knowledge when teaching a thinking person but should stress interpersonal skills when teaching a feeling person.

Age   Age provides information on the person's developmental status. Simple questions to school-age children and adolescents will elicit information on what they know. Observing children in play provides information about their motor and intellectual development as well as relationships with other children. For the elderly person, conversation and questioning may reveal slow recall or limited psychomotor skills and learning difficulties. For additional information, see "Special Teaching Strategies" later in this chapter.

Health Beliefs and Practices   A client's health beliefs and practices are important to consider in any teaching plan. The health belief model described in Chapter 13 provides a predictor of preventive health behavior. However, even if a nurse is convinced that a client's health beliefs should be changed, doing so may not be possible because so many factors are involved in a person's health beliefs.

Education   Clients' education will probably influence their present knowledge as well as the teaching method that is most effective. Although some research indicates that education does not always affect learning, the client's ability to read or write does affect the teaching style.

DIAGNOSING

Nursing diagnoses pertinent to a client's learning needs are all grouped under the diagnostic category of **Knowledge deficit.** It is extremely important that the nurse specify which exact deficits individual clients manifest. Examples include the following:

- **Knowledge deficit: low-calorie diet** related to newly ordered therapy
- **Knowledge deficit: diabetic diet** related to prescribed treatment
- **Knowledge deficit: preoperative care** related to impending surgical procedure
- **Knowledge deficit: medications** related to language differences
- **Knowledge deficit: home safety hazards** related to denial of declining health
- **Knowledge deficit: substance abuse** related to lack of motivation to acquire information

PLANNING

Developing a teaching plan is accomplished in a series of steps. Involving the client at this time promotes the formation of a meaningful plan and stimulates client motivation. The client who participates in the formulation of the teaching plan is more likely to achieve the desired outcomes.

Determining Teaching Priorities

The client's learning needs must be ranked according to priority. The client and the nurse should do this together, with the client's priorities always being considered. Once a client's priorities have been addressed, the client is generally more motivated to concentrate on other identified learning needs. Nurses can also use theoretical frameworks to establish priorities, such as Maslow's hierarchy of needs. See Chapter 4.

Setting Learning Objectives

The terms *goals* and *objectives* are used interchangeably by some educators and distinguished by others. Used interchangeably, they can be considered as both immedi-

ate and long-term aims to be accomplished in a learning situation. However, goal is often the more general term, describing a general, long-range intended outcome of learning, whereas objective is used to mean a specific immediate, short-range intended measurable outcome of a learning situation.

The setting of goals and objectives is done by the client (or support persons) and the nurse. Objectives relate to immediate client needs, such as perineal care after birth of a baby. Goals relate to long-term needs, such as an obese new mother's need to lose weight (in which case the goal may be a specific weight loss through diet and exercise).

The objectives for learning should be both specific and observable in terms of behavior. A specific objective might be "to take 60 mg furosemide (Lasix) upon identifying ankle edema." An objective needs to be stated in terms of client behavior, not nurse behavior: for example, "Will write his own diets as instructed" (client behavior), not "To teach the client about his diet" (nurse behavior). See Table 19–2 for a list of behavioral (observable) verbs and nonbehavioral verbs.

Objectives should contain three types of information: performance, conditions, and criteria (Mager 1975, p. 21) *Performance,* or behavior, describes what the learner will be able to do after mastering the objective. The objective must reflect an observable activity. The performance may be visible, e.g., walking, or invisible, e.g., adding a column of figures. However, it is necessary to be able to deduce whether an unobservable activity has been mastered from some performance that represents the activity. Therefore, the performance of an objective might be written: "Writes the total for a column of figures in the indicated space" (observable), not "Adds a column of figures" (unobservable).

TABLE 19–2 *Selected Verbs for Objectives*

Behavioral Verbs	Nonbehavioral Verbs
Defines	Knows
Identifies	Understands
Chooses	Appreciates
Demonstrates	Feels
Differentiates	
Applies	
Compares	

In some instances it is necessary to state the *conditions* under which a performance is to be carried out so that the objective is clear. For example, "Walks to the end of the hall and back without crutches" describes a performance clearly; "without crutches" is a condition of the objective. Nurses always need to determine the conditions in which an activity will be carried out. Then the objectives for the learning plan can reflect those conditions. For example, if Mr. Jones lives alone and must irrigate his own colostomy, then "Irrigates his colostomy *independently* as taught" is the correct objective.

Criteria state the standards of performance that are considered acceptable. Each objective should specify a standard against which the performance can be measured. Examples include speed, quality, and accuracy. Learners need to understand the criteria so that they can evaluate their performance validly.

Selecting Teaching Strategies

The method of teaching chosen by the nurse should be suited to the individual, to the material to be learned, and to the teacher. For example, the person who cannot read needs material presented in other ways; a discus-

TABLE 19-3 *Selected Teaching Strategies*

Strategy	Major Type of Learning	Characteristics
Explanation or description (e.g., lecture)	Cognitive	Teacher controls contents and pace. Feedback is determined by teacher. May be given to individual or group. Encourages retention of facts.
One-to-one discussion	Affective, cognitive	Encourages participation by learner. Permits reinforcement and repetition at learner's level. Permits introduction of sensitive subjects.
Answering questions	Cognitive	Teacher controls most of content and pace. Teacher must understand question and what it means to learner. Can be used with individuals and groups. Teacher sometimes needs to confirm whether question has been answered by asking learner, e.g., "Does that answer your question?"
Demonstration	Psychomotor	Often used with explanation. Can be used with individuals, small or large groups. Does not permit use of equipment by learners.
Group discussion	Affective, cognitive	Learner can obtain assistance from supportive group. Group members learn from one another.
Practice	Psychomotor	Allows repetition and immediate feedback. Permits "hands-on" experience.
Printed and audiovisual materials	Cognitive	Forms include books, pamphlets, films, programmed instruction, and computer learning. Learners can proceed at their own speed. Nurse can act as resource person, need not be present during learning.
Role playing	Affective, cognitive	Permits expression of attitudes, values, and emotions. Can assist in development of communication skills. Involves active participation by learner.
Modeling	Affective, psychomotor	Nurse sets example by attitude, psychomotor skill.

sion is usually not the best strategy for teaching to give an injection; and a teacher using group discussion for teaching should be a competent group leader. Some people are visually oriented and learn best through seeing; others learn best through hearing and having the skill explained. These attributes should be considered during the planning phase. If this fact is not identified until the teaching plan has been implemented, the plan may need revising. See Table 19–3 for selected teaching strategies.

Choosing Content

The content to be taught is determined by the objectives. For instance, "Identify appropriate sites for insulin injections" means the nurse must include content about the body sites suitable for insulin injections.

There are many sources for content information. Nurses will have some knowledge as a result of their own education. Pamphlets, books, and journals can also assist nurses and clients. In addition, clients can learn a great deal from peers. For example, the client who has recently had a colostomy often can learn a great deal from a person who has had a colostomy for several years. Self-help groups function on this premise.

Audiovisual aids (film strips, films, posters, line drawings) often are helpful for client learning. It is important, however, that the nurse review these aids before presenting them to clients, for sometimes they are out of date, or they differ in content from other materials (even minimal differences can be confusing to clients).

Ordering Learning Experiences

Some health agencies have developed teaching guides for lessons that nurses commonly give. The guides save nurses time in constructing their own guides. They also standardize content and assist staff in remembering it. Whether the nurse is implementing a plan devised by another or developing an individualized teaching plan, some guidelines can help the nurse order the learning experience.

■ Start with something the learner is concerned about, e.g., before learning how to administer insulin to himself, an adolescent wants to know how he can adjust his life-style and still play football.

■ Begin with what the learner knows and proceed to the unknown. This gives the learner confidence. Sometimes a nurse does not know the client's knowledge or skill base and needs to elicit this information either by asking questions or by having the client fill out a form, such as a pretest.

■ Any area of learning that is anxiety provoking should be taught first. A high level of anxiety can impair concentration in other areas. For example, a woman highly anxious about turning her husband in bed might not be able to learn about bathing him until she has successfully learned to turn him.

■ Teach the basics first, then proceed to the variations or adjustments. It is very confusing to learners to have to consider every possible adjustment and variation before the basic concepts are understood. For example, when teaching a female client how to insert a retention catheter, it is best to teach the basic procedure before teaching any adjustments that might be needed if the catheter stops draining after insertion.

IMPLEMENTING

The nurse needs to be flexible in implementing any teaching plan, since the plan may need revising, e.g., because the client tires sooner than anticipated, the client is faced with too much information too quickly, the client's needs change, or external factors intervene. For instance, the nurse and the client, Mr. Brown, may have planned for him to learn to administer his own insulin at a particular time, but when the time comes the nurse finds that he wants additional information before actually giving himself the insulin. In this case, the nurse alters the teaching plan and discusses the desired information, provides written information, and defers teaching the psychomotor skill until the next day.

It is also important for nurses to use teaching techniques that enhance learning and to consider any barriers to learning. See Table 19–4 for barriers to learning. When implementing a teaching plan, the nurse may find the following eight guidelines helpful.

1. The optimal time for each session depends largely on the learner. Some people, for example, learn best at the beginning of the day, when they are most rested; others prefer late afternoon, when no other activities are scheduled.

2. The pace of each teaching session also affects learning. Nurses should be sensitive to any signs that the pace is too fast or too slow. A client who appears confused or does not comprehend material when questioned may be finding the pace too fast. When the

TABLE 19-4 Barriers to Learning

Barrier	Explanation	Nursing Implications
Acute illness	Client requires all resources to cope with illness.	Defer teaching until client is less ill.
Pain	Pain decreases ability to concentrate.	Deal with pain before teaching.
Age	Vision, hearing, and motor control can be impaired in the elderly.	Allow for sensory and motor deficits in teaching.
Prognosis	Client can be preoccupied with illness and unable to concentrate on new information.	Defer teaching to a better time.
Biorhythms	Mental and physical performances have a circadian rhythm.	Change time of teaching to suit client.
Emotion (e.g., anxiety, denial, depression)	Emotions require energy and distract from learning.	Deal with emotions first and possible misinformation.
Language and ethnic background	Client may not be fluent in the nurse's language.	Obtain services of an interpreter or nurse with appropriate language skills.
Iatrogenic barriers	The nurse may set up barriers by appearing condescending or hurried or ignoring client cues.	Establish a helping relationship and be sensitive to client's needs.

client appears bored and loses interest, the pace may be too slow, the learning period may be too long, or the client may be tired.

3. An environment can detract from or assist learning; e.g., noise or interruptions usually interfere with concentration, whereas a comfortable environment promotes learning. Environmental characteristics that should be considered are: lighting, temperature, sound, ventilation, visibility, and a chair or support for the learner.

4. Teaching aids can foster learning. Posters and displays, for example, can help focus a learner's attention. To ensure the transfer of learning, the nurse should use the type of supplies or equipment that the client will eventually use.

5. Learning is more effective when the learners discover the content for themselves. Ways to increase learning include stimulating motivation and stimulating self-direction, e.g., by providing specific objectives, giving feedback, and helping the learner derive satisfaction from learning. Nurses can maximize learner satisfaction by setting realistic goals with the learner.

6. Repetition—e.g., summarizing content, rephrasing (using other words), and approaching the material from another point of view—reinforces learning.

7. It is helpful to employ "organizers" to introduce material to be learned and to present it at a higher level of abstraction, generality, or inclusiveness (Rorden 1987, p. 120). Advanced organizers provide a means of relating unknown material to known material and generating logical relationships. The details that follow such an introduction are then seen within its framework, and the details have added meaning.

8. Using a layperson's vocabulary enhances communication. So often nurses use terms and abbreviations that have meaning to other health professionals but make little sense to clients. Even words such as *urine* or *feces* may be unfamiliar to clients, and abbreviations such as "RR" (recovery room) or "PAR" (post-anesthesia room) are often misunderstood.

Special Teaching Strategies

There are a number of special teaching strategies that nurses can use: client contracting, group teaching, behavior modification, and various accelerated strategies.

Client Contracting   Client contracting involves establishing a contract with a client that specifies certain objectives and when they are to be met. The contract, drawn up and signed by the client and the nurse, specifies not only the learning objectives but also the responsibilities of the client and the nurse, and the teaching plan. The agreement allows for freedom, mutual respect, and mutual responsibility. For additional information about client contracting see Chapter 15.

Group Teaching

Group instruction is economical and it provides members with an opportunity to share with and learn from others. A small group allows for discussion in which everyone can participate. A large group often necessitates a lecture technique.

It is important that all members involved in group instruction have a need in common, e.g., prenatal health, preoperative instruction. It is also important that sociocultural factors be considered in the formation of a group. Whereas middle-class Americans may value sharing experiences with others, people from a culture such as Japan may consider it inappropriate to reveal their thoughts and feelings.

Behavior Modification

The behavior modification system for changing behavior has as its basic assumptions that human behaviors are learned and can be selectively strengthened, weakened, eliminated, or replaced and that a person's behavior is under conscious control. Under this system, desirable behavior is rewarded and undesirable behavior is ignored. The client's response is the key to behavior change. For example, clients trying to quit smoking are not criticized when they smoke, but they are praised or rewarded when they go without a cigarette for a certain period of time. For some people a learning contract is combined with behavior modification.

Some pertinent features of behavior modification are the following:

- Positive reinforcement—e.g., praise—is used.
- The client participates in the development of the learning plan.
- Undesirable behavior is ignored, not criticized.
- The expectation of the client and the nurse is that the task will be mastered, i.e., the behavior will change.
- Success is maximized through positive reinforcement; failure and the threat of failure are minimized.

Teaching Throughout the Life Span

Infants and Toddlers

The primary caregiver, i.e., the parent, is the best person to teach the infant or toddler. Infants learn by exploring their environment with their senses. An infant's routines normally should not be changed, unless they involve something that is making the infant ill. Predictable routines help infants feel secure. When teaching toddlers before surgery, the nurse should make sure they are able to hold the mask or the equipment with which they will come into contact later. Toddlers like to explore, e.g., handle equipment. They also need to be reassured that their parents have seen the room in which they will "wake up," because then the children know their parents will be able to find them.

Toddlers who reply "no" when they are being taught a new activity such as brushing their teeth are asserting their independence; this does not mean they will not learn. Better results will usually be produced if the nurse postpones the teaching to another time and repeats the lesson rather than arguing with the toddler.

Preschoolers

Most preschoolers want to learn. They have limited verbal abilities and like to explore, just as toddlers do. Most preschoolers like to practice procedures such as bandaging; such activity helps them deal with their fears.

Preschoolers like to ask questions, but the nurse's answers should be short and at a level that can be understood. Preschoolers like explanations, and they worry about such things as providing a blood specimen because the nurse "may take all my blood." The nurse should emphasize that treatment is not punishment.

School-Age Children

School-age children know more about their bodies than do preschoolers. Since their attention span is short, they learn best in brief stages. They usually like to handle objects and to draw pictures and color in books. Although their vocabulary is limited, they are learning new things. A school-age child's day is often filled with short projects.

School-age children love to ask why. They require explanations that meet their needs and that use words they understand. Children at this age should be encouraged to express their feelings, including fear about dying. School-age children love to do things the "right way," and any changes they consider as not "right" they often do not accept.

Adolescents

Adolescents may prefer to learn in the absence of their parents. Although they do have knowledge about their bodies, some of it may be incorrect. Adolescents learn best when they see immediate benefit to themselves. For example, an adolescent who understands that taking his medicine regularly will permit him to continue playing football is more likely to follow through than if he is told the medication will prevent heart problems when he is in his forties.

Young and Middle-Aged Adults

Young adults often take health for granted ("It won't happen to me"), and they may not be interested in learning about other people's problems. However, when young adults understand how something affects them, learning is facilitated. Young adults not living at home may find it unacceptable to be dependent on parents for health matters, and they may prefer a friend or the nurse to help them through a health problem.

Middle-aged adults are usually aware of the problems that can result from unhealthy life-styles. This is the period when changes in life-style are often indicated. Some middle-aged people change despite difficulty, and others still believe "it won't happen to me."

Elderly Adults

Healthy elderly adults can learn new techniques and procedures and usually desire to do so if it will mean their continued health and independence. Recent research has shown that there is no general decline in intelligence with age.

Teaching methods should be geared to the older person's memory. Those who, for example, have difficulty with recent memory should be taught by methods that take this into consideration. In addition, like people of other ages, elderly people must be motivated to learn. People who have always assumed responsibility for their own health will probably be better motivated to change life-style and learn skills designed to improve health than will people who have had others assume this responsibility. Also, elderly people who prefer dependence may find it difficult to learn health practices that promote independence.

Teaching methods should also consider the individual's past learning methods. Visualization using pictures may be preferable to discussion. The acuity of an elderly person's senses is an important consideration in this regard. The following physiologic changes commonly occur in old age (Kick 1989, pp. 682–84).

- Reaction time is longer, but a decrease in speed is often compensated by an increase in accuracy.
- High-pitched sound is often difficult to discriminate.
- Background noises such as a fan can interfere with hearing.
- Visual acuity is decreased.

- Color discrimination may be less acute, e.g., red, yellow, blue, and orange are less readily read on white paper.
- The senses of taste and smell and fine discrimination in touch, pressure, and temperature are less acute.
- Cerebral function can be compromised by decreases in oxygenation, cerebral blood flow, and hemoglobin.
- Recent memory recall may be more difficult than recall of events long past.

EVALUATING

Evaluating is an ongoing and terminal process in which the client, the nurse, and often the support persons determine what has been learned. Both short-term objectives and long-term goals need to be evaluated. Learning is measured against the predetermined objectives. Thus, the objectives serve not only to direct the teaching plan but also to provide criteria for evaluation. For example, the objective "Selects foods that are low in carbohydrates" can be evaluated by asking the client to name such foods or to select low-carbohydrate foods from a list.

The best method for evaluating depends on the type of learning. In cognitive learning, asking questions of the client is one way to determine what has been learned. The acquisition of psychomotor skills is best evaluated by observing the client carry out a procedure, such as changing a dressing or carrying out a urinary self-catheterization. Affective learning is more difficult to evaluate. Whether attitudes or values have been learned may be inferred by listening to the client's responses to questions and by the way the client speaks about relevant subjects and by observing the client's behavior. For example, has an obese client learned to value health sufficiently to follow a reducing diet? Do clients who state that they value health actually stop smoking?

Following evaluation, the nurse may find it necessary to modify or repeat the teaching plan if the objectives have not been met or have been met only partially. For the hospitalized client, follow-up teaching in the home may be needed.

It is important for nurses to evaluate their own teaching. This should include a consideration of all factors—the timing, the teaching strategies, the amount of information, whether it was helpful, etc. The nurse may find, for example, that the client was overwhelmed with too much information, was bored, or was motivated to learn more.

The following guidelines (Smitherman 1981, pp. 141–44) can assist nurses in the evaluative process:

- Forgetting is normal and should be anticipated. Nurses can suggest to clients that they write down information they might forget. Often, clients are provided printed instructions, because such information may be easily forgotten.

- Both the client and the teacher should evaluate the learning experience. The learner may tell the nurse what was helpful, interesting, etc. Questionnaires and videotapes of the learning sessions can also be helpful.

- Behavior change does not always take place immediately after learning. Often individuals will accept change intellectually first and then may change their behavior only periodically. If the new behavior is to replace old behavior, it must emerge gradually; otherwise, the old behavior may prevail. Nurses can assist clients with behavior change by allowing for client vacillation and by providing encouragement.

DOCUMENTATION

Documentation of the teaching process is essential, for this provides a legal record that the teaching took place and communicates the teaching to other health professionals. According to Omdahl, client teaching has been identified as "the most underdocumented skilled service because most nurses in home care do not recognize the scope and depth of the teaching they do" and "tend to view much of their teaching as commonsense suggestions" (Omdahl 1987, p. 1033).

The record should include the client's achievements. A specific client teaching record or the nurse's notes can be used. The client's reaction to the teaching should also be included, and this reaction should be incorporated into further planning. Documentation of the responses of support persons are also important to include.

The record of the teaching process should include written teaching plans, nursing Kardexes, and planning sessions with other health team members. Documentation of the teaching/learning process serves several other functions as well: reference for client learning and support-person learning; reevaluation of the teaching plan; reinforcement of identified areas of learning need; and revision of the teaching strategies (Corkadel and McGlashan 1983, pp. 14–15).

OTHER INSTRUCTIONAL ACTIVITIES OF PROFESSIONAL NURSES

Nurses are frequently called upon to provide instructional activities to individuals or groups in addition to direct client/nurse interaction. Such professional instructional situations include: (1) the instruction of client support persons, including parents, spouse, children, and significant others; (2) orientation of new employees; (3) in-service employee instruction regarding new policies or techniques; (4) community education programs for student groups, parent groups, senior citizens groups, or groups with specific health care interests, such as heart disease, cancer, AIDS, pregnancy, and nutrition; and (5) clinical instruction and supervision of nursing or other allied health students.

Regardless of the learner, the basic principles of teaching learning apply:

- Be knowledgeable about the subject matter
- Assess the learners' needs
- Provide a supportive instructional environment
- Define the teaching goals and objectives in learner directed, measurable terms
- Use content-appropriate instructional methods and materials
- Provide evaluative feedback to the learner.

CHAPTER HIGHLIGHTS

▶ Learning is represented by a change behavior.

▶ Bloom identified three learning domains: cognitive, affective, and psychomotor.

▶ A number of factors facilitate learning, including motivation, readiness, active involvement, and success at learning.

▶

CHAPTER HIGHLIGHTS *(continued)*

▸ Factors such as extreme anxiety, certain physiologic processes, and cultural barriers impede learning.

▸ Teaching is a system of activities intended to produce learning. Rapport between the teacher and the learner is essential for effective teaching.

▸ Assessment relative to the preparation of a teaching plan must include identification of the client's learning needs and relevant client data such as readiness to learn, motivation, socioeconomic factors, learning style, age, and health beliefs and practices.

▸ Readiness is an important aspect of assessment *prior* to teaching.

▸ Learning objectives guide the content of the teaching plan and are written in terms of client behavior.

▸ Teaching strategies should be suited to the client, the material to be learned, and the teacher.

▸ A teaching plan is a written plan and must be revised when the client's needs change or the teaching strategies prove ineffective.

▸ Evaluation of the teaching/learning process is an ongoing and terminal process.

▸ Documentation of client teaching is essential to communicate the teaching to other health professionals and to provide a record for legal purposes.

▸ Nurses are involved in instructional activities for allied health personnel, professional colleagues, community groups, and students.

LEARNING ACTIVITIES

■ Identify the most frequently required instructional topics for clients on your clinical nursing unit. Who carries out this instruction? Do you have standard teaching plans for these instructional topics? Are there specific instructional materials conveniently available to support client instruction in these topics?

■ Select one of the topics identified above. Develop a standard teaching plan for the topic, including: (1) description of the instruction; (2) learning goals; (3) specific measurable learning objectives; (4) instructional outline; (5) instructional methods and learning materials, e.g., handouts, pamphlets, videotapes, films, books; and (6) evaluation of the learner, program, and teacher.

■ Keep a log for one week listing all teaching/learning activities in which you participate as a nurse teacher. Include formal and informal instructional activities. Include client teaching as well as others within the hospital and the community. What percent of your time is spent in health-teaching activities?

READINGS AND REFERENCES

SUGGESTED READINGS

Kick, E. September 1989. Patient teaching for elders. *Nursing Clinics of North America* 24:681–87.
    Kick introduces this article by briefly explaining two myths about the elderly: older people experience a decline in mental abilities, and older people cannot learn. An overview of four ways in which aging affects learning is provided. Kick discusses how older persons learn and concludes the article with information about instructional settings.

Robinson, Y. K. January 1986. Teaching adults: Some issues in adult education for health education. *Physiotherapy* 72:49–52.
    Discusses adults as learners, including a list of ten beliefs about an andragogical humanistic approach to adult learning. The author sees learning as a cooperative effort on the part of the teacher and the learner, and describes participatory and group learning as well as individual differences and cognitive style and change.

Tripp-Reimer, T. September 1989. Cross-cultural perspectives on patient teaching. *Nursing Clinics of North America* 24:613–19.
    Tripp-Reimer states at the beginning of this article that "individual health behavior largely is culturally patterned." The author maintains that nurses should carry out a cultural

assessment and a cultural negotiation before establishing a teaching plan. The author also points out that nurses should establish rapport and assess the problem and readiness to learn. Throughout the article Tripp-Reimer describes the significance of considering cultural values.

RELATED RESEARCH

Brown, S. A. July/August 1988. Effects of educational interventions in diabetes care: A meta-analysis of findings. *Nursing Research* 37:223–29.

Streiff, L. D. Summer 1986. Can clients understand our instructions? *Image: Journal of Nursing Scholarship* 18:48–52.

Vessey, J. A. September/October 1988. Comparison of two teaching methods on children's knowledge of their internal bodies. *Nursing Research* 38:262–87.

SELECTED REFERENCES

Armstrong, M. L. September 1989. Orchestrating the process of patient education: Methods and approaches. *Nursing Clinics of North America* 24:597–604.

Bloom, B. S., editor. 1956. *Taxonomy of educational objectives.* Book 1, *Cognitive domain.* New York: Longman, Inc.

Corkadel, L., and McGlashan, R. January/February 1983. A practical approach to patient teaching. *The Journal of Continuing Education in Nursing* 14:9–15.

Cross, K. P. 1988. *Adults as learners.* San Francisco: Jossey-Bass.

DeYoung, S. 1990. *Teaching nursing.* Redwood City, Calif.: Addison-Wesley Publishing Co.

Edwards, L. 1990. Health education. In Edelman, C. L., and Mandle, C. L. *Health promotion throughout the lifespan.* 2d ed. St. Louis: C. V. Mosby Co., pp. 173–191.

Fox, V. August 1986. Patient teaching: Understanding the needs of the adult learner. *AORN Journal* 44:234–42.

Gessner, B. A. September 1989. Adult education: The cornerstone of patient teaching. *Nursing Clinics of North America* 24:589–95.

Guinée, K. K. 1978. *Teaching and learning in nursing.* New York: Macmillan Publishing Co.

Johnson, E. A., and Jackson, J. E. September 1989. Teaching the home care client. *Nursing Clinics of North America* 24:687–93.

Kick, E. September 1989. Patient teaching for elders. *Nursing Clinics of North America* 24:681–86.

Knowles, M. S. 1980. *The modern practice of adult education:* From pedagogy to andragogy. Chicago: Follett.

———. 1984. *Andragogy in action.* San Francisco: Jossey-Bass.

Laird, M. August 1975. Techniques for teaching pre- and postoperative patients. *American Journal of Nursing* 75:1338–40.

Lawrence, G. 1982. *People types and tiger stripes: A practical guide to learning styles.* Gainesville, Florida: Center for Applications of Psychological Type, Inc.

Lewin, K. 1951. *Field theory in social science.* New York: Harper and Row.

Mager, R. F. 1975. *Preparing instructional objectives.* 2d ed. Belmont, California: Fearon Publishers, Inc.

Nuttleman, D. November 1977. Instructional objectives. *Supervisor Nurse.* 77:35–44.

Omdahl, D. J. August 1987. Preventing home care denials. *American Journal of Nursing* 87:1031–33.

Phillips, J. A., and Hekelman, F. P. September/October 1983. The role of the nurse as a teacher: A position paper. *Nephrology Nurse* 5:42–46.

Pohl, M. L. 1981. *The teaching function of the nursing practitioner.* 4th ed. Dubuque, Iowa: Wm. C. Brown Co.

Redman, B. K. 1988. *The process of patient education.* 6th ed. St. Louis: C. V. Mosby Co.

Rorden, J. W. 1987. *Nurses as health teachers: A practical guide.* Philadelphia: W. B. Saunders Co.

Smith, C. E., editor. 1987. *Patient education: Nurses in partnership with other health professionals.* Orlando Florida: Grune & Stratton.

Smitherman, C. 1981. *Nursing actions for health promotion.* Philadelphia: F. A. Davis Co.

Thurlow, J. G. Spring 1990. Tools for patient education. *Gastroenterological Nursing* 12:286–88.

Tyson, J. 1984. Before we educate. *Diabetes Educator* (special issue) 10:23–24.

Ward, D. B. January 1986. Why patient teaching fails. *RN* 49:45–47.

CHAPTER

20

Managing and Directing

CONTENTS

THE NURSE AS LEADER AND MANAGER

The professional nurse often assumes the roles of leader and manager. These two roles are often linked; that is, managers must have leadership abilities and leaders will often manage, but the two roles are uniquely different.

Nurses are role models to all who interact with them: clients, nursing colleagues, nursing students, physicians, health professionals, and members of the community. The ability to advocate for the client is linked to

the nurse's leadership ability. Leadership activities may not only be related to professional practice, but may also include the application of nursing knowledge to personal concerns. Nurses as members of the community provide leadership in matters related to health because of their special knowledge of risk factors and health promotion behaviors. This leadership behavior is exemplified in nursing involvement in organizations such as Mothers Against Drunk Drivers (MADD) (founded by a nurse), the American Cancer Society, the American Heart Association, and so on. Nurses also demonstrate leadership activity in programs for the homeless, the elderly, victims of AIDS, child welfare, and environmental protection programs.

The nurse assumes management functions in several ways. As manager and provider of client care, the nurse coordinates the various health professionals who provide service to the client, including those in X ray, pharmacy, respiratory therapy, physical therapy, social work, or occupational therapy. The nurse may also assume a situational role of manager as head nurse, nursing supervisor, and so on. In this management role the nurse directs and evaluates the nursing and non-nursing staff members.

As discussed in Chapter 3, the nurse can be a leader in the care of the individual client, the client family, groups of clients, professional colleagues, or society at large. The purposes of nursing leadership vary according to the level of application and include (a) improving the health status of individuals or families, (b) increasing the effectiveness and level of satisfaction among professional colleagues who provide care, and (c) improving the attitudes of citizens and legislators toward the nursing profession and their expectations of it (Leddy and Pepper 1989, p. 336).

Leadership Styles

Three leadership styles have been described: Autocratic or authoritarian, democratic, and laissez-faire. The three styles are often blended in a selective combination to fit the situation, the needs of the leader, and the needs of the group, rather than implemented continuously in pure form. More recent leadership styles include participative (diffused) leadership, and situational leadership.

In *autocratic leadership,* the leader exerts strong control over the group and makes the decisions. The leader may be benevolent or dictatorial. This style presupposes that the group is incapable of making its own decisions. The leader determines policies and gives orders and directions to the members. Autocratic leadership generally has negative connotations and often results in group dissatisfaction. There are times, however, when autocratic leadership may be most effective. When decisions are necessary in an urgent situation, such as a cardiac arrest, a unit fire, or a mass casualty event, one person must assume the responsibility to make decisions without incurring challenges or negotiation from other team members. When group members are unable or do not wish to participate in making a decision, the autocratic style will effect resolution of the problem and enable the individual or group to move on. This style can also be effective

when a project must be completed quickly and efficiently.

In *democratic leadership,* the leader participates as a facilitator, encouraging group discussion and decision making. This supportive style increases group productivity and satisfaction. It presupposes that group members are capable of making decisions, are motivated to do so, and value independence. Democratic leadership generally has positive connotations, but requires time for consultation and collaboration. It may not always be the most effective or efficient method if an urgent decision is required or if members lack skills and information to make decisions. It is important that the nurse utilizing the democratic leadership style provide necessary information for the group to make appropriate decisions.

Democratic leadership is based on the following principles:

- Every group member should participate in decision-making.

- Freedom of belief and action is allowed within reasonable bounds that are set by society and by the group.

- Each individual is responsible for himself or herself and for the welfare of the group.

- There should be concern and consideration for each group member as a unique individual. (Tappen 1989, p. 34)

In *laissez-faire leadership,* the leader participates minimally and often only on request of the members. This style is described as a "hands-off" approach. It recognizes the group's need for autonomy and self-regulation. It is most effective after a group has made a decision, is committed to it, and has the expertise to implement it. The leader acts as a resource person and consultant.

Participative leadership is an approach to group leadership in which functions are distributed. Inherent in this concept is the recognition that the leadership function is not held irrevocably by one person but rather is distributed among the group members. To clarify this concept, Francis and Young (1979, p. 63) distinguish the role of group manager (the formal head of the group) from that of group leader. Managers have special responsibilities and functions that are recognized by the organization and are vital to the group's performance as an energizing and creative force. However, group leadership is a broad function. Different members assume leadership in their areas of strength to suit the tasks at hand.

Participative leaders are guided by the following principles (Richards 1987, p. 114):

- Leadership is not concentrated, but is diffused throughout the group.
- Formal or designated leadership is situational, and other members may perform functions equal in importance to or more important than those of the formal leader.
- The more members who function as leader, the better, because the act of leadership develops initiative, creativity, and responsibility.
- Leadership is a set of learned behaviors.

Situational leadership theory encourages managers to combine leader task behavior, leader relationship behavior, and follower maturity levels into four options of leadership style (Teasley 1987, p. 112):

1. High task–Low relationship
2. High task–High relationship
3. Low task–High relationship
4. Low task–Low relationship

Task behavior refers to leadership activities that set goals and define role expectations. The leader explains how, what, when, and where the task must be done. For example, a nurse would use this style when teaching a client about self-administration of prescribed medication.

Relationship behavior is concerned with communications between the leader and follower. It involves mutual listening, supporting, informing, and facilitating so that people see various aspects of mutual problems and get acquainted through general conversation in a social atmosphere. For example, a vice president of nursing may hold regular coffee or lunch sessions with nursing coordinators or supervisory staff.

Follower maturity level refers to the follower's state of job and psychologic functioning (high to low) for specific activities in particular situations. This involves assessment of job maturity and psychologic maturity. Assessment of job maturity requires a description of the person's education, experience, and capability of performing a particular function. Assessment of psychologic maturity requires a description of the person's performance motivation and willingness to accept responsibility for a specific assignment.

To choose the best leadership style for a specific follower on a particular occasion, the leader must first assess the follower's maturity level and match it with the appropriate style. The leader must be competent in performing all four styles listed above.

A high task–low relationship leadership style may be used when the followers have a low job maturity level.

For example, a leader helps nursing staff adopt a new computer system with which they are unfamiliar. A high task–high relationship leadership style may be used when the staff, now more familiar with the system, is revealing consistent errors or problems with the system. Here, the leader empathizes with the followers and reteaches them. A low task–high relationship style would be necessary in situations that create frustration and call for participation and communication. Low task–low relationship leadership styles are used when a follower has a high job maturity level, i.e., is proficient, interested, and motivated. In this situation, the leader may delegate certain activities and be available as a consultant. A situational leadership style can improve job performance, help followers develop professionally, and promote competence in the leader.

Effective leadership is a learned process. Much has been written about effective leadership style; some descriptive statements are listed in the accompanying box.

Effective Leaders

- Use a leadership style that is natural to them
- Use a leadership style appropriate to the task and the members
- Assess the effects of their behavior on others and the effects of others' behavior on themselves
- Are sensitive to forces acting for and against change
- Express an optimistic view about human nature
- Are energetic
- Are open and encourage openness, so that real issues are confronted
- Facilitate personal relationships
- Plan and organize activities of the group
- Are consistent in behavior toward group members
- Delegate tasks and responsibilities to develop members' abilities, not merely to get tasks performed
- Involve members in all decisions
- Value and use group members' contributions
- Encourage creativity
- Encourage feedback about their leadership style

MANAGEMENT PRACTICES

Nurses function differently in various types of organizations. An organization may be autocratic, with one person having primary knowledge and power while other

persons are subordinate. Bureaucratic organizations control through policy, structured jobs, and compartmentalized actions. Other organizations decentralize control and emphasize self-direction and self-discipline of members. Another organization may be a component of a system that interacts interdependently and adapts dynamically to change. This organization is particularly useful for the nurse who manages the care of individuals, families, and communities. On a larger scale, the nurse-manager must work in the organizational framework of the employing agency.

Authority is the right to act and command. It is an integral component of managing. Authority is conveyed through leadership actions; it is determined largely by the situation, and it is always associated with responsibility and accountability.

Accountability means assuming responsibility for one's actions and accepting the consequences of one's behavior. Accountability can be viewed within a hierarchical systems framework, starting at the individual level, through the institutional/professional level, and then to the societal level (Sullivan and Decker 1988, p. 5). At the individual or client level, accountability is reflected in the nurse's ethical integrity. At the institutional level, it is reflected in the statement of philosophy and objectives of the nursing department and nursing audits. At the professional level, it is reflected in standards of practice developed by national or provincial nursing associations. At the societal level, it is reflected in legislated nurse practice acts.

Delegation is the sharing of responsibility and authority with others and holding them accountable for performance (Sullivan and Decker 1988, p. 251). Because it is often impossible to provide all of the nursing care needed by a group of clients, the nurse as a delegator must assign aspects of the client's care to other nursing personnel. Delegation is a major tool in making the most efficient use of time. Delegation is a high-level implementation skill. The nurse as a delegator must have the following information: (a) needs of the client and family, (b) goals of the client, (c) nursing activity that can help the client meet the goals, and (d) skills and knowledge of various nursing personnel.

The nurse-delegator must also determine how many nursing personnel are needed. This information may be indicated on the client's records. Other sources of this information are the client, the charge nurse, other nursing personnel, and the nurse-delegator's own judgment. Nurses may require assistance to give client care quickly in certain situations. Assistance may also be necessary to ensure client safety.

After establishing that assistance is required, the

nurse-delegator must identify what type of help is needed, how long help is required, when it is required, and what assistance is available. The nurse must arrange for assistance, usually by asking the appropriate person on the unit, before beginning the nursing activity. Delegation does not mean that a nurse-delegator performs nursing activities appropriate to personal knowledge and skills. An important aspect of delegation is the development of the potential of nursing personnel. By knowing the background, experience, knowledge, skills, and strengths of each person, a nurse can delegate responsibilities that help develop each person's competence. Nursing personnel to whom aspects of care have been delegated need to be supervised and evaluated. The amount of supervision required is highly variable, depending on the knowledge and skills of each person. As the person who assigns the activity and observes the performance, the nurse-delegator contributes to the evaluation process. Because individual motivation varies, the nurse-delegator needs to realize that not all persons perform equally. Thus, standards of performance must be evaluated against written job descriptions, rather than by comparing one person to another. It is essential, too, for the nurse-delegator to realize that people require ongoing feedback about their performance. Feedback should be given in an objective manner and include both positive and negative input.

Characteristics of effective nurse managers as described by Sullivan and Decker (1988, p. 576) are listed in the accompanying box.

NURSING MANAGEMENT SYSTEMS

Over the years, different types of nursing management systems have been used to manage the care of individuals or groups of clients. They include case method, functional nursing, team nursing, primary nursing, and case management.

Case Method

The case method, also referred to as total care, is one of the earliest models. This method is client-centered. One nurse is assigned to and is responsible for the comprehensive care of a client or group of clients during an 8- or 12-hour shift. Historically, in some situations the nurse lived in the client's home and provided home care in addition to care during hospitalization. During its popularity in the 1920s, the case method "emphasized following physicians' orders" (Marriner-Tomey 1988, p. 146.)

For each client, the nurse assesses needs, makes nursing plans, formulates diagnoses, implements care, and evaluates the effectiveness of care. In this method, a client has consistent contact with one nurse during a shift but may have different nurses on other shifts. The case method, considered the precursor of primary nursing, continues to be used in a variety of practice settings. With the shortage of nursing personnel during World War II, however, the case method could no longer be the chief mode of client care. To meet staff shortages, managers hired personnel with less educational preparation than the professional nurse, and developed on-the-job training programs for auxiliary helpers. The total care method became unfeasible in such situations, and the functional method was developed in response.

Functional Method

This system of assignment, which evolved from concepts of scientific management used in the field of business administration, focuses on the jobs to be completed. In this task-oriented approach, personnel with less preparation than the professional nurse fulfill less complex care requirements. It is based on a production and efficiency model that gives authority and responsibility to the person assigning the work. Clearly defined job descriptions, procedures, policies, and lines of communication are required. The functional approach to nursing is economical and efficient and permits centralized direction and control. Its disadvantages are fragmentation of care (the client receives care from several different categories of personnel) and the possibility that non-quantifiable aspects of care, such as meeting the client's emotional needs, may be overlooked.

Team Nursing

In the early 1950s, Eleanor Lambertson (1953) and her colleagues proposed a system of team nursing to overcome the fragmentation of care resulting from the task-oriented functional approach and to meet the increasing demands for professional nurses created by advances in technologic aspects of care. Team nursing is the delivery of individualized nursing care to clients by a nursing team led by a professional nurse. A nursing team consists of registered nurses, licensed practical nurses, and often nurses' aides. This team is responsible for providing coordinated nursing care to a group of clients during an 8- or 12-hour shift. Compared to the functional system, team nursing emphasizes humanistic values and responds to the needs of both clients and employees. Individualized client care on a personal level rather than task-oriented care on an impersonal level is emphasized. Employees are stimulated to learn and develop new skills by the professional nurse leader, who instructs them, supervises them, and provides assignments that offer the potential for growth.

Basic to team nursing are the team conference, the nursing care plan, and leadership skills. The conference, led by the professional nurse team leader, includes all personnel assigned to the team. Discussing the needs of clients, establishing goals, individualizing the plan of care, instructing personnel, and following up are all under the direction of the team leader. In essence, the team leader has a management role that requires a high degree of competence in coordination and leadership.

Although the team nursing approach has worked effectively in many health care agencies, certain weaknesses have been observed in some settings. The client may still perceive care as fragmented if the team leader does not establish a satisfactory relationship with the client. Teams may not have the appropriate health care personnel, and team members may not have the expertise to meet the needs of a particular client population. Ideally, the team should include several professional nurses. Often, there is only one professional nurse, who must assume the role of team leader. When there are no professional nurses assigned to a unit, technical nurses, who have natural leadership ability but are not educationally prepared to fulfill the leadership role required of a team leader, are assigned to this role. In some situations the leader may use a functional mode of delivering care.

Primary Nursing

Primary nursing, a system in which one nurse is responsible for total care of a number of clients 24 hours a day, 7 days a week, was introduced at the Loeb Center for Nursing and Rehabilitation, in the Bronx, New York, under the leadership of Lydia Hall (1963). It is a method of providing comprehensive, individualized, and consistent care.

Primary nursing uses the nurse's technical knowledge and management skills. The primary nurse assesses and prioritizes each client's needs, identifies nursing diagnoses, develops a plan of care with the client, and evaluates the effectiveness of care. Associates may provide some care, but the primary nurse acts as coordinator and communicates information about the client's health to other nurses and health professionals. Primary nursing encompasses all aspects of the professional role, including teaching, advocacy, decision-making, and continuity of care. The primary nurse is the first-line manager of the client's care.

Case Management System

Case management is a more recent nursing care delivery system in which case managers are responsible for a case load of clients throughout their hospitalization. These managers may be associated with case loads in a variety of ways, for instance (a) with specific physicians and their clients, (b) with clients geographically within a unit or units, and (c) by diagnosis category. The case management system maintains the philosophy of primary nursing and often requires a graduate of a bachelor's or master's program to implement high-level professional practice.

COMPUTERS IN NURSING

In the next century, most nurses will use computers in many aspects of their professional practice. Computers can organize, analyze, and store different kinds of information or data in a rapid, accurate, and easily retrievable manner. "User-friendly" computers are already of great help to the nurse in assessing, diagnosing, planning, implementing, and evaluating nursing care. The nurse educator and the nurse manager have also discovered the usefulness of computers in managing staffing, budgeting, enhancing instruction, producing grade reports, writing papers, and improving productivity. In fact, computer skills and knowledge will soon be expected and perhaps required for a great many positions. Those who ignore this technologic revolution may be left behind.

As previously stated in this chapter, the nurse is the manager of client care. Hospital information flows to and through nursing departments. Nurses must take an active role in the design, development, and implementation of computer systems to enhance the quality of client care while at the same time increasing accuracy and efficiency. Professional nurses who understand the conceptual framework of computer applications will find the computer extraordinarily useful in their professional practice.

In the past, hospital computer applications have been administrative. Tasks such as client billing, maintaining financial records, and long-term planning are necessary aspects of the business side of the hospital. As computers get smaller, less costly, more powerful, and easier to use, they will be used increasingly in other areas of the health care system. Today it is common to find a microcomputer system or computer terminal in the nurse's station. Small bedside computer terminals are used in

Client name :	Martha Johnson	**Rm number**	403
Admission date :	05/25/91		
Sex :	F	**Religion :**	Catholic
Age :	58	**Date of birth :**	03/13/33
Admitting physician :	Dr. Raymond Atkins		
Medical diagnosis :	Diabetes		
Primary nurse :	Judy Foster, R.N.		
Allergies :	Penicillin	**Diet :**	1500 c ADA
Risk factors :	Hearing aid	**Vital signs :**	T.I.D.
Nursing diagnosis :	Impairment of skin integrity related to pruritus.		
Long-term goals :	Client will experience improved skin integrity within 48 hours.		

Short-term goals	**Nursing interventions**	**Evaluation**
Given the prescribed care, client will experience decreased itching sensation	1. Infrequent baths. 2. Use cool water. 3. Soap substitute. 4. Blot skin dry. DO NOT RUB! 5. Lubricate skin with lotion after bath.	
Client will understand and implement health teaching.	1. Explain phenomenon of itching. 2. Teach avoidance of excessive warmth. 3. Teach need for increased humidity.	

Figure 20-1 Computer-generated nursing care plan.

coronary care, burn care, and other special care areas to monitor vital signs, laboratory data, nursing admission data, and continuous nursing care planning. These computers are networked to computers throughout the hospital, including the unit nurse's station, the laboratory, and the pharmacy. In the future, nurses in community health and home care may use portable computers to facilitate client record keeping.

Using the Computer to Plan Care

Automated client care systems allow "on-line" (i.e., directly connected to the computer) use of standardized nursing care plans (see Figure 20–1). After analyzing the assessment database and identifying the client's nursing diagnoses, nurses are able to create a care plan easily, customize it for each client, type in additions as needed, evaluate and update information at any time, and retrieve data appropriate to each specific nursing diagnosis. Specific ways in which an automated client care plan can facilitate the role of the nurse include the following:

1. Entry of nursing assessments is simplified; e.g., the nurse can touch a computer screen that displays assessment possibilities.

2. Laboratory data can be ordered by entering a request at a computer workstation.

3. Laboratory results can be retrieved in a shorter time with less paperwork.

4. The system facilitates complete and legible medication orders.

5. The system promotes consistent physician's orders (verbal orders are not accepted).

6. The nursing implications of a physician's order can be sent to the nurse. Client preparation needs for a particular test can be listed automatically in the client's nursing care plan.

7. The use of nursing diagnosis is facilitated; a common format can be used.

8. Current information can be updated easily. Discontinued medication orders can be detected easily, making all information timely, legible, and complete.

Using the Computer as a Consultant

The term *expert system* will no doubt become familiar to those in the health care professions over the next decade. An expert system is a computer-based model (using some of the principles of an exciting area of computer science called artificial intelligence) that strives to simulate the way human experts in a particular discipline gather data and make decisions. The human expert, for example, a clinical nurse specialist, is an important part of the design of these systems. In effect, the clinical nurse specialist is fulfilling a consulting role through the computer.

COMMES (Creighton On-Line Multiple Modular Expert Systems) is an artificial intelligence system that can simulate a consultation with a professional nurse. To do so, the system must have a current knowledge base and be able to mimic professional decision-making skills while avoiding the risk of providing incorrect or inappropriate data (Ryan 1985). Some expert systems are, in many ways, merely computer data bases that allow retrieval of data in various ways. It is quite likely that in the

near future, expert systems will not only contain the information of a human considered an expert in a particular field but also, like that human expert, be able to analyze logically and make decisions. In this way, the "system" can begin to provide assistance in educational settings, hospital settings, and emergency settings and facilitate client care of consistent quality.

Using the Computer as a Research Tool

Nursing research is also made easier by the computer's ability to access information in client records. Many hospitals maintain extensive computerized records. If access to these data is permitted, the nurse researcher can gather information that may be important in a particular study or project. For example, a researcher interested in determining what interventions were most successful in caring for clients with the nursing diagnosis "impaired skin integrity" can retrieve the care plans containing this information from the computer-based record. In addition, other key variables, such as the client's age, background, and sex, can be obtained and used to facilitate the analysis of the research problem. Collecting these data manually (if they were available at all) would take a long time.

Research is also facilitated by the availability of computerized literature retrieval systems such as Medline, CINAHL, and so on. Also available are computerized systems such as SPSS and Statsoft for statistical analysis of data.

Using the Computer for Administrative Tasks

The particular needs of the nursing administrator or manager can often be met by a hospital's computer system. The director of nurses or the division head of client services in a hospital needs data related to staffing, nurse scheduling, budgeting, and the evaluation of client services. If the appropriate information is stored in a computer-based information system, the manager can generate reports on the acuity levels of clients on each unit. These can be used to devise a formula for determining both the appropriate skill levels and the number of nurses required per shift and per floor. In addition, the scheduling of personnel is often made difficult by changing shifts, different skill levels, vacations, weekends, legal coverage requirements, and so on. Computer-based scheduling models can save much time and provide options that can be difficult to discover if the information is handled manually.

Using the Computer for Education

In the educational setting, the computer is becoming increasingly important, both as a teaching tool and as a resource for improving faculty and student productivity. It is likely that the use of the computer in these ways will increase dramatically over the next few years. Two factors contributing to the potential increase in computer use in education are (1) increasing availability of computer-assisted instructional (CAI) programs and interactive videodisc computer programs, and (2) the change to a computerized format for the nursing licensing examination (NCLEX).

For the student and practicing nurse, computers can be used for:

- Remediation or reinforcement of material already presented in the classroom
- CPR instruction/certification
- Cognitive and psychomotor skill practice
- Enrichment activities
- Practice of clinical decision-making
- Determination of advanced placement standing
- Formative and summative evaluation
- Presentation of new material
- Word-processing to improve writing/composition skills

Computers may also be used for client education programs. Instruction can be presented in an interactive, non-threatening, individualized, and private manner. As people become more proficient with computer and electronic gaming (e.g., Nintendo, home computers), these "fun" approaches to client health education will become more popular.

For faculty, computers can help with record-keeping, test construction, library information retrieval, word-processing, and development of new educational programs to enhance learning.

The Nurse's Role in Developing Computer Systems

Nurses can play many roles to integrate the computer into their environment. One method is to become more comfortable with, knowledgeable about, and an advocate of the use of microcomputers. In addition (and perhaps more importantly), nurses need to become involved with the planning, design, and implementation of any computer systems that affect their profession. In most cases, health care applications are designed by persons or groups with computer expertise, who often lack skill in and knowledge of the application area in which they plan to put the computer to use. Sometimes, these developers seek out the active participation of those who will use the implemented system every day. Many times, no such attempt is made. It is essential that nurses demand involvement in the design of any systems that will eventually affect them and/or their clients. Otherwise, they run the risk of having to work with a computer system designed by someone unfamiliar with their needs. The likelihood of such systems being successful without this involvement is remote.

MENTORS AND PRECEPTORS

The term *mentor* is defined by Ardery (1990) as "an experienced guide, adviser, or advocate who assumes responsibility for promoting the growth and professional advancement of a less experienced individual—the protege." Most nursing literature describes the nurse-mentor relationship as important for career development in nursing administration or nursing education. The concept of mentoring should also be encouraged to assist the nurse's professional growth from new graduate to experienced nurse. The nurse then, in turn, may choose to mentor those who follow.

In the clinical area, the term *preceptor* is used to describe mentoring relationships in which the experienced nurse assists the "new" nurse in improving her clinical nursing skill and judgment. The preceptor also instills understanding of the routines, policies, and procedures of the institution and the unit.

Mentors provide support. Often the mentor relationship is one of teacher-learner as the mentor instructs the protege in the expected role, introduces the protege to those who are important to the achievement of goals, listens to and helps the protege evaluate his/her ideas in light of institutional policy, and challenges the protege to advance his or her professional practice.

Nurses who wish to improve and advance their professional practice, whether in education, administration, or clinical practice, should seek mentors to assist them. Mentors are usually of the same sex, 8 to 15 years older, and have a position of authority in the organization.

They are usually knowledgeable individuals who are willing to share their knowledge and experience. Mentors often choose proteges because of their leadership and/or managerial qualities.

NETWORKING

In order to function effectively in all nursing roles, but especially in leadership and management roles, the nurse needs to network with other professionals. Network development builds linkages with people throughout the profession, both within and outside the work environment. Getting to know people helps build a trust relationship which can facilitate the achievement of professional goals. It is easier to access people you know than it is to access strangers. This provides for the exchange of ideas, knowledge, and information. Tappen (1989, p. 73) states "the sharing of information and opportunities with fellow professionals can have a synergistic effect: The nurse can increase her energy, supply of information, and influence by sharing it."

Nurses can develop networks by (a) attending local, regional, and national conferences, (b) taking classes for continuing education or toward an academic degree, (c) joining the alumni association and attending alumni meetings, (d) attending professional organization meetings, (e) keeping in touch with former teachers and co-workers, and (f) socializing with professional colleagues (O'Leary, Wendelgass, and Zimmerman 1986, pp. 14–15). Keeping an updated card file of colleagues and keeping in touch socially can keep the network fresh.

GROUP DYNAMICS

The nurse as leader and manager works with groups and may be responsible for managing people in groups. Chapter 18 contains introductory information about group interaction and classification, and discusses many of the client-based health care groups, e.g., teaching groups, self-help groups, self-awareness/growth groups, and therapy groups. It also presents material on the characteristics of effective groups, group dynamics, and group self-evaluation. The group dynamics discussion that follows focuses on two types of groups that nurse managers may encounter: task groups and work-related social support groups.

Task Groups

The task group is one of the most common types of work-related groups to which nurses belong. Examples are health care planning committees, nursing service committees, nursing team meetings, nursing care conference groups, and hospital staff meetings. The focus of such groups is the completion of a specific task, and the format is defined at the outset by the leader and/or members. The methods used to perform the task vary according to the task.

The leader of a task group, usually called the chairperson, must be accepted by the members as an appropriate leader, and therefore should be an expert in the area of task emphasis. The chairperson's role is to identify the specific task, clarify communication, and assist in expressing opinions and offering solutions. Committee members are generally selected in terms of their individual functional role and employment status, rather than in terms of their personal characteristics. Member participation is determined by the task. A target date for termination of the group is usually set in advance.

Work-Related Social Support Groups

Many nurses experience high levels of vocational stress. Social support groups can help reduce stress if various types of support are provided to buffer the stress. Richman and Rosenfeld (1987, p. 205) delineate four types of social support (listed in order of importance) that effective support groups must provide to buffer stress:

1. *Technical challenge.* Group members who know about the work of others can encourage and challenge members to be more creative and enthusiastic about their work and to achieve more.

2. *Share social reality.* Group members act as sounding boards and verify perceptions of the social context with other members who have similar priorities, values, and perspectives.

3. *Emotional challenge.* Group members provide emotional challenge to each other when they question whether others are doing their best to achieve goals and overcome obstacles.

4. *Listening.* Group members share the joys of success and the frustration of failure through active listening without giving advice or making judgments. This type of social support is best given outside of the work-related support group, since mere reflective listening is counterproductive for stress reduction. It is difficult for members to combine listening support with other types of support.

CHAPTER HIGHLIGHTS

▶ Purposes of leadership vary according to the level of application.

▶ Three leadership styles have been described: autocratic, democratic, and laissez-faire. The three styles are often blended in order to best fit the situation. Group leadership styles include participative and situational. Nurses should know which style is most consistent with their behavior and learn to incorporate aspects of other styles into their practice.

▶ Nurse managers work in the organizational framework of the employing agency. Principles of management include authority, accountability, and delegation.

▶ Nursing management systems that have been or are currently being used to provide client care include (a) case method, (b) functional method, (c) team nursing, (d) primary nursing, and (e) case management.

▶ The use of the computer in nursing and health care is expanding and demands that nurses take an active role in developing computer application systems.

▶ Mentors and preceptors are important in the support and professional development of beginning nurses. Nurses should seek out mentoring relationships to enhance career growth.

▶ Networking is the establishment of professional linkages in order to obtain information, share ideas, and facilitate the accomplishment of professional goals. Nurses can develop professional networks throughout their career in a variety of settings including school, work, professional organizations, and social groups.

▶ Nurse managers may use the principles of group dynamics to direct task groups and work-related social support groups.

LEARNING ACTIVITIES

■ After reviewing the leadership styles outlined, determine which style is most consistent with your nursing practice. How can you incorporate behaviors of the other styles in your practice to enable you to be a more effective leader?

■ Review the different types of nursing management systems. Which system is utilized to provide client care in your nursing area? Are there nursing units in your organization that use other systems? Identify specific rationales for the use of the different nursing management systems in modern nursing practice.

■ Review your own nursing career. Have you had mentor or preceptor relationships? Have you kept in touch with nurses who have helped you develop your professional self? What networking have you done? List nurses who have influenced your professional practice who remain a part of your professional network.

READINGS AND REFERENCES

SUGGESTED READINGS

Marriner-Tomey, A. 1988. *Guide to nursing management.* 3d ed. St. Louis: C. V. Mosby Co.
This book is designed to teach the management process and to supply the practicing nurse with practical information about nursing administration. The management process—plan, organize, staff, direct, and control—is presented in detail and applied to nursing. The book incorporates management sources from business and the social sciences.

Sullivan, E. J., and Decker, P. J. 1988. *Effective management in nursing.* 2d ed. Menlo Park, Calif.: Addison-Wesley Publishing Co. This text provides an in-depth analysis of concepts related to nursing management and leadership. Topics included are productivity, change, ethics in management, time management, motivation, problem solving and decision making, staffing, training, performance appraisal, budgeting, collective bargaining, conflict resolution, stress management, computers in health care, and quality assurance.

Tappen, R. M. 1989. *Nursing leadership and management: Concepts and practice.* 2d ed. Philadelphia: F. A. Davis Co. This book provides a detailed discussion of basic and advanced concepts of nursing leadership and management. Leadership and management theories are presented along with components of effective leadership and management. Other topics include critical thinking, planning, decision making, financial management, time management, computer applications, collective bargaining, motivation, communication, evaluation, accountability, quality assurance, and staff development.

REFERENCES

Ardery, G. 1990. Mentors and proteges: From ideology to knowledge. In McCloskey, J. C., and Grace, H. K., editors. *Current issues in nursing.* 3d ed. St. Louis: C. V. Mosby Co.

Ball, M. J., and Hannah, K. J. 1984. *Using computers in nursing.* Reston, Va.: Reston Publishing Co.

DeYoung, L. 1985. *Dynamics of nursing.* 5th ed. St. Louis: C. V. Mosby Co.

Ellis, J. F., and Hartley, C. L. 1988. *Nursing in today's world: Challenges, issues, and trends.* 3d ed. Philadelphia: J. B. Lippincott Co.

Epstein, C. 1982. *The nurse leader: Philosophy and practice.* Reston, Va.: Reston Publishing.

Francis, D., and Young, D. 1979. *Improving work groups: A practical manual for team building.* San Diego, Calif.: University Associates.

Hall, L. November 1963. A center for nursing. *Nursing Outlook* 11:805–6.

Hollie, M. L., and Blatchley, M. E. Winter 1989. Teaching leadership with role theory. *Nursing Connections* 2:53–61.

Kelly, L. Y. 1987. *The nursing experience: Trends, challenges, and traditions.* New York: Macmillan Publishing Co.

Kelly, L. Y. 1991. *Dimensions of professional nursing.* 6th ed. New York: Pergamon Press.

Kemp, V. H. 1986. An overview of change and leadership. In Hein, E. C., and Nicholson, M. J., editors. *Contemporary leadership behavior: Selected readings.* 2d ed. Boston: Little, Brown and Co.

Kozier, B., Erb, G., and Olivieri, R. 1991. *Fundamentals of nursing: Concepts, process and practice.* 4th ed. Redwood City, Calif.: Addison-Wesley Publishing Co.

Lambertson, E. 1953. *Nursing team organization and functioning.* New York: Teachers College Press.

Larson, D. May 1991. Integration of computer technology into curriculum. Workshop. Miami, Florida.

Leddy, S. and Pepper, J. M. 1989. *Conceptual bases of professional nursing.* 2d ed. Philadelphia: J. B. Lippincott Co.

Marriner-Tomey, A. 1988. *Guide to nursing management.* 3d ed. St. Louis: C. V. Mosby Co.

Monheim, F. J. January/February 1989. Encouraging the growth of computer applications in nursing. *Computers in Nursing* 7:35, 34.

O'Leary, J. G.; Wendelgass, S. T.; and Zimmerman, H. E. 1986. *Winning strategies for nursing managers.* Philadelphia: J. B. Lippincott Co.

Richards, M. B. November 1987. Developing "participative leaders." *Nursing Management* 18:113–15.

Richman, J. M., and Rosenfeld, L. B. Summer 1987. Stress reduction for hospice workers: A support group model. *Hospice Journal* 3:205–21.

Ryan, S. A. March/April 1985. An expert system for nursing practice: Clinical decision support. *Computers in Nursing* 3:77–84.

Salmon, M. E., and Vanderbush, P. 1990. Leadership and change in public and community health nursing today. In McCloskey, J. C., and Grace, H. K., editors. *Current issues in nursing.* 3d ed. St. Louis: C. V. Mosby Co.

Smith, G. R. July/August 1985. Unionization for nurses: An issue for the 1980's. *Journal of Professional Nursing* 1:192–201.

Sullivan, E. J., and Decker, P. J. 1988. *Effective management in nursing.* 2nd ed. Menlo Park, Calif.: Addison-Wesley Publishing Co.

Tappen, R. M. 1989. *Nursing leadership and management: Concepts and practice.* 2d ed. Philadelphia: F. A. Davis Co.

Teasley, D. November 1987. Situational leadership for nurses. *Nursing Management* 18:112–13.

Wilson, H., and Kniesl, C. R. 1988. *Psychiatric nursing.* 3d ed. Menlo Park, Calif.: Addison-Wesley Publishing Co.

Yura, H.; Ozimek, D.; and Walsh, M. B. 1981. *Nursing leadership: Theory and process.* New York: Appleton-Century-Crofts.

Healthy Aging

CONTENTS

THE ELDERLY CLIENT

The elderly client, for purposes of this book, is the person over 65 years of age. Because of advances in medical and related sciences and health promotion and protection, an increasing number of people are living to an advanced age. In 1960, life expectancy at birth was about 70 years; i.e., the average person born in 1960 could expect to live about 70 years. By 1987, life expectancy had increased to 71.5 years for males and 78.3 years for females (U.S. Bureau of the Census 1989 p. 71). Because of increasing life expectancy, it may be helpful to divide late adulthood into three periods: 65–74 years, the "young-old," 75–84 years, the "middle-old"; and 85 years and older, the "old-old."

The "young-old" refers to that group that is generally still independent and active. They may be working in a full- or part-time capacity, and often do not yet require a large number of dependent health services. The "middle-old" refers to that group that is usually experiencing one or more chronic health problems related to the aging process. They experience more difficulty with independent care and have a greater need for health and social services. The "old-old" are sometimes referred to as the frail elderly. This group is usually dependent on others for some or all of their care. The majority of residents of nursing homes or other extended care facilities are in this age group.

Gerontology, the study of all aspects of the aging process, includes biologic, psychologic, and sociologic fac-

TABLE 21-1   *Biologic Theories of Aging*

Biologic Theory	Description
Genetic theory	Aging results from biochemical changes programmed into the DNA molecule in each cell.
Immunologic slow virus theory	The immune system becomes less effective with age, and viruses that have incubated in the body become able to damage body organs.
Autoimmune theory	The production of autoimmune antibodies increases, and they attack the body cells.
Cross-link theory	As cells age, chemical reactions create strong bonds, especially in collagen tissues. These bonds cause loss of elasticity, stiffness, and eventual loss of function.
Stress theory	Aging results from cellular loss due to wear and tear on the body. Regeneration of body tissues eventually cannot keep pace with wear and tear, and the body is unable to maintain a stable internal environment.
Free-radical theory	Unstable free radicals (groups of atoms) result from the oxidation of organic materials, such as carbohydrates and proteins. These radicals cause biochemical changes in the cells, and the cells cannot regenerate themselves.
Program theory	The organism is capable of a predetermined number of cell divisions, after which the cells die.

tors. *Nursing gerontology* refers to the scientific study of the nursing care of the elderly (Yurick, Spier, Robb, and Ebert 1989, p. 5). Nursing practice that focuses on the care of the elderly requires basic nursing knowledge and skills combined with specialized knowledge of the diverse needs of the aging population.

In the past decade, workers in the field of gerontology have dedicated themselves with renewed enthusiasm to answering the question "Why do we age?" According to Hayflick (1988, p. 87), little progress has been made in providing an answer to this question. Hayflick suggests that "perhaps aging simply means that we are running short on reserve capacity" (1988, p. 77). More theories about the aging process have proliferated. Table 21–1 lists some of these well-known theories. Biologic theories of aging are either intrinsic or extrinsic. Extrinsic theory encompasses factors in the environment; intrinsic theory addresses factors within the body.

Physical Changes

As the person ages, a number of physical changes occur; some are visible, some are not.

Appearance   Obvious changes occur in the integument with age. A decrease in sebaceous gland activity, combined with the inability of the aged skin to retain fluid, results in dryness of the skin. Itching may increase because of dryness and the deterioration of nerve fibers and sensory endings. Lentigo senilus (brown "age

spots") commonly appear on the hands and arms and, in some instances, on the face. These are the result of the clustering of melanocytes. The skin also becomes paler and blotchy and loses its elasticity. Baldness and hair loss is thought to be due to the destruction of the tissue layer that produces hair follicles (Murray and Zentner 1989, p. 505). The loss of hair color is due to a decrease in the number of functioning pigment-producing cells. Fingernails and toenails become thickened and brittle, and in women over 60, facial hair increases.

The ways people respond to these changes vary among individuals and cultures. For example, one person may feel distinguished with gray hair, while another may feel embarrassed by it. Most women dislike their facial hair because hirsute women do not conform to the feminine cultural ideal of North Americans.

The integumentary changes accompany progressive losses of underlying adipose and muscle tissue, muscle atrophy, and loss of elastic fiber, creating a wrinkled and wasted appearance. Bony prominences become visible, a double chin develops, and lower eyelids appear puffy. In elderly women, the breasts become smaller and may sag; if large and pendulous, they may cause chafing where the skin surfaces touch. Loss of subcutaneous fat also decreases the elderly person's tolerance of cold.

Body Temperature   Body temperature is lower in the elderly adult because of a decrease in the metabolic rate. It is not uncommon for an elderly adult to have a temperature of 35 C (95 F), particularly in the early morning when the body's metabolism is low. Therefore, a temperature of 37.5 C (99.5 F) can represent a marked fever in some elderly people, although it represents only a mild fever in most young adults. It is important that the normal temperature of each individual person be known as a baseline for assessing changes.

The elderly client is more likely to experience hypothermia or hyperthermia. Hyperthermia may be manifested as either heat stroke or heat exhaustion. One of the body's normal compensating reactions to a fall in heat production is the contraction of the surface blood vessels and shivering. Because elderly adults have a diminished shivering reflex and do not produce as much body heat from metabolic processes, they tolerate prolonged exposure to cold poorly. At the other extreme, the body compensates for higher temperatures by slowing down muscular activity to produce less heat and by dilating surface blood vessels and sweating to increase losses of body heat. Older people, however, often have sluggish sweating and circulatory mechanisms and therefore cannot cope with heat as well as younger people. For example, they do not tolerate working in moderately high temperatures for prolonged periods. It is therefore important for the elderly adult to have a constant, comfortable environmental temperature. Many elderly persons who feel cold in rooms with a "normal" temperature wear extra clothes.

Sensory/Perceptual Changes

Changes in *vision* associated with aging include the obvious changes around the eye, such as the shrunken appearance of the eyes due to loss of orbital fat, the slowed blink reflex, and the looseness of the eyelids, particularly the lower lid, due to poorer muscle tone. Other changes result in loss of visual acuity, less power of adaptation to darkness and dim light, decrease in accommodation to near and far objects, loss of peripheral vision, and difficulty in discriminating similar colors. Visible changes in the eye include a loss of corneal luster, and arcus senilis, an opaque, white ring surrounding the cornea usually related to the deposit of fat granules in the cornea. The degenerative changes in the eyes beginning in middle age lead to the relative inflexibility of the lens, called *presbyopia*.

As the lens of the eye ages, it becomes more opaque and less elastic. By the age of 80 all elderly people have some lens opacity (cataracts) that reduces visual acuity and causes glare to be a problem. Surgical removal of cataracts is common at this age. Accompanying this are changes in the ciliary muscles, which control the shape of the lens. These changes reduce the power of the lens to adjust to near and far vision. The diameter of the pupil is reduced, and the amount of light entering the eye is thereby restricted. This slows the reaction time to decreases in light or illumination, a problem compounded at night with driving. Reduced blood supply due to arteriosclerosis can diminish retinal function. Reduced peripheral vision also is thought to be a result of arteriosclerosis.

The loss of *hearing* due to senescent change is called *presbycusis*. These changes begin in middle adulthood and continue through later life. Up to 40% of those over 65 years of age and up to 90% of those over 80 are hearing impaired (Lichtenstein, Bess, and Logan 1988, pp. 2875–78). Presbycusis comes about through changes in the structure of the inner ear: changes in nerve tissues in the inner ear and a thickening of the eardrum. Gradual loss of hearing is more common among men than women, perhaps because men are more frequently in noisy work environments. Hearing loss is usually greater in the left ear than the right and greater in the higher frequencies than the lower. Thus, older adults with hearing loss usually hear speakers with low, distinct voices best. Older adults may have more difficulty compensating for hearing loss than the young, who pay closer attention to the lip movements of the speaker. It is important that sensory/perceptual changes in vision and hearing not be misinterpreted as confusion or disorientation.

Older persons have a poorer sense of *taste and smell* and are less stimulated by food than the young. The number of taste buds in the tongue decreases, and the olfactory bulb (responsible for smell perception) at the base of the brain atrophies. Because taste and smell contribute significantly to appetite, decrease in these senses often results in poor nutrition in the elderly client. Additionally, problems may arise with overuse of salt and sugar as the client attempts to season foods because of altered taste sensations.

Loss of skin receptors takes place gradually, producing an increased threshold for *sensations of pain and touch*. The elderly person may not be able to distinguish hot from cold or the intensity of heat. Stimuli causing severe pain in a younger person may cause only minor sensation or pressure in the elderly.

Cardiopulmonary Changes

Respiratory efficiency is reduced with age. There is a decrease in vital capacity related to flattening of the diaphragm, atrophy of respiratory muscles, and skeletal changes, including calcification of costal cartilage and demineralization of bone resulting in kyphosis. The A-P diameter of the chest increases, causing a "barrel-chested" appearance. There is a greater volume of residual air left in the lungs after expiration and a decreased capacity to cough efficiently because of weaker expiratory muscles. Mucous secretions tend to collect more readily in the respiratory tree because of decreased ciliary activity. Thus, susceptibility to respiratory infections is notable in elderly adults.

Dyspnea occurs frequently with increased activity, such as running for a bus or carrying heavy parcels up stairs. This dyspnea occurs in response to an oxygen debt in the muscles. Intense exercise is followed by short, heavy, rapid breathing, which is an attempt to repay this oxygen debt in the muscles. Although this response is normal, it occurs more quickly in the aged because delivery and diffusion of oxygen to tissues is often diminished by changes in both respiratory and vascular tissues.

Blood pressure measurements often indicate a significant increase in systolic and a slight increase in diastolic pressures. This is a result of the inelasticity of the systemic arteries and an increase in peripheral resistance. There is an increased incidence of postural hypotension. There are no changes with age in the heart rate at normal rest. However, the heart rate of the aged person is slow to respond to stress and slow to return to normal after periods of physical activity.

The *working capacity of the heart* is diminished with age. This is particularly evident when increased demands are made on the heart muscles, such as during periods of exercise or emotional stress. The valves of the heart tend to become harder and less pliable, resulting in reduced filling and emptying abilities. In addition, the pumping action of the heart is reduced due to changes in the coronary (cardiac) arteries, which supply progressively smaller amounts of blood to the heart muscle. These changes are evidenced by shortness of breath on exertion and pooling of blood in the systemic veins. Electrocardiogram changes that occur as a result of the physiologic changes include atrial arrhythmias, bradycardia, bundle branch blocks, and extra systoles. When listening to heart sounds during physical examination, the nurse may hear systolic murmurs related to calcification of the mitral and aortic valves.

Changes in the *arteries* occur concurrently. The elasticity of smaller arteries is reduced by the thickening of their walls and increased calcium deposits in the muscular layer. Reduced arterial elasticity often results in diminished blood supply to, for instance, the legs and the brain, resulting in pain on exertion in the calf muscles (intermittent claudication) and dizziness, respectively.

Changes in Digestion

The digestive system is significantly less impaired by aging than are other body systems. Gradual decreases in digestive enzymes occur; examples are ptyalin in salivary secretions, which converts starch; pepsin and trypsin, which digest protein; and lipase, a fat-splitting enzyme.

There is also a decrease in the number of absorbing cells in the intestinal tract and a rise in gastric pH. These factors lower the absorption rate, slowing the absorption of nutrients and drugs. The muscle tone of the intestines also decreases, causing a decrease in peristalsis and elimination. These changes in muscle tone, digestive juices, and intestinal activity may lead to *indigestion, constipation,* and *malnutrition* in the older adult.

Changes in Urinary Elimination

The excretory function of the kidney diminishes with age, but usually not significantly below normal levels unless a disease process intervenes. Blood flow can be reduced by arteriosclerotic changes, impairing renal function. With age, the number of functioning nephrons (the basic functional units of the kidney) decreases to some degree, thus impairing the kidney's filtering abilities.

More noticeable changes are those related to the bladder. Complaints of urinary urgency, frequency, and dribbling in men are usually related to enlargement of the prostate. Elderly women complain of stress incontinence, frequency, and urgency, all resulting from weakened muscles supporting the bladder and the urethral sphincter. The capacity of the bladder and its ability to empty completely diminish with age. This explains *nocturnal frequency* and the *retention* of residual urine, predisposing the elderly adult to bladder infections.

Changes in Sexual Activity and Reproductive Organs

Sexual drives persist into the seventies, eighties, and nineties, provided that health is good and an interested partner is available. Interest in sexual activity in old age depends, in large measure, on interest in sexual activity earlier in life (Thienhaus 1988, p. 63). That is, people who are active in young and middle adulthood will remain active during their later years. However, sexual activity does become less frequent. Many factors may play a role in the ability of the elderly person to engage in sexual activity. For example, society does not look favorably on sexual feelings in the elderly. Physical problems such as diabetes, arthritis, and heart and respiratory conditions may also affect the elderly person's energy or physical ability to participate in sexual activity. In addition, several medications are known to impair sexual ability in men.

Degenerative changes in the gonads are very gradual in men. The testes can produce sperm well into old age, although there is a gradual decrease in the number of sperm produced. The production of testosterone is reduced, the prostate hypertrophies, and the penile arteries and veins sclerose. This results in a slowed erection and ejaculation and a decreased intensity of ejaculation. The penis decreases in size and the testicles hang lower in the scrotum. There is also thinning and graying of the pubic hair.

In women, the degenerative changes in the ovaries are characterized by the abrupt cessation of menses in middle age, during menopause. Changes in the gonads of elderly women result from diminished secretion of estrogen. Some changes, such as the shrinking of the uterus and ovaries, go unnoticed. The breasts atrophy, and the vagina narrows and shortens and its mucosa becomes thin, dry, and pale. Normal vaginal lubricating secretions are reduced, sometimes resulting in dyspareunia (painful intercourse), which often necessitates the use of lubricating jellies.

Neuromusculoskeletal Changes

With aging there is *gradual reduction in the speed and power of skeletal or voluntary muscle contractions*. The capacity for sustained muscular effort is also decreased. Great individual differences in muscular efficiency are apparent throughout life. Exercise can strengthen weakened muscles, and up to about age 50 the skeletal muscles can increase in bulk and density. After that time, there is a steady decrease in muscle fibers, ultimately leading to the typical wasted appearance of the very old person. Thus, elderly adults often complain about their lack of strength and how quickly they tire. Activities can still be carried out, but at a slower pace. Often balance is impaired with age. Prolonged muscular efforts may be sustained by older people provided they take judicious rest pauses and avoid capacity or peak performance.

A person's reaction time is slowed with age because of the diminished conduction speed of nerve fibers. Reaction time can be delayed further by decreased muscle tone as a result of diminished physical activity. Elderly people compensate for this reaction difference by being exceptionally cautious, for instance, in their driving habits, which exasperate some impatient younger drivers.

Slight loss in overall stature occurs with age due to atrophy of the discs between the spinal vertebrae. This can be exaggerated by muscular weakness resulting in a stooping posture and *kyphosis* (humpback of the upper spine). *Osteoporosis,* a decrease in bone density, along with increased brittleness of bone, makes the elderly adult prone to serious fractures, some of which are spontaneous. Since the incidence of osteoporosis is higher in elderly women, the effects of the menopause on the skeleton are being investigated. Causes of osteoporosis are thought to be lack of activity and inadequate calcium intake or inability to metabolize calcium.

Some degenerative joint changes occur, which make movement stiffer and more restricted. Stiffness is aggravated by inactivity; for example, if persons sit too long, their joints become stiff and they have difficulty standing and walking. A continuous program of physical activity and proper nutrition will slow bone density loss and decrease muscle atrophy and stiffness.

Psychosocial Development

A number of theories explain psychosocial aging. According to *disengagement theory,* aging involves mutual withdrawal (disengagement) between the older person and others in the elderly person's environment. This withdrawal relieves the elderly person of some of society's pressures and gradually reduces the number of people with whom the elderly person interacts. According to *activity theory,* the best way to age is to stay active physically and mentally, and according to *continuity theory,* people maintain their values, habits, and behavior in old age. A person who is accustomed to having people around will continue to do so, and the person who prefers not to be involved with others will more likely disengage. This theory accounts for the great variety of behavior seen in elderly people.

According to Erikson, the developmental task at this time is *ego integrity versus self-despair*. People who attain ego integrity view life with a sense of wholeness and derive satisfaction from past accomplishments. They view death as an acceptable completion of life. According to Erikson, people who develop integrity accept "one's one and only life cycle" (Erikson 1963, p. 263). By contrast, people who despair often believe they have made poor choices during life and wish they could live life over. Robert Butler sees integrity as bringing serenity and wisdom, and despair as resulting in the inability to accept one's fate. Despair gives rise to feelings of frustration, discouragement, and a sense that one's life has been worthless (Butler 1963, p. 65).

Acknowledging that the "young-old" and the "old-old" differ not only in physical characteristics but also in psychosocial responses, many people have difficulty with Erikson's singular developmental task. Peck (1968) proposes three developmental tasks of the older adult in contrast to Erikson's task of ego integrity versus despair. Kart, Metress, and Metress (1978, p. 180) further clarify these three tasks and suggest how they should be achieved. First, elderly people must establish new activities so that the loss of accustomed roles is less keenly felt. Second, they must select activities compatible with the physical limitations of old age. Third, individuals may make contributions that extend beyond their own lifetimes, thereby providing a meaning for life.

Havighurst (1974) has identified specific developmental tasks for the individual during later years, and Duvall (1977) has specified developmental tasks for the elderly family. There are many similarities between the two lists, and they are therefore integrated as follows:

- Making satisfactory living arrangements (Havighurst, Duvall)
- Establishing comfortable routines (Duvall)
- Adjusting to retirement and reduced income (Havighurst, Duvall)
- Maintaining love, sex, and marital arrangements (Duvall)
- Adjusting to decreasing physical strength and health (Havighurst)
- Safeguarding physical and mental health (Duvall)
- Remaining in touch with other family members (Duvall)
- Establishing an explicit affiliation with one's age group (Havighurst)
- Meeting civic and social obligations (Havighurst)
- Keeping active and involved (Duvall)
- Finding meaning in life (Duvall)
- Finding meaning in death (Duvall)
- Adjusting to the death of spouse (Havighurst)

Retirement   Today, a majority of the people over 65 are unemployed. Most industries and professions make retirement mandatory, although this policy is currently being questioned. Some who are self-employed continue to work as long as they are healthy. Work offers these people a better income, a sense of self-worth, and the chance to continue long-established routines. Some need to work for economic reasons.

Retirement can be a time when projects or recreational activities deferred for a long time can be pursued. Retired people are no longer governed by an alarm clock and can get up when they please. The enjoyment of staying up later is another luxury. Few elderly people, however, spend much time resting or sleeping. Being

accustomed to activity most of their lives, most elderly find many outlets, jobs, community projects, volunteer services, intellectual or recreational pursuits, or hobbies such as stamp collecting or fishing. Travel opportunities are expanding.

The life-style of later years is to a large degree formulated in youth. This fact was recognized by Robert Browning: "Grow old along with me! / The best is yet to be, / The last of life, for which the first was made." People who attempt suddenly to refocus and enrich their lives at retirement usually have difficulty. Those who learned early in life to live well-balanced and fulfilling lives are generally more successful in retirement. The woman who has been concerned only with the accomplishments of her children or the man who has been concerned only with the paycheck and his job status can be left with a feeling of emptiness when children leave and the job no longer exists. The later years can foster a sense of integrity and continuity, or they can be years of despair.

Economic Change   The financial needs of elderly people vary considerably. Though most need less money for clothing, entertainment, and work, and although some own their homes outright, costs continue to rise, making it difficult for some to manage. Food and medical costs alone are often a financial burden. When older people speak about their greatest need, often it is not happiness or health, but money. Money allows them to be independent and look after themselves.

Problems with income are often related to low retirement benefits, lack of pension plans for many workers, and the increased length of the retirement years. Elderly members of minority groups have greater financial problems than elderly whites. Elderly women of all ages have lower incomes than men, and the oldest women are the poorest. Women, as a group, receive less from pensions, less from income, and less from government sources (Yurick, Spier, Robb, and Ebert 1989, p. 304–5).

Nurses should be aware of the costs of health care. For example, while assisting a client to plan a diet, the nurse must consider which foods the client can afford to buy. The nurse or the client can request the physician to order lower-priced medications. In addition, the supplies used in a client's care should be as economical as possible.

Relocation   During late adulthood, many people experience relocation. A variety of factors may lead to this decision. The house or apartment may be too large or too expensive. The work involved in maintaining the house may become burdensome or impossible for the aged person or couple. Some elderly persons with decreased mobility want living arrangements that are all on one floor or need more accessible bathroom facilities.

Making the decision to move is often a very stressful one. The elderly person may be moving to an apartment, which may mean leaving the comfort of the family home and the neighbors and friends of several decades. Some need to move nearer to their children for general support and supervision. For many, this decision is difficult and stressful. For others, relocation is voluntary. The person may be seeking a more moderate climate with better recreational facilities geared to a more leisurely life-style. Adjustment will be much easier for the elderly person making a voluntary move.

A small percentage of the elderly, between 5% and 7%, must relocate to long-term care facilities or nursing homes. The decision to enter a nursing home is frequently made when elderly persons can no longer care for themselves, often because of problems of mobility and memory impairment. An increasing number of nursing home residents are in the very old age group (85 years and over), and most are women (Fulmer 1988, p. 544).

The facilities in nursing homes differ in many ways and offer varying degrees of independence to the residents. All provide meals but vary in giving other services, such as assistance with hygiene and dressing, physical therapy or exercise, recreational activities, transportation services, and medical and nursing supervision.

Between independent living arrangements in private homes or apartments and dependent care in nursing homes are a variety of residential options that are being utilized to house and care for the elderly. Some of these programs are more successful than others. The options include multigenerational residences, shared housing, adult congregate living facilities (ACLFs), domiciliary care, foster care, and boarding homes. In *multigenerational residences,* families share their homes with elderly relatives or nonrelated elders. A large number of elderly are living with adult children and their families. *Shared housing* matches older persons who own their own single-family residence with elderly persons who are looking for independent housing arrangements. The benefits are mutual as the elderly residents of shared housing share expenses and provide each other mutual support. *Adult congregate living facilities* (ACLFs) or *domiciliary care* are homes that provide structured support services in a noninstitutional setting. *Foster care* provides housing for the elderly client in a family setting that provides support in shared family activites, meals, and household tasks. The elderly resident may be totally independent or slightly disabled. Often, the elderly person assists in the supervision of children after school before the parents get home from work. *Boarding home care* provides the elderly resident with a room, meals, and communal living with others who are usually also elderly. There are similarities between foster care and boarding home care depending on the geographic location and the specific functional abilities of the elderly resident. Housing decisions for the elderly should be a collaborative decision between the client, his family, and the health care professional. Criteria for appropriate placement are usually based on the client's wishes, with the goal of promoting independence consistent with his functional ability.

Nurses in hospitals should find out whether a client is being discharged to a nursing home, to home, or to some other housing arrangement. Many nursing homes provide nursing services to clients and require appropriate information to provide for continuity of care. Clients returning home or to another facility, however, may require the assistance of a home care nurse.

Facing Death and Grieving   Well-adjusted aging couples usually thrive on companionship. Many couples rely increasingly on their mates for this company and may have few outside friends. Great bonds of affection and closeness can develop during this period of aging together and nurturing each other. When a mate dies, the remaining partner inevitably experiences feelings of loss, emptiness, and loneliness. Many are capable and manage to live alone; however, reliance on younger family members increases as age advances and ill health occurs. Some widows and widowers remarry, particularly the latter, because widowers are less inclined than widows to maintain a household.

Women face bereavement and solitude more often than men, since women usually live longer. The brevity of life is constantly reinforced by the death of friends. It is a time when one's life is reviewed with happiness or regret. Feelings of serenity or guilt and inadequacy can arise. Independence established prior to loss of a mate makes this adjustment period easier. A person who has some meaningful friendships, economic security, ongoing interests in the community, or private hobbies and a peaceful philosophy of life copes more easily with bereavement. Successful relationships with children and grandchildren are also of inestimable value. Facing death is discussed in Chapter 27.

Nurses can sometimes help clients who are alone a great deal to adjust their living arrangements or life-style so that they have more companionship. Moving to a retirement home that has other people in similar circumstances and organized social activities is one example. Many communities provide social centers for the elderly, for example, drop-in centers or community centers that offer day trips for seniors. Nurses can refer clients to services and encourage them to obtain companionship.

Cognitive Development

Piaget's phases of cognitive development end with the formal operations phase. However, considerable research on cognitive abilities and aging is currently being conducted. Researchers generally believe that there is minimal change in intellectual capacity of the healthy aging person (Murray and Zentner 1989, p. 519).

Intellectual capacity includes perception, cognitive agility, memory, and learning. *Perception,* or the ability to interpret the environment, depends on the acuteness of the senses. If the aging person's senses are impaired, the ability to perceive the environment and react appropriately is diminished. Perceptual capacity may be affected by changes in the nervous system as well. Cognitive ability, or the ability to know, is related to perceptual ability. An older man, for example, may know that he will be retiring next year but be unable to plan for retirement. He cannot accept the knowledge psychologically because his work provides his sense of worth, self-esteem, and identity.

Changes in cognitive structures occur as a person ages. It is believed that there is progressive loss of neurons. In addition, blood flow to the brain decreases, the meninges appear to thicken, and brain metabolism slows. Experts do not agree whether the brain decreases in weight with age, although it is thought that the brain loses about 7% of its mass by 80 years of age (Murray and Zentner 1989, p. 505). As yet, little is known about the effect of these physical changes on the cognitive functioning of the older adult. Neurofibrillary tangles have been found in the hippocampal cortex, the area of the brain concerned with memory. Neuritic plaques are also found in the aging brain. Neurofibrillary tangles and neuritic plaques could account for some of the functional changes found in normal aging people.

Memory is also a component of intellectual capacity and is closely related to learning. The three-stage memory model divides memory into the sensory, primary, and secondary stages. Sensory memory is the momentary perception of stimuli by the senses. Information from the senses is then stored temporarily in the memory stores (e.g., visual information is stored in visual memory). Some of this information is then passed into primary memory. Primary memory, or short-term memory, is what one has in mind at a given moment. For information to be retained, it must enter secondary memory. Secondary memory, or long-term memory, contains all the information one knows, from minutes to years.

Research regarding the effects of aging on human memory has been carried out over the last several decades. These studies generally agree that despite age-related changes in the sensory organs, visual or auditory memory does not substantially decline with age (Ciocon and Potter 1988, p. 43). It is believed, however, that the elderly are able to remember information better when it is presented visually. Primary memory, which includes the ability both to retain and to retrieve information, is also considered to remain substantially unchanged with age. Secondary memory, however, is reported to decline with age. Older people have some impairment in their ability to enter new information into secondary memory; once it has been entered into secondary memory, moreover, they have some difficulty in bringing the information out of memory stores [Ciocon and Potter 1988, p. 45).

Older people need additional time for learning, largely because of the problem of retrieving information. Motivation is also important. Older adults have more difficulty than younger ones in learning information they do not consider meaningful. It is suggested that the older person remain mentally active to maintain cognitive ability at the highest possible level. Lifelong mental activity, particularly verbal activity, helps the older person retain a high level of cognitive function and may help maintain long-term memory. Cognitive impairment that interferes with normal life is not considered part of normal aging. A decline in intellectual abilities that interferes with social or occupational functions should always be regarded as abnormal. Family members should be advised to seek prompt medical evaluation.

Dementia   *Dementia* is a decline in memory and other cognitive abilities, in comparison to the individual's performance in the past. The onset of dementia is slow and is often denied or hidden by the client and family members. Some dementias, such as those caused by depression, infection, or thyroid disturbance, are reversible if treated promptly. The return of cognitive function for the person with a reversible dementia depends on prompt diagnosis and treatment. The large majority of older persons diagnosed with dementia will be found to have irreversible brain disease. The most common type of irreversible dementia in old age is *Alzheimer's disease* (AD), which accounts for 60% to 70% of all the cases. Other common types include multi-infarct dementia (10%), caused by repeated strokes, and Parkinson's disease (5%) (Rowe and Besdine 1988, pp. 377–81).

Dementia is recognized as a major public health problem in the United States, affecting approximately 5% of the population from 65 to 74 years of age, and more than 30% of those over age 80. Of the elderly residing in the community, 10% experience intellectual impairment; in the nursing home population, between 50% and 75% of the clients are affected with cognitive impairment that is thought to be dementia of the Alzheimer type (Rowe and Besdine 1988, pp. 377–81).

Alzheimer's disease affects about 3 million people in the United States. By the year 2030, that number is expected to rise to nearly 5 million. The monetary cost of care for AD clients is estimated at $30 billion annually in the United States. The symptoms of AD have been grouped into three or four stages and may vary somewhat from client to client. The most prominent symptoms are cognitive dysfunctions, including decline in memory, learning, attention, judgment, orientation, and language skills. The symptoms are progressive, and all victims experience a steady decline in cognitive and physical abilities, lasting between 7 and 15 years and ending in death. In the last stage, the client requires total assistance, is unable to communicate, is incontinent, and may be unable to walk.

Although several theories are being investigated, the cause of AD is not known. Some of the causative theories include accumulation of aluminum deposits in the neurons, changes in the immune system, active and latent viruses, and defects in the neurotransmitter system. Currently, definite diagnosis can be made only on autopsy, where the physical changes specific to AD can be validated. Scanning techniques, such as PET (positron emission tomography) and MRI (magnetic resonance imaging) are currently aiding physicians in following the clinical progression of AD. Recently, a protein designated A68 has been detected in the brain of AD victims and from the spinal fluid of AD clients. In addition, A68 is also associated with neurofibrillary tangles. If the results of further studies on A68 support these initial findings, a routine laboratory test could be developed that makes early and accurate diagnosis of AD possible.

There is no cure or specific treatment for AD. Several drugs have been developed, but none has been shown consistently to retard or reverse the progression of the disease. It is hoped that one experimental drug, tetrahydroaminocridine (THA), will allow the brain cells to function more efficiently, thereby improving cognitive function. Research is currently under way.

It is estimated that about one million people with AD are cared for in the home. The burden of care is frequently on women—wives and daughters—who are themselves aging. It has frequently been observed that "Alzheimer's causes more damage to the family than any other disease" (Burggraf and Stanley 1989, pp. 332–33). The nurse's responsibility is to provide supportive nursing care, accurate information, and referral assistance, if placement in a nursing care facility becomes necessary.

Moral Development

According to Kohlberg, moral development is completed in the early adult years. Most old people stay at Kohlberg's conventional level of moral development (see Chapter 11), and some are at the preconventional level. An elderly person at the preconventional level obeys rules to avoid pain and the displeasure of others. At stage 1, a person defines good and bad in relation to self, whereas older persons at stage 2 may act to meet another's needs as well as their own. Elderly people at the conventional level follow society's rules of conduct in response to the expectations of others. They value conformity, loyalty, and social order (Edelman and Mandle 1986, p. 548).

Rybash, Roodin, and Hoyer studied the kinds of moral problems elderly people face. These researchers found that the moral concerns of the elderly are more interpersonal than social or legalistic. For example, an elderly man is more likely to be concerned with the moral problems involving a member of his family than with the moral problems posed by his occupation or a friend's extramarital affair (Rybash, Roodin, and Hoyer 1983, p. 253).

Spiritual Development

Murray and Zentner (1989, p. 525) write that the elderly person with a mature religious outlook strives to incorporate views of theology and religious action into thinking. Elderly people can contemplate new religious and philosophical views and try to understand ideas missed previously or interpreted differently. The elderly person also derives a sense of worth by sharing experiences or views. In contrast, the elderly person who has not matured spiritually may feel impoverishment or despair as the drive for economic and professional success wanes.

The older person's knowledge becomes wisdom, an inner resource for dealing with both positive and negative life experiences. Many elderly persons have strong religious convictions and continue to attend church services. Involvement in religion often helps the elderly person to resolve issues related to the meaning of life, to adversity, or to good fortune (Yurick, Spier, Robb, and Ebert 1989, p. 207). The "old-old" person who cannot attend formal services often continues religious participation in a more private manner. Many elderly persons watch television evangelists and some, being vulnerable to fund raising ventures, send money that they can ill afford to spare to these organizations.

According to Fowler and Keen (1985), some people enter the sixth stage of spiritual development, *universalizing*. People whose spiritual development reaches this level think and act in a way that exemplifies love and justice.

HEALTH PROMOTION AND PROTECTION

Guidelines for assessment of growth and development of the older adult are shown in the box below. Assessment activities may include measurement of weight, height, and vital signs; observation of the skin for hydration status or presence of lesions; examination of visual acuity using the Snellen chart; examination of hearing acuity using the whisper, Weber, and Rinne tests; and questions about the following:

ASSESSMENT GUIDELINES
The Older Adult

Does the older adult:

- Adjust to the physiologic changes related to aging?
- Manage retirement years in a satisfying manner?
- Have satisfactory living arrangements and income to meet changing needs?
- Participate in social and leisure activities?
- Have a social network of friends and support persons?
- View life as worthwhile?
- Have high self-esteem?
- Have the abilities to care for self or to secure appropriate help?
- Gain support from value system or spiritual philosophy?
- Adapt life-style to diminishing energy and ability?
- Accept and adjust to the death of significant others?

- Usual dietary pattern
- Any problems with bowel or urinary elimination
- Activity/exercise and sleep/rest patterns
- Family and social activities and interests
- Any problems with reading, writing, or problem solving
- Adjustment to retirement or loss of partner

According to recent research, much of the decline in health that was previously considered to be due to "old age" is due to chronic illnesses resulting from unhealthy life-styles and poor health habits rather than aging itself (Smith 1988, p. 48). To retard the aging process, the older person must learn self-care techniques related to health promotion and disease prevention. Studies indicate that older persons are concerned about their health and are interested in information and behavioral strategies directed toward improving it (Smith 1988, p. 48). To assist the older adult in promoting health, the nurse may wish to discuss some or all of the following topics.

Health Maintenance Visits and Immunization

The older adult should have routine health assessments that may involve a yearly physical examination including a urinalysis and stool test for occult blood, yearly visual examination, audiometry if hearing ability is at risk, yearly dental assessment, yearly mammogram, Pap test every year if in high-risk group or every 3 years if not, and yearly testicular and prostate examination. Some physicians may also recommend a sigmoidoscopy every 5 years and certain blood tests (e.g., blood lipids) on a regular basis.

The older adult should receive a diphtheria and tetanus booster every 10 years; for those at risk for hepatitis, hepatitis B vaccine is also recommended. Clients with a history of chronic respiratory or cardiac disease are usually encouraged to receive immunizations against pneumococcal pneumonia and influenza.

Safety

Accident prevention is a major concern for elderly people. Because vision is limited, reflexes are slowed, and bones are brittle, climbing stairs, driving a car, and even walking require caution. Driving, particularly night driving, requires caution because accommodation of the eye to light is impaired and peripheral vision is diminished. Older persons need to learn to turn the head before changing lanes and should not rely on side vision, for example, when crossing a street. Driving in fog or other hazardous conditions should be avoided.

Fires are a hazard for the elderly person with a failing memory. The older person may forget that the iron or stove is left on or may not extinguish a cigarette completely. Because of reduced sensitivity to pain and heat, care must be taken to prevent burns when the person bathes or uses heating devices.

Many elderly persons suffer and die each year from hypothermia. A lowered metabolism and loss of normal insulation from thinning subcutaneous tissue decrease the elderly client's ability to retain heat. Health promotion should focus on teaching the elderly client to

- Dress warmly with layered clothing and protect head and hands when going outdoors in cold weather

- Use extra blankets at night and keep feet warm with woolen socks, which are safer than hot-water bottles

- Eat a balanced diet, including high-energy foods such as fats and carbohydrates

- Learn to monitor the household thermostat and be sure that adequate home heating fuel is available

Because older clients who take analgesics or sedatives may become lethargic or confused, they should be monitored regularly and closely. Other measures to induce sleep should be used whenever possible. Nurses can help elderly clients make the home environment safe. Specific hazards can be identified and corrected; e.g., hand rails can be installed on staircases. The nurse teaches the importance of taking only prescribed medications and contacting a health professional at the first indication of intolerance to them.

Guidelines for accident prevention for the older adult are detailed in the box on the following page.

Nutrition

The older adult requires the same basic nutrition as the younger adult. However, fewer calories are needed by the older adult because of the lower metabolic rate and the decrease in physical activity. The older adult should consume about 1200 calories per day. This figure may vary for each person according to the level of individual activity.

A major problem of the elderly is the loss of teeth due to poor dental care and periodontal disease. Poorly fitting dentures may also be a concern. These factors coupled with a decrease in salivation may cause difficulty in chewing and limit the type of food the older person can eat. As a result, the older person may avoid foods that require extensive chewing, such as meats or fresh fruits, and nutritional deficiencies may result.

A decrease in the thirst sensation, combined with a self-imposed limitation of fluids to compensate for incontinence, may result in an inadequate intake of fluids in elderly clients. The nurse should instruct the older adult that about 8 glasses of water a day is needed to maintain kidney function, soften stools, prevent dehydration, and moisturize skin.

Common problems related to diet include undernutrition and overnutrition. Undernutrition may result from a variety of physical and psychosocial factors. The elderly client may be eating empty calories rather than nutritious food, eating alone, or suffering from chronic diseases that affect food intake and metabolism, such as malignant disorders, alcoholism, or depression. Elderly clients frequently have dietary deficiencies of vitamins A, B, and C and iron. In the United States, 40% of the people over 60 years of age suffer from iron deficiency anemia from insufficient iron intake and poor absorption and utilization of iron (Schuster and Ashburn 1986, p. 808). The nurse should assess the dietary habits of the elderly client and ascertain that intake of foods rich in these vitamins is adequate.

Decreased exposure to sunlight and changes in the intestines and liver that interfere with metabolism are thought to contribute to vitamin D deficiency and bone disorders. Osteomalacia is marked by "softening of the bones," which become bent and deformed. Osteoporosis causes bones to become porous and less dense, resulting in an increased susceptibility to fracture and collapse (Andreasen and Conley 1987, p. 176). To prevent these problems, the nurse must take special care to ensure that older adults ingest sufficient amounts of vitamin D and calcium. Outdoor activities should also be encouraged to increase exposure to sunlight, a natural source of vitamin D, as well as to enhance overall well-being.

Overnutrition may result from lifelong eating patterns coupled with a lack of exercise. Retirement from work or problems with mobility due to chronic disease may also compound the problem. Other reasons cited for overeating include past habits, occupation, anxiety or nervousness, difficult life situations, mental illness, glandular imbalance, and grief or loss (Saxon and Etten 1987, pp. 195–96). Overeating may lead to chronic illness such as heart disease, high blood pressure, arteriosclerosis, and diabetes.

Guidelines for promoting nutritional health of older adults include the following:

- Encourage regular visits to the dentist to have dentures repaired or replaced to ensure chewing ability.

Accident Prevention for the Older Adult

Preventing falls:

- Make sure all rooms, hallways, and stairwells are adequately lit.
- Have an easily accessible light switch next to the bed.
- Leave a night light on in the hallway or bathroom.
- Get out of bed slowly, i.e., sit before standing and stand briefly before walking, to prevent dizziness from orthostatic hypotension.
- Install grab bars in the bathroom near the toilet and tub.
- Make sure rugs and carpets are firmly attached to floors and stairs.
- Make sure that electrical cords are secured against baseboards to prevent tripping.
- Keep indoor and outdoor walkways and stairs in good repair.
- Install sturdy slip-resistant hand railings along stairs.

Preventing burns:

- Check the temperature of bath water and heating pads. Run cold water before hot water.
- Lower thermostats of water heaters to provide warm rather than very hot water.
- Avoid smoking in bed or when sleepy.
- Install smoke alarms.
- Place a hand fire extinguisher in a convenient area of the home, e.g., the kitchen.
- Smother kitchen grease fires with a large lid or baking soda.
- Avoid wearing loose-fitting clothing when cooking.
- Do not overload electric circuits and keep electrical appliances in good repair.
- Keep passageways to outside doors unobstructed.

Preventing pedestrian accidents:

- Wear reflective or light-colored clothing at night.

- Cross streets at intersections with cross walks and traffic lights when possible; do not cross major streets in the middle of the block.
- Be sure to look both ways before stepping from the curb.

Preventing automobile accidents:

- Have regular eye examinations to assess vision, acquire appropriate refractive corrections, and detect other problems early.
- Wear good-quality gray or green sunglasses during daytime driving to reduce glare.
- Keep car windows clean and windshield wipers in good condition.
- Place mirrors on both sides of the car and always check rearview and side mirrors before changing lanes.
- Always look behind your vehicle for people or obstacles before backing up.
- Avoid smoking when driving, especially at night. Smoke can reduce visibility.
- Follow your physician's restrictions, if any, about when and where to drive.
- Learn the effects of prescribed medications on driving ability.
- Do not drink and drive.
- Stop periodically to stretch your muscles and rest your eyes.
- Leave car windows partially open and set the radio and fans low so that you can hear sirens and horns.
- Have your ability to drive periodically re-evaluated.
- Keep your automobile in good repair and keep headlights, tail lights, and turn signals clean so they are visible to others.

- Advise having several small meals per day and smaller portions of all foods.

- Encourage use of leaner cuts of meat and broiling or baking foods instead of frying them.

- Advise substituting fruit for rich pastry and using low-fat milk and cheese.

- Encourage the client to take an interest in food preparation and serving for themselves or their spouses.

- Review diet restrictions, and find ways to make meals appealing within these guidelines.

- Discuss the food budget of the elderly client, and suggest more economical and nutritious choices, if appropriate.

- If food preparation is not possible for the older client, suggest community resources such as Meals on Wheels.

Elimination

Constipation is a common problem in the elderly population. Many elderly believe that "regularity" means a bowel movement every day. Those who do not meet this criterion often seek over-the-counter preparations to relieve what they believe to be constipation. Elderly clients should be advised that normal patterns of bowel elimination vary considerably. Normal for some may be every other day, for others twice a day. Adequate roughage in the diet, adequate exercise, and 6 to 8 glasses of fluid daily are essential preventive measures for constipation. A cup of hot water or tea at a regular time in the morning is helpful for some. Responding to the gastrocolic reflex is also an important consideration.

The older adult should be warned that consistent use of over-the-counter preparations is thought to cause rather than cure constipation. In a few cases, moreover, they can cause serious problems such as appendicitis. Laxatives may also interfere with the body's electrolyte balance and decrease the absorption of certain vitamins. The reasons for constipation can range from life-style habits to serious malignant disorders. The nurse should evaluate any complaints of constipation carefully for each individual. A change in bowel habits over several weeks with or without weight loss, pain, or fever should be referred to a physician for a complete medical evaluation.

A decline in bladder capacity, plus weaker muscle tone, results in an increase in frequency as well as urgency in many older persons. The nurse should be aware of these changes and teach the elderly person appropriate strategies to prevent embarrassment due to incontinence. Toilet facilities should be accessible, and elderly persons should be instructed to give themselves enough time to get to the bathroom and remove their clothing. Bladder training exercises as well as a regular toilet schedule may also be helpful adjuncts.

Many older people learn to deal with nocturnal frequency by restricting their fluid intake in the latter part of the evening, particularly those fluids that stimulate voiding, such as coffee or alcohol. Eventually most men require prostatic surgery to relieve increasing urinary frequency throughout the day, and some women require vaginal surgery for cystoceles or rectoceles. Both of these conditions produce pressure and reduce bladder capacity, thereby creating urinary urgency and frequency.

Weakness in muscle tone in the ureters and bladder also increases the elderly person's risk for urinary tract infections (UTI). Preventive measures, such as increasing fluid intake, including juices that produce an acid ash such as cranberry juice, and preventing contamination of the urinary tract should be included in the teaching plan. Elderly clients should seek medical evaluation for any of the symptoms of UTI (e.g., burning on urination, frequency, and sometimes fever).

Activity and Exercise

A regular program of moderate exercise is recommended for elderly adults. Walking, golfing, gardening, bowling, and bicycling are common activities. These can be performed at a leisurely pace. It is important that exercise not be too strenuous and that rest periods be taken as needed. Rapid breathing and accelerated heartbeat should disappear within a few minutes after exercise; exercise should refresh rather than fatigue. People who are too disabled to engage in active exercise can implement a program of isometric exercises to maintain joint mobility and muscle tone.

Perhaps the most significant physical benefit of regular exercise for the older adult is a decrease in the risk for cardiovascular disease. In addition, exercise maintains bone calcification, helps to maintain muscle tone throughout the body, and reduces muscle tension and muscle pain.

The nurse should suggest some safety precautions for the elderly client beginning an exercise program. These include (1) wearing proper shoes with nonstick soles; (2) avoiding slick surfaces; (3) exercising or walking in safe, well-lighted areas; (4) being aware of adverse symptoms of exercise, such as dizziness, shortness of breath, or irregular heartbeat; and (5) beginning any exercise program slowly to allow the body time to adjust.

RESEARCH NOTE

Does Walking Reduce Fatigue?

The researchers involved in this study wanted to determine whether a short outdoor walk would be beneficial to the ambulatory nursing home resident. Although the answer would at first seem obvious, the authors found that some ambulatory elderly individuals living in nursing homes walk less frequently than their counterparts of comparable age and health status living in retirement villages. In fact, an alarming 81% of the sample surveyed reported that they had never walked outside. Most of the nursing home residents who went outside sat in rockers on the porch.

Thirty-two ambulatory and mentally alert individuals 60 to 93 years of age participated in the study. Subjects in Group A (16 patients) were residents of a nursing home. Group B comprised 16 individuals of similar age and health state residing in a retirement village nearby. Within each group, some subjects were assigned a walking protocol, while others simply continued their normal routines.

The findings revealed several significant differences between the groups. The nursing home residents who participated in the walking regimen reported significantly lower fatigue scores at the end of three weeks. The nursing home residents in the nonwalking group actually reported an increased feeling of fatigue. The fatigue scores of the walking and nonwalking groups at the retirement village were not very different, since daily outdoor walking was already a part of their usual routine.

The researchers acknowledge that the sample size was small. Yet, they feel it is conclusive that the nursing home residents who participated in the three-week walking regimen felt significantly less fatigued than both their counterparts in the retirement village and those in the groups that did not walk.

Implications: When health status and safety conditions permit, regular outdoor walking should be instituted as a standard intervention for all nursing home residents who are ambulatory, even if walkers or canes are necessary.

S. H. Gueldner and J. Spradley. Outdoor walking lowers fatigue, *Journal of Gerontological Nursing,* October 1988, 14:6–12.

Some physicians may recommend an exercise stress test to determine the type and intensity of exercise program that is best for the individual client. During a stress test, blood pressure and heart rhythm are continuously monitored while the client exercises, either on a treadmill or on a bicycle.

Rest and Sleep   The aging process affects the length of sleep, distribution of sleep throughout a 24-hour period, and the sleep stage patterns (Schuster and Ashburn 1986, p. 510). Elderly adults tend to take somewhat longer to get to sleep, wake up frequently during the night, stay in bed longer to make up for missed sleep, and wake up feeling tired. The amount of deep sleep (Stage IV), as well as REM sleep, also decreases, compounding feelings of fatigue. The amount of sleep needed by the elderly client varies. In general, most healthy older adults require about the same amount of sleep as they did during the middle adult years.

Elderly clients who complain of insomnia or difficulty sleeping at night should have a thorough assessment of their activities during the day, including exercise, naps, television time, social activities, meals, and snacks. For many elderly retired this assessment may reveal several periods of dozing or napping, especially when watching television. An adjustment of the client's daily schedule to increase periods of activity—whether social, recreational, or exercise—and to decrease sedentary times, may help the client achieve a longer sleep period during the nighttime hours. Encouraging usual bedtime rituals such as reading before bed, drinking a glass of milk, or a soothing bath may also enhance nighttime sleep. A medication assessment may suggest that the client's use of prescribed or over-the-counter drugs are interfering with nighttime sleep, thus indicating the need for an adjustment in the medication schedule.

Maintaining Independence and Self-Esteem

Most elderly people thrive on independence. It is important to them to be able to look after themselves even if they have to struggle to do so. Although it may be difficult for younger family members to watch the elder completing tasks in a slow, determined way, aging persons need this sense of accomplishment. Children might notice that the aging father or mother with failing vision cannot keep the kitchen as clean as before. The aging father and mother may be slower and less meticulous in carpentry tasks or gardening. To maintain the elderly adult's sense of self-respect, nurses and family members need to encourage them to do as much as possible for themselves, provided that safety is maintained. Many young people err in thinking that they are helpful to older people when they take over for them and do the job much faster and more efficiently.

Aging people need to be recognized for their unique individual characteristics. It can be difficult to recognize these differences, since elderly people have less energy than the young to show how they are different. Perhaps this is one reason elderly people tend to talk about past accomplishments, jobs, deeds, and experiences.

Nurses need to acknowledge the elderly client's ability to think, reason, and make decisions. Most elderly people are willing to listen to suggestions and advice, but they do not want to be ordered around. The nurse can support a decision by an elderly client even if eventually the decision is reversed because of failing health.

Older people appreciate thoughtfulness, consideration, and acceptance of their waning abilities. For example, having dinner out in a well-lighted restaurant or not expecting grandmother to babysit for too many hours, if at all, are actions that recognize the diminished vision and energy of older people. The values and standards held by older people need to be accepted, whether they are related to ethical, religious, or household matters.

Elder Abuse

Older adults who are unable to care for themselves are often cared for by family members, usually a daughter or spouse. Caring for a spouse or a parent often causes a great deal of strain and frustration in a relationship and may lead to violence and abuse. It is estimated that over one million elderly Americans are abused annually. The victims of abuse are likely to be white, female, and over 70 years of age. In addition, most victims of abuse are afflicted with substantial mental or physical impairments.

The types of abuse used against the elder include (1) psychologic abuse, such as yelling and screaming; (2) physical abuse, such as hitting, slapping, or restraining for long periods of time; (3) financial abuse, such as taking the older adults' money or forcing them to sign over their assets; and (4) neglect, such as withholding food, medication, or basic care.

The perpetrator of abuse is usually the spouse or the child of the victim. Caregivers who abuse their elderly family members are often middle-aged or older or have emotional problems such as alcoholism; in some cases,

three or four generations may be sharing living quarters. Caregivers are often placed in the stressful situation of administering care to parents who treat them like children. Many elderly people use guilt to control their children's lives and do not give them the privacy and respect that they need. The cost of medical care may also be a burden for the caregiver, as well as the stress involved in 24-hour responsibility for another person.

To prevent abuse, the nurse should spend time counseling families prior to their making the decision to care for their elderly parent. The nurse should also be aware that ongoing support is needed for the caregiver as well as for the elderly client. Frequent visits should be made to the home of an elderly client to assess the home situation for factors that may lead to an abusive situation. The elderly in general are unwilling and/or often unable to report abuse. They may feel guilty that they have raised a child who has mistreated them, or they may feel that they have no other place to go. In some cases, the abused persons may be cognitively impaired and unable to advocate in their own behalf.

The nurse who suspects an abusive situation has an obligation to report it. Nurses should be familiar with the laws of their particular state regarding reporting of suspected or known abuse. The legally competent adult cannot be forced, however, to leave the abusive situation and in many cases may decide to stay. If the elderly client is not legally competent, court proceedings to attain guardianship can be initiated.

Drug Use and Misuse

When those who are now elderly were growing up, few pills or other cures were available to treat physical or emotional problems. In the past several decades, however, major progress has been made in the pharmaceutical industry. As a result, hundreds of prescription and nonprescription drugs are available to the public. Elderly adults frequently suffer from one or more chronic diseases that often require medication. Episodes of acute illness may require additional medications. The complexities involved in the self-administration of medication may lead to a variety of misuse situations, including taking too much or too little medication, combining alcohol and medication, combining prescribed medications with over-the-counter drugs, taking medications at the wrong time, or taking someone else's medication. Other potential misuse situations occur when elderly people have more than one physician prescribing medications and fail to tell each doctor what has been previously prescribed.

It is important for the nurse to remember that there are significant changes in the pharmacodynamics of drugs in the elderly. Absorption, distribution, metabolism, and excretion of drugs are all delayed. This contributes to a potential increase in drug effect that may result in symptoms of drug overdose as well as an increase in drug-drug interactions and drug-nutrient interactions. To prevent drug misuse, the nurse should assess the drug history of the elderly person carefully and determine a realistic teaching plan.

Elderly clients should be given written instructions, in large print and in language that they can understand. In addition, the side effects of each drug should be listed and reviewed with the client. In simple terms, elderly clients should be taught the importance of maintaining a schedule for important medications (e.g., digitoxin, insulin) and the risks involved in skipping a dose or "running out" of pills. Forgetful persons may need to use a pill organizer to ensure accurate medication ingestion. The nurse should also discuss any over-the-counter drugs the elderly client may use and explain potential risks and side effects of self-medication and multiple medications. In some cases, the nurse can offer conservative measures, such as relaxation techniques or soothing baths, to replace tranquilizers or pain medications. Health promotion activities, such as diet and exercise, may also be helpful adjuncts to reduce the need for medications for chronic disease.

Alcoholism

The estimates of alcohol abuse among elderly Americans vary from 5% to 20% of the population (Burnside 1988, p. 1009). In general, people tend to consume less alcohol as they get older. Elderly alcoholics include those who began drinking alcohol in their youth and those who began excessive alcohol use later in life. Alcoholics who begin drinking later in life do so to help them cope with the changes and problem of their older years. Many late-onset alcoholics are widowers.

Chronic drinking has major effects on all body systems, causes progressive liver and kidney damage, damages the stomach and related organs, and slows mental response, frequently leading to accidents and death. Alcohol interacts with various drugs, altering the normal effect of the medication on the body. Some medications have an increased effect when taken with alcohol (such as anticoagulants and narcotics), whereas the action of other medications (such as antibiotics) is inhibited. For the elderly person who has a chronic illness and takes many medications, the combination of drugs and alcohol can lead to serious drug overdose.

Elderly alcoholic clients should not be stereotyped or prejudged by the nurse. Rather, they should be accepted, listened to, and offered help. The nurse should assess the number and type of alcoholic beverages consumed as well as the pattern and frequency of consumption. It is important that the nurse discuss any medications the client is taking and review the side effects and interaction effects of alcohol and medication. The role of the nurse is to act as a client advocate and facilitate the treatment of the drinking problem and the prevention of complications.

CHAPTER HIGHLIGHTS

▶ The life expectancy of North Americans is increasing, so that late adulthood is now divided by some into three periods: "young-old" (65–74 years); "middle-old" (75–84 years); and "old-old" (85 years and over).

▶ A number of theories strive to account for the biologic aging process: genetic, immunologic slow virus, autoimmune, cross-link, stress, free-radical, and program theories.

▶ Psychosocial theories about aging include the disengagement, activity, and continuity theories.

▶ A number of physical changes occur with aging and involve most body systems: the integument, body temperature, and the sensory/perceptual, neuromusculoskeletal, cardiopulmonary, digestive, urinary, and reproductive systems.

▶ The older adult usually has to adjust to many psychosocial changes. Included are retirement (which necessitates financial and social adjustments), relocation, increasing dependence on others, and coping with death and grief.

CHAPTER HIGHLIGHTS *(continued)*

▸ There is minimal change in the intellectual abilities of the healthy elderly person. Of the three types of memory (sensory, primary, and secondary), secondary memory has been found to decline with aging.

▸ A decline in memory and cognitive abilities (dementia) caused by such factors as depression, infection, and thyroid disorder are reversible if prompt diagnosis and treatment are obtained. Dementia caused by Alzheimer's disease, repeated strokes, and Parkinson's disease are irreversible at this time.

▸ The moral concerns of elderly people tend to be interpersonal rather than social or legalistic.

▸ Spiritual maturity can provide the elderly person with inner resources for dealing with life experiences.

▸ Much of the decline in health during late adulthood is due to chronic illnesses resulting from unhealthy lifestyles and poor health habits, rather than the aging process itself.

▸ Health promotion and protection activities of the older adult focus on regular health maintenance visits and immunization; accident prevention; ensuring adequate nutrition; prevention of elimination problems; encouraging appropriate exercise, rest, and sleep; and maintaining the person's self-esteem and independence to the maximum potential.

▸ Elder abuse, drug use and misuse, and alcoholism are situations that require sensitive assessment and counseling by the nurse.

LEARNING ACTIVITIES

■ Assess the demographics of aging in your community. What percentage of your community is "young-old," "middle-old," and "old-old"? What services are available for the elderly in your community for financial assistance, social interaction, nutritious meals, health care, recreation, safety, and security?

■ Interview a client from each of the elderly age groups. What physical, psychologic, social, and developmental needs does each client have? How would you intervene to meet these needs? What differences do you observe between the three clients? What similarities?

■ Contact the National Institute on Aging for information and client education materials related to the aging process, including materials on current research on aging, health problems of aging, and self-care.

National Institute on Aging
U.S. Department of Health and Human Services
Information Center
2209 Distribution Circle
Silver Spring, Maryland 20910
    or
National Institute on Aging
Public Information Office
Federal Building, 6th floor
Bethesda, Maryland 20892

READINGS AND REFERENCES

SUGGESTED READINGS

Andresen, G. P. June 1989. A fresh look at assessing the elderly. *RN* 52:28–40.
  Physiologic changes in the elderly are related to genetic inheritance, health history, life-style, environment, and social factors. Because of these factors, the elderly population will have great diversity in what is considered "normal aging." The author presents a review of each body system in both text and charts, including clinical assessment, cause, and related nursing interventions. Andresen also provides laboratory values for the elderly client but cautions that findings must be interpreted carefully and always in light of the client's total health profile.

Resnick, B. M. May/June 1989. Care for life . . . even if a life care community is utopia, the move can be a dramatic change. Here's how to smooth the transition. *Geriatric Nursing* 10:130–32.

More than 150,000 elders live in over 600 life-care communities in the United States. A life-care community offers its residents the convenience of a comfortable, independent living situation with the guarantee of a nursing home bed when needed. Although the move is planned by the older adult, nursing care is needed to help ease the transition. The author suggests several strategies such as (1) initial nursing assessment to determine potential problems, (2) group support to allow the residents to build on each other's strengths, and (3) teaching the older adult the symptoms of stress they might experience.

Smith, D. L. September/October 1988. Health promotion for older adults. *Health Values* 12:46–51.

This article reviews recent health promotion programs focusing on the elderly population. These programs typically offer a combination of health education, fitness training, and preventive health screenings. The author proposes that health promotion for elderly adults must be taken seriously to prevent the disability as well as the costs incurred by the increases in chronic illness.

RELATED RESEARCH

Gueldner, S. H., and Spradley, J. October 1988. Outdoor walking lowers fatigue. *Journal of Gerontological Nursing* 14:6–12.

Ruffing-Rahal, M. January/February 1989. Ecological well-being: A study of community dwelling older adults. *Health Values.* 13:10–19.

Steinke, E. Summer, 1988. Older adults' knowledge and attitudes about sexuality and aging. *Image: Journal of Nursing Scholarship* 20:93–5.

Thomas, B. December 1988. Self esteem and life satisfaction. *Journal of Gerontological Nursing* 14:25–30.

SELECTED REFERENCES

Andreasen, M. E. and Conley, D. M. July/August 1987. Let the sun shine in. *Geriatric Nursing* 8:174–77.

Bates, B. 1991. *A guide to physical examination and history taking.* 5th ed. Philadelphia: J.B. Lippincott Co.

Burggraf, V., and Donlon, B. 1985. Assessing the elderly: System by system, 2 parts. *American Journal of Nursing.* September, pp. 974–984, October, pp. 1103–1112.

Burggraf, V., and Stanley, M. 1989. *Nursing the elderly: A care plan approach.* Philadelphia: J.B. Lippincott Co.

Burnside, I. M. 1988. *Nursing and the aged: A self-care approach.* 3d ed. New York: McGraw-Hill.

Butler, R. 1963. The life review: An interpretation of reminiscence in the aged. *Psychiatry* 26:65.

Caliandro, G., and Judkins, B. 1988. *Primary nursing practice.* Glenview, Ill.: Scott, Foresman & Co.

Christian, J. L. and Greger, J. L. 1988. Nutrition for living. Menlo Park, Calif: Benjamin/Cummings.

Ciocon, J., and Potter, J. October 1988. Age related changes in human memory: Normal and abnormal. *Geriatrics* 43:43–48.

Disparti, J. 1988. Nutrition and self-care. In Caliandro, G., and Judkins, B., editors. pp. 134–50. *Primary nursing practice.* Glenview, Ill.: Scott, Foresman & Co.

Duvall, E. 1977. *Family development.* 5th ed. Philadelphia: J.B. Lippincott Co.

Ebersole, P., and Hess, P. 1990. *Toward healthy aging: Human needs and nursing response.* St. Louis: C.V. Mosby Co.

Edelman, C., and Mandle, C. L. 1986. *Health promotion throughout the life span.* St. Louis: C. V. Mosby Co.

Erikson, E. H. 1963. *Childhood and society.* 2d ed. New York: W. W. Norton and Co.

———. 1982. *The life cycle completed: A review.* New York: W. W. Norton and Co.

Fowler, J., and Keen, S. 1985. *Life maps: Conversations in the journey of faith.* Waco, Texas: Word Books.

Fulmer, T. 1988. The older adult. In Caliandro, G., and Judkins, B., editors. pp. 543–57. *Primary nursing practice.* Glenview, Ill.: Scott, Foresman & Co.

Godkin, M.A., Wolf, R.S., and Pillemer, K.A. 1989. A case-comparison analysis of elder abuse and neglect. *International Journal of Aging and Human Development* 28(3):207–225.

Hales, D. 1989. *An invitation to health.* 4th ed. Menlo Park: Benjamin/Cummings.

Havighurst, R. 1974. *Developmental tasks and education.* 3d ed. New York: David McKay Publisher.

Hawkins, W. E.; Duncan, D. F.; and McDermott, R. J. May 1988. A health assessment of older Americans: Some multidimensional measures. *Preventive Medicine* 17:344–56.

Hayflick, L. October 1988. Why do we live so long? *Geriatrics* 43:77–87.

Hogstel, M., and Kashka, M. January/February 1989. Staying healthy after 85. *Geriatric Nursing.* 19:16–18.

Job, S., and Anema, M. December 1988. Elder care: Ethical dimensions. *Journal of Gerontological Nursing* 14:16–19.

Kart, C. S.; Metress, E. S.; and Metress, J. F. 1978. *Aging and health: Biologic and social perspectives.* Menlo Park, Calif.: Addison-Wesley Publishing Co.

Kohlberg, L. 1971. *Recent research in moral development.* New York: Holt, Rinehart and Winston.

Lenihan, A. A. July/August 1988. Identification of self care behaviors in the elderly: A nursing assessment tool. *Journal of Professional Nursing* 4:285–88.

Lichtenstein, M.; Bess, F.; and Logan, S. May 1988. Validation of screening tools for identifying hearing impaired elderly in primary care. *Journal of the American Medical Association* 259:2875–78.

McCracken, A. L. October 1988. Sexual practice by elders: The forgotten aspect of functional health. *Journal of Gerontological Nursing* 14:13–18.

Murray, R. B., and Zentner, J. P. 1989. *Nursing assessment and* health promotion strategies through the life span. 4th ed. Norwalk, Conn.: Appleton & Lange.

Nesbitt, B. July 1988. Nursing Diagnosis: Age related changes. *Journal of Gerontological Nursing* 14:6–12.

Peck, R. 1955. Psychological developments in the second half of life. In Anderson, J., editor. *Psychological aspects of aging.* Washington, D.C.: American Psychological Association.

———. 1968. Psychological development in the second half of life. In Neugarten, B. L., editor. *Middle age and aging.* Chicago: University of Chicago Press.

Pender, N. J. 1987. Health promotion and nursing practice. 2d ed. Norwalk, Conn.: Appleton & Lange.

Portnow, J., and Houtmann, M. 1987. *Home care for the elderly.* New York: McGraw-Hill Book Co.

Rathbone-McCuan, E., and Voyles, B. 1982. Case detection of abused elderly parents. *American Journal of Psychiatry* 139:2, February.

Reed, A. T., and Birge, S. J. July 1988. Screening for osteoporosis. *Journal of Gerontological Nursing* 14:18–20.

Rowe, J., and Besdine, R. 1988. *Geriatric Medicine.* 2d ed. Boston: Little, Brown and Co.

Rybash, J.; Hoyer, W.; and Roodin, P. 1986. *Adult cognition and aging.* New York: Pergamon Press.

Rybash, J. M.; Roodin, P. A.; and Hoyer, W. J. 1983. Expres-sions of moral thought in later adulthood. *Gerontologist* 23:254–59.

Saxon, S. V., and Etten, M. J. 1987. *Physical change and aging: A guide for the helping professions.* 2d ed. New York: Tiresias Press.

Schuster, C. S., and Ashburn, S. S. 1986. *The process of human development: A holistic approach.* 2d ed. Boston: Little, Brown and Co.

Scura, K. W. October 1988. Audiological assessment program. *Journal of Gerontological Nursing* 14:19–25.

Smith, D. L. September/October 1988. Health promotion for older adults. *Health Values* 12:46–51.

Thienhaus, O. J. August 1988. Practical overview of sexual function and advancing age. *Geriatrics* 43:63–67.

U.S. Bureau of the Census. 1989. *Statistical abstract of the United States,* 109th ed. U.S. Government Printing Office, Washington, D.C.

Utley, Q. E.; Hawkins, J. E.; Igou, J. F.; and Johnson, F. F. June 1988. Giving and getting support at the wellness center. *Journal of Gerontological Nursing* 14:23–25.

Webster, J. A. December 1988. Key to healthy aging: Exercise. *Journal of Gerontological Nursing* 14:8–15.

Yurick, A.; Spier, B.; Robb, S.; and Ebert, N. 1989. *The aged person and the nursing process.* Norwalk, Conn.: Appleton & Lange.

Self-Concept and Role Relationships

IMPORTANCE OF A HEALTHY SELF-CONCEPT

Self-concept, self-esteem, and *self-image* are essential to a person's mental and physical health. Individuals with a positive self-concept or high self-esteem are better able to develop and maintain warm interpersonal relationships and resist psychologic and physical illness. A healthy self-concept enables a person to find happiness in life and to cope with life's disappointments and changes. Failure to achieve a positive self-image presents major obstacles in the treatment of common disorders such as depression, eating disorders, postvictimization syndrome (abuse or rape), and crisis reactions. One of the nurse's major responsibilities is to identify persons with a negative self-concept or low self-esteem and to assist them in developing a more positive view of themselves. People who do not have a healthy self-concept are less able to live as fully or be as happy as they might be. People with an unhealthy self-concept generally express feelings of worthlessness, self-dislike or self-hatred, and, on some occasions, hatred for others. They often feel sad or hopeless and are drained of energy.

Self-concept or self-esteem influences a person in these ways (Sanford and Donovan 1984, p. 3):

- It affects everything one thinks, says, or does.
- It affects how others in the world see and treat one.
- It affects the choices one makes, such as who one will be involved with and what to do with one's life.
- It affects one's ability to give and receive love.
- It affects one's ability to take action to change things that need to be changed.

The nurse's own self-concept is also important. Nurses who have difficulty meeting their own needs have difficulty meeting the needs of clients. Nurses who feel positive about themselves are better equipped to meet the needs of others. Such nurses feel good, look good, are effective and productive, and respond to people (including themselves) in healthy and positive ways.

CONCEPT OF SELF AND SELF-ESTEEM

The terms *self-concept, self-image, self-esteem, self-worth, sense of self-worth, self-respect,* and *self-love* are often used interchangeably. *Self-concept* has been referred to as the *cognitive* component of the self system, and *self-esteem* as the *affective* component (Hamachek 1978). In other words, **self-concept** is "how I *see* myself," and **self-esteem** is "how I *feel about* myself." Stanwyck (1983, p. 11), however, maintains that these two constructs are inseparable, since self-esteem is based on self-concept. To Stanwyck, self-esteem is "how I feel about how I see myself," even though most researchers use the terms interchangeably.

Three positions of self-concept have been delineated (Burns 1979, p. 50):

1. *Cognized self,* or self as known to the individual: "How I am," or, "How I perceive me."
2. *Other self,* or social self: "How I perceive others perceiving me."
3. *Ideal self:* "How I would like to be."

People who value most "how I perceive me" can be termed "me-centered." They try hard to live up to their own expectations and compete only with themselves,

not others. In contrast, "other-centered" people have a high need for approval from others and try hard to live up to the expectations of others, constantly comparing, competing, and evaluating themselves in relation to others. They tend to avoid personal shortcomings, are unable to assert themselves, and continually fear disapproval. The healthy self-concept, therefore, is me-centered and is formed without reference to other persons.

Global and Specific Self-Concept

The term **global self** refers to the aggregate beliefs and images one holds about oneself. It is the most complete description that individuals can give of themselves at any one time. It is also a person's frame of reference for experiencing and viewing the world. Some of these beliefs and images represent statements of fact, for example, "I am a woman"; "I am a mother"; "I am black"; "I am short"; "I am a student"; "I am poor." Others refer to less tangible aspects of self, for instance, "I am stupid"; "I am competent"; "I am clumsy"; "I am lovable"; "I am no good"; "I am shy"; "I am strong"; "I am outgoing."

Each separate image and belief one holds about oneself has a bearing on self-concept. However, self-concept is not simply a sum of its parts, for the various images and beliefs persons hold about themselves are not given equal weight and prominence (Sanford and Donovan 1984, p. 9). Each person's self-concept is like a collage. At the center of the collage are the beliefs and images that are most vital to the person's identity and self-esteem. They constitute **core self-concept.** For example: "I am competent/incompetent"; "I am pretty/ugly"; "I am rich/poor"; "I am male/female." Images and beliefs that are less important to the person are on the periphery. For example: "I am left-/right-handed"; "I am athletic/unathletic"; "I am a good/poor cook"; "I have brown/blue eyes."

According to Goldin (1985, p. 33), people base their self-concept on how they perceive and evaluate themselves in these areas:

- Vocational performance
- Intellectual functioning
- Personal appearance and physical attractiveness
- Sexual attractiveness and performance
- Being liked by others
- Ability to cope with and resolve problems
- Independence
- Particular talents

Self-esteem categories for children include the following (Stanwyck 1983, p. 12):

- School performance
- Peer relationships
- Family relationships
- Emotional well-being
- Physical self-perception

A person's self-perception in any of these areas becomes a self-fulfilling prophecy: Individuals actually behave as they perceive themselves (Goldin 1985, p. 34).

Components of Self-Concept

The North American Nursing Diagnosis Association suggests four components of self-concept: body image, role performance, personal identity, and self-esteem (Kim, McFarland, and McLane 1989, p. 47).

Body Image   The image of physical self, or **body image,** is how a person perceives the size, appearance, and functioning of the body and its parts. It includes clothing, make-up, hairstyle, jewelry, and other things intimately connected to the person, e.g., artificial limb or wheelchair. A person's body image develops partly from others' attitudes and responses to that person's body. Cultural and societal values also influence a person's body image. For instance, Western societies value beauty, youth, and wholeness. Generally, a person has developed a stable body image over a long time; thus, actual or potential threats to alterations in body image can create considerable anxiety.

Role Performance   Throughout life people undergo numerous role changes. A **role** is a set of expectations about how the person occupying one position behaves toward a person occupying another position (Roy 1984, p. 285). Expectations, or standards of behavior, are set by society or the smaller group to which the person belongs. Each person usually has several roles, e.g., husband, parent, brother, son, employee, friend, golf club member. Some roles are assumed for only limited periods, e.g., client/nurse, student/instructor, and the sick role.

To act appropriately, people need to know who they are in relation to others and what society expects for the positions they hold. When there is **role ambiguity,** expectations are unclear, and people do not know what to do or how to do it and are unable to predict the reactions of others to their behavior. This creates confusion and stress. To relate or interact appropriately with others, people also need to know the role positions that others occupy.

Role performance relates what a person does in a particular role in relation to the behaviors expected of that role. **Role mastery** means that the person's behaviors meet social expectations. Failure to master a role creates frustration and feelings of inadequacy, often with consequent lowered self-esteem.

Self-concept is also affected by role strain and role conflicts. Persons undergoing **role strain** are frustrated because they feel or are made to feel inadequate or unsuited to a role. Role strain often is associated with sex role stereotypes. For example, women in occupations traditionally held by men may be thought less knowledgeable and less competent than men in the same roles. As a result, these women feel the need to surpass the level expected for role mastery by male counterparts.

Role conflicts arise from opposing or incompatible expectations. In an *interpersonal conflict,* different people have different expectations about a particular role. For example, a mother's parents may have different expectations about how the mother should care for her children. In an *interrole conflict,* one person's or group's role expectations differ from the expectations of another person or group. For example, a woman who works in an office 8 hours a day may have a role conflict if her husband expects her to be home with the children. In a **person-role conflict,** role expectations violate the beliefs or values of the role occupant. For example, a woman who values her right to choose abortion will have a conflict if this right is denied.

Personal Identity   A person's personal or **self-identity** is the conscious sense of individuality and uniqueness that is continually evolving throughout life. People often view their identity in terms of name, sex, age, race, ethnic origin or culture, occupation or roles, talents, and other situational characteristics (e.g., marital status and education). People usually first identify themselves by name and occupation or roles. When interactions progress beyond the superficial, other characteristics may be revealed, e.g., special talents or interests. Self-identity also includes a person's beliefs and values, personality, and character. For instance, is the person outgoing, friendly, reserved, generous, kind, honest, ruthless, selfish? Self-identity, thus, encompasses both the tangible and factual, such as name and sex, and the intangible, such as values and beliefs. In brief: Identity is what distinguishes self from others.

Self-Esteem The way one perceives and structures one's self-concept can result in either positive or negative self-esteem. There are two types of self-esteem: global and specific (Sanford and Donovan 1984, p. 9). **Global self-esteem** is how much the person likes his or her perceived self as a whole. **Specific self-esteem** is how much a person approves of a certain part of himself or herself (Sanford and Donovan 1984, p. 9). Global self-esteem is influenced by specific self-esteem. For example, if a man values his looks, then how he looks will strongly affect his global self-esteem. By contrast, if a man places little value on his cooking skills, then how well or badly he cooks will have little influence on his global self-esteem.

Maintenance and Evaluation of Self-Esteem

By the time people reach adulthood, their *basic* self-concept and *basic* level of self-esteem are relatively well established, and they already have some idea about their **perceived self,** i.e., how they see themselves and how they are seen by others. In addition, they have an idea about their **ideal self,** i.e., how they should be or would prefer to be. Sometimes this ideal self is realistic; sometimes it is not. When perceived self is close to ideal self, people do not wish to be much different from what they believe they already are. When there is a discrepancy between ideal self and perceived self, this can be an incentive to self-improvement. However, when the discrepancy is large, low self-esteem can result.

Basic self-esteem refers to the foundation for self-esteem that is established during early life experiences, usually within the family. However, an adult's functional level of overall self-esteem may change markedly from day to day and moment to moment. *Functional self-esteem* is a result of the person's ongoing evaluation of interactions with people and objects. Functional self-esteem can exceed basic self-esteem, or it can regress to a level below that of basic self-esteem. Severe stress—for example, prolonged illness or unemployment—can substantially lower a person's basic self-esteem.

Perceptions of self (both as is and as desired) generally arise from self-evaluation in accordance with certain criteria. Four basic criteria by which people judge themselves are

1. *Power*—the ability to influence significant others and control events that are personally important
2. *Significance*—the acceptance, attention, and affection of others who communicate to the person a clear sense of being valued and cared about as a worthwhile human being
3. *Competence*—successfully meeting demands for achievement, particularly personally important goals
4. *Virtue*—adherence to moral and ethical standards

Self-evaluation is usually a covert mental process. Frequently, people label themselves negatively or project failures into the future. Positive self-credit is usually less frequent.

DEVELOPMENT OF SELF-ESTEEM

Four elements of experience that are pertinent to the development of self-esteem are (a) significant others, (b) social role expectations, (c) crises of psychosocial development, and (d) communication/coping style (Stanwyck 1983, p. 13).

Significant Others The crucial role of social interaction in the development of self-esteem is recognized by most social psychologists. Because some people exert more influence than others on the development of an individual's self-esteem, Sullivan's term *significant other* has been generally accepted (Sullivan 1950). A **significant other** is an individual or group that takes on special importance for the development of self-esteem during a particular life stage. Significant others may include parents, siblings, peers, teachers, and the like. During various stages of development one or several significant others may be identified. Through social interaction with significant others and the resultant interpreted feedback on the perceptions of others, one develops attitudes toward oneself. Put more simply, "as a person is judged by others, so he comes to judge himself" (Burns 1979, p. 184). Many components of a person's self-evaluation are established early in life under the influence of significant others. These values often get so strongly reinforced that they are difficult to change later, even though it may benefit the person to do so.

Social Role Expectations At the various stages of life, people are strongly influenced by general societal expectations regarding role-specific behavior. The larger society and smaller societal groups have expectations that differ in clarity and are communicated with varying degrees of force. Expectations differ by age, sex, socioeconomic status, ethnicity, and career identification. Smaller societal groups such as the family, school, armed forces, work groups, and recreational groups also expect certain behaviors and performance levels of people. Success in meeting such expectations has profound implications for self-esteem.

Because North American society is highly achievement oriented, everything a person does is evaluated, e.g., earning capacity, social skills, performance at school, athletic performance, and sexual performance. A high level of performance is rewarded; poor performance is belittled. As a result people tend to focus on their failures and shortcomings rather than on their strengths. In many instances a person's actual performance is superior to the person's *perception* of that performance. Compliance with the social expectations for role-specific behavior therefore leads to judgments of personal worth; noncompliance often leads to judgments of personal worthlessness.

Crises of Psychosocial Development

Throughout life people face certain developmental tasks that, if not successfully achieved, may lead to problems with self, self-concept, and self-esteem. The eight psychosocial stages described by Erikson (1963) provide a convenient and familiar theoretic framework with obvious implications for self-esteem. The success with which a person copes with these developmental crises largely determines the development of self-concept. Inability to cope results in self-concept problems, at the time and often later in life. See Table 22–1 for behaviors indicating successful and unsuccessful resolution of these developmental crises.

Communication/Coping Styles

A person's choice of strategies to cope with a stress-producing situation is important in determining how successfully a person adapts to that situation and whether self-esteem is maintained, enhanced, or decreased. Reactions to stressful situations that threaten self-esteem include problem-solving reactions, assertive reactions, and defensive reactions.

Problem-solving reactions

Problem solving is a conscious, action-oriented response in which the person uses cognitive skills to deal with a stressor. First the person cognitively appraises the threatening situation by asking questions such as these:

- What is the exact nature of the threatening situation?
- What unfavorable consequences can I expect from the situation should it occur?

- What courses of action can I use to cope with the threat?
- What courses of action are most likely to succeed, i.e., cause the least personal loss or problem?

After a realistic appraisal, the person chooses the most effective course of action, e.g., talking to a friend, calling a crisis center, doing nothing, or seeking out professional help.

Assertive reactions

Everyday interpersonal interactions can produce stress. In such situations, assertive behavior is useful. **Assertiveness** involves expressing oneself openly and directly without hurting others. It provides feelings of control and self-confidence for the communicator and is based on the belief that each person is important. Assertive people are able to present their feelings and values, stand up for themselves, and claim their rights. Assertiveness is prerequisite to building self-esteem. Because it enables the person to cope with a stressful event actively, it enhances self-esteem.

Assertiveness with individuals and groups facilitates

- Prompt coping with problems
- Achievement of group goals
- Communication of power within oneself
- Communication of competence and self-confidence
- Reduction of anxiety or tenseness in key situations

Assertive behavior can be described as falling between nonassertiveness and aggressive behavior on a continuum. Nonassertive or passive persons appear hesitant and unsure of themselves. Their feelings are hidden, for fear of hurting others or being hurt. Because nonassertive persons do not ask or know how to ask, they often do not obtain what they want and thus become frustrated. After a time, this frustration often results in explosively aggressive behavior, which helps the person feel better, but only briefly. Through **aggressiveness,** at the other extreme, people can make their feelings known, but often at others' expense. Although this behavior can result in change, it can be harmful to the individual eventually, as others respond negatively to the aggressive behavior.

Nurses, too, can benefit from using assertive responses. The example that follows illustrates the different types of responses in a typical nursing situation.

Situation
Charge nurse: Miss Eammons, why can't you ever take your blood pressures on time? This is the fourth day this week that they have not been taken.

TABLE 22-1 *Examples of Behaviors Associated with Erikson's Stages of Psychosocial Development*

Stage: Developmental Crisis	Behaviors Indicating Positive Resolution	Behaviors Indicating Negative Resolution
Infancy: Trust vs mistrust	Requesting assistance and expecting to receive it Expressing belief of another person Sharing time, opinions, and experiences	Restricting conversation to superficialities Refusing to provide a person with information Being unable to accept assistance
Toddlerhood: Autonomy vs shame and doubt	Accepting the rules of a group but also expressing disagreement when it is felt Expressing one's own opinion Easily accepting deferment of a wish fulfillment	Failing to express needs Not expressing one's own opinion when opposed
Early childhood: Initiative vs guilt	Starting projects eagerly Expressing curiosity about many things Demonstrating original thought	Imitating others rather than developing independent ideas Apologizing and being very embarrassed over small mistakes Verbalizing fear about starting a new project
Early school years: Industry vs inferiority	Completing a task once it has been started Working well with others Using time effectively	Not completing tasks started Not assisting with the work of others Not organizing work
Adolescence: Identity vs role confusion	Asserting independence Planning realistically for future roles Establishing close interpersonal relationships	Failing to assume responsibility for directing one's own behavior Accepting the values of others without question Failing to set goals in life
Early adulthood: Intimacy vs isolation	Establishing a close, intense relationship with another person Accepting sexual behavior as desirable Making a commitment to that relationship, even in times of stress and sacrifice	Remaining alone Avoiding close interpersonal relationships
Middle-aged adults: Generativity vs stagnation	Being willing to share with another person Guiding others Establishing a priority of needs, recognizing both self and others	Talking about oneself instead of listening to others Showing concern for oneself in spite of the needs of others Being unable to accept interdependence
Elderly adults: Integrity vs despair	Using past experience to assist others Maintaining productivity in some areas Accepting limitations	Crying and being apathetic Not accepting changes Demanding unnecessary assistance and attention from others

Aggressive response

Nurse: It's not my fault they are late. You're always interrupting my work with extra duties.

Nonassertive response

Nurse: Yes, I'm sorry. We've been short staffed, and I have a very heavy load.

Assertive response

Nurse: I didn't know that all the blood pressures were late. I'd like to check that further. Could we discuss this in your office before you leave today?

The assertive techniques shown in the accompanying box can help the nurse.

Three assertive methods of coping with criticism are fogging, negative assertion, and negative inquiry (Smith 1975, pp. 104–32). *Fogging* is agreeing in principle to a statement made by another. In this technique, the nurse listens carefully to the criticism and accepts it without becoming defensive or anxious.

Client: You can't do anything right.

Nurse: You're not satisfied with my work, Mr. Milos.

Negative assertion is the assertive expression of those attributes that are negative about oneself:

Client: You didn't give that injection well.

Nurse: I didn't give it very smoothly.

Negative inquiry asks for additional information about the critical statements:

Charge nurse: You look messy today.

Nurse: What do you mean?

Charge nurse: You look untidy.

Nurse: Do you mean my uniform is wrinkled?

To learn assertiveness, nurses can take workshops or study articles on the subject.

Defensive reactions   Defensive responses are generally used when other responses have been unsuccessful in adapting to the stressful event and anxiety or other feelings remain high. Specific defensive coping behaviors are called ego-defense mechanisms. These are discussed in Chapter 23.

ASSESSING

Assessing problems related to self-concept is normally indicated if (a) the client or support persons present cues that could reflect problems or (b) the client's illness

CLINICAL GUIDELINES
Assertive Techniques

- Include positive and negative information in a statement: "I like your plan, but. . . ."

- Start the statement with "I," and avoid generalizations such as "we all believe" or "it seems like a good idea."

- Express your own beliefs and rights: "I believe that. . . ."

- Express your thoughts and feelings directly to reinforce your identity: "I feel you are. . ." or "I want you to. . . ."

- When replying negatively, state, "I won't . . ." not "I can't. . . ." The latter implies lack of power, whereas the former communicates assumption of responsibility.

- Make assertive statements:
  a. Simple assertive: "I think. . . ."
  b. Empathic assertive: "I realize you are very tired, but. . . ."
  c. Confrontive assertive: "You said you could bathe Mr. Greene, but you didn't. . . ."
  d. Soft assertive: "I am very grateful you did that for me, and I think. . . ."
  e. Persuasive assertive: "I agree with most of what you said, but I also think. . . ."

When an individual says something that the nurse perceives as negative or a "put-down," the following assertive responses can be given to provide time:

- "I need to think about this for a few minutes."

- "It seems to me that . . ." and a clear statement of personal feelings.

- Silence as an answer, giving no verbal response.

is one often associated with self-concept problems. Problems with self-concept and self-esteem are frequently manifested by expressions of anxiety, fear, anger, hostility, guilt, and/or powerlessness. Behaviors reflecting excessive role conflict may also indicate the need for meaningful intervention by nurses.

A trusting client-nurse relationship is essential for an effective assessment of self-concept. Clients tend not to share personal feelings unless the nurse has established an empathetic, nonjudgmental relationship. Potential disclosure of personal data can be threatening. Some people, particularly those with low self-esteem, may

Physical Self

- How do you feel about your personal appearance (or physical features)?

- What do others say about your personal appearance (or physical features)?

- How would you describe your physical movements?

- What changes in your body do you expect as a result of this illness (or surgery, or treatment)?

- What changes have you noticed in how your body looks (or functions)?

- How have important persons in your life (e.g., spouse, parent, partner) reacted to changes in your body?

- How do you think the important people in your life will react to the anticipated change in your body?

Personal Self

- How would you describe your personal characteristics? or, How do you see yourself as a person?

- What do you like about yourself?

- How do others describe you as a person?

- What do you do well?

- What are your personal strengths, talents, and abilities?

- What would you change about yourself if you could?

- Does it bother you a great deal if you think someone doesn't like you?

- Is it difficult for you to say no when you want to say no?

- How do you feel about your educational accomplishments?

- Do you ever feel inadequate with certain people? Who?

- How easily can you express your opinion when it differs from that of others?

- Do you make friends easily?

- Generally, do you feel liked by your peers and coworkers?

- How do you feel about your occupation?

- Do you feel appreciated by your employer?

fear that the nurse will not accept or like them if they reveal their true performance capabilities, thoughts, and feelings.

The nursing assessment involves four areas: (a) self-perception or self-awareness, (b) role performance and relationships, (c) major stressors and coping strategies, (d) behaviors suggestive of low self-esteem.

Self-Perception

Assessment of self-perception involves (a) determining the client's perceptions of physical and personal self and (b) observing for nonverbal cues that reflect the client's self-perception.

To determine the client's perception of *physical self,* or body image, the nurse either listens to comments the client makes about the physical self or asks the client the questions shown in the accompanying box. Responses such as "I feel ugly," "I'm awkward and clumsy," "I can't do anything now," "No one will like me now," and "I'm afraid my husband won't love me any more" indicate that the client's self-esteem is threatened or low. The client is focusing on particular disabilities or shortcomings and blocking out accurate perception of the total self.

In regard to *personal self,* some people may volunteer clearly self-deprecating or over-critical comments indicating low self-esteem—e.g., "People don't like me," or "I'm no good." For other clients, the nurse may consider asking some of the questions shown in the box in the left column.

Nonverbal behaviors—such as body posture, movements, gestures, tone of voice, speech pattern, and general appearance—tend to be more spontaneous than verbal messages and can provide important clues to the person's self-concept. Nonverbal cues that can indicate low self-esteem include stooped shoulders, lack of attention to hygiene or grooming, avoiding eye contact, hesitant speech, and withdrawing from social interaction. Nonverbal cues can help the nurse confirm the reliability of the client's verbal messages.

Role Relationships

The nurse assesses the client's satisfactions and dissatisfactions associated with role responsibilities and relationships: family roles, work roles, student roles, social roles. Family roles are especially important to clients, since family relationships are particularly close. Relationships can be supportive and growth-producing or, at the opposite extreme, highly stressful if violence and

ASSESSMENT INTERVIEW
Role Relationships

Family Relationships

- Tell me about your family.
- What is home like?
- Who are you closest to in the family?
- Who are you most distant from in the family?
- What are your relationships like with your other relatives?
- What are your responsibilities in the family?
- How well do you feel you accomplish what is expected of you?
- What about your role or responsibilities would you like changed?
- Do you see yourself as frequently getting the short end of things and coming out second best?
- Are you proud of your family members?
- Do you feel your family members are proud of you?
- Tell me how you spend your time each day.

Work Roles and Social Roles

- Do you like your work?
- How do you get along at work?
- What about your work would you like to change if you could?
- How do you spend your free time?
- Are you involved in any community groups?
- Are you most comfortable alone, with one other person, or in a group?
- Who is most important to you?
- Whom do you seek out for help?

Stressors Affecting Self-Concept and Self-Esteem

Body-Image Stressors

- Loss of body parts, e.g., amputation, mastectomy, hysterectomy
- Loss of body functions, e.g., from heart disease, renal disease, spinal cord injury, cerebrovascular accident, neuromuscular disease, arthritis, declining mental or sensory abilities
- Disfigurement, e.g., through pregnancy, severe burns, facial blemishes, colostomy, ileostomy, tracheostomy, laryngectomy

Role Stressors

- Loss of parent, spouse, child, or close friend
- Change or loss of job
- Retirement
- Divorce or separation
- Illness
- Hospitalization
- Ambiguous role expectations
- Conflicting role expectations
- Inability to meet role expectations

Identity Stressors

- Change in physical appearance
- Declining physical, mental, or sensory abilities
- Inability to achieve goals
- Relationship concerns
- Sexuality concerns
- Unrealistic ideal self
- Membership in a minority group

abuse permeate relationships. Assessment of family role relationships may begin with structural aspects such as number in the family group, ages, and residence location. For more information on the family, see Chapter 16. To obtain data related to the client's family relationships and satisfaction or dissatisfaction with work roles and social roles, the nurse might ask some of the questions shown in the Assessment box above, keeping in mind, however, that questions need to be tailored to the individuals and their age and situation.

Major Stressors and Coping Strategies

The nurse needs to identify stressors that challenge the client's self-worth. Most people face numerous stress-producing events simultaneously. Illness and hospitalization can compound the effects. Common stressors that influence a client's self-concept and self-esteem are shown in the box above.

When stressors are identified, the nurse needs to determine how the client perceives the stressor. A positive, growth-oriented perception of stressful events reinforces self-worth; a negative, hopeless, defeatist perception leads to decreased self-esteem. The nurse also should identify the client's coping style and determine whether or not this style is effective by asking the client such questions as these:

■ When you have a problem or face a stressful situation, how do you usually deal with it?

■ Do these methods work?

Behaviors Suggesting Low Self-Esteem

Some of the verbal and nonverbal behaviors that can indicate altered self-concept or low self-esteem were dis-cussed earlier in this section. Other behaviors associated with low self-esteem are listed in the box below.

People with low self-esteem generally exhibit illogical and *distorted thinking.* Some cognitive therapists (Ellis and Harper 1975, p. 100; Beck 1979, p. 54) assert that illogical and distorted thinking causes or perpetuates low self-esteem. Common types of irrational, illogical, or muddled thinking include the following (Crouch and Straub 1983, p. 72).

■ *Catastrophizing,* the tendency to think the worst. For example, the person says, "If something bad can happen it will," or, "Things are bad now, but they will get worse."

■ *Minimizing and maximizing,* the tendency to minimize the positive, to overlook partial successes, to magnify the significance or meaning of the negative, and to emphasize mistakes.

Behaviors Associated with Low Self-Esteem

The client:

■ Avoids eye contact

■ Stoops in posture and moves slowly

■ Is poorly groomed and has an unkempt appearance

■ Is hesitant or halting in speech

■ Is overly critical of self, e.g., "I'm no good," "I'm ugly," or "People don't like me."

■ May be overly critical of others

■ Is unable to accept positive remarks about self

■ Encourages reprimands from others, to punish self

■ Apologizes frequently

■ Verbalizes feelings of hopelessness, helplessness, and powerlessness, such as "I really don't care what happens," "I'll do whatever anyone wants," "Whatever is destined will happen."

■ Verbalizes feelings of worthlessness, such as "Nobody cares about me," "I'm just a burden to everyone," "I'm not worth all that trouble."

■ Verbalizes feelings of guilt, such as "It's all my fault," "I am to blame."

■ Withdraws from or changes social involvements or relationships

■ Fails to complete or follow through with activities

■ Avoids initiating conversation or interaction with others

■ Exhibits self-destructive behavior, such as excessive use of alcohol, drugs

■ Has negative feelings about own body, e.g., avoids looking at or touching body part, or hides body part; emphasizes previous appearance or function; talks excessively about loss or change

■ Is indecisive, e.g., "I can't make up my mind what to do," "I don't understand what's happening."

■ Cannot solve problems effectively and does not ask for help

■ Displays overdependence, e.g., asks for assistance unnecessarily, seeks attention by speaking loudly, asks irrelevant questions, seeks approval and praise

■ Displays lack of energy, e.g., "I feel tired all the time."

■ Verbalizes inability to cope

■ Expresses or manifests anxiety, fear, anger

■ Does not meet role expectations

- *Black-and-white thinking,* the tendency to attribute things to one of two extremes. Things are either perfect or no good. Activities must be performed without mistake or the performance is a failure.

- *Overgeneralization,* the tendency to believe that something that applied in one situation or that happened once will apply in all situations.

- *Self-reference,* the tendency to believe that what others are thinking, saying, or doing relates to self. The person believes that others are highly concerned with that person's thoughts and actions and are particularly aware of the person's shortcomings and mistakes.

- *Filtering,* the tendency to support beliefs or conclusions by selectively pulling certain details out of context and neglecting other facts. Usually, it is the negative details that are selected while positive facts are neglected.

DIAGNOSING

Nursing diagnoses for clients with problems related to self-concept include **Body image disturbance,** the state in which one experiences or is at risk of experiencing a disruption in the way one perceives one's body image; **Personal identity disturbance,** the inability to distinguish self from nonself; **Altered role performance,** the disruption in the way one perceives one's role performance; and **Self-esteem disturbance,** the state in which one experiences or is at risk of experiencing negative feelings or self-evaluation about oneself or one's capabilities.

The diagnosis of **Self-esteem disturbance** is subcategorized into **Chronic low self-esteem** and **Situational low self-esteem. Chronic low self-esteem** applies to clients with long-standing negative self-evaluation or feelings about self or their own capabilities. **Situational low self-esteem** applies to clients who previously had a positive self-evaluation but have developed negative self-evaluation or feelings about self in response to a loss or change.

Because the diagnosis of **Personal identity disturbance** requires further development and research, it is recommended that the student use other diagnoses at this time.

Other diagnoses that relate to self-concept include **Ineffective individual coping, Social isolation, Powerlessness, Sexual dysfunction, Anticipatory grieving,** and **Dysfunctional grieving.** These diagnoses are discussed in other chapters of this book.

Examples of contributing factors for selected diagnoses follow.

Body image disturbance related to:

- Loss of body part (e.g., amputation, mastectomy)
- Loss of body function (e.g., from heart disease, spinal cord injury, neuromuscular disease)
- Disfigurement (e.g., pregnancy, severe burns, colostomy)
- Delayed development of secondary characteristics
- Extreme thinness or obesity

Altered role performance related to:

- Change in physical or mental capacity
- Newly assumed work and family roles
- Multiple life stressors

Chronic low self-esteem related to:

- Loss of body function
- Infant or childhood deprivation
- Unrealistic parental expectations
- Unrealistic personal expectations

Situational low self-esteem related to:

- Loss of body part or function
- Divorce
- Loss of job
- Termination of relationship

Powerlessness related to:

- Inability to perform activities of daily living secondary to neuromuscular disease
- Inability to perform role responsibilities secondary to progressive debilitating disease

Ineffective individual coping related to:

- Death of parent
- Inadequate personal resources and social support
- Divorce and change in financial status
- Need for mutilating surgery

PLANNING

The nurse's focus when planning is to assist the client to set goals that reflect a positive resolution of the problem or stressors identified in the nursing diagnosis. Goals should emphasize strengths rather than weaknesses or impairments. Broadly speaking, goals may be stated as follows. The client:

- Increases awareness of strengths and weaknesses.
- Improves feelings of self-worth.
- Perceives and responds to stressors in a constructive manner.
- Improves interpersonal relationships.

Two types of self-image goals can be considered: tangible and personality (Goldin 1985, p. 35). Tangible goals are those that can be measured by objective means, for example, to improve personal appearance, educational level, and fund of information. Personality goals are more subjective in nature, for example, to increase assertiveness, to enhance ability to reach out for new friendships, to become more independent and self-sufficient, to develop self-pride. Once goals for changing self-image are set, the process of modifying self-image begins.

Nursing strategies to help clients meet goals related to self-concept may include helping clients to (a) identify areas of strength, (b) learn to communicate more clearly, and (c) develop more positive thoughts and images about themselves. Planning also involves establishing outcome criteria by which to measure goal achievement. Examples of outcome criteria follow.

The client with **Body image disturbance:**

- Describes changes in thoughts and feelings about self.
- Verbalizes acceptance of changes that have occurred.
- Looks at, touches, and discusses changed body part.
- Continues preexisting socialization pattern.
- Engages in appropriate role functions.
- Engages in recreational activities appropriate to limitations.
- Maximizes use of remaining strengths.
- Uses all available resources to improve functioning (or appearance) of body part.
- Accepts offers of help.

The client with a **Self-esteem disturbance:**

- Demonstrates an improvement in personal appearance.
- Verbalizes realistic perceptions of self.
- Identifies at least five positive personal attributes.
- Shares feelings about self with significant others.
- Compares ideal self and perceived self.

- Uses appropriate assertive and communication skills.
- Demonstrates use of active rather than passive language pattern (e.g., says, "I choose to" or "I choose not to").
- Demonstrates increased social contacts and friendship networks.
- Expresses satisfaction with own achievements.
- Engages in positive talk about self.
- Analyzes own behavior and its consequences.
- Discusses options and alternatives when trying to solve problems.
- Identifies ways of exerting control and influencing outcomes.

The client with **Altered role performance:**

- Verbalizes realistic perception and positive acceptance of self in changed role.
- Verbalizes understanding of role expectations and obligations associated with role.
- Develops realistic plans for adapting to new role or role changes.

IMPLEMENTING

Assisting people with self-concept disturbances requires skills in communicating and in developing helping relationships (see Chapter 18). Helping clients with self-concept disturbances is akin to promoting health, as discussed in Chapter 15. The client assumes responsibility for implementing the plans. The nurse provides information, education, and ongoing support; suggests strategies to encourage behavioral change; and implements techniques that help the client gain a realistic and acceptable view of self. Selected interventions to help clients with self-concept disturbances follow. Numerous community self-improvement programs are also available, many of which emphasize the need for individuals to take charge of their lives, to take responsibility for their actions, to think positively rather than negatively, and to become more assertive.

It is important for both the nurse and the client to realize that changes in self-concept require an extended period of time. Although varying from person to person, this may take several months or years. It is essential for the client to learn that self-concept or self-image is not etched in stone; it can change and improve in progressive small steps, particularly if the client desires such change.

Identifying Areas of Strength

Healthy people often perceive their problems and weaknesses more clearly than their assets and strengths. Average well-functioning persons with some college education, when asked to write down their strengths, are able to list only five or six; however, the same persons can list three to four times as many problems or areas of weakness (Otto 1965, p. 34).

Because people with low self-esteem tend to focus on their limitations, they may list even fewer strengths and many more problems. When a client has difficulty identifying personality strengths and assets, the nurse must provide the client with a framework to follow. Interests, abilities, and past accomplishments and experiences need to be included. Such an inventory has the following advantages.

- It can result in a more well-rounded self-concept and more positive self-esteem.

- It can help mobilize health and regenerative processes.

- It can help the person to become more aware of the strengths of others and thus facilitate relationships. The person begins to see others' previously unrecognized strengths or "good side."

Developing Behavior Specificity

Many people overgeneralize and think in unspecific ways. The nurse can assist clients to think more clearly and to become more behavior specific in language and thought. Crouch and Straub (1983, p. 71) offer the following strategies for developing behavior specificity.

1. *Define goals clearly.* For example, in response to the question "How would you like to feel differently about yourself?" the client may give an unspecific, subjective, and unmeasurable answer such as "better," "happier," or "not so uptight." To help the client, the nurse needs to bring unspecific answers into focus. This can be done by inquiring, for example, "How will you know you are better?" or "What do you mean by 'uptight'?" or "If I were to observe you now in your usual activities and then after you had made these changes, how could I tell you had achieved them?" Open-ended questions that probe into the who, what, how much, when, where, and how of thought and behavior help the client and the nurse develop a clearer understanding of the individual, the problem, and the goals.

When formulating goals, and strategies for achieving them, and nurse needs to assess the client's ideal self and perceived self, along with the amount of discrepancy between them. Teaching clients about perceived self and ideal self can assist them in exploring areas in which they may be unduly biased. It is also of value for subsequent exploration and assessment. For example, if clients express discouragement about their behavior in a situation, the nurse could say, "Ideally, how do you think you should have acted or reacted?" and then "How do you perceive you actually acted?" Some situations involve complications that are beyond the person's control; such questioning will help clarify that for the client.

2. *Help the client think clearly.* Clients with low self-esteem tend to think negatively and irrationally. For example, a client with low self-esteem who has followed through on homework for three out of seven days might say, "There was no excuse; I failed," or "I didn't follow through; I can't do anything right." When responding, the nurse should avoid contradicting the client but need not accept the client's evaluation as accurate. The nurse might ask, "What exactly did you not follow through with?" or "How does not doing the homework perfectly mean you can't do anything right?"

Changing Language Patterns

Helping clients to change language patterns from passive phrases to more active phrases can help them assume greater responsibility for their power. Examples of passive phrases and alternate active phrases follow:

It makes me . . . (passive)
I choose to . . . *or* I do. (active)

I have to . . . (passive)
I want to . . . (active)

I can't . . . (passive)
I won't . . . *or* I choose not to . . . (active)

Changing language patterns does not alter a person's beliefs, but the process of recognizing and modifying language helps the person consider habitual as well as alternate ways of thinking and believing. To encourage the use of more active language, the nurse may have the client initially listen for passive language without modifying it and then deliberately notice passive language and modify it. It is also important for clients to gain awareness of their overall feeling states when using passive or active language.

Encouraging Positive Self-Evaluation

Persons with high self-esteem express positive self-evaluation more frequently than negative self-evaluation. Persons with low self-esteem, by contrast, frequently make negative self-evaluations and rarely give themselves positive feedback. Therefore, clients with low self-esteem need help in developing more positive thoughts and images about themselves. Strategies include modeling, praise or recognition, positive self-feedback, and visualization.

Modeling   The nurse can model positive self-statements for the client by saying such things as "I did a good job painting my recreation room last weekend," or "I am improving my cooking," or "I am proud of the produce I'm getting from my vegetable garden."

Praise   To help the client make the transition to self-recognition, the nurse provides honest, positive feedback. For example, the nurse might say, "I think you did a really fine job," or "It sounds like you worked very hard and have done well."

Positive Self-Feedback   To help clients begin making positive self-statements, the nurse may implement some of the following strategies.

1. Ask the client: "Tell me some things you have done recently that you feel good about," or "Tell me some things you like about yourself."
2. Ask clients to develop a list of accomplishments they feel good about and a list of characteristics they like about themselves. Accomplishments, behaviors, and characteristics that hold high significance for the person are preferred, since they incorporate a sense of competence, virtue, and power. Frequent reference to this list or to one attribute on the list is encouraged.
3. Reduce negative self-feedback through thought-stopping techniques. For example, every time the client begins to think negatively about self, ask the client to say mentally, "Stop," or "No," or "Think about now," and then attend to the details of the present experience.

Visualization   Because strong positive images or expectations often become self-fulfilling, visualization, or imagery procedures, can be used to enhance self-esteem. Positive images of desired changes are consciously imagined. This can be a powerful tool for achieving goals and gaining a positive self-concept. To strengthen goals with visualization, the client:

1. Sets a positive goal or image, such as "I am talking with someone at a party" or "I am saying to my family that I need some help from them to be able to manage work and home responsibilities."
2. Relaxes and slowly repeats the goal-phrase several times.
3. Closes the eyes and visualizes the goal-phrase on a written page.
4. Envisions self as having accomplished the goal.

Because a person's receptivity to positive suggestions is greater when that person is deeply relaxed, deep-breathing exercises, progressive relaxation techniques, meditation, and self-hypnosis are often introduced before imagery techniques are used in individual and group self-involvement programs. The nurse may refer clients to specific community programs.

Enhancing Self-Esteem in Children and Adolescents

The roles of parents and teachers are of great significance in determining children's self-concept. Children are able to grow in self-confidence, personal competence, and independence if they can develop five basic attitudes, involving (a) security and trust, (b) identity, (c) belonging, (d) purpose, and (e) personal competence (Reasoner 1983, p. 55). Parents and teachers have specific roles and responsibilities in helping children develop these five basic attitudes. The nurse can be instrumental in helping parents learn their supportive role.

Security and Trust   This first step in the development of self-esteem can be achieved by providing the child with well-defined limits, i.e., what is expected in terms of behavior and what has to be done to get approval. Limits need to be enforced consistently by all involved adults. Inconsistency tends to create anxiety and weakens feelings of security. Rules or standards need to be reasonable and broad enough to serve as general guidelines in new situations, such as in a neighbor's house, a friend's yard, or school classroom. Standards needs to be established for the treatment of others, respect for the property of others, the value of honesty, and routines such as getting ready for school in the morning, doing homework, completing chores, and going to bed at night.

Systems such as checklists, charts, and calendars can serve as reminders of what is expected and also enable children to monitor their own performance. Conforming to expectations builds positive self-esteem. Self-monitoring builds a sense of pride and provides opportunities for positive recognition as opposed to only negative feedback for uncompleted chores.

Preparing the child for what to expect if standards are *not* met is also effective in encouraging desired behavior and discouraging misbehavior. Restricting privileges tends to be more effective than scolding or lecturing and helps children learn the consequences of their behavior.

To feel secure, children also need to believe that the adults responsible for them are dependable and can be counted on. Adults, therefore, must serve as role models for appropriate behavior.

Identity

The second step in developing self-esteem is a strong sense of identity. Children need to feel they are unique. A child's identity is strengthened when the child is given positive feedback, recognition of strengths, love and acceptance, and help in assessing strengths and shortcomings.

Children need positive feedback from the people of greatest significance to them: parents, grandparents, older siblings, teachers, and close friends. The kind of feedback given can be more significant than the child's actual level of performance. Positive feedback enhances a child's sense of identity and self-concept. No feedback is likely to make a child hesitant and unsure in new situations. Predominantly negative feedback can give a child a negative self-image.

Adults foster a strong self-concept by recognizing a child's strengths. Parents and teachers who focus on the child's shortcomings and devote extra time to only those areas considered weak contribute to the child's negative feelings. Adults need to point out the child's special talents and qualities, such as an attractive smile, skill at playing games, desire to help others, and a strong sense of right and wrong.

Before they can accept themselves, children need to feel loved and accepted. Adults can demonstrate this by taking time to be with the child, to listen, to read, to play, or to just be there. Physical contact—a hand on the shoulder, or a hug—usually conveys warmth and caring more tellingly than words.

Children need to learn to assess their own level of performance and to build confidence in their own judgment. Even though positive feedback from others is always important, children also need to learn to rely on their own judgment. They can be encouraged to evaluate their performance through test results, grades, or other objective measures.

Belonging

Feeling socially accepted is important to children. Just as children need to feel unique, so do they need to feel just like everyone else. They need to dress the same, talk the same, and be in the same club. A sense of belonging can be developed through a family that is united. The family unit enables children to learn how to function as group members, to learn that they cannot always be first or have their way, and to learn that they need to handle their own share of responsibilities. In the family unit and in groups, children learn sensitivity and concern for others. Parents and group leaders can foster this concern by encouraging children to express empathy for others and to find ways to help others. Learning how to be of service to others and how to be a friend builds a sense of belonging and reduces feelings of alienation.

Purpose

Children need a sense of purpose to provide direction to their lives and a basis for success, fulfillment, and, therefore, a positive self-concept. Adults can help a child develop a sense of purpose by setting reasonable expectations, by helping the child set realistic goals, by conveying faith and confidence in the child's ability to achieve the goals, and by helping the child expand interests, talents, and abilities.

Children tend to work toward expectations that are set for them by parents or teachers, especially if the goals are within their capabilities and the adults are confident the children can achieve them. If expectations are too high or too low, motivation is reduced. Expectations that are long-term and relatively general put less pressure on the child and tend to enhance motivation (Reasoner 1983, p. 60). For example, expecting a child to improve general math skills is more motivating and less stressful than expecting an A on the next math test. To encourage children to try new challenges and reach new levels of performance, adults can expose children to new experiences. For instance, watching a demonstration on how to cook Chinese food, observing a highly skilled gymnast's performance, or talking with a fireman can help children identify their own goals. The more opportunities children have, the more likely they will be motivated to learn and to acquire new skills.

Children need to help to be specific in defining what they want to learn or how to solve a problem. Parents can help by assisting children to identify the sequence of steps needed to achieve a goal or solve a problem. When a child sets a goal, involved adults should convey faith in the child's ability to achieve the goal. Children who sense a parent's or teacher's confidence in them tend to increase their efforts toward, and their chances for, success.

Personal Competence   A sense of personal competence grows out of a sequence of successes. This gives the child a feeling of being able to cope with problems or meet goals. Children with a sense of personal competence have a positive approach to solving problems, tend to achieve success, and feel responsible for their own actions. Children who lack a sense of personal competence are overwhelmed by problems and may attribute lack of success to fate or being victimized. Parents can foster a feeling of competence by helping the child achieve the goals. To do this, the parent needs to do the following:

1. Develop a plan of action by having the child list the steps to be taken or review alternatives for achieving the goals. Parents should avoid prescribing what to do. Directing tends to foster dependency rather than independence. The child needs the freedom to make final decisions on how a plan should proceed.

2. Provide encouragement and support while monitoring the child's progress. From time to time, the parent needs to check on the child's progress, helping assess what might still need to be done, fostering consideration of other resources, or—most important—praising the child's efforts and achievement.

3. Provide feedback that will help the child determine whether the goal has been achieved. This should include more sharing of the joy of accomplishment and factual comparative information than judgment or praise, although some children value an extrinsic reward more highly. However, children need to learn to become less dependent on extrinsic or tangible rewards. Excessive praise also can make some children more dependent rather than less dependent (Reasoner 1983, p. 62).

Enhancing Self-Esteem in Older Adults

There is a wide variation in the way older adults perceive themselves; most, however, benefit from having their independence fostered. Low self-esteem is often associated with the dependence that accompanies the declining physical and mental capacities related to aging. The nurse can foster the older adult's independence and a more positive self-concept by doing the following (Hirst and Metcalf 1984, p. 76):

1. Encourage clients to participate in planning their care, and involve them in decision making. For example, encourage clients to choose what to wear or what activities to participate in, and consult them about food preferences.

2. Encourage clients to collect numerous objects around them. These establish one's territory or physical space as one's own.

3. Ask permission before putting the client's clothing (e.g., dressing gown, nightclothes) or other objects into the client's locker or closet. To do so without permission would deny the existence of the client's personal space and can be perceived as disrespectful.

4. Listen to what the client is saying. Elderly people need to know their comments are valued.

5. Allow the client sufficient time to complete an interaction or activity. Older adults are often slow to respond. Attempts to hurry their responses can create anxiety and embarrassment and can lower self-esteem.

6. Receive contributions of thanks or appreciation (e.g., candy or fruit) graciously and sincerely. Having something to contribute helps older adults maintain or enhance their self-esteem.

RESEARCH NOTE

Can the Elderly Increase Their Life Satisfaction and Self-Esteem?

The purpose of this study was to investigate whether elderly black females could be provided with a means for improving their perceptions of life satisfaction and self-esteem through regular practice of meditation/relaxation skills. The results of study indicated that the group who participated did report greater life satisfaction and self-esteem than the group that did not participate.

Implications: Nurses can help elderly clients improve their life satisfaction and self-esteem.

B. L. Thomas, Self-esteem and life satisfaction, *Journal of Gerontological Nursing,* December 1988, 14:25–30, 35–36.

EVALUATING

To evaluate the achievement of client goals, the nurse obtains data relevant to the outcome criteria established in the planning phase. To elicit such data, the nurse requires communication and interviewing skills such as listening attentively and asking open-ended questions.

Observation skills are also essential for evaluating changes in behavior and appearance.

Examples of evaluative statements are "Client verbalized feelings of anger about his paralysis," "Client listed five of her strengths," and "Client described three situations in which he used active language rather than passive language this past week."

CHAPTER HIGHLIGHTS

▶ A healthy self-concept, or positive self-esteem, is essential to a person's physical and psychologic well-being.

▶ Self-concept is sometimes referred to as the cognitive component of the self system and self-esteem as the affective component.

▶ Self-concept and self-esteem are closely related, since self-esteem is "how I feel about how I see myself."

▶ Components of self-concept include body image, role performance, personal identity, and self-esteem.

▶ A person's self-perception can differ from the person's perception of how others see the person and from how the person would like to be.

▶ From the hour of birth, interactions with significant others create the conditions that influence self-esteem throughout life.

▶ When individuals are able to conceptualize the self, they begin a lifelong process of deciding whether and to what extent they are valuable and worthy.

▶ Individuals who grow up in families whose members value each other are likely to feel good about themselves.

▶ Most individuals feel good about themselves in some ways and bad about themselves in other ways.

▶ The development of self-esteem can be seen as a process of establishing a sense of security, a sense of identity, and a sense of belonging.

▶ When children feel secure and accepted, they can be encouraged to set goals for themselves.

▶ If adults help children to accomplish goals that are important to them, children begin to develop a sense of personal competence and independence.

▶ Four elements of experience that affect the development of self-esteem are significant others, social role expectations, psychosocial development crises, and communication/coping styles.

▶ Adults base their self-concept on how they perceive and evaluate their performance in the areas of work, intellect, appearance, sexual attractiveness, particular talents, ability to cope and to resolve problems, independence, and interpersonal interactions.

▶ An individual's functional level of overall self-esteem may change markedly from day to day and moment to moment.

▶ Because a healthy self-concept is basic to health, one of the nurse's major responsibilities is to assist clients whose self-concept is disturbed to develop a more positive and realistic image of themselves.

▶ A trusting client-nurse relationship is essential for the effective assessment of a client's self-concept, for providing help and support, and for motivating client behavior change.

LEARNING ACTIVITIES

- Utilizing the assessment instruments of self-perception and role relationships on pages 416 and 417, analyze your own self-perception and role relationships. How does your view of self-perception and role relationships enhance your professional self as a nurse? What factors may be detrimental to your professional growth? How might you improve your self-perception and role relationships in order to achieve professional goals?

- Interview a client using the Self-Perception and Role Relationships Assessment instruments on pages 416 and 417. Identify the strengths of self perception and role relationships in your client. What are the weaknesses in self-perception? In role relationships? How might the nurse intervene to enhance the client's self-perception? Role relationships?

READINGS AND REFERENCES

SUGGESTED READINGS

Meissner, J. E. February 1980. Semantic differential scales for assessing patients' feelings. *Nursing 80* 10:70–71.

This article presents a semantic differential scale on which clients are asked to check the boxes that most closely describe their feelings, e.g., "lonely," "nervous," "indifferent," "calm," and "dejected."

Self-esteem and health. August 1983. *Family and Community Health* 6: entire issue.

Articles in this issue deal with self-esteem and physical health, self-esteem throughout the lifespan, the evaluation of self-esteem, and the enhancement of self-esteem in children, adolescents, and adults.

RELATED RESEARCH

Baird, S. E. January/February 1985. Development of a nursing assessment tool to diagnose altered body image in immobilized patients. *Orthopedic Nursing* 4:47–54.

Thomas, B. L. December 1988. Self-esteem and life satisfaction. *Journal of Gerontological Nursing* 14:25–30, 35–36.

Volden, C.; Langemo, D.; Adamson, M.; Oechsle, L. February 1990. The relationship of age, gender, and exercise practices to measures of health, life-style and self-esteem. *Applied Nursing Research* 3:20–26.

SELECTED REFERENCES

Barry, P. D. 1989. *Psychosocial nursing assessment and intervention: Care of the physically ill person.* 2d ed. Philadelphia: J. B. Lippincott Co.

Beck, A. T. 1979. *Cognitive theory of depression.* New York: The Guilford Press.

Burns, R. B. 1979. *The self concept in theory, measurement, development, and behavior.* London: Longman Group Ltd.

Carpenito, L. J. 1989. *Nursing diagnosis: Application to clinical practice.* 3d ed. Philadelphia: J. B. Lippincott Co.

Crouch, M. A., and Straub, V. August 1983. Enhancement of self-esteem in adults. *Family and Community Health* 6: 65–78.

Ellis, A., and Harper, R. A. 1975. *A new guide to rational living.* North Hollywood, Calif.: Wilshire Book Co.

Erikson, E. H. 1963. *Childhood and society.* 2d ed. New York: W. W. Norton and Co.

Goldin, J. November/December 1985. The influence of self-image upon the performance of nursing home staff. *Nursing Homes* 34:33–38.

Hamachek, D. E. 1978. *Encounters with self.* 2d ed. New York: Holt, Rinehart and Winston.

Hirst, S. P., and Metcalf, B. J. February 1984. Promoting self-esteem. *Journal of Gerontological Nursing* 2:72–77.

Husted, G. L., Miller, M. C., Wilczynski, E. M. May 1990. 5 ways to build your self-esteem. *Nursing 90* 20:152, 154.

Kim, M. J.; McFarland, G. K.; and McLane, A. M. 1989. *Pocket guide to nursing diagnoses.* 3d ed. St. Louis: C. V. Mosby Co.

Mixson, K. November/December 1989. How to enhance our self-esteem. *Advanced Clinical Nursing* 4:12–14.

Muhlenkamp, A. F., and Sayles, J. A. November/December 1986. Self-esteem, social support, and positive health practices. *Nursing Research* 35:334–38.

Nelson, P. B. February 1990. Intrinsic/extrinsic religious orientation of the elderly: Relationship to depression and self-esteem. *Journal of Gerontological Nursing* 16:29–37.

Norris, J., and Kunes-Connell, M. December 1985. Self-esteem disturbance. *Nursing Clinics of North America* 20:745–61.

Oldaker, S. M. December 1985. Identity confusion. Nursing diagnoses for adolescents. *Nursing Clinics of North America* 20:763–73.

Otto, H. A. August 1965. The human potentialities of nurses and patients. *Nursing Outlook* 13:32–35.

Reasoner, R. W. August 1983. Enhancing self-esteem in children and adolescents. *Family and Community Health* 6:51–64.

Roy, S. C. 1984. *Introduction to nursing. An adaptation model.* 2d ed. Englewood Cliffs, N.J.: Prentice-Hall, Inc.

Sanford, L. T., and Donovan, M. E. 1984. *Women and self-esteem.* New York: Penguin Books.

Smith, M. J. 1975. *When I say no, I feel guilty.* New York: Bantam Books.

Stanwyck, D. J. August 1983. Self-esteem through the life span. *Family and Community Health* 6:11–28.

Sullivan, H. S. 1950. *The interpersonal theory of psychiatry.* New York: W. W. Norton and Co.

Sundeen, S. J.; Stuart, G. W.; Rankin, E. A. D.; and Cohen, S. A. 1989. *Nurse-client interaction.* 4th ed. St. Louis: C. V. Mosby Co.

CHAPTER

23

Stress Tolerance and Coping

CONCEPT OF STRESS

In recent years, stress has become a household word. Parents refer to the stress of raising children; working people talk of the stress of their jobs. In many areas of nursing practice, stress is identified as a major factor in high turnover rates and job dissatisfaction. Stress is a universal phenomenon. All people experience it. The concept of stress is important because it provides a way of understanding the person as a unified being who responds in totality (mind and body) to a variety of changes that take place in daily life.

Stress can have physical, emotional, intellectual, social, and spiritual consequences. Usually, the effects are mixed because stress affects the whole person. Physically, stress can threaten a person's physiologic homeo-

429

stasis. Emotionally, stress can produce negative or non-constructive feelings about self. Intellectually, stress can alter a person's perceptual and problem-solving abilities. Socially, stress can alter a person's relationships with others. Spiritually, stress can change a person's general outlook on life. Many illnesses, including hypertension, duodenal ulcers, bronchial asthma, and coronary heart disease, have been linked to stress.

Stress as a Stimulus

Stress may be defined as a stimulus, a life event (sometimes called a "life change") or set of circumstances causing a disrupted response (Lyon and Werner 1987) that increases the individual's vulnerability to illness. Holmes and Rahe (1967) assigned a numerical value to

---

RESEARCH NOTE

Can Ethical Dilemmas of Nursing Practice Contribute to Stress and Burnout?

Martin surveyed 75 nurses who were primary caregivers of persons with AIDS. The instruments used in this study were the AIDS Ethical Dilemma Scale, the Maslach Burnout Inventory (MBI), and the COPE Inventory. The focus of the study was to relate the ethical dilemmas experienced by nurses caring for AIDS patients to burnout and coping mechanisms. The findings suggest that ethical dilemmas posed in caring for AIDS patients are stressful. Fifty percent of the nurses surveyed reported a high degree of emotional exhaustion on the MBI. The findings also suggest that nurses who had more nursing experience were able to use more effective coping mechanisms in stressful situations.

Implications: Nurses facing ethical dilemmas in practice need to identify what issues are presenting the dilemma. They also need to identify their positive coping strategies and use them when confronting stressful situations. Nurses working in care areas that have a high degree of ethical dilemmas should form support groups to deal effectively with those issues and prevent harmful stress and burnout.

D. Martin. Effects of ethical dilemmas on stress felt by nurses providing care to AIDS patients. *Critical Care Nursing Quarterly,* 12:4 March 1, 1990, 53–57.

---

43 life changes or events. The scale of stressful life events is used to document a person's relatively recent experiences, such as divorce, pregnancy, and retirement. In this view, both positive and negative events are considered stressful.

Since 1967, similar scales have been developed. Burgess and Lazare (1976, p. 58) caution people in the use of such scales. They emphasize that the degree of stress the event presents can be highly individual. For example, a divorce may be highly traumatic to one person and cause relatively little anxiety to another. What is important is that research has shown that people who have a high level of stress are often more prone to illness and have lowered ability to cope with illness and subsequent stress.

Stress as a Response

Stress may also be defined as a response, the disruption caused by a noxious stimulus or stressor (Lyon and Werner 1987). In this definition of stress, reactions rather than events are the focus. The response view was developed by Hans Selye (1956, 1976). He defined stress as "the nonspecific response of the body to any kind of demand made upon it" (1976, p. 1). Regardless of the cause, situation, or psychologic interpretation of a demanding situation, Selye's stress response is characterized by the same chain or pattern of physiologic events. This nonspecific response was called the *general adaptation syndrome (GAS)* or *stress syndrome.*

To differentiate the cause of stress from the response to stress, Selye created the term *stressor* (1976, p. 51) to denote any factor that produces stress and disturbs the body's equilibrium. Because stress is a state of the body, it can be observed only by the changes it produces in the body. This response of the body, the stress syndrome or general adaptation syndrome, occurs with the release of certain adaptive hormones and subsequent changes in the structure and chemical composition of the body. Body organs affected by stress are the gastrointestinal tract, the adrenals, and the lymphatic structures. With prolonged stress, the adrenals enlarge considerably; the lymphatic structures, such as the thymus, spleen, and lymph nodes, atrophy and deep ulcers appear in the lining of the stomach. In addition to adapting globally, the body can also react locally, i.e., one organ or a part of the body reacts alone. This is referred to as the *local adaptation syndrome,* or *LAS.* One example of the LAS is inflammation. Selye proposed that both the GAS and the LAS have three stages (1976, p. 38): alarm reaction, resistance, and exhaustion.

Alarm Reaction (AR)

The initial reaction of the body is the alarm reaction, which alerts the body's defenses against the stressor, whether the stressor is heat, bacteria, or a verbal or physical attack from someone. Selye divided this stage into two parts: the shock phase and the countershock phase.

During the shock phase, the stressor may be perceived consciously or unconsciously by the person. In any case, the autonomic nervous system reacts, and large amounts of epinephrine (adrenaline) and cortisone are released into the body. The person is then ready for fight or flight. This primary response is short lived, lasting from 1 minute to 24 hours.

The second part of the alarm reaction is called the countershock phase. During this time, the body changes produced during the shock phase are reversed. It is, therefore, during the shock phase of the alarm reaction that a person is best mobilized to react.

Stage of Resistance (SR)

During the second stage in the GAS and LAS syndromes, the body's adaptation takes place. In other words, the body attempts to cope with the stressor and to limit the stressor to the smallest area of the body that can deal with it.

Stage of Exhaustion (SE)

During the third stage, the adaptation that the body made during the second stage cannot be maintained. This means that the ways used to cope with the stressor have been exhausted. If adaptation has not overcome the stressor, the stress effects may spread to the entire body. At the end of this stage, the body may either rest and return to normal, or death may be the ultimate consequence. The end of this stage depends largely on the adaptive energy resources of the individual, the severity of the stressor, and the external adaptive resources that are provided, such as oxygen.

Selye's general adaptation syndrome encompasses a range of physiologic responses to stressors in the body as a whole. See Figure 23–1. Stressors stimulate the sympathetic nervous system, which in turn stimulates the hypothalamus. The hypothalamus releases corticotropin-releasing hormone (CRH), which stimulates the anterior pituitary gland to release adrenocorticotropin (ACTH). During stress, the adrenal medulla, which is functionally related to the sympathetic nervous system, secretes epinephrine and norepinephrine in response to sympathetic stimulation. Significant body responses to epinephrine include the following:

1. Increased myocardial contractility, which increases cardiac output and blood flow to active muscles

2. Bronchial dilation, which allows increased oxygen intake

3. Increased blood clotting

4. Increased cellular metabolism

5. Increased fat mobilization to make energy available and to synthesize other compounds needed by the body

The principal effect of norepinephrine is decreased blood to the kidneys and increased secretion of renin. Renin hydrolyzes one of the blood proteins to produce *angiotensin,* which tends to increase the blood pressure by constricting arterioles. The sum of all these adrenal hormonal effects permits the person to perform far more strenuous physical activity than would otherwise be possible.

Stress as a Transaction

Lazarus's Model

Transactional theories of stress are based on the work of Lazarus (1966), who states that the stimulus theory and the response theory do not consider individual differences. Neither explains which factors lead some persons and not others to respond effectively nor interprets why some persons are able to adapt over longer periods than others. According to Lazarus, "Stimulus definitions focus on events in the environment such as natural disasters, illness, or termination of employment. This approach assumes that certain situations are normatively stressful but does not allow for individual differences in the evaluation of events. Response definitions refer to a state of stress; the person is spoken of as reacting with stress, being under stress, and so on. Stimulus and response definitions have limited utility, because a stimulus gets defined as stressful only in terms of a stress response" (Lazarus and Folkman 1984, p. 21).

Although Lazarus recognizes that certain environmental demands and pressures produce stress in substantial numbers of people, he emphasizes that people and groups differ in their sensitivity and vulnerability to certain types of events, as well as in their interpretations and reactions. For example, in terms of illness, one person may respond with denial, another with anxiety, and still another with depression. To explain variations among individuals under comparable conditions, the Lazarus model takes into account cognitive processes that intervene between the encounter and the reaction, and the factors that affect the nature of this process. In contrast to Selye, who focuses on physiologic re-

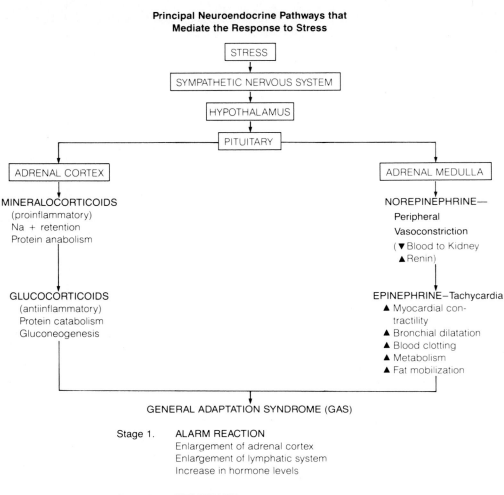

**Principal Neuroendocrine Pathways that
Mediate the Response to Stress**

STRESS

↓

SYMPATHETIC NERVOUS SYSTEM

↓

HYPOTHALAMUS

↓

PITUITARY

ADRENAL CORTEX	ADRENAL MEDULLA

MINERALOCORTICOIDS
(proinflammatory)
Na + retention
Protein anabolism

NOREPINEPHRINE—
Peripheral
Vasoconstriction
(▼ Blood to Kidney
▲ Renin)

GLUCOCORTICOIDS
(antiinflammatory)
Protein catabolism
Gluconeogenesis

EPINEPHRINE–Tachycardia
▲ Myocardial con-
   tractility
▲ Bronchial dilatation
▲ Blood clotting
▲ Metabolism
▲ Fat mobilization

GENERAL ADAPTATION SYNDROME (GAS)

Stage 1.   ALARM REACTION
   Enlargement of adrenal cortex
   Enlargement of lymphatic system
   Increase in hormone levels

Stage 2.   RESISTANCE
   Shrinkage of adrenal cortex
   Lymph nodes closer to normal size
   Hormone levels sustained

Stage 3.   EXHAUSTION
   Enlargement/dysfunction of
      lymphatic structures
   Increase in hormone levels
   Depletion of adaptive hormones

A stress syndrome, termed the General Adaption Syndrome
(GAS) by Hans Selye, evolves in three stages. Stages 1 and 2 are
continuously repeated throughout a lifetime cycle. If resistance
cannot be sustained, exhaustion (Stage 3), with its altered psycho-
physiological functioning, occurs.

Figure 23-1 Physiologic response to stress: general adaptation syndrome.   *Source:* Physiologic responses of the general adaptation syndrome. From M. J. Smith
and H. Selye, Stress: Reducing the negative effects of stress, *American Journal of Nursing,* November
1979, 79:1954. Used by permission.

sponses, Lazarus includes mental and psychologic components or responses as part of his concept of stress.

The Lazarus *transactional stress theory* encompasses a set of cognitive, affective, and adaptive (coping) responses that arise out of person-environment transactions. The person and the environment are inseparable; each affects and is affected by the other. Stress is defined as a particular relationship between the person and the environment that is appraised by the person as taxing or exceeding the person's resources and endangering well-being (Lazarus and Folkman 1984, p. 19). The individual responds to perceived environmental changes by adaptive or coping responses. *Cognitive appraisal* is an evaluative process that determines why and to what extent a particular transaction or series of transactions between the person and the environment is stressful. Coping is the process through which the individual manages the demands of the person-environment relationship that are appraised as stressful and the emotions they generate (Lazarus and Folkman 1984, p. 19).

Nuernberger's Model   Nuernberger (1981, p. 69) believes that there is an adaptive pattern of responding beyond the arousal mechanism of the sympathetic nervous system. This other response, based on stimulation of the parasympathetic nervous system, is one of inhibition. He calls this response the *general inhibition syndrome* or *possum response*. To Nuernberger (1981, p. 71), healthy nonstress functioning is represented by a balance between the two parts of the autonomic nervous system: sympathetic and parasympathetic branches. Stress is a state of internal imbalance reflecting the unrelieved dominance of either arousal by the sympathetic nervous system (fight-or-flight response) or inhibition by the parasympathetic nervous system (possum response). The effects of excessive stimulation of or dominance by either of these systems are evinced as a localized response in a specific organ or as a generalized response pattern. Both responses are designed for self-protection.

Nuernberger maintains that the presence of either arousal or inhibition does not in itself constitute stress. Stress occurs only when arousal is not balanced by relaxation or when relaxation (inhibition) is not balanced by activity. Prolonged or intense parasympathetic imbalances are associated with such diseases as asthma or depression. Prolonged sympathetic imbalances are associated with, for example, cardiovascular disease.

Nuernberger (1981, p. 81) writes that the primary source of stress is not the external environment; it is a person's internal state of mind; it is the emotional and perceptual factors that form a person's basic personality. The greatest source of hypothalamic arousal is the cerebral cortex in response to repetitive thought patterns and apprehensions about unresolved past, present, or future events that people associate with potentially painful or negative consequences in their lives.

Nuernberger defines emotional stress as the result of a mental process: It is a state of autonomic imbalance generated as a reaction to the perception of some kind of threat, pain or discomfort. This perception involves an interpretation of selected sensory stimuli, which is colored, or structured, by memories of past pain. It is also involved with the anticipation that this pain will occur in the future as a consequence of present sensory stimuli and environmental conditions. It is sustained by indecisiveness, the inability to resolve the threat" (Nuernberger 1981, p. 86).

MANIFESTATIONS OF STRESS

Manifestations of the stress experience, both physiologic and psychologic, may be considered coping strategies or mechanisms. *Coping* is the immediate response of a person to a threatening situation. In contrast, *adaptation* is the final response or change that occurs. According to Lazarus and Folkman (1984, p. 141), coping refers to constantly changing cognitive and behavioral efforts to manage specific external and/or internal demands that are appraised as taxing or exceeding the resources of a person.

Coping may be described as dealing with problems and situations, or contending with them successfully. A *coping strategy* (coping mechanism) is an innate or acquired way of responding to a changing environment or specific problem or situation. In nursing literature, effective and ineffective coping are often differentiated. *Effective coping* results in adaptation; *ineffective coping* results in maladaptation. Although coping behavior may not always seem appropriate, the nurse needs to remember that coping is always purposeful.

Coping strategies vary among individuals and are often related to the individual's perception of the stressful event. A person's coping strategies often change with a reappraisal of a situation. There is never only one way to cope. Some people choose avoidance; others confront a situation as a means of coping. Still others seek information or rely on religious beliefs as a means of coping. Bell (1977, p. 137) places coping strategies into two groups: long term and short term. Long-term coping strategies can be constructive and realistic. For example, in certain situations talking with others about the problem and trying to find out more about the situation are long-term strategies.

Short-term coping strategies can reduce stress to a tolerable limit temporarily but are in the long run ineffective ways to deal with reality. They may even have a destructive or detrimental effect on the person (Bell 1977, p. 137). Examples of short-term strategies are using alcoholic beverages or drugs, daydreaming and fantasizing, and relying on the belief that everything will work out.

Physiologic Manifestations

Physiologic manifestations, such as increased heart rate and blood pressure, muscle tension, mental alertness or lassitude, and diaphoresis, may or may not occur in clients experiencing stress, depending on the way the client perceives the stressful event and on the effectiveness of his or her coping strategies. There is considerable evidence that a person's cognitive coping strategies mediate blood pressure and heart rates. For example, when a person cognitively attends to the stressor or threat, there is a decrease in heart rate.

Psychologic Manifestations

Psychologic manifestations include anxiety, anger, cognitive behaviors, verbal and motor responses, and unconscious ego defense mechanisms. Some of these coping patterns are helpful; others are a hindrance, depending on the situation and the length of time they are used or experienced. Indeed, anxiety is often considered to be a response to a stressful event rather than a coping mechanism, since it may impede action to remove the stressor.

Anxiety, a common reaction to stress, can be experienced at the conscious, subconscious, or unconscious levels. It differs from fear in four ways:

1. Its source is not identifiable; the source of fear is identifiable.
2. It is related to the future, i.e., an anticipated event. Fear is related to the present.
3. It is vague, whereas fear is definite.
4. It is the result of psychologic or emotional conflict; fear is the result of a discrete physical or psychologic entity.

All people experience anxiety to some degree most of the time. Mild or moderate anxiety is needed to accomplish developmental tasks and motivate goal-directed behavior. In this sense, anxiety is an effective coping strategy. Excessive anxiety, however, often has destructive effects.

Anxiety may be manifested on four different levels:

1. *Mild anxiety,* which produces a slight arousal state that enhances perception, learning, and productive abilities. Most healthy persons experience mild anxiety, perhaps as a feeling of mild restlessness that prompts a person to seek information and ask questions.

2. *Moderate anxiety,* which increases the client's arousal state to a point where the person expresses feelings of tension, nervousness, or concern. Perceptual abilities are narrowed. Attention is focused more on a particular aspect of a situation than on peripheral activities.

3. *Severe anxiety,* which consumes most of the person's energies and requires intervention. Perception is further decreased. The person, unable to focus on what is really happening, focuses on only one specific detail of the situation generating the anxiety.

4. *Panic,* which is an overpowering, frightening level of anxiety causing the person to lose control. It is less frequently experienced than other levels of anxiety. The perception of a panicked person can be altered to the point where the person distorts events. See Table 23–1 for signs of these levels.

Anger, another response to stress, is commonly manifested in altered voice tone as a communication to desist from some action or other. Verbal expression of anger can therefore be considered a signal to others of one's internal psychologic discomfort and a call for assistance to deal with perceived stress. In contrast, *hostility* is usually marked by overt antagonism and harmful or destructive behavior; *aggression* is an unprovoked attack or a hostile, injurious, or destructive action or outlook; and *violence* is the exertion of physical force to injure or abuse. Verbally expressed anger differs from hostility, aggression, and violence, but it can lead to destructiveness and violence if the anger persists unabated.

Clearly expressed verbal communication of anger, when the angry person tells the other person about the anger and carefully identifies the source, is constructive. This clarity of communication gets the anger out into the open so that the other person can deal with it and help to alleviate it. The angry person "gets it off his chest" and

TABLE 23-1 *Signs of Mild, Moderate, and Severe Anxiety*

Sign	Mild	Moderate	Severe (Panic)
Verbalization changes	Expresses feelings of increased arousal and concern Increased questioning or information seeking	Expresses feelings of tension, apprehension, nervousness, or concern Verbalized expectation of danger Voice tremors and pitch changes Increased rate and quantity of verbalization	Expresses feelings of severe dread, apprehension, nervousness, concern, helplessness, and isolation Absence of verbalization Inappropriate verbalization, e.g., false cheerfulness or laughing while discussing a serious subject
Motor activity changes	Mild restlessness	Pacing Hand tremor or shakiness Increased muscle tension	Immobilization Purposeless activity Increased muscle tension Rigid posture Fixed or scattered perceptual focus
Perception and attention changes	Increased awareness Increased attending Ability to focus on most of what is really happening	Narrowed focus of attention Ability to focus on most of what is really happening	Intellectualizing about a subject, e.g., explaining the pathophysiology of leukemia rather than describing own feelings Intent and fearful watching of everything going on Inability to focus on what is really happening Inability to focus on reality, e.g., denial, saying "I don't want to talk about it"
Respiratory and circulatory changes	Nil	Rapid pulse Increased respiratory rate	Tachycardia Palpitations Hyperventilation
Other changes	Nil	Diaphoresis Sleep or eating disturbances, e.g., insomnia, somnolence, overeating, or anorexia Irritability	Diaphoresis Dilated pupils Pallor Clammy hands and skin Dry mouth Sullenness, withdrawal

Sources: Compiled from M. Gordon, *Manual of nursing diagnosis* (New York: McGraw-Hill, 1982), pp. 153–60; and Anxiety: recognition and intervention (programmed instruction) *American Journal of Nursing* September 1965, 65:129–52. Copyright © 1965 The American Journal of Nursing Company; M. J. Kim, G. K. McFarland, and A. M. McLane, *Pocket guide to nursing diagnoses,* 3d ed. (St. Louis: C. V. Mosby Co., 1989), p. 4; and L. J. Carpenito, *Nursing diagnosis: Application to clinical practice,* 3d ed. (Philadelphia: J. B. Lippincott Co., 1989).

prevents an emotional buildup. Constructive expressions of anger have three elements (Duldt 1981, p. 516):

1. *Alerting,* the act of engaging another's attention
2. *Describing,* the process of delineating the source of the angry person's feelings, i.e., what has happened here and now
3. *Identifying,* the act of seeking a response and support from others

Unclear communication of anger is destructive. It is similar to constructive expressions only in the alerting behavior. Then the person fails to describe the source of the feelings adequately and denies any responsibility for the anger by blaming others or by generalizing to other people or past situations. Thus, those in the presence of the angry person are unable to respond helpfully.

Cognitive Manifestations

Cognitive manifestations of stress include problem solving, structuring, self-control or self-discipline, suppression, fantasy, and prayer. *Problem solving* involves thinking through the threatening situation, using specific steps, similar to those of the nursing process, to arrive at a solution. The person assesses the situation or problem, analyzes or defines it, chooses alternatives, carries out the selected alternative, and evaluates whether the solution was successful.

Structuring is the arrangement or manipulation of a situation so that threatening events do not occur. For example, a nurse can structure or control an interview with a client by asking only direct, closed questions. This strategy avoids information or questions that may be threatening to the nurse's knowledge or values. Structuring, however, can be productive in certain situations.

Self-control (discipline) is assuming a manner and facial expression that convey a sense of being in control or in charge, no matter what the situation is. When self-control prevents panic and harmful or nonproductive actions in a threatening situation, it is a helpful response that conveys strength. Self-control carried to an extreme, however, can delay problem solving and prevent a person from receiving the support of others, who may perceive the person as handling the situation well, as cold, or as unconcerned.

Suppression is consciously and willfully putting a thought or feeling out of mind: "I won't deal with that today. I'll do it tomorrow." This response relieves stress temporarily but does not solve the problem.

Fantasy or daydreaming is likened to make-believe.

Unfulfilled wishes and desires are imagined as fulfilled, or a threatening experience is reworked or replayed so that it ends differently from reality. Experiences can be relived, everyday problems solved, and plans for the future made. The outcome of current problems may also be fantasized. Fantasy responses can be helpful if they lead to problem solving, but they can be destructive and nonproductive if a person uses them to excess and retreats from reality.

Prayer often involves identifying and describing the problem, suggesting solutions, and reaching out for support and help. If the problem-solving steps lead to action, prayer can be a constructive response, aside from the support and meaning the person derives from it.

Verbal and Motor Manifestations

Verbal or motor manifestations of stress may be the first responses evident. Among these responses are crying, verbal abuse, laughing, screaming, hitting and kicking, and holding and touching. *Crying* releases tension in situations perceived as painful, joyful, or sad and when the situation cannot yet be managed cognitively. As a response, crying tends to be more socially acceptable in women and in certain cultures, for instance, among Hispanics or Mediterranean people. People often cry when they perceive that others care. Crying is beneficial as a release of tension and if it is followed by problem solving. It is not helpful without problem solving.

Verbal abuse is another release mechanism most often expressed toward stress-producing objects and events, such as nonfunctional equipment, misplaced or lost items, and rainy weather. *Laughing* is also an anxiety-reducing response that can lead to constructive problem solving. People may laugh at small incidents and at the way they handled a situation.

Screaming is a response to fear or intense frustration and anger. One may scream in response to a person appearing suddenly out of the dark or in response to a family member who keeps planning other activities to avoid cleaning the garage. Screaming, like other verbal responses, reduces tension but can be harmful if the person is unable to control it and becomes hysterical. The hysterical, frightened person needs to be moved to a quiet place and assured that the threat is over. The hysterical, frustrated person needs assistance to deal with the situation with a more effective coping strategy, e.g., problem solving.

Hitting and kicking are spontaneous responses to physical threats. Adults who are socialized to control such responses toward people may direct them toward objects by pounding a table with a fist or kicking a wastebasket. Preschoolers, however, have not matured enough to develop control and may, for example, hit or kick a nurse who is administering an injection. Hitting or kicking can be helpful in reducing tension provided the person or object is not damaged and provided they lead toward cognitive coping techniques.

Holding and touching are often responses to joyful, painful, or sad events. Holding or touching another is a gesture of support and comfort. Holding and touching responses vary considerably, however, among cultures and among individuals in a culture. Verbal communication can also convey caring. "Crisis lines" or close friends often provide meaningful and supportive verbal communication that conveys caring over the telephone or in person.

Unconscious Ego Defense Mechanisms

Unconscious *ego defense mechanisms* are psychologic defensive (adaptive) mechanisms or, in the words of Sigmund Freud (1946), mental mechanisms, which develop as the personality attempts to defend itself, establish compromises among conflicting impulses, and allay inner tensions. Defense mechanisms are the working of the unconscious mind to protect the person from anxiety. They can be considered precursors to conscious cognitive coping mechanisms that will ultimately solve the problem. Like some verbal and motor responses, defense mechanisms release tension. Table 23–2 describes these mechanisms and lists examples of their adaptive and maladaptive use.

FACTORS INFLUENCING THE MANIFESTATIONS OF STRESS

The degree to which a stressor affects an individual depends on the nature of the stressor, perception of the stressor, number of simultaneous stressors, duration of exposure to the stressor, experiences with a comparable stressor (Byrne and Thompson 1978, p. 3), age, and support people available. The *nature of the stressor* refers to its magnitude. Obviously, a fall from the roof of a building is more stressful than a fall from a chair. Similarly, angry remarks from a loved one are more stressful than those from a stranger.

Perception of the stressor (what the stressor means to the person) can be as important as the actual magnitude of the stressor. Because perception is a subjective phenomenon, there are wide differences in how people regard a stressor. Being late can create a greater stress response in a punctual person than a nonpunctual person.

The *number of stressors* a person is experiencing at one time can greatly affect the responses. This often explains why a stressor that the nurse considers small can elicit a disproportionate response. The client uses up his coping strategies as he expends them on multiple problems before he has a chance to renew himself.

The *duration of exposure to the stressor* can also influence the manifestations of stress. If the duration of the stressor extends a person's stage of resistance beyond the person's coping powers, the person becomes exhausted and can eventually die.

Previous *experience with a comparable stressor* can be useful both in predicting how the person will react and in reducing stress in the current situation. A person who has successfully adjusted to a situation once before is more likely to do so again in a similar situation than a person who is adjusting to the situation for the first time. Such people are strengthened by knowledge that they handled the situation successfully before. Determining what a particular event means to a person can help the nurse plan care.

The *age* of the individual affects response and adaptation to stressors. Infants, for example, have poorly developed immune mechanisms and cannot tolerate large fluid losses. Elderly people may have declining physical and mental resources to cope with increased stressors. *Support people* can assist a person coping with stress to maintain psychologic and physical integrity. They provide emotional support, often help in decision making, and, by sharing the experience, can relieve the intensity of the stress response.

Friedman and Rosenman (1974) identify two *personality types:* type A and type B. They point out that type A personalities are very prone to cardiovascular disease, whereas type B personalities do not usually develop it. The most pervasive cardiovascular disease is hypertension: the higher a person's blood pressure, the higher the risk of developing hardening of the arteries, which results in heart attacks and strokes. See the box on page 440 for behavior patterns typical of both personality types.

Type A personalities are under constant pressure to perform and are hurried, impatient, and sometimes hostile. Type B personalities are relaxed, free from the urgencies of time, and able to enjoy work or play. Nuernberger (1981, p. 12) identifies another personality type, called type C, the coping personality. This personality

text continues on p. 440

TABLE 23-2 *Unconscious Ego Defense Mechanisms*

Mechanism	Description	Adaptive Use	Maladaptive Use
Denial	Blocking painful or anxiety-producing aspects of reality out of consciousness. Reality is either completely disregarded or transformed so that it is no longer threatening.	A man does not acknowledge that he has cancer even though the physician has told him the results of the biopsy. A child insists his mother is not dead, just "out of town for a few days."	A woman who has had a heart attack refuses to acknowledge illness and does not follow prescribed therapy.
Rationalization	Often referred to as the "sour-grapes" or "half-truth" mechanism. Good reasons, acceptable to the conscious mind, are given for behavior or circumstances instead of the real reason. The person often disparages some goal that in reality the person would like to attain.	A student who fails an examination because she doesn't understand the material says that the teacher did not clarify the material sufficiently or she did not prepare adequately. A client whose work is interrupted by illness prematurely gives up the work and says he wouldn't have been successful in that field anyway.	A man always gives reasons for not attaining his goals and refuses to accept self-responsibility for not achieving them.
Compensation	Substituting an activity for one that the person really would like to do or cannot do.	A short man shows aggressive, dominating traits to suggest strength and authority that his stature does not convey. A boy who cannot participate in athletics studies hard and attains high grades.	A woman abuses alcohol and drugs to make up for feelings of inadequacy.
Repression	Excluding from consciousness desires, impulses, thoughts, memories, and strivings that conflict with self-image or that involve guilt, shame, or lowering of self-esteem. The painful events cannot be recalled or recognized. Repression is the underlying basis of all defense mechanisms.	A woman forgets a repugnant work assignment. A young woman who was raped and was brought to the outpatient clinic by her roommate says she feels very anxious but cannot remember the events of the past few hours.	A woman excludes a number of events from memory (amnesia).
Regression	Adopting behavior that was comforting earlier in life to overcome the discomfort and insecurity of the present situation.	A toilet-trained preschooler begins bed-wetting after his mother returns home with a new baby. A hospitalized elderly woman becomes more dependent on the nurse than is physically warranted.	A teenager assumes the fetal position for prolonged periods or plays with the genitals.
Sublimation	Redirecting libidinal drives (sexual and aggressive) into socially acceptable channels.	A person channels, to a limited degree, a sex drive into athletic activity, work, poetry, or music.	A person has extreme difficulty in communicating with others.

▶

TABLE 23-2 *(continued)*

Mechanism	Description	Adaptive Use	Maladaptive Use
		A man who is fired goes to the gym and punches a punching bag to express rage at his boss.	
Identification	Assuming the attitudes, ideas, and behavior patterns of another person or persons; it is an important growth mechanism for children. It is unconscious and differs from imitation, which is conscious.	A teenager changes her hairstyle to that of an idolized movie star. After having surgery, a young boy decides to become a doctor.	A man imitates socially unacceptable or harmful behavior.
Projection	Attributing to others characteristics and feelings that one does not want to admit are one's own.	A woman criticizes a neighbor for being a terrible gossip when in fact the woman herself gossips. A wife with illicit sexual wishes claims that all husbands are unfaithful and not to be trusted.	A person fails to take any responsibility for own behavior.
Conversion	Transforming a mental conflict into a physical symptom.	Before taking a math exam, a young girl develops a headache. A woman develops a "lump in her throat" at a sad event.	A man experiences paralysis of his punching arm to avoid letting his anger get out of control and punching his boss. A girl develops an inability to speak in the context of protecting a sexually abusive father. A pregnant woman develops pathologic vomiting to express the forbidden desire not to have the baby.
Displacement	Transferring an emotion or feeling from the actual object to a less dangerous or threatening substitute.	A child directs hostility toward a parent to a teacher. A woman who has had an unpleasant experience with a man with red hair reacts strongly against all men with red hair.	A man is verbally or physically aggressive toward all authority or oppressive figures.
Reaction formation	Acting oppositely to what the person truly feels.	A woman shows great interest and concern for her mother-in-law, whom she dislikes. A man strongly criticizes pornographic literature when he has a desire to read it.	A young woman is always unnaturally sweet and loving and is unable to consider the possibility of being angry. A person with strong sadistic tendencies becomes an ardent opponent of surgical research on animals.

Source: Adapted with permission from P. Solomon and V. I. Patch. *Handbook of Psychiatry* 3d ed. (Los Altos, Calif.: Lange Medical Publications, 1974), pp. 500–505. Copyright © Lange Medical Publications.

sustains considerable stress but has learned to cope with it. Nuernberger believes many people are type C, since most people share some of the characteristics of types A and B.

HOMEOSTASIS AND ADAPTATION

The concept of homeostasis was first introduced by W. B. Cannon (1939) to describe the relative constancy of the internal processes of the body, such as blood oxygen and carbon dioxide levels, blood pressure, body temperature, blood glucose, and fluid and electrolyte balance. To Cannon, the word *homeostasis* did not imply something stagnant, set, or immobile; it meant a condition that might vary but remained relatively constant.

Cannon viewed the human being as separate from the external environment and constantly endeavoring to maintain physiologic *equilibrium,* or balance, through adaptation to that environment. *Homeostasis,* then, is the tendency of the body to maintain a state of balance or equilibrium while continually changing.

Physiologic Homeostasis

Physiologic homeostasis means that the internal environment of the body is relatively stable and constant. All cells of the body require a relatively constant environment to function; thus, the body's internal environment must be maintained within narrow limits. Homeostatic mechanisms have four main characteristics:

1. They are self-regulating.
2. They are compensatory.

3. They tend to be regulated by negative feedback systems.

4. They may require several feedback mechanisms to correct only one physiologic imbalance.

Self-regulation means that homeostatic mechanisms come into play automatically in the healthy person. However, if a person is ill, or if a respiratory organ such as a lung is injured, the homeostatic mechanisms may not be able to respond to the stimulus as they would normally. Homeostatic mechanisms are *compensatory* (counterbalancing), because they tend to counteract conditions that are abnormal for the person.

Feedback is the mechanism by which some of the output of a system is "fed back" into the system as input. This input influences the behavior of the system and its future output. *Negative feedback* inhibits change; *positive feedback* stimulates change. Most biologic systems are controlled by negative feedback to bring the system back to stability. This type of feedback system senses and counteracts any deviations from normal. The deviations may be greater or less than the normal level or range. Negative feedback is a common control mechanism for hormone levels. For example, an increase in the production of parathyroid hormone is stimulated by a drop in blood calcium, but, when parathyroid hormone is increased and raises the level of blood calcium, its production is then inhibited. Several negative feedback systems may be required to correct one physiologic imbalance. For example, with hypoxia (shortage of oxygen), the concentration of red blood cells increases and the heart rate becomes faster to transport the blood and available oxygen around the body adequately.

The two major homeostatic regulators are the autonomic nervous system and the endocrine system. In addition, the cardiovascular system, the renal system, the respiratory system, and the gastrointestinal system are important in maintaining homeostasis.

Psychologic Homeostasis

The term psychologic homeostasis refers to emotional or psychologic balance or a state of mental well-being. It is maintained by a variety of mechanisms. Each person has certain psychologic needs, such as the need for love, security, and self-esteem, that must be met to maintain psychologic homeostasis. When one or more of these needs is not met or is threatened, certain coping mechanisms are activated to protect the person and provide psychologic homeostasis.

Psychologic homeostasis is acquired or learned through the experience of living and interacting with others. In addition, societal norms and culture influence behavior. Some prerequisites for a person to develop psychologic homeostasis can be summarized:

- A stable physical environment in which the person feels safe and secure. For example, the basic needs for food, shelter, and clothing must be met consistently from birth onward.

- A stable psychologic environment from infancy onward, so that feelings of trust and love develop. Growing children and adolescents also need kind but firm and consistent discipline, encouragement, and support to be their own unique selves.

- A social environment that includes adults who are healthy role models. Children learn the customs and values of society from these individuals.

- A life experience that provides satisfactions. Throughout life, people encounter many frustrations. People deal with these better if enough satisfying experiences have occurred to counterbalance the frustrating ones.

Adaptation

Adaptation is the basis of homeostasis and resistance to stress. To adapt is to modify to meet new, changing, or different conditions. Because it is a phenomenon of all living things, adaptation is studied in many disciplines, such as plant biology, physics, psychology, education (personality adaptation), biochemistry, psychiatry, and ecology. In all disciplines, adaptation denotes interaction and change. The change is viewed as positive, for the better, or healthy.

Modes of Adaptation Human adaptation occurs in three interrelated modes: physiologic, psychologic, and sociocultural.

Physiologic Mode *Physiologic* or *biologic adaptation* occurs in response to increased or altered demands placed on the body and results in compensatory physical changes (e.g., increased muscle size and strength following prolonged exercise, increased capacity of the heart and lungs after prolonged exercise, and immunity to a specific disease following the invasion of a specific microorganism).

Psychologic Mode *Psychologic adaptation* involves a change in attitude and behavior, e.g., coping strategies, toward emotionally stressful situations. Examples include changing a life-style pattern (such as eating a balanced diet, exercising regularly, or balancing leisure time with work), using problem solving in decision making instead of anger or other nonconstructive responses, and stopping smoking.

Adaptation in the psychologic mode may also be maladaptive. For example, abusing alcohol and constantly giving in to others to avoid their anger are maladaptive.

Sociocultural Mode   *Sociocultural adaptation* involves changes in the person's behavior in accordance with the norms, conventions, and beliefs of various groups, such as family, society, ethnic group, religious group, professional group, and economic group (e.g., becoming socialized into a profession or military group, or living in a new country and learning to speak the language).

Developmental Mode   Developmental adaptation occurs in response to developmental stressors (see Table 23–3), at the level of knowledge, experience, and skill that the individual has attained. For example, a child who has not developed coping strategies is less able to adapt than an adult. An infant whose physical systems are not sufficiently developed is less able to adapt to changes in environmental temperatures.

Characteristics of Adaptive Responses   All adaptive responses, whether physiologic, psychologic, or sociocultural, have common characteristics:

1. All adaptive responses are attempts to maintain homeostasis.
2. Adaptation is a whole body or total organism response.
3. Adaptive responses have limits. Physiologic adaptive responses are more limited than psychologic or social responses.
4. Adaptation requires time. A person adapts to an inadequate cardiac output that occurs gradually because the heart increases its pumping rate and the size of the ventricles. In the psychologic realm, people are able to think more rationally in controlled or expected situations than in emergencies.
5. Adaptability varies from person to person. The person who is physically healthy has greater resources to adapt. The person who is flexible, responds readily to change, and uses a wide range of coping strategies is more likely to adapt than the person who does not tolerate change and responds in a limited way.

TABLE 23-3   *Selected Stressors Associated with Developmental Stages*

Developmental Stage	Stressors
Child	Resolving conflict between independence and dependence
	Beginning school
	Establishing peer relationships and adjustments
	Coping with peer competition
Adolescent	Accepting changing body physique
	Developing heterosexual or other relationships
	Achieving independence
	Choosing a career
Young adult	Getting married
	Leaving home
	Managing a home
	Getting started in an occupation
	Continuing one's education
	Rearing children
Middle adult	Accepting physical changes of aging
	Maintaining social status and standard of living
	Helping teenage children to become independent
	Adjusting to aging parents
Older adult	Accepting decreasing physical abilities and health
	Accepting changes in residence
	Adjusting to retirement and reduced income
	Adjusting to death of spouse and friends

6. Adaptive responses may be inadequate or excessive. For example, the inflammatory response to bacterial invasion may not be sufficient to overcome an infection without antibiotic therapy. Inflammation in response to allergies can be excessive and create other problems.
7. Adaptive responses are egocentric and tiring because they require body energy and tax physical and psychologic resources. Adapting can consume a person's energy to the point that the person overlooks

the needs of others and fails to give the support they require.

ASSESSING

How a person perceives and responds to stressors is highly individual. Vulnerability to stressors is largely related to previous learning, stage of development, life events, health, and coping methods. The nurse can help the client recognize stress and support effective coping strategies or teach the client new and more effective ways of handling stress.

Assessment relative to a client's stress and coping patterns includes (a) a stress and coping pattern history and (b) clinical examination of the client for indicators of stress. Questions to elicit data about the client's stress and coping patterns are shown in the accompanying box. In addition, the nurse should be aware of expected developmental transitions (predictable tasks that must be accomplished if the person is to grow psychologically as well as physically). This knowledge helps the nurse identify additional stressors that are present and the client's response to them. See Table 23–3.

Indicators of stress were discussed earlier in this chapter. See Table 23–1 for descriptions of levels of anxiety. Observe the client also for verbal, motor, and cognitive manifestations. Remember, however, that clinical signs and symptoms may not occur when cognitive coping is effective.

ASSESSMENT INTERVIEW
Stress and Coping Patterns

- On a scale of one to ten, how would you rate the stress you are experiencing in the following areas?
  a. Home
  b. Work or school
  c. Finance
  d. Recent illness or loss of loved one
  e. Your health
  f. Family responsibilities
  g. Ethnic or cultural group
  h. Religion
  i. Relationships with friends
  j. Relationship with parents or children
  k. Relationship with partner
  l. Recent hospitalization
  m. Other (specify)
- How long have you been dealing with the above stressor(s)?
- How do you usually handle stressful situations?
  a. Cry?
  b. Get angry?
  c. Become verbally abusive?
  d. Talk to someone (who)?
  e. Withdraw from the situation?
  f. Structure and control others or situation?
  g. Go for a walk or physical exercise?
  h. Try to arrive at a solution?
  i. Pray for wisdom and courage?
  j. Other (specify)?
- How does your usual coping strategy work?

DIAGNOSING

Several nursing diagnoses may apply to clients who are experiencing stress and having difficulties in coping with that stress. According to the NANDA definition, the nursing diagnosis **Anxiety** is a "state in which the individual experiences feelings of uneasiness (apprehension) and activation of the autonomic nervous system in response to a vague, nonspecific threat" (Carpenito 1989, p. 128). When the nurse assesses that the client manifests physiologic symptoms of anxiety (e.g., increased heart rate, diaphoresis, trembling), emotional symptoms (e.g., apprehension, nervousness, tension), and cognitive symptoms (e.g., inability to concentrate, forgetfulness, lack of awareness of surroundings), the nurse can be reasonably sure that the client is anxious.

Fear is "a state in which an individual or group experiences a feeling of physiological or emotional disruption related to an identifiable source that is perceived as dangerous" (Carpenito 1989, p. 324). Unlike the anxious person, the fearful person can identify the specific threat. According to Carpenito (1989, p. 324), **Fear** and **Anxiety** often coexist in clinical practice.

Ineffective individual coping is a "state in which the individual experiences or is at risk of experiencing an inability to manage internal or environmental stressors adequately because of inadequate resources (physical, psychological, or behavioral)" (Carpenito 1989, p. 242). This diagnosis is appropriate when the nurse assesses that the client is not meeting role expectations, is using defense mechanisms inappropriately, or verbalizes an inability to cope. As with most nursing diagnoses, the etiology may be physiologic, psychologic, situational, or maturational. **Ineffective family coping** is discussed in Chapter 16.

Decisional conflict is the "state in which an individual or group experiences uncertainty about a course of action when the choice involves risk, loss, or challenge" (Carpenito 1989, p. 277). This diagnosis applies when the client verbalizes uncertainty about choices or undesired consequences of alternative actions being considered and vacillates between choices or delays decision making.

Examples of these diagnoses and possible contributing factors follow.

Anxiety related to:

- Perceived threat to self-concept
- Threat of dying
- Change in health status
- Actual or perceived loss of loved one
- Maturational crisis (e.g., parenting, career development, retirement)
- Change in environment (e.g., hospital, nursing home)
- Change in socioeconomic status
- Conflict about essential values

Fear related to:

- Perceived changes in body integrity (e.g., loss of body part, disfigurement)
- Separation from family or other support persons
- Language barrier
- Pain and perceived inability to cope

Ineffective individual coping related to:

- Changes in body (e.g., loss of body part)
- Inadequate support system
- Unrealistic perceptions
- Inadequate coping method
- Work overload
- Impairment of nervous system
- Chronic pain

Decisional conflict (specify) related to:

- Knowledge deficit
- Conflict with personal values/beliefs

- Unclear values/beliefs
- Ethical dilemma
- Disagreement with significant others

PLANNING

The nurse develops plans in collaboration with the client and significant support persons when possible, according to the client's state of health (e.g., ability to return to work), level of anxiety, support resources, coping mechanisms, and sociocultural and religious affiliation. The nurse with little experience intervening with clients undergoing stress may wish to consult with a clinical specialist or more experienced nurse to develop effective plans. Nurse and client set goals to change the existing client responses to the stressor or stressors. Examples of possible goal statements for some of the sample nursing diagnoses are shown in the accompanying box.

Nursing interventions for achieving the goals planned may include

- Minimizing anxiety or mediating anger
- Identifying the coping mechanisms most useful to the client
- Identifying meaningful support persons who can help the client
- Planning stress reduction measures, such as physical exercise, rest periods, or time management, or provid-

---

Goal Statements: Stress

- The client experiences reduction in level of anxiety.
- The client resolves anxiety concerning the loved one's death.
- The client is able to cope with multiple life changes.
- The client receives adequate support for coping.
- The family is able to cope with existing economic problems.
- The family is able to cope with the ongoing effects of one of its member's prolonged disability.

---

ing referral for advanced stress reduction techniques, such as yoga.

Examples of outcome criteria to measure goal achievement and the effectiveness of nursing interventions follow.

The client experiencing **Anxiety:**

- Verbalizes awareness of feelings of anxiety.
- Keeps a log of incidents that arouse anxiety, frustration, or time urgency.
- Reports an increase in psychologic and physiologic comfort.
- Experiences a reduction in the manifestations of anxiety (specify).
- Uses adaptive coping methods to reduce anxiety (e.g., relaxation techniques; time management strategies; direct, open discussion; problem-solving skills).
- Avoids blaming others and expecting others to change.

The client experiencing **Fear:**

- Discusses fears.
- Reports an increase in psychologic and physiologic comfort.
- Experiences reduction in manifestations indicative of fear (e.g., tension, apprehension, panic).
- Has blood pressure and heart rate within normal range, relaxed muscles, and normal pupil size.
- Describes effective and ineffective coping patterns.
- Identifies own coping resources.

The client with **Ineffective individual coping:**

- Identifies ineffective coping behaviors and consequences.
- Verbalizes awareness of own coping.
- Identifies personal strengths (skills, knowledge, abilities) to cope with threats.
- Seeks new knowledge and skills to resolve stressful event(s).
- Reports decrease in emotional responsiveness.
- Demonstrates increased objectivity, ability to solve problems, and assertiveness.
- Uses appropriate coping resources (e.g., support systems, problem-solving and decision-making skills, professional help, spiritual values).
- Performs usual family, social, and work roles.

The client with **Decisional conflict:**

- Verbalizes fears and concerns regarding choices and responses of others.
- Identifies and assesses available alternatives.
- Recognizes consequences of available alternatives.
- Makes decisions compatible with personal values and life-style.
- Seeks support as needed for decision making.

IMPLEMENTING

Although stress accompanies every disease and illness, it is also highly individual; a situation that to one person is a major stressor may not affect another. Some methods to help reduce stress will be effective for one person; other methods will be appropriate for a different person. A nurse who is sensitive to clients' needs and reactions can choose those methods of intervention that will be most effective for each individual.

Minimizing Anxiety

One way to reduce or perhaps eliminate anxiety is for the nurse and client to establish goals that are attainable. Clients must first recognize that they are anxious. This recognition is best brought about in an atmosphere of warmth and trust. Sometimes anxious clients react negatively to nurses because of personal frustration. It is important for nurses to understand this response and react to the behavior in a calm, accepting, and confident manner.

After clients realize that they are anxious, it is important to discuss all the possible reasons for their anxiety. Perley (1984, p. 362) categorizes three underlying states of mind associated with anxiety: *helplessness,* such as that in the person who has recently had a stroke and is unable to perform previous functions; *isolation,* such as that in an adolescent who fears rejection because of a sexually transmitted disease; and *insecurity,* such as that in a person who is worried about being unable to earn a living or pay medical bills. When clients can identify the cause of their anxiety, they may find it helpful to explore the cause with the objective of learning better coping strategies. General nursing guidelines to minimize the client's anxiety and stress follow:

1. *Support the client and family at a time of illness.* By conveying caring and understanding, the nurse can help clients reduce their stress. Feeling that someone else cares is a source of support to stressed people. Often families require time to talk about their

worries and anxieties before they can feel assured and less stressed.

2. *Orient the client to the hospital or agency.* The nurse helps the client adjust to the role change from, for example, independent wage earner to relatively dependent client. The nurse can help family members by giving information, for instance, about visiting hours and specific unit policies.

3. *Give the client in a hospital some way of maintaining identity.* A person's name and clothes are important parts of the person's uniqueness as an individual. Nurses can help clients maintain identity by addressing them by the name they prefer and by assisting them to wear their own clothes in a hospital setting, when this is possible.

4. *Provide information when the client has insufficient information.* Fear of the unknown and incorrect information can frequently cause stress. Stressed clients often misunderstand facts related by health personnel. Additional information or clarification can allay stress.

5. *Repeat information when the client has difficulty remembering.* Nurses can assist clients by repeating information when it is requested and assisting people to apply it when they so desire. This problem is particularly prevalent among elderly people who are stressed by a change of setting as well as by their illness.

6. *Encourage the client to participate in the plan of care.* Loss of the right to determine their own destiny can be very stressful to some people, particularly adults who function independently or who assume responsibility for others in their daily lives.

7. *Give the client time to express feelings and thoughts.* Allow time for clients to describe their feelings and worries if they wish. Nurses should be sensitive to clients' needs and neither probe with prying questions nor be too busy to listen.

8. *Ensure that expectations are within the client's capabilities.* Whatever the activity, whether an exercise or recreation, the nurse should make sure that it is possible for the client to accomplish it. If an activity is beyond the client's ability, the client is likely to be more stressed by not achieving the goal.

9. *Be sensitive to specific situations and experiences that increase anxiety and stress for clients.* For example, a man might appear highly stressed each time he receives an intramuscular injection. A careful remark by the nurse about the stress may elicit

information that the nurse can use to assist the client.

10. *Assist a client to make a correct appraisal of a situation.* Sometimes, through a lack of knowledge or misinterpretation of a sequence of events, people draw incorrect conclusions. Having valid information might relieve the client's stress.

11. *Provide an environment in which a person can function independently to some degree without assistance.* It may be difficult and stressful for an adult to assume the dependent client role even for a short time. By restoring some degree of independent functioning, such as by adapting eating utensils so that clients can feed themselves, nurses can lower clients' stress levels.

12. *Reinforce positive environmental factors and recognize negative ones to help reduce stress.* Dwelling on problems and difficulties increases stress, but focusing on what can be accomplished positively usually decreases stress.

13. *Arrange for other clients with similar experiences to visit.* Clients with colostomies or similar conditions may be highly stressed and feel that they will never be able to live a normal life again. Meeting another person who has successfully adjusted to a colostomy can lower the stress greatly.

14. *Bring clients and their support persons into contact with people in community agencies who can help them make valid plans.* Social workers are familiar with discharge planning and arrangements that a client may need to make. Often people are stressed needlessly because they do not know what help is available to them in the community.

15. *Communicate competence, understanding, and empathy rather than stress and anxiety.* When a nurse conveys stress or anxiety, the client and support persons may be concerned about the nurse's ability to function where the client's health and life are involved. To reduce a client's stress, nurses need to know themselves well and be able to function in a nondefensive manner that conveys competence and empathy.

Mediating Anger

Often nurses find clients' anger difficult to handle. Caring for the client who is angry is difficult for two reasons (Gluck 1981, p. 9):

1. Clients rarely state "I feel angry or frustrated" and rarely indicate the reason for their anger. Instead,

they may refuse treatment, become verbally abusive or demanding, may threaten violence, or become overly critical. Their complaints rarely reflect the cause of their anger.

2. Anger from clients can elicit fear and anger in the nurse, who may respond in a manner that intensifies the client's anger even to the point of violence. The majority of nurses respond in a way that reduces their own stress rather than the client's stress (Gluck 1981, p. 11).

Responses whose major purpose is to reduce the nurse's stress include defending, providing reassurance, offering advice or persuading, and retaliating aggressively. For example, this response to a client's demands is defensive: "I can't take care of everyone at once! We've been very busy this evening." This response does not recognize the client's problem and increases the client's tension and anger. A reassuring response, such as "You'll feel better as soon as you are up and about," is a way to recognize the problem and calm the client; however, it does not encourage the person to talk about the problem. Responses meant to offer advice or persuade often begin with the words "Yes, but, . . ." By offering advice or persuading, nurses focus on their own values and ideas, thus increasing the client's sense of powerlessness. Aggressive responses indicate disapproval of the client's behavior. For example, a nurse might say, "What do *you* want *now?* Some people here are a lot sicker than you and need my help."

Responses that reduce the client's anger and stress include offering help, apologizing, asking relevant questions, and conveying understanding. For example, the nurse might respond by saying, "I guess it's pretty frustrating being alone and having to wait for others to do things for you." Gluck (1981, p. 10) suggests that nurses wishing to provide understanding responses to clients follow these guidelines:

1. Focus on the feeling words of the client.

2. Note the general content of the message.

3. Restate the feeling and content of what the client has communicated.

4. Observe the client's body language.

5. Ask yourself, "If I were in the client's shoes, what would I be feeling?"

In addition to these general guidelines for minimizing stress, several health promotion strategies (see Chapter 15) are often appropriate as interventions for clients with stress-related nursing diagnoses. Among these are physical exercise, optimal nutrition, adequate rest and sleep, time management, and relaxation techniques.

STRESS MANAGEMENT TECHNIQUES

Many stress management techniques are used in current practice. These include movement and proprioception therapies such as exercise and progressive relaxation; cognitive therapies such as humor, guided imagery, meditation, and yoga; and sensory therapies such as massage, biofeedback, therapeutic touch, and music therapy. Some of these therapies may be initiated and implemented independently by the nurse; others may require specialized education. Nurses can also inform clients about the availability of community classes provided by other health professionals.

Exercise and Recreation

Participating in sports, dancing, running, swimming, bicycling or other high-energy activities can be very effective in releasing stress-related tension. Similar to other strategies for dealing with stress, exercise has both physiologic and psychologic benefits. Physiologically, exercise promotes cardiovascular endurance, increases muscular strength and tone, improves efficiency in handling oxygen, and reduces blood pressure and pulse rate. The stimulation of the production of endorphins and enkephalins relieves pain and causes a feeling of well-being.

Exercises for specific areas of the body such as the neck and back muscles can relieve tension and reduce feelings of stress. Total body relaxation exercises can reduce stress and refresh the individual.

Other recreational activities such as walking, hobbies, painting, playing a musical instrument, and other creative or diversional activities can help in relieving stress. A change of pace or scenery can relieve stress immediately; taking a brief walk outside; listening to music for a few minutes; looking out the window at a garden, window box, flower or tree. Murray and Zentner (1989) suggest that recreational activities should be emotionally rewarding, i.e., they should provide enjoyment. They should be performed voluntarily rather than out of a sense of obligation, and done outside of ordinary routines. Additionally, they should be attention absorbing but they should not be profit motivated.

Exercise and other recreational activities provide the individual with a momentary escape from the stressors of life. Following such activities, the individual is physically and psychologically refreshed and often more able to face life's crises and solve life's problems.

Humor

Humor is defined as the ability to discover, express, or appreciate the ludicrous or absurdly incongruous, to be amused by one's own imperfections or the whimsical aspects of life, and to see the funny side of an otherwise serious situation (Murray and Huelskoetter 1983, pp. 192). According to Simon (1989) humor has both psychologic and physical benefits. Psychologically, humor relieves tension and anxiety, reduces aggression, and distracts from sadness or guilt. This promotes a feeling of relaxation and well-being. The physiologic benefits include alternating states of stimulation and relaxation. During laughter, stimulation causes increases in respiratory rate, heart rate, muscular tension, and oxygen exchange. A state of relaxation follows laughter, during which heart rate, blood pressure, respiration, and muscle tension decrease. Humor stimulates production of catecholamines and hormones, and increases pain tolerance by releasing endorphins (Fry, 1979).

Fay's research (1983) indicated that individuals most effective in coping with stress had the greatest ability to appreciate humor. Martin and Lefcourt (1983) found that humor had a moderating effect on stress; however, research by Safranek and Schill (1982) has not supported this notion.

Humor also enhances communication by allowing the individual to offer feedback and suggestions in a non-threatening manner. Humor can help to convey a sense of empathy to another, express warmth and affection, and encourage learning (Murray and Huelskoetter 1983, pp. 192).

Massage

The major purpose for the use of massage is to relieve muscle tension and enhance relaxation, but it may also be performed to improve muscle and skin functioning, to relieve insomnia, and to decrease pain. A variety of strokes or movements may be used singly or in combination depending on the outcome desired. These include *effleurage* (stroking), friction, pressure, *petrissage* (kneading), vibration, and percussion.

Historically, the back massage has been used by nurses to enhance or induce relaxation before sleep or to stimulate skin circulation in association with hygienic measures. Michaelson's (1978) back massage technique includes eight steps that demonstrate how a combination of massage strokes may be used:

- Effleurage of the entire back
- Friction strokes next to the spine
- Petrissage of the shoulders
- Hand pressure movements up the back
- Effleurage and petrissage of the upper back and shoulders
- Pressure strokes along the spinal column
- Circular movements over the lower back
- Light effleurage movements over the entire back.

More research is required to validate the use of massage for specific clients in terms of the amount of pressure or types of strokes to use, length of the therapy, and the effects of gender of the nurse and client.

Shiatsu Massage

Shiatsu massage is a highly specialized form of massage designed to relieve muscle tension and fatigue. It is the application of firm, gentle pressure to the acupuncture points of the body and therefore is sometimes referred to as acupressure. Shiatsu aims to restore the balance of true Qi (pronounced "chee"), a balance of the constantly flowing life energy forces of *yang* and *yin*. True Qi circulates around the body through 12 main channels called meridians, which correspond to 12 organs, including the lungs, heart, and stomach. Clients can use shiatsu on themselves to relieve minor ailments. For example, a frontal headache may be relieved by applying firm pressure behind the head at the base of the skull.

Progressive Relaxation

Relaxation techniques have been used extensively to reduce high levels of stress and chronic pain. Using relaxation techniques enables the client to exert control over the body's responses to tension and anxiety. For many years, nurses on maternity units have encouraged women in labor to relax and breathe rhythmically. These techniques, however, can be useful for many other clients to reduce anxiety, reduce pain, or promote health.

Progressive relaxation requires that the client (a) tense and then relax successive muscle groups, and (b) focus attention on discriminating the feelings experienced when the muscle group is relaxed in contrast to when it was tense. Jacobsen (1938), the originator of the progressive relaxation technique, found that tension of a muscle group before its relaxation actually achieved a greater degree of relaxation than simply commanding oneself to relax. This technique can result in decreased body oxygen consumption, metabolism, respiratory rate, cardiac rate, muscle tension, and systolic and diastolic blood pressures.

Three requisites to relaxation are correct posture, a mind at rest, and a quiet environment. The client must be positioned comfortably, with all body parts supported, joints slightly flexed, and no strain or pull on muscles (e.g., arms and legs should not be crossed). To rest the mind, the client is asked to gaze slowly around the room, e.g., across the ceiling, down the wall, along a window curtain, around the fabric pattern, and back up the wall. This exercise focuses the mind outside of the body and creates a second center of concentration. To relax the face, the client is encouraged to smile slightly, let the lower jaw sag, and lightly place the tip of the tongue against the inner upper teeth.

Procedures for teaching progressive relaxation vary. The method for relaxing muscle groups, the specific muscle groups to be relaxed, the number of sessions involved, and the role of the instructor (taped versus live instructions) may differ. Tension of muscle groups is often maintained for a period of 5–7 seconds and is followed by relaxation of the muscle group at a predetermined cue. To achieve maximum relaxation, various positive and affirmative phrases are used by the instructor, such as, "Let all the tension go" and "Enjoy the feelings as your muscles become relaxed and loose." Murray and Huelskoetter (1983, p. 413) recommend the total body relaxation technique outlined in the accompanying box.

Guided Imagery

Guided imagery involves the use of self-chosen or instructor-suggested positive images to achieve specific health-related goals. Imagery is "the formation of a mental representation of an object that is usually only perceived through the senses" (Sodergren 1985, p. 104). Images can have visual, auditory, olfactory, gustatory, or tactile-proprioceptive qualities. For examples of the different types of images, see Table 23–4. Images often evoke more than one sense. For example, the image of waves breaking upon a shore may combine the visual picture with the sound of the waves and the smell of the salt air.

Imagery can be used to enhance other forms of medical and nursing therapies to improve the body's response to therapy (e.g., chemotherapy and radiation

---

A Total Body Relaxation Technique

- Inhale. Send breath down to your toes and relax them. Send breath to the soles of your feet and ankles, and relax them. Exhale. Your feet are now fully relaxed.

- Inhale. Send breath to the muscles of your lower legs from the ankles to the knees and relax them. First the left leg; then the right leg. Exhale. Feel the relaxation from your toes to the tops of your legs.

- Inhale. Send breath to your buttocks and groin and relax them. Exhale.

- Inhale. Send breath to your stomach and lower back muscles. Relax them. Exhale.

- Inhale. Send breath to your chest and upper back muscles. Relax them. Exhale.

- Inhale. Send breath to your shoulders to the tips of your fingers. Relax them. Exhale.

- Inhale. Send breath to your forehead, cheeks, eyelids, and jaw muscles. Let jaw drop. Feel a comfortable letting go as these muscles are relaxed. Let this feeling of deep relaxation spread to your neck, throat, and tongue muscles. Exhale.

- Breathe very slowly and easily throughout this exercise, allowing breathing to match rhythms of the relaxed body.

Source: R. B. Murray and M. M. W. Huelskoetter. 1983. *Psychiatric/mental health nursing: Giving emotional care.* Englewood Cliffs, N.J.: Prentice-Hall, p. 413.

TABLE 23-4 *Types of Images*

Type	Example
Visual	A valley scene with its many shades of greenery
Auditory	Ocean waves breaking rhythmically upon a beach
Olfactory	Freshly baked bread
Gustatory	A juicy hamburger
Tactile-proprioceptive	Stroking a soft, furry cat

therapy). It may also be used to assist in acute and chronic pain control, and to augment relaxation techniques.

Biofeedback

Biofeedback is a technique that brings under conscious control bodily processes normally thought to be beyond voluntary command. In the past, most physiologic processes were considered involuntary. However, it has been discovered that many of these processes are partially subject to voluntary control. Studies show that muscle tension, heartbeat, blood flow, peristalsis, and skin temperature, for example, can be controlled voluntarily. The feedback is usually provided through temperature meters that indicate skin temperature changes or an electromyogram (EMG) that shows the electric potential created by the contraction of muscles. Reduced EMG activity reflects muscle relaxation. Biofeedback teaches clients to achieve a generalized state of relaxation characterized by parasympathetic dominance and antagonistic to the pattern of physiologic arousal manifested in stress-related disorders.

Meditation

Meditation is a cognitive strategy derived from Eastern spiritual disciplines. Originally it was viewed as a religious practice. In the Western world, however, it may be used as an intervention to relieve anxiety, to expand awareness or consciousness, and to improve overall health. As a stress management technique, health care professionals focus on the physiologic effects that meditation can produce, i.e., reduced heart rate, decreased oxygen consumption, decreased blood pressure, increased skin resistance, and increased regularity and amplitude of alpha brain waves (Shapiro 1980, p. 159).

Because many types of meditation exist, the techniques used to achieve the desired outcome vary widely. In one type of meditation, referred to as *concentrative meditation,* the person focuses his or her attention on one particular object (e.g., a candle) or repeats the words of a mantra so that all other objects and stimuli in the environment are excluded. In another type of meditation, referred to as *"opening up"* or *"mindfulness" meditation,* the person attempts to remain open to all stimuli. Various other types of meditation integrate elements of both techniques. For example, a person may focus on his or her breathing pattern (Zen meditation) or

on a mantra (transcendental meditation) but be willing to allow other thoughts to "come up," watch those thoughts, and then return to the original focus.

Although meditation is regarded as an effective stress management technique for many people, this technique may not be indicated for certain clients. For example, a person with Type A personality may have difficulty mastering such a passive technique. A hypotensive person with a diastolic blood pressure below 90 mm Hg may experience light-headedness and dizziness. In addition, a prolonged duration of meditation has been reported to cause hallucinations and loss of reality contact in some individuals (Snyder 1985, p. 177).

Yoga

Yoga is a traditional Indian science that helps a person coordinate body and mind more effectively. It promotes tranquillity of mind and increases resistance to stress. Integrated yoga, described by Patanjali 2500 years ago, incorporated the following methods (Udupa 1983, p. 135):

1. *Yama.* This refers to improvement in social behavior and is achieved by five noble practices: (a) nonviolence (both physical and psychologic), (b) truthfulness, (c) nonstealing, (d) self-restraint in every sphere of life, and (e) nonhoarding.

2. *Niyama.* This refers to improvement in personal behavior and is achieved by (a) maintaining a purity of body and mind, (b) developing a habit of contentment, (c) practicing austerity in every sphere of life, (d) studying relevant literature, and (c) practicing dedication to God daily.

3. *Physical postures.* There are many yoga postures, e.g., cobra posture and plough posture. They are meant to improve the bodily health, especially the functions of various organs, such as the heart, lungs, liver and organs of the gastrointestinal tract, kidneys, and endocrine system. People may assume 10 to 15 yogic postures, including stationary exercises, for all parts of the body for a period of about 15 minutes daily.

4. *Breathing exercises.* In this important part of yogic exercise, one inhales fresh air to the maximum capacity through one nostril, holds the breath for a while, and exhales through the other nostril, practicing deep expiration. Done 20 times or more daily, this exercise improves the oxygenation of all the organs and tissues of the body. Better circulation of oxygen-

ated blood in the body in turn relaxes the person.

5. *Control of the sense organs*. This aspect of yoga involves restraining the activities of all the sense organs with the ultimate goal of restraining the mind. It is achieved by minimizing the stimulation of the sense organs and leading as simple a life as possible.

6. *Concentration of the mind*. Learning to avoid all distractions and concentrate on any object involves tremendous perseverance and willpower. Concentrating on an object of one's choice helps to calm any mental excitement and to induce tranquillity and serenity of the mind.

7. *Mediation*. Research shows that the regular practice of integrated yoga can not only prevent the development of various psychosomatic disorders but also improve a person's resistance and ability to endure stressful situations effectively. Studies on normal individuals indicate that the regular practice of yogic postures leads to psychologic improvement, increased intelligence and memory quotients, and decreased pulse rate, blood pressure, respiration, and body weight (Ibid).

Therapeutic Touch

Therapeutic touch (TT) is a process by which energy is transmitted or transferred from one person to another with the intent of potentiating the healing process of one who is ill or injured. It is derived from, but not the same as, the "laying on of hands" associated with Eastern, European, and religious philosophies. Delores Krieger (1979), who coined the term *therapeutic touch,* refers to TT as a healing meditation, since the primary act of the nurse (healer) is to "center" the self and to maintain that center (mental concentration and focusing) throughout the process.

Basic to therapeutic touch are the concepts that the human being has an energy field, or, more properly, *is* an energy field (human field) and that energy can be intentionally channeled from one person to another. The human field extends beyond the level of the skin and is perceptible to the trained sense (primarily touch) of a healer. This energy field can be most clearly "felt" within several feet of the body. An everyday experience that may demonstrate this field phenomenon is the feeling of having one's space invaded when someone stands too close in a crowded elevator, even though there is no physical contact.

The body and the environment are considered open systems and constantly exchange energy and matter.

The pattern and organization of the human field are constantly affected by the flow of energy from the environment. In situations of disease, illness, or pain, the pattern and organization of the field are disrupted; there may be a loss of energy, a disruption in the flow, an accumulation, or a blockage (Wright 1987, p. 708).

The therapeutic touch process consists of the following four steps (Snyder 1985, p. 203):

1. *Centering* is a meditative step in which the person directs attention inward to achieve a sense of detachment, sensitivity, and balance.

2. *Assessing* is a head-to-toe scanning process in which the palms of both hands of the nurse are held two to three inches over the client's skin surface. This process can be performed by one nurse or two. One nurse scans the client's front while the second nurse simultaneously scans the client's back. The purpose of the assessment is to detect asymmetric differences in the client's energy flow, such as heat, cold, tingling, congestion, pressure, emptiness, or other sensations.

3. *Unruffling* is a process in which an identified congestive energy field is "unruffled," or mobilized, to make the client's energy field more receptive and to enhance the transfer of energy from the nurse to the client. This is accomplished by moving the hands (palms facing the client) in a sweeping motion from the area where pressure was perceived down along the long bones of the body.

4. *Transferring energy* is the process in which occurs the actual transference of energy from the nurse to the client. The nurse must know which form of energy to use, how to modulate energy, and where to apply energy. The form of energy has different effects, and is related to colors: blue energy is sedating; yellow energy is stimulating and energizing; and green energy is harmonizing. These energy forms are modulated by mentally visualizing the color, e.g., visualizing light through a blue stained-glass window. Energy may be applied directly over an identified area of congestion, or to one of the *chakras* (special channels that serve as entry areas for energy from the environment). These are located in the thoracic or solar plexus. Energy transference helps restore the balance of the energy field and provides additional energy to promote self-healing.

Music Therapy

Music therapy may be prescribed to achieve various

goals, such as reality orientation in the elderly, stimulation or increased movement, activity reduction, relief or distraction from acute or chronic pain, decreased anxiety levels, and increased feelings of well-being. To reduce anxiety, soothing music is generally considered most appropriate. However, the personal preference of the client must be considered when planning the therapy. Both rock and roll and classical music have been effective in reducing anxiety (Synder 1985, p. 219).

Before implementing music therapy, nurses need a knowledge of music and the effects that particular types of music can produce. Attention needs to be given, for example, to the type of music to use, when to use it, and for how long. Merely placing a radio at a client's bedside does not constitute music therapy.

EVALUATING

To evaluate the achievement of client goals, the nurse collects data in accordance with the outcome criteria established earlier. Evaluation activities may include the following:

- Observing the client for absence or reduction of manifestations of fear and/or anxiety
- Measuring blood pressure and pulse rate
- Listening to the client's reports of increased physiologic or psychologic comfort, decreased emotional responsiveness, or verbalizations of fears and concerns
- Asking the client about personal strengths or coping resources identified
- Questioning the client about effective and ineffective coping responses and consequences
- Discussing situations in which the client has used specific adaptive coping methods and the client's perception of their effectiveness
- Asking the client about specific resources used, including support persons

Examples of evaluative statements indicating goal achievement are "The client identified four personal strengths as requested to cope with threats to self," "The client cited two examples in which problem solving and assertiveness were used in a stressful situation rather than her usual emotional reaction of anger," and "The client attended a time-management seminar on July 20, 1992 and stated it was valuable."

STRESS MANAGEMENT FOR NURSES

Nurses, like clients, are susceptible to experiencing anxiety and crises. In recent years, more attention has been given to the occupational stress nurses experience. Nursing practice involves many stressors related to both clients and the work environment. Kinzel (1982, p. 55) devised a 20-item, 24-hour scale to help nurses measure their stress levels. All 20 items fall into five main categories: inadequate knowledge, inadequate support from peers and supervisors, dealing with death, poor communication, and salary and staffing problems. The purpose of such a scale is to make nurses aware of the source of negative feelings and frustration on the job, to help them make adjustments, and to support colleagues.

Nurses can manage stress by using all of the techniques discussed for clients. In addition, Hamilton (1984), Scully (1980), and Wilson (1989) suggest the following:

1. First recognize that you are stressed. Become attuned to feelings of being overwhelmed, fatigue, angry outbursts, and physical illness. Also be aware of increases in smoking, drinking coffee, or other substance abuse and determine whether you are distancing yourself from client interaction.

2. When attuned to your reactions to stress, determine when the reactions occur.

3. When attuned to your stress and when it occurs, determine alternative actions to deal with it constructively. Some suggestions follow:
   a. Plan a daily relaxation program with meaningful quiet times to reduce tension.
   b. Establish an activity program to direct energy outward.
   c. Become more assertive to overcome feelings of powerlessness in relationships with others. Learn to say no.
   d. Manage time better by delegating to others and combining tasks.
   e. Take a course in biofeedback, yoga, meditation, or some other advanced relaxation technique.
   f. Learn to accept failures and learn from them.
   g. Learn to ask for help, and share your feelings with colleagues.
   h. Learn to support your colleagues in times of need. Give them a chance to "ventilate" feelings and listen to their concerns.
   i. Learn to handle problems constructively instead of defensively.

j. Accept what cannot be changed. There are certain limitations in every situation.

k. If working in an intensive care or similar unit (ICU), establish a structured emotional support group. These groups are identified by various names: ventilation groups, discussion forums, or regular staff meetings for the purpose of dealing with feelings and anxieties generated in the work setting. See Work-Related Social Support Groups in Chapter 20, page 384.

CHAPTER HIGHLIGHTS

▸ Stress is a state of physiologic or psychologic tension that affects the whole person—physically, emotionally, intellectually, socially, and spiritually.

▸ A person's response to stressors varies according to the way the stressor is perceived, its intensity and duration, the number of stressors, previous experience, coping mechanisms used, support people available, and age.

▸ A common psychologic response to stress is anxiety, which is manifested in a variety of cognitive, verbal, and motor responses that reduce tension.

▸ Unconscious psychologic defense mechanisms, such as denial, rationalization, compensation, and sublimation, also protect the individual from tension.

▸ Both physiologic and psychologic responses to stressors can be adaptive or maladaptive.

▸ Physiologic homeostasis is maintained by coordinated functioning of the autonomic nervous, endocrine, respiratory, cardiovascular, renal, and gastrointestinal systems.

▸ Psychologic homeostasis, or emotional well-being, is acquired or learned through the experience of living and interacting with others.

▸ Adaptation is a process of change that occurs in response to stress. It occurs in three interrelated modes: physiologic, psychologic, and sociocultural.

▸ Coping is a more immediate response to stress than adaptation.

▸ Coping strategies can be either effective or ineffective and may result in adaptation or maladaptation, respectively.

▸ The nurse can help clients recognize stress and support clients' effective coping mechanisms.

▸ Nursing interventions for stress are aimed at reducing anxiety, at promoting clients' physical and mental well-being so that they handle stress more effectively, and at helping clients learn more effective coping mechanisms.

▸ The nurse, too, is prone to occupational stress and needs to learn effective stress-management techniques.

LEARNING ACTIVITIES

■ Assess your nursing unit for sources of stress for clients and visitors, nursing personnel, and physicians. Unit stressors may be physical, such as noise levels, or psychological, such as staff relationships. List the unit stressors and identify interventions for reducing or eliminating each stressor. Develop a plan for implementing these interventions. (Don't forget that change is a stressor, so don't implement too many changes at one time.)

■ Assess your own ability to cope with stress. Make a list of stressors in both your personal and professional life. Prioritize your list from highest stressors to lowest stressors. List personal strategies that have been effective for you in coping with stress. Do you need additional or new coping strategies? Select one new coping strategy and develop a plan to incorporate it into your personal stress management system.

READINGS AND REFERENCES

SUGGESTED READINGS

Leidy, N. K. October 1989. A physiologic analysis of stress and chronic illness. *Journal of Advanced Nursing* 14:868–76.

The author briefly reviews the history of stress research, explains the general adaptation syndrome (GAS) and relates it to nursing practice. In summary, Leidy writes that "Selye's principles of stress adaptation and GAS provide a useful framework for understanding the physiologic processes involved in the stress-illness relationship."

Wilson, L. K. December 1989. Professional growth section. High-gear nursing: How it can run you down and what you can do about it. *Nursing 89* 19:81–2, 84, 86, 88.

The author points out that the nurse's reaction to stress can cause burnout. The warning signs of stress mentioned include feeling overwhelmed, fatigue, angry outbursts and depression, forgetfulness and disorganization, guilt, and self-sacrifice. The ways to cope with stress include developing a "can do" attitude, becoming more assertive, managing time better, and nurturing oneself and each other.

RELATED RESEARCH

Dewe, P. J. April 1989. Stressor frequency, tension, tiredness and coping: Some measurement issues and a comparison across nursing groups. *Journal of Advanced Nursing* 14:308–20.

McGrath, A.; Reid, N.; and Boore, J. 1989. Occupational stress in nursing. *International Journal of Nursing Studies* 26(4):343–58.

Martin, D. March 1, 1990. Effects of ethical dilemmas on stress felt by nurses providing care to AIDS patients. *Critical Care Nursing Quarterly,* 12:53–57.

SELECTED REFERENCES

Bell, J. M. March/April 1977. Stressful life events and coping methods in mental-illness and wellness behaviors. *Nursing Research* 26:136–40.

Breakwell, G. M. August 1990. Are you stressed out? *American Journal of Nursing* 90:31–33.

Burgess, A. W., and Lazare, A. 1976. *Community mental health: Target populations.* Englewood Cliffs, N.J.: Prentice-Hall.

Byrne, M. L., and Thompson, L. F. 1978. *Key concepts for the study and practice of nursing.* St. Louis: C. V. Mosby Co.

Cannon, W. B. 1939. *The wisdom of the body.* 2d ed. New York: Norton Publishing Co.

Carpenito, L. J. 1989. *Nursing diagnosis: Application to clinical practice.* 3d ed. Philadelphia: J. B. Lippincott Co.

Detherage, K. S., and Johnson, S. S. 1990. Stress reduction and crisis intervention. In Edelman, C. L., and Mandle, C. L. *Health promotion: Throughout the lifespan.* St. Louis: C. V. Mosby Co.

Dossey, B. M., Keegan, L., Guzzetto, C. E., and Kolkmeier, L. G. 1988. *Holistic nursing: A handbook for practice.* Rockville, Md.: Aspen Publishers, Inc.

Duldt, B. W. September 1981. Anger: An occupational hazard for nurses. *Nursing Outlook* 29:510–18.

Ebersole, P., and Hess, P. 1990. *Toward healthy aging: Human needs and nursing response.* St. Louis: C. V. Mosby Co. pp. 709–710.

Fay, R. 1983. The defensive role of humor in the management of stress. Dissertation Abstracts International 44:1219B.

Freud, S. 1946. *The ego and the mechanisms of defense.* New York: International Universities Press.

Friedman, M., and Rosenman, R. 1974. *Type A behavior and your heart.* Greenwich, Conn.: Fawcett Publications.

Fry, W. 1979. Humor and the human cardiovascular system. In Mindness, H. and Turek, J., editors: *The study of humor.* Los Angeles: Antioch University.

Gluck, M. March 1981. Learning a therapeutic verbal response to anger. *Journal of Psychiatric Nursing and Mental Health Services* 19:9–12.

Hamilton, J. M. July/August 1984. Effective ways to relieve stress. *Nursing Life* 4:24–27.

Holmes, T. H., and Rahe, R. H. August 1967. The social readjustment rating scale. *Journal of Psychosomatic Research* 11:213–18.

Horowitz, J. A. Nurse-client relationship. In Edelman, C. L., and Mandle, C. L. 1990. *Health promotion: Throughout the lifespan.* St. Louis: C. V. Mosby Co.

Jacobsen, E. 1938. *Progressive relaxation.* Chicago: University of Chicago Press.

Johnson, J. E., and Lauver, D. R. January 1989. Alternative explanations of coping with stressful experiences associated with physical illness. *Advances in Nursing Science* 11:39–52.

Kinzel, S. L. March/April 1982. What's your stress level? *Nursing Life* 2:54–55.

Krieger, D. May 1975. Therapeutic touch: The imprimature of nursing. *American Journal of Nursing* 75:784–87.

———. 1979. *The therapeutic touch: How to use your hands to help or heal.* Englewood Cliffs, N.J.: Prentice-Hall.

Lazarus, R. S. 1966. *Psychological stress and the coping process.* New York: McGraw-Hill.

Lazarus, R. S., and Folkman, S. 1984. *Stress, appraisal, and coping.* New York: Springer Publishing Co.

Lyon, B. L., and Werner, J. 1987. Stress. In Fitzpatrick, J. J. and Taunton, R. L., editors. *Annual Review of Nursing Research.* New York: Springer Publishing Co. vol 5, pp. 3–22.

Martin, R. A., and Lefcourt, H. M. Sense of humor as a moderator of the relation between stressors and moods. *Journal of Perspectives of Social Psychology* 45(6):1313–1324.

Michaelson, D. C. July 1978. Giving a great back rub. *American Journal of Nursing.* 78:1197–99.

Monat, A., and Lazarus, R. S. (editors). 1985. *Stress and coping:*

An anthology. 2d ed. New York: Columbia University Press.

Murray, R. B., and Huelskoetter, M. M. 1983. *Psychiatric/mental health nursing: Giving emotional care.* Englewood Cliffs, N.J.: Prentice-Hall, Inc.

Murray, R. B., and Zentner, J. P. 1989. *Nursing assessment and health promotion strategies through the life span.* 4th ed. Norwalk, Conn.: Appleton & Lange.

NANDA approved nursing diagnostic categories for clinical use and testing. Summer 1988. *Nursing Diagnosis Newsletter* 15:1–3.

Nuernberger, P. 1981. *Freedom from stress.* Honesdale, Pa.: The Himalayan International Institute of Yoga Science and Philosophy.

Perley, N. Z. 1984. Problems in self-consistency: Anxiety. In Roy, C., editor. *Introduction to nursing: An adaptation model.* Englewood Cliffs, N.J.: Prentice-Hall.

Safranek, R. and Schill, R. 1982. Coping with stress: Does humor help? *Psychological Reports* 51:1908.

Scully, R. May 1980. Stress in the nurse. *American Journal of Nursing* 80:912–14.

Selye, H. 1956. *The stress of life.* New York: McGraw-Hill.

——— . 1976. *The stress of life.* Rev. ed. New York: McGraw-Hill.

Shapiro, Jr., D. H. 1980. Meditation and holistic medicine. In Hastings, A. C., Fadiman, J., and Gordon, J. S., editors. *Health for the whole person.* Boulder, Colo.: Westview Press, 1980, pp. 159–165.

Simon, J. M. 1988. The therapeutic value of humor in aging adults. *Journal of Gerontological Nursing* 14:8–13.

Simon, J. M. 1989. Humor techniques for oncology nurses. *Oncology Nursing Forum* 16(5):667–670.

Sodergren, K. M. 1985. Guided imagery. In Snyder, M. pp. 103–24. *Independent nursing interventions.* New York: John Wiley and Sons.

Snyder, M. 1985. *Independent nursing interventions.* New York: John Wiley and Sons.

Udupa, K. N. 1983. Yoga and meditation for mental health. In Bannerman, R. H., Burton, J., and Wen-Chieh, C., eds. Traditional medicine and health care coverage. Geneva: World Health Organization.

Wilson, L. K. December 1989. Professional growth section. High-gear nursing: How it can run you down and what you can do about it. *Nursing 89.* 19:81–2, 84, 86, 88.

Wright, S. M. September 1987. The use of therapeutic touch in the management of pain. *Nursing Clinics of North America* 22:705–13.

Ethnic and Cultural Values

CONCEPTS OF ETHNICITY AND CULTURE

Definitions

Ethnicity is the condition of belonging to a specific ethnic group. An *ethnic group* is a set of individuals who share a unique cultural and social heritage passed on from one generation to another (Henderson and Primeaux 1981, p. xx). Ethnicity thus differs from race. *Race* denotes a system of classifying humans into subgroups according to specific physical characteristics, including skin pigmentation, stature, facial features, texture of body hair, and head form (Henderson and Primeaux 1981, p. xix). The three racial types that are commonly recognized are Caucasoid, Negroid, and

Mongoloid. However, because of the mixture of races, the three groups meld together, and there are many commonalities among groups.

Culture should not be confused with race or ethnic group. *Culture* is the beliefs and practices that are shared by people and passed down from generation to generation. Anthropologists have traditionally divided it into material culture and nonmaterial culture. *Material culture* consists of objects (such as dress, art, religious artifacts, or eating utensils) and the ways these are used. *Nonmaterial culture* consists of beliefs, customs, languages, and social institutions. Races have different ethnic groups, and the ethnic groups have different cultures. It is therefore important to understand that not all white or black people have the same culture. North America is inhabited by people of many different ethnic groups and cultures. Their cultural beliefs and practices can affect health and illness and thus become an important consideration for nurses.

Large cultural groups often have cultural subgroups or subsystems. A subculture is usually composed of people who have a distinct identity and yet are also related to a larger cultural group. A subcultural group generally has ethnicity, occupation, or physical characteristics in common with the larger cultural group. Examples of cultural subgroups are occupational groups (e.g., nurses), societal groups (e.g., feminists), and ethnic groups (e.g., Cajuns, who may be black, French, or German but who share French Acadian heritage and customs). A *bicultural group* is a group of people who embrace two cultures, life-styles, and sets of values (Chen-Louie 1980, p. 4).

Culture as a concept is a universal experience, but no two cultures are exactly alike. Two important terms identify the differences and similarities among peoples of different cultures. *Culture universals* are the common features or attributes of behavior or life pattern that are similar among different cultures. *Culture specifics* are the practices, values, beliefs, and behavior patterns that are special or unique to a given culture. For example, most cultures have ceremonies to celebrate the passage from childhood to adulthood; this practice is a culture universal. However, different cultural groups celebrate this important life event in very different ways. In Latin cultures, the "quince" party, which celebrates a girl's fifteenth birthday, signifies that the young girl has now become a woman. In some African tribes, ritual circumcision is performed as part of the ceremony that marks the passage from boyhood to manhood. In the Jewish culture, the bar mitzvah (for boys) and the bas mitzvah (for girls) are celebrations of the passage to adulthood. These are examples of culture specifics.

Two other terms commonly used with reference to ethnicity and culture are *dominant group* and *minority group*. A dominant group is "a collectivity within a society which has a preeminent authority to function as guardians and sustainers of the controlling value system and as prime allocators of rewards in the society" (Schermerhorn 1970, p. 13). A minority group or minority is a "group of people who, because of their physical or cultural characteristics, are singled out from the others in the society in which they live for differential and unequal treatment, and who therefore regard themselves as objects of collective discrimination" (Wirth 1945, p. 347). A dominant group is often the largest group in a society, for example, the white middle-class of the United States. However, the dominant group is not always the largest; for example, white South Africans are the dominant group and black South Africans are the minority group, yet the blacks far outnumber the whites.

Not uncommonly, people of a minority group often lose the cultural characteristics that distinguish them from the dominant group. This process is referred to as *cultural assimilation* or *acculturation*. Sometimes mutual cultural assimilation occurs, e.g., Chinese people coming to a North American community learn to speak English, and the people in the community learn to cook Chinese dishes.

Ethnocentrism is the belief that one's own culture is superior to all others. This can be seen in the comparison of the values and behavior of other cultures to those of one's own culture, using one's own culture as the standard. Although all people are subject to ethnocentrism, it is important for nurses to be consciously aware of ethnic and cultural differences and to accept these as appropriate. These differences should not be viewed as good or bad. Many immigrants to the United States and Canada maintain their ethnic and cultural identities in terms of their dress, language, customs, and rituals; accepting these is basic to accepting the client as an individual.

Stereotyping is assuming that all members of a culture or ethnic group are alike. For example, one may assume that all Italians express pain volubly or that all Chinese people like rice. Stereotyping may be based on generalizations founded in research, or it may be unrelated to reality. For example, research indicates that Italians are likely to express pain verbally; however, a particular Italian client may not verbalize pain. Stereotyping that is unrelated to reality may be positive or negative and is frequently an outcome of racism. *Racism* is the assumption of inherent racial superiority or inferiority and the consequent discrimination against certain races. An example of positive stereotyping is "All Jewish people are very clever." An example of negative stereotyping is "All Native Americans are alcoholics." Stereotyping can cause problems in nursing practice, especially if the nurse plans care based on stereotyping rather than on individual assessment of the client.

Ethnoscience is "the systematic study of the way of life of a designated cultural group with the purpose of obtaining an accurate account of the people's behavior and how they perceive and interpret their universe" (Leininger 1970, p. 168). Ethnoscientists attempt to provide an inside view of a culture from the way the people of the culture talk about it. They study and classify data about a cultural or subcultural group so that their report is meaningful to both people within the culture and people outside the culture who try to understand it. Emphasis is placed on the person's point of view, the person's vision, and the person's world.

Nurses can apply much of the knowledge gained by ethnoscientists, specifically about the health-illness behavior systems of people from cultural backgrounds different from their own. In the past decade or more, the client's personal view of illness has received recognition and emphasis. Nurses have, as a result, implemented methods to discover how well clients understand their illnesses, how clients perceive they can be helped by health personnel, and how illness has affected them and their families. In recent years, cultural views affecting health practices and beliefs have been receiving greater recognition. The fact that health beliefs and practices vary among cultures and the implications of this fact for nursing have also received greater attention. To provide effective nursing services to clients, nurses need data about the client's personal and cultural views regarding health and illness. When developing care plans, nurses need to consider the client's world and daily experiences. To make valid assessments, nurses need to try to see and hear the world as their clients do. Specific cultural data can provide scientific generalizations about health and illness behavior in different cultures. Clients' needs and behaviors can be better understood when particular health norms are identified.

Characteristics of Culture

- *Culture is learned.* It is not instinctive or innate. It is learned through life experiences after birth.
- *Culture is taught.* It is transmitted from parents to children over successive generations. All animals can learn, but only humans can pass culture along. Language is the chief vehicle of culture.

- *Culture is social.* It originates and develops through the interactions of people.
- *Culture is adaptive.* Customs, beliefs, and practices change slowly, but they do adapt to the social environment and to the biologic and psychologic needs of people. As life conditions change, some traditional forms in a culture may cease to provide satisfaction and are eliminated. For example, if it has been customary for family members of different generations to live together (extended family), yet education and employment may require children to leave their parents and move to other parts of the country, the extended family norm then changes.
- *Culture is integrative.* The elements in a culture tend to form a consistent and integrated system. For example, religious beliefs and practices influence and are influenced by family organization, economic values, and health practices.
- *Culture is ideational.* Ideational means forming images or objects in the mind. The group habits that are part of culture are to a considerable extent ideal norms or patterns of behavior. People do not always follow those norms. The norms of their culture may in fact be different from the norms of society as a whole.
- *Culture is satisfying.* Cultural habits persist only as long as they satisfy people's needs. Gratification strengthens habits and beliefs. Once they no longer bring gratification, they may disappear.

DIVERSITY OF NORTH AMERICAN SOCIETY

The populations of the United States and Canada are a mixture of many ethnic groups and cultures. In the United States, white Americans make up 79% of the total population; minority groups, 21%. The minority population can be further broken down as shown in Figure 24–1. In Canada, British Canadians make up 25.3% of the total population; French Canadians, 24.4%. See Figure 24–1.

The provision of quality nursing care to all North Americans is a desired goal. Because of the multicultural, multiethnic nature of American society, it is essential that consideration be given to the unique needs of ethnic and cultural groups. The following general considerations can help nurses develop an awareness and sensitivity to some of these specific needs.

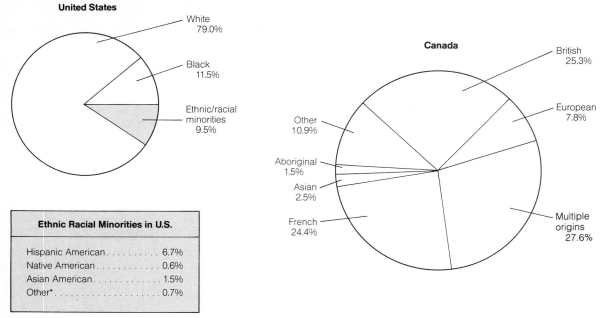

United States

White
79.0%

Black
11.5%

Ethnic/racial
minorities
9.5%

Ethnic Racial Minorities in U.S.	
Hispanic American	6.7%
Native American	0.6%
Asian American	1.5%
Other*	0.7%

*Some Hispanic Americans are also included in "Other."

Canada

British
25.3%

European
7.8%

Other
10.9%

Aboriginal
1.5%

Asian
2.5%

Multiple
origins
27.6%

French
24.4%

Figure 24-1 Estimates of the distribution of population by ethnic/racial origin based on statistical abstract of the United States (1989) and the Canadian 1990 census. *Sources* U.S. Department of Commerce, Bureau of the Census, *Statistical abstract of the United States,* 109th ed (Washington, D.C.: Government Printing Office, 1989), pp. 4–11, 15–57. Statistics Canada, January 1990, Census of Canada, Focus on Ethnic Diversity in Canada, Catalog 98-132, Minister of Supplies and Services, Ottawa, Canada.

Male-Female Roles

Most cultures are patriarchal; i.e., the man is the dominant figure. The degree of dominance of men is variable; when men are highly dominant, women are usually passive. An example of a patriarchal society is the Islamic culture of Iran, where women must be veiled in public and all important decisions are left to the men.

In contrast, the Native American culture is matriarchal, i.e., the woman is the dominant person in the family. Knowing who the decision maker or dominant person in a family is helps nurses understand the meaning of illness to a family and its decision-making process relative to health care. In Mexican American families, the father generally holds the primary power, whereas in Jewish American families, the mother is generally "the power behind the throne" (Friedman 1981, p. 271).

Language and Communication Patterns

People of an ethnic or cultural group may speak the language of their group fluently and not the language of the country. This is particularly true of certain women who,

because they stay in the home, have limited interaction with people outside the family. Even the mother of a family who has been in the United States for 30 years may know very little English. This is also true of elderly immigrants or refugees, who may have little or no interaction with people of the dominant culture until they become ill. The degree to which people learn the language of a new country is highly variable. Some people may become fluent in English very quickly, while others may learn only enough English to get along in their daily activities. When people in the latter group become ill, they are frequently unable to describe their symptoms or answer a health questionnaire. Even if they have learned the language of their new home, they may have difficulty remembering or using the new language when under the stress of illness. If nurses do not establish that there is a language barrier, a client's needs may not be met. Most health agencies have interpreters to help nurses and clients.

Language barriers can be particularly frustrating and anxiety-producing when a person is ill and can neither state problems nor understand instructions. It is most difficult for people to convey their emotions about threatening situations in a second language, a crucial factor in cases of emotional and psychiatric illness. Language barriers also arise between people using the same language. The idiomatic English of a regional or cultural group may not be readily understood outside the group. For example, *belly* can mean the abdomen or the entire cavity from the nipple line to the pubic area.

Communication patterns also differ among subcultures. For example, Native Americans commonly do not say goodbye before they leave. Swedish people talk more freely over shared food, and most cultures talk more slowly than the dominant American culture (Wold 1981, p. 143).

An additional aspect of communication is body language. Facial gestures, eye contact, hand gestures, and body positioning are all part of communication. Different cultures place different meaning on these aspects of body language. For example, the Anglo-American usually places high value on maintaining eye contact. The Anglo-American may interpret a person's failure to maintain eye contact to mean that the individual is not trustworthy, is lying, or is trying to hide something. Conversely, the Native American may consider continuous eye contact insulting or disrespectful. "Staring into the eyes of a person is likened to controlling the person's spirit" (Wilson 1983, p. 278).

Territoriality and Personal Space

Both territoriality and personal space are influenced by an individual's culture and ethnicity. *Territoriality* is the pattern of behavior arising from an individual's feeling that certain spaces and objects belong to that person. *Personal space* is the distance a person prefers to maintain from others when interacting with them. In general, people of Arabic, Southern European, and African origins frequently sit or stand relatively close to each other when talking, whereas people of Asian, North European, and North American countries are comfortable talking farther apart. For additional information about territoriality and personal space, see Chapter 18.

Time Orientation

The middle-class in the United States and in Canada tends to be oriented to the future. People plan for the future, establish long-term goals, and are increasingly concerned about preventing future illness. In daily life, people are oriented to the time of day; meals are taken at a specified time, and clients have appointment times with many health care professionals. The nurse is also highly attuned to time; medications are given at specific times, and work begins and ends at specified times.

However, not all cultures are future oriented. People of other cultures, e.g., Asians, may be oriented to the past. This orientation is illustrated by ancestor worship and the influence of ancient beliefs such as Confucianism on the present. Other cultures, such as the Native American, are very much oriented to the present. Many Native American homes do not have clocks, and the people live one day at a time with little concern for the future. Hispanic Americans often value relationships with others and the present more than the future.

An individual's orientation to time may affect punctuality for health care appointments, compliance with self-medication regimens, and reporting onset of illness or other health concerns. The nurse needs to inform clients when timing is important in self-care situations.

Family

The minority client's concept of family can differ from that of white middle-class culture. The minority group family may include the extended family (the nuclear family plus uncles, aunts, grandparents, cousins, and godparents). An associated concept is that family members are most important and must be helped at all costs. When health care is offered to such persons, it is important to consider the needs of the whole family. Sometimes, priorities in such families are detrimental to the health of one of its members. For example, a mother may not think that purchasing elastic stockings for her own ankle edema is as important as purchasing food for an unemployed relative. The home health care nurse in this instance may have to see that the relative's food needs are met before dealing with the mother's health needs.

Cultures that value the needs of the extended family as much as personal needs may also hold the belief that personal and family information must stay within the family. Some cultural groups, e.g., the traditional Chinese family, are very reluctant to disclose family information to outsiders, including physicians and nurses. This attitude can present difficulties for psychiatrists and mental health workers who view family interaction patterns as the locus of emotional problems.

Food and Nutritional Practices

The food people eat and the customs associated with food vary widely among subcultures and ethnic groups. For example, the staple food of Asians is rice; of Italians, pasta; and of Eastern Europeans, wheat bread. Even families who have been in the United States or Canada for several generations often continue to eat the food of their country (Christian and Greger 1985, p. 213).

Hospitalized clients often have very little choice about the food they are served. The nurse can encourage family members to bring in special meals if the client's health allows. Instructions about meal planning for clients requiring special diets at home may have to be given to younger family members who are fluent in English or given by a health worker of the same culture who can act as an interpreter.

When clients are learning about a special diet, nurses must be sensitive to the cultural meanings of food and to the foods a client is accustomed to. For example, it is unwise to recommend a service such as Meals on Wheels if the service is unable to supply the foods to which the client is accustomed, e.g., bean sprouts and vegetables for the Japanese client and fish and rice for the Chinese client.

SUSCEPTIBILITY TO DISEASE

Because of genetic and life-style influences, some ethnic and cultural groups in American society are more susceptible to certain diseases than the general population. Generally, bicultural groups in a lower socioeconomic area have a higher incidence of acquired diseases, such as infections. The following diseases are more prevalent in certain groups than in the general population:

- *Sickle-cell* disease affects approximately 50,000 Americans of African and Mediterranean descent. It affects both males and females equally. It is estimated that between 8% and 10% of the black population in the United States has the sickle cell trait. The inherited recessive trait is a defect in the hemoglobin molecule. Both parents must have the gene for sickling hemoglobin for their children to be affected clinically. In people with sickle-cell disease, the red blood cells have a 20-day life, in contrast to the normal 120-day life. The symptoms and severity of the disease are variable, depending on the syndrome. Some people are very ill and have a series of crises, while others live fairly long and normal lives (Richardson and Milne 1983, p. 417).

- *Hypertension* is more prevalent among black and other nonwhite Americans than white Americans, and the incidence is highest in Taiwan and Japan, two highly industrialized nations. It is also more common in recent immigrants to the United States. The pattern of incidence suggests that stress, obesity, and salt intake are implicated in hypertension (Overfield 1985, p. 114).

- *Diabetes mellitus* is a major health problem of Native Americans. It occurs at an early age, i.e., teens, and the rate of death from diabetes is 3 to 4 times higher among Native Americans than the general population. The incidence may be related to a diet high in refined carbohydrate and fats and low in traditional foods, as well as a sedentary life-style (Overfield 1985, p. 153).

- A number of *cancers* vary racially in their incidence; however, diet and some other environmental factors appear to be better predictors of cancer than race (Overfield 1985, p. 91). In the United States, white women have a higher incidence of breast cancer than black women. Skin cancers of all types are less common among blacks than whites; this is thought to be due to the added protection dark pigmentation provides against the sun's rays. Although digestive tract cancers show high and low incidences relative to specific geographic areas and racial groups, diet rather than genetic factors are probably the cause (Overfield 1985, pp. 91–93).

- Differences among races have been found in *alcohol metabolism*. Many Asians and Native Americans convert alcohol into acetaldehyde more rapidly and convert acetaldehyde to acetic acid more slowly than the general population does. Therefore, these Asians and Native Americans experience a rapid onset of and prolonged exposure to high blood acetaldehyde levels, which cause many of the symptoms of alcohol intoxication (Overfield 1985, pp. 83–84).

- Certain *dermatologic conditions* are more common among blacks than whites. Keloid formation, an exaggerated wound healing process of the skin, is commonly found in blacks. Keloids develop following skin trauma, e.g., surgical incision and burns (Bloch 1976, p. 28).

CULTURAL RESPONSE TO PAIN

In many cultures based on the Judeo-Christian ethic, pain may be considered a punishment for bad deeds; the individual is, therefore, to tolerate without complaint in order to atone for sins. In some Middle Eastern and African cultures, self-infliction of pain is a sign of mourning or grief. In other groups, pain may be anticipated as a part of the ritualistic practices of passage ceremonies, and therefore tolerance of pain signifies strength and endurance. The meaning of pain will affect the individual's perception of pain, tolerance of painful stimuli, and the expression of or reaction to pain.

Chapman and Jones (1944), Zborowski (1952, 1969), Weisenberg (1975), and Flannery (1981) have studied the perception and manifestations of pain in different cultural groups. Responses to pain range from stoic denial or objective reporting to social withdrawal to emotional expressions of crying, screaming, writhing, and complaining. Individuals of some groups want to endure their pain privately, whereas others of different groups want the sympathy and support of family members, loved ones, and caregivers.

Nurses must consider the methods used by individuals of different cultures for effective pain control or relief. Examples of methods of pain management that originated in non-Western cultures are the Chinese use of acupuncture and the Hindu use of yoga and meditation. Herbal remedies for pain were used in ancient Egyptian and Chinese cultures. Therapeutic touch, or "healing" touch, is related to the ancient "laying on of hands" and is still practiced today in some modern cultures. Religious rituals may provide comfort for the client in pain. Cultural healers that may be helpful in the relief of pain include shamans, curanderos, and espiritos.

It is important that nurses be aware of their own attitudes toward pain and not impose their beliefs about pain and pain expression on clients. Ludwig-Beymer (1983) states that the majority of nurses in America are white, middle-class women of European descent who place a high value on self-control in response to pain. Overt expressions of pain such as crying or screaming should not be viewed as "bad," nor should quiet stoicism in response to pain be considered "good," rather the expression of pain should be viewed within its cultural context. The goal of nursing is to identify when the client is experiencing pain and to intervene promptly to relieve discomfort.

Management of the client's pain should be done in collaboration with the client. Nursing awareness of and support for cultural behaviors related to pain can further alleviate discomfort as the client gains a feeling of acceptance.

FOLK HEALING AND TRADITIONAL WESTERN MEDICINE

People of many cultures use *folk medicine* as an alternative to traditional Western health care. The reader may recall special teas or "cures" that were used by older family members to prevent or treat colds, fevers, indi-gestion, and other common health problems. People continue to use chicken soup as a treatment for "flu." Health care professionals are often unaware of the practices of folk medicine in their community because clients are embarrassed or afraid to relate the methods they use to prevent or treat illness. An additional concern about the use of such methods is the possible delay in treating a major health problem.

An important component of folk healing is the identification of the cause of illness. Many cultures attribute the cause of illness to evil spirits or evil curses. It therefore becomes the healer's role to cast out the evil spirits or to remove the curse. It is important to note that cultural healers often base their practices in religious or other spiritual belief systems. Examples of folk healing beliefs and practices are voodoo, root medicine, and "laying on of hands."

Why do individuals use these nontraditional folk healing methods? Folk medicine, in contrast to traditional health care, is thought to be more humanistic. The consultation and treatment take place in the community of the recipient, frequently in the home of the healer or the recipient. It is less expensive than traditional health care, as the health problem is identified primarily through conversation with the client and the family. The healer often prepares the treatments, e.g., teas to be ingested, poultices to be applied, or charms or amulets to be worn. A frequent component of treatment is some ritual practice on the part of the healer or the recipient to cause healing to occur. Because folk healing is more culturally based, it is often more comfortable and less frightening for the client. Table 24–1 presents a comparison of the characteristics of folk medicine and traditional health care.

When folk healing practices have failed, the client may turn to traditional Western medicine for treatment. It is important for nurses to determine what folk treatments clients have used and what benefits were obtained without demeaning the clients or their health beliefs. The client may still be wearing a healing charm or amulet or wish to continue the folk treatment while accepting traditional treatment. Nurses should determine whether there are any medical contraindications to continuing their healing practices. If there are no contraindications, permitting clients to maintain their practices may promote their well-being.

Some folk healing practices that were previously dismissed by practitioners of traditional Western medicine are gaining more interest as their effectiveness is recognized. Acupuncture, for example, is gaining more acceptance as its contributions to pain management are being demonstrated. This encourages continued research into

TABLE 24-1 *Characteristics of Folk Medicine versus Traditional Western Health Care*

Folk Medicine	Traditional Health Care
Humanistic	Scientific
Familiar, practical, concrete	Unfamiliar, abstract
Holistic	Fragmented
Caring	Curing
Socioculturally based	Technologically based
Prevention oriented	Treatment oriented
Occurs in the home	Occurs in institutions/hospitals
Inexpensive	Expensive

other folk healing practices to determine their possible use in traditional Western health care.

CULTURAL AND ETHNIC GROUPS IN NORTH AMERICA

This section outlines some selected cultural and ethnic characteristics of significance to nurses. It is important to remember, however, that many people in ethnic and cultural subgroups do not conform to all the practices of their group. This is especially true of second- and third-generation family members, who may be assimilated into the dominant cultural group. Table 24–2 on pages 466–469 presents a summary of the impact of culture on health and illness.

Native Americans

In the United States and Canada, the responsibility for health services for Native Americans rests with the federal government. There are, however, differences in health care practices in various geographic locations in the United States. For example, Native Americans living in the eastern states and in most urban areas are not covered by the services of the Indian Health Service, whereas Native Americans living on reservations in the

western states are eligible for such services (Spector 1985, pp. 190–91).

Because about 200 different tribes of Native Americans exist in the United States, each with its own language, folkways, religion, mores, and patterns of interpersonal relationships, caution needs to be taken in generalizing about Native American culture. In terms of health care, this variability needs to be considered. For example, the Native American who lives in isolation on a reservation may hold to traditional beliefs of cure provided by the tribal medicine man, while the urban Native American who lives away from the reservation may respond more to the values of modern medicine provided by the majority culture. It is not uncommon for Native Americans to accept both kinds of health practices concurrently.

Various tribal groups differ in their traditional values and beliefs. Henderson and Primeaux (1981, pp. 73–74) list the following characteristics, which apply in general to traditional Native Americans:

- *Orientation to present.* Native Americans tend to live in the present and are not concerned about the future, whereas non-Native Americans tend to be future oriented.

- *Major concern with finishing a task.* Native Americans are more concerned about finishing a task rather than about being punctual. In the past, many Native American tribes had no word for time.

- *Giving.* The Native American who gives to others is highly respected. In some tribes, accumulating goods and saving money are not approved.

- *Respect for age.* Leadership positions are often given to the elderly rather than the young.

- *Cooperation.* A high value is placed upon working together rather than on competition.

- *Harmony with nature.* Native Americans believe in living in harmony with nature and taking from it only what one needs to live.

- *Integration into the extended family.* The Native American extended family may include three generations in one household and includes other households of relatives. The elderly are often the official and symbolic leaders.

Native Americans are sometimes assumed to be inattentive because they may not make direct eye contact when speaking with another person. This practice is based on their respect for the other person's privacy and the other person's soul. Some Native Americans believe that direct eye contact is disrespectful, intrudes on individual privacy, and may even take the other's soul away.

Associated with this belief is the Native American's commitment to autonomy. Each person has the right to speak only for himself or herself, and each person's actions should be self-initiated. Thus, the nurse may have difficulty obtaining a client's history from close family members. Family members may believe they have no right to give personal information about another; they do not mean to be uncooperative but are following an unwritten ethical code.

Native Americans accept that they will die as part of the life cycle and do not worry about how or when or why. They know they will join another world of long-ago ancestors when the Spirit intends. Funerals generally take place in the home and are associated with a large feast and gifts for relatives of the deceased. Burial rituals according to tribal tradition are important to many Native Americans.

Associated with burial is the belief of wholeness. Thus, some Native Americans may want to reclaim amputated limbs and retain them for burial when the person dies. Native Americans also fear the spirits of the dead. It is important to the dying Native American client and family that people, e.g., relatives, be present at the death.

Family   During illness, the client is comforted by visits from relatives and friends. Visits convey caring and enduring bonds of support. Being present is generally more important than talking, and it is not uncommon for large numbers of people to congregate. Most often, one person likes to remain near the client for long periods. The Native American's kinship system can be confusing to nurses of other cultures. A child, for example, may have several mothers or several sets of brothers or sisters who are not direct relatives but are considered such. These people are all-important to the ill client. The aged, particularly, are looked upon for counsel and wisdom. Friendship ties are strong and can be as meaningful as those of the family or extended family in sustaining the client's recuperative powers.

Health Beliefs   Native Americans believe that a state of health exists when a person is in total harmony with nature. Each rock, tree, animal, flower, and person is equally respected, and all are seen to coexist in harmony. The earth is considered a living organism that has a will and desire to be well, but, just as human beings, may be healthy or not. It is believed that when people harm the earth they harm themselves, and vice versa. Thus, Native Americans believe they should treat the body and the earth with respect.

Many Native Americans view illness not as an altered physiologic state but as an imbalance between the person who is ill and the natural or supernatural forces around the person. Causes of illness relate to this concept. Native Americans believe that if one interferes with this harmony by abusing or offending another person or thing, one may become ill. Even bad thoughts or wishes, such as jealousy or anger, may cause illness. In addition, supernatural or spiritual forces may be involved. In the Papago tribe of southern Arizona, for example, many persons believe that ghosts of the dead, returning as owls or other animals of night, bring sickness. All animals are believed to have supernatural powers, which they can use to send sickness (Winn 1976, p. 281).

Native Americans do not relate disease causation to germ theory. A survey of Native American registered nurses from 23 tribes revealed that none of these tribes had a word for *germ* (Henderson and Primeaux 1981, p. 243). This trait makes it difficult for Native Americans to understand the cause of tuberculosis, for example. Some Navajo Native Americans believed that the signs and symptoms caused by tuberculosis were the result of lightning. Using the wood of a tree struck by lightening for firewood or other purposes would cause abscesses to develop in the lungs (Wauneka 1976, p. 236).

Health Practices   Various curative and preventive rituals may be conducted to restore balance when illness occurs. Some of these may be carried out by medicine men, others by family members. Sacred foods, such as cornmeal, may be sprinkled on people's shoulders before they enter a home to prevent disease from entering the home. This sacred food or other substance, such as tobacco or feathers, may be sprinkled around an ill person's bed. It is important for nurses to provide privacy for such ceremonies and to inquire about how long the substance is to be left in place, how to dispose of it, and, if it must be disturbed, exactly how and where the nurse may do so. Items such as herbs or mixtures are frequently placed near the client on the bedside stand or on the bed; some may be worn by the client. Nurses need to acquire permission from the client, family, or medicine man, if these have to be removed.

Healing ceremonies, sometimes referred to as *sings* or *prayers,* may be requested. These vary in length from 30 minutes to 9 days. Space and privacy need to be provided for such ceremonies. In the hospital, the sing usually lasts less than 1 hour. A medicine man may also be

(text continues on p. 470)

TABLE 24-2   Comparison of Health-Related Factors and Subcultures

	Definition of Health	Cause of Illness—Is Prevention Possible; If so, How?	Name of Healer, Healing Practices	Problems of Entry to Health Care System	Communication Patterns	Sexuality and Family Life	Beliefs about Death
Navajo (Native American)	Harmony between individual, earth, and supernatural, as well as the ability to survive difficult circumstances[1,2]	Disease is disharmony and can be caused by violating taboo or attack by witch; illness prevented through elaborate religious rituals; do not believe in germ theory[1,2]	Medicine man, who is more than average human being, is therefore influential figure; medicine man diagnoses and treats problem; treatments include yucca root, massage, herbs, and chanting; his chant states person will get well, and person believes him[1,2]	Language; will first visit medicine man; general beliefs are not compatible with health care system and structure; problems also include money and past experiences of disrespect; fear of spirits of dead may influence decision to leave hospital early[1,2]	Time of silence after each speaker to show respect and reflection on what they said; little eye contact; time orientation not very strict; recording of conversation invasion of privacy[1,2]	Family, extended family, and tribal ties strong; cooperation emphasized; consider children as individuals as soon as they can talk, therefore can make own decisions[1,2]	Fear of spirits of dead; children and family should be with dying person[1]
Hispanic American	Gift from God, also good luck; can tell healthy person by robust appearance and report of feeling well[1,3,4]	Illness is punishment from God for wrongdoing, to be suffered; it can be prevented by eating well, praying, being good, and working; wearing medals may help; physical illness is an imbalance between "hot"	Healer called *curandero*; cures hot illness with cold medicine and reverse; classification of hot and cold diseases varies; penicillin is hot medicine; massages and cleanings are common[4]	Language; will first go to woman for advice, then if needed, to "señora," then to curandero, then to physician; many migrant workers are Hispanic, and frequent moves may make access to medical care difficult;	Confidentiality and modesty important; too many questions are insulting; it is more acceptable to make tentative statement to which they can respond; time orientation not strict; politeness essential[1,3-5]	High degree of modesty, may prefer home births for this reason; men are breadwinners, women homemakers; women are healers, men make all decisions[1,3-5]	Afterlife of heaven and hell exists

466

TABLE 24-2 *Comparison of Health-Related Factors and Subcultures (continued)*

	Definition of Health	Cause of Illness—Is Prevention Possible; If so, How?	Name of Healer, Healing Practices	Problems of Entry to Health Care System	Communication Patterns	Sexuality and Family Life	Beliefs about Death
		and "cold" properties of body[1,3,4]		belief that hospital is place to go to die causes underuse of system; modesty may result in woman bringing friend to physician with her[1,3,4]			
Traditional black American	Harmony with nature, no separation of mind and body[4]	Disease is disharmony caused by spirits and demons; it can be prevented through good diet, rest, cleanliness, and laxatives to clean out system; some use of copper and silver bracelets for prevention	Some belief in voodoo still prevalent; religious healing practiced[4,6]	May seek folk or religious healer first; money and type of service affect decision; emergency room frequent entry point; black women have high "noncompliance" rate[4,6]	Racism toward blacks still prevalent; common names for symptoms should be known by health worker; time orientation not strict	Matriarchy prevalent; almost 30% of black families have woman head of household; therefore women make decisions[4,6]	Death is passage from evils of this world to another state; blacks have shorter life expectancy than national average[6]
Chinese American	Balance of yin and yang (negative and positive energy forces); healthy body is gift from parents and ancestors[4,7,8]	Illness caused by imbalance of yin and yang, which may be due to overexertion or prolonged sitting; disease is prevented through	Acupuncture and moxibustion (which is a therapeutic application of heat to skin) restore balance of yin and yang; herbal remedies such as ginseng	Language; traditional Chinese physicians were paid to keep their clients well and cared for sick without fees because illness indicated they had failed	Open expression of emotions not acceptable; therefore might not complain about pain or symptoms; client may smile when they do not understand[4,7]	Women subservient to men; patriarchal family; ancestor worship and respect for obedience for parents observed; divorce considered disgrace[1,4,5]	Reincarnation[7]

TABLE 24-2 *Comparison of Health-Related Factors and Subcultures (continued)*

	Definition of Health	Cause of Illness—Is Prevention Possible; If so, How?	Name of Healer, Healing Practices	Problems of Entry to Health Care System	Communication Patterns	Sexuality and Family Life	Beliefs about Death
		better adaptation to nature[4,7]	used for many illnesses; healer is called physician[4,7]	in their job; Chinese physicians are available in community and may encourage clients to use Western physician; family spokesman may accompany client to Western physician[4,7]			
Culture of poverty	Functional definition; if you can work, you are healthy[5,9]	Belief that illness is not preventable; fatalism common; future orientation minimal because present problems are too great[1,5,9]	Will often rely on folk healers and remedies because of belief and problems gaining access to health care system[5]	Use of public funding may limit access and type of care; present time orientation and beliefs about prevention may cause delay in obtaining care; inability to afford health insurance; may lose day's pay to go to physician[5,9]	May use slang and language of subculture; may view providers as authoritarian; time orientation not strict[5]	Many single-parent families with woman head of household[9]	Depends on culture and religion
Health care culture	Optimal level of functioning; more than absence of disease; physical,	Scientific approach to cause of illness; prevention involves periodic	Healing done by physician, usually takes place in office or hospital;	Physician is main access to system; focus is basically curing illness rather	Widespread use of jargon and specialized language; large percentage of workers from	Hierarchy, with physicians making decisions	Death usually means workers have failed to do their job; elaborate

TABLE 24-2 Comparison of Health-Related Factors and Subcultures (continued)

Definition of Health	Cause of Illness—Is Prevention Possible; If So, How?	Name of Healer, Healing Practices	Problems of Entry to Health Care System	Communication Patterns	Sexuality and Family Life	Beliefs about Death
emotional, social, and mental health included[5]	physical examinations, laboratory studies, inoculations, as well as avoiding smoking and overeating[4]	treatments based on scientific knowledge and are frequently embarrassing or uncomfortable; often emotional component of disease is ignored[4]	than prevention; encouragement given to population to seek care as soon as symptoms appear; consider health care system as only provider	middle class; often expect gratitude for care given; time orientation strict; written records kept[4]		means are used to keep people alive; ethical and legal questions are being discussed and tested

[1] Data from A. T. Brownlee, *Community, culture, and care: A cross-cultural guide for health workers* (St. Louis: C. V. Mosby Co., 1978).
[2] Data from R. Wood, The American Indian and health. In *Ethnicity and health care* (NLN pub. no. 14–1625, 1976), pp. 29–35.
[3] Data from H. Gonzales, Health care needs of the Mexican American family. In *Ethnicity and health care*. (NLN pub. no. 14–1625, 1976), pp. 21–28.
[4] Data from R. Spector, *Cultural diversity in health and illness* (New York: Appleton-Century-Crofts, 1985).
[5] Data from R. Murray and J. Zentner, *Nursing assessment and health promotion through the life span* (Englewood Cliffs, N.J.: Prentice-Hall, 1975).
[6] Data from B. Martin, Ethnicity and health care: Afro-Americans. In *Ethnicity and health care* (NLN pub. no. 14–1625, 1976), pp. 47–55.
[7] Data from R. Wang, Chinese Americans and health care. In *Ethnicity and health care* (NLN pub. no. 14–1625, 1976). pp. 9–18.
[8] Data from G. Channing, What is a Christian Scientist? In Rosten, L., editor: *A guide to religions of America* (New York: Simon & Schuster, 1955).
[9] Data from M. Fromer, Community health care and the nursing process (St. Louis: C. V. Mosby Co., 1979).

Source Adapted from Joanne Gingrich-Crass, Structural variables: Factors affecting adaptation, in S. J. Wold, *School nursing: A framework for practice* (St. Louis: C. V. Mosby Co.) pp. 136–41. Copyright 1981 by Susan Wold, RN, MPH. Reprinted by permission of the author.

requested to perform curative rituals, which vary with the signs and symptoms of the client.

Health Problems

The leading causes of death in the Native American population are accidents, suicide, diabetes, alcoholism, and homicide (Primeaux 1977, pp. 58–59). At least one-third of the Native American population is poverty-stricken. Associated with this income level are poor living conditions, malnutrition, tuberculosis, and high maternal and infant death rates. Native Americans have the highest infant mortality rate in the United States, even though their birth rate is almost twice that of the general population. This mortality rate is attributed to the high incidence of diarrhea in young babies and the harsh environment in which they live (Spector 1985, p. 187).

Nursing Implications

When caring for Native American clients, nurses need to consider the following:

- Although most Native Americans recognize the value of Anglo-Western health care, many continue to use traditional medicine and cures either independently or in conjunction with such care.
- Native Indian medicine and religion cannot be separated. Native Americans make no distinction between physical and mental illness or the mind and the body. They live the concept of wholeness.
- Tribal healing ceremonies and practices are highly ritualistic, religious ways to deal with sickness and death.
- Tribal rituals that include extended "family" members are the way that Native Americans share all aspects of life.
- Each tribe assigns symbolic meanings to foods or other substances.
- Such characteristics as not looking others in the eye should not be interpreted as disrespect, inattention, lack of interest, or avoidance.
- Nurses attempting communication with Native Americans need to be aware of the following factors:
  a. It is the custom for the person to speak only for himself or herself.
  b. Use of extensive questions during history taking may be construed as an intrusion on individual privacy. The history taker may need to rely on observation techniques and make declarative statements to elicit information from the client, such as, "You have an obvious cough that keeps you awake at night."
  c. Note taking may pose a barrier to communication, since Native Americans tend to value conversation, story telling, and listening.
  d. Native Americans often use a very low tone of voice, and the listener is expected to pay attention.

Black Americans

Black culture in America is a composite of the cultures of many black groups, all of which trace their roots to Africa. With the arrival of the first African slaves in Jamestown, Virginia, in 1619, a history of deprivation for blacks on this continent began. Even after slavery was abolished, black people endured severe economic and social deprivation. The struggles to overcome these deprivations continue today. More recently, black immigrants have come to the United States from Jamaica, Haiti, and other islands of the Caribbean, fleeing oppression and seeking economic opportunity. Black American culture is more similar to white American culture now than it was 300 years ago.

There is a large black middle class and a large black lower class. There are strong kinship bonds in both low-income and more prosperous black families. These families provide financial support, assist with child care, and serve as buffers against racism and discrimination during children's growing years. A black family may show much cohesion and sharing, particularly in times of trouble.

Often a significant member of a black family must be consulted before important decisions are made. This person may be a father, mother, aunt, son, or grandparent. Nurses need to be sensitive to the fact that a decision may not be made until this person is consulted.

When black Americans who are not familiar with the health care system enter it, they may show defensive behaviors such as hostility and suspicion. These attitudes are often adopted in expectation of being demeaned in some manner. It is important for nurses to recognize the reasons for these responses and learn to relate to all clients as worthy human beings.

Family

Middle-class black households tend to have two parents, and often both parents work to maintain a middle-class life-style. Children of middle-class black families often feel the need to achieve. Many plan to attend college to maintain or advance their position in the community.

Lower-income blacks often live in extended families, i.e., grandparents, aunts, uncles live in the house with the parents and children. Single-parent families in financial difficulty may depend on government programs for income. Black families frequently have extended support systems. LaFargue (1980, p. 1637) states that part of the survival strategy of blacks in the urban north is to immerse themselves in a domestic circle of kinfolk who will help them.

Health Beliefs   Black Americans may believe traditionally that health is maintained by proper diet, which includes a hot breakfast. Some believe that laxatives are important to keep the system running and open (Spector 1985, p. 147). A person who is a practicing Black Muslim does not eat pork or pork products.

It is important for nurses to understand the values held by a black client and that person's definition of health. Traditional definitions in black culture stem from the African view of life as a process rather than a state. All things, whether living or dead, were believed to influence each other (Spector 1985, p. 142). Health meant being in harmony with nature; illness was a state of disharmony. Therefore, illness could be treated in a number of ways, including reliance on the power of a "healer." These beliefs and practices may or may not apply to a particular black client. However, nurses should be aware of any cultural differences and take these into consideration when planning care. See also Table 24–2. In LaFargue's study, blacks defined illness as "feeling bad" or "inhibition of physical activity" (LaFargue 1972, p. 54).

Health Practices   The poor black client may not seek help until a health problem is serious for many reasons, e.g., "finances, child care problems, fear of hospitals, possibility of becoming a 'guinea pig,' and fear of death" (White 1977, p. 30), reasons often cited by poor clients regardless of ethnicity. Many black families in rural areas of the South continue to use folk health practices (Henderson and Primeaux 1981, p. 210) and home remedies. Voodoo and witchcraft are practiced to a minor extent. (Disease, for instance, may be attributed to a hex.) Spiritualists or sorcerers may sometimes be consulted, or clients may vacillate between Western physicians and witch doctors or spiritualists who can remove spells. Historically, churches have been a bulwark of support for blacks, hence religious practices and Bible reading often continue during hospitalization. Often the black clergy can help bridge the gap between the black client and health professionals because they have "the understanding of the rituals, folkways, and mores" of black culture (Smith 1976, p. 12).

Health Problems   The major health problems of blacks in the United States are hypertension, sickle-cell disease, and cancers of the lungs, oral cavity, larynx,

pharynx, esophagus, and urinary bladder. The increase in cancer in these areas is thought to be largely due to the increase in smoking (Orque et al. 1983, p. 106). Poverty among blacks leads to relatively high morbidity and mortality rates among infants and mothers, even though these rates have declined since 1960 (National Center for Health Statistics 1985, p. 2).

Obesity is a greater problem among black women than white women. Approximately 60% of black females 45 to 75 years were overweight in 1975 to 1980 (National Center for Health Statistics 1985, p. 9). The incidence of hypertension in blacks is twice that of whites. The onset is earlier in life, the severity is greater, and there are more premature deaths than in the white population (Boyle 1989, p. 225).

Nursing Implications   Nursing implications relative to the care of the black client include: skin and hair care, assessing skin color, communication, and food preferences.

Many black people are very much aware of any signs of racial discrimination. A sensitive nurse should be alert to actions or behavior that may be interpreted as discriminatory and intervene as the client's advocate.

Some black clients speak black English, a highly rhythmic and stylized speech. It differs from standard English in its pronunciation and syntax and in the connotations of some words. Black English has also been called black dialect, black Creole, soul talk, Afro-American speech, Ebonics, and Afro (Orque et al. 1983, p. 86). Refugees from Haiti speak Creole, French and African dialect. Because this language is primarily spoken rather than written, communication with this group can be difficult.

Black clients may favor a traditional rural Southern diet, an urban middle-class diet, or a combination of the two. Soul food is the traditional diet of the Southern black. Pork is the chief meat. Hominy grits, black-eyed peas, and mustard and collard greens are also consumed. To these are often added cabbage, rice, white potatoes, okra, macaroni, and noodles (Orque et al. 1983, pp. 95–96). Nurses can often assist blacks who are accustomed to eating soul food to adapt special diets to their tastes.

Asian Americans

The term *Asian American* refers to four primary ethnic groups: Chinese, Japanese, Koreans, and Vietnamese. Recently, the term *Pacific Asian* has been used to include people originally from the Pacific islands, such as the Philippines, Samoa, and Guam, as well as the other Asian countries.

It is difficult to classify many Asians because they are of mixed national parentage. For example, the person's parents may be Chinese and Korean or Japanese and Filipino. In addition, most Asians view themselves as belonging to particular subgroups and ethnic groups and generally dislike being viewed as a member of another group. For example, the Chinese Americans and Japanese Americans in Hawaii consider themselves different from the "mainlanders," i.e., those in the United States.

Because of the wide diversity of groups of Asians, full coverage of their views is beyond the scope of this book. This section focuses primarily on Chinese health beliefs and practices, since the traditions of many other Asians derive in part from them. The health beliefs and practices of Japanese Americans, Vietnamese Americans, and Filipino Americans will be considered briefly in separate sections. First, however, some general, traditional Asian values and behaviors are outlined, but the student must recognize that a wide range of behaviors exists among and within groups.

General Traditional Asian Values and Beliefs
Chang (1981, pp. 260–75) outlines the following general Asian values and behaviors:

- Traditionally, the Asian household consisted of the extended kinship family, in which grandparents, parents, siblings, uncles, aunts, and cousins lived together. Although such households are rare in North America today, members of traditional families often maintain strong emotional bonds. It is not unusual, therefore, for hospitalized Asians to have many family members visit them.

- The traditional Asian family is male dominated. Elderly persons who live with the family are usually the husband's parents. Asian women historically occupied an inferior position to men, and sons were more welcome in a family than daughters. Even in modern families, sons may receive preferential treatment. It is wise, therefore, for nurses to ascertain the opinion of the father, or in his absence the eldest son, on health care issues requiring decision making.

- Traditionally, there is unquestioning respect for and deference to authority. It is expected that each individual will maintain filial piety (devotion and loyalty to family authority). Asian families are considered a continuum from past to future. Membership includes not only the present generation but also the ancestors and the unborn. Failure to comply with familial authority, duty, and obligations, to pay obedience to the family, and to engage in behavior that gives the family and the ethnic group a good name results in feelings of shame and guilt.

- Interactions in the Asian family tend to be less verbal than those of the white middle-class family, and praise of self or of members of one's own family is considered bad manners. This behavior of Asians is often misconstrued as lack of self-esteem or as belittling of family members. This does not imply that nurses should not offer appropriate praise; but they should accept a self-deprecating response as a cultural variant.

- Asians strongly emphasize harmony and avoidance of conflict in groups. In contrast to the behavior of whites, who may consider the individual most important, the behavior of Asians may be best not for the individual but for the situation and for others in the group. Often, behavior is quiet, obedient, unassertive, reticent, agreeable, and reserved. For example, an individual may remain quiet or simply nod the head, often to avoid conflicts in ambiguous, embarrassing, or anxiety-producing situations. This behavior may be more apparent in Asian women because of their socialization. Asians avoid direct confrontations in which one of the parties must lose face; to do so, they may blame themselves for a mistake even when facts indicate that it was the other person's error.

- Asian respect for those in positions of authority such as doctors, teachers, and nurses, often evokes a yes response that is different from the American connotation of the word. Asians tend to answer yes to be polite and to mean, "I don't want to cause embarrassment." For example, in response to a nurse's question, "Is that clear?" an Asian may say yes because it is considered impolite to say "No, it is not clear"; that response may imply that the nurse is either confused or unable to communicate. It is wise, therefore, for nurses to ask questions that require more than a yes-or-no answer.

- Outward signs of feelings are discouraged. Asians are taught patterns of self-control and bravery even in situations of emotional conflict, hardship, and pain. Nurses must be aware of these attitudes when assessing pain and assisting Asians during emotional crises. Often, Asians express feelings of caring by their physical presence and attendance in times of illness rather than by an outward verbal expression of feelings.

- Asians characteristically avoid attracting special attention to themselves. This inconspicuousness is related to their culture, which emphasizes harmony, consideration of others' rights and feelings, avoidance of behavior that would dishonor the family, and respect for and obedience to those in authority.

Chinese Americans

The Chinese in the United States and Canada are largely concentrated on the west coasts of the countries, on the east coast of the United States, and in large cities such as New York and Chicago. The Chinese population can be considered in three groups: immigrants from rural China who arrived in North America 40 to 50 years ago (who still are largely oriented to Chinese folk medicine), new immigrants from several Asian countries and Hong Kong (who often practice a mixture of Chinese folk and Western medicine), and native North American descendants of nineteenth-century Chinese immigrants (who are oriented to Western medical practices but still may be influenced by their elders in regard to health care).

Family

Prior to the revolution in China, the Chinese family was patriarchal and patrilineal (tracing descent through the paternal line). Respect for ancestors and parents and obedience to the family were important. The Chinese family was frequently an extended one, with several generations living in one household. Family clans formed of people of the same bloodline with the same surnames were strong social organizations. People who came to North America 40 to 50 years ago set up the same traditional families.

Following the revolution, traditional family practices and superstitions became less evident in China and among immigrants. Although family ties continue to be strong, the nuclear family is now more common than the extended family in Chinese-American society. In many Asian families, at least two people are employed full time; they often use their income to support the extended family (Wang 1976, pp. 33–41).

Health beliefs

Chinese folk medicine originated with Taoist philosophy. It proposes that the universe and health are regulated by two forces, the *yin* and the *yang*. The yin is a negative, female force; some of its characteristics are darkness, cold, and emptiness. The yang represents the positive, maleness, light, warmth, and fullness. When these two energy forces are in balance, health exists. A person with too much yin is nervous and predisposed to digestive disorders. Too much yang, on the other hand, causes dehydration, fever, and irritability.

The Chinese do not consider their bodies to be personal property. The body is viewed as a gift provided by parents and ancestors, and it thus must be cared for. Various parts of the body are controlled by yin and yang. The inside, the front part of the body, and five solid organs *(ts'ang)* that collect and store secretions—i.e., the liver, heart, spleen, lungs, and kidneys—are controlled by yin. The outside, the back part of the body, and five hollow organs *(fu)* that excrete—i.e., the gallbladder, stomach, large and small intestines, and bladder—are controlled by yang. Yin stores the vital strength of life; yang protects the body from outside forces. A person who does not balance yin and yang properly will have a short life. Illness occurs when an imbalance of yin and yang exists. The sole cause of disease is considered to be disrupted harmony.

Chinese staples are tofu and polished rice. In addition vegetables such as *bok choy, gai lan,* spinach, Chinese cabbage, and mustard greens are favored. Many Chinese do not tolerate milk or cheese well.

Health practices

Some Chinese-American clients follow both Western and Chinese medical advice at the same time. This can produce problems if the therapies are not correlated. For example, a client may be receiving two forms of the same drug, one from an herbalist and one from the Western physician, thus taking a double dose. Chinese clients should be encouraged to tell a doctor whether they are taking or receiving other therapy.

Pregnant women often observe folk medicine practices (e.g., the use of soy sauce may be restricted so that the baby's skin will not be very dark). In Chinese folk medicine, herbs and acupuncture are used. A folk medicine diagnosis is made chiefly by observing, questioning, listening to the body, and taking the pulse. The prescription is a combination of herbs, which are obtained from a Chinese pharmacy. Acupuncture is used chiefly to treat muscular and skeletal disorders and diseases characterized by excessive yang. Needles are inserted into the body at specific points along certain internal channels, which are called meridians. The internal organs are believed to be connected to the skin points and to the meridians; the acupuncture helps to balance the energy that flows within them.

The concept of yin and yang also applies to the balance of a meal. Yin is cold and includes fruits, vegetables, cold drinks, and hot (in temperature) melon soup. Yang is hot and includes, for example, soups containing ginger and scrambled eggs. In Chinese culture, the concepts of hot and cold have nothing to do with the temperature of the food. A Chinese client who is ill with a hot disease, such as an eye infection, may wish to eat cold foods rather than hot foods in order to get well.

Chinese people of the older generations may also believe that their blood is not replaceable. Therefore, they are often very reluctant to give blood even for a blood test. Like many other people, the elderly Chinese often believe that a hospital is a place to go to die rather than to get well.

Following are some differences between Western practice and Chinese folk medicine (see also Table 24–2, earlier).

- One dose of an herbal medicine is thought to cure a person or make the person feel better. Thus, the Chinese client may be puzzled by a multiplicity of medicines prescribed in multiple doses.

- Herbs are generally boiled in water for a prescribed time before being ingested rather than prepared as capsules or pills.

- Chinese clients may change physicians during an illness in order to find the best cure. When they do so, they may not tell the former doctor because they do not want the doctor to lose face.

- Some Chinese do not understand or react well to painful diagnostic procedures. They believe that a physician should be able to make a diagnosis solely on the basis of a physical examination. Many may leave the Western health care system to avoid distasteful procedures.

- Most Chinese believe that it is best to die with the body intact. This belief originates with Confucius, who taught that only those who at the end of their lives return their physical bodies whole and sound shall be truly revered. As a result, Chinese clients may refuse surgery and donation of organs after death.

- Ginseng is a highly valued herb used as a general strength tonic for the pregnant woman (Chung 1977, p. 71).

Health problems   Specific health problems more prevalent among the Chinese than the general population are eye problems, tuberculosis, dental caries, malnutrition, and mental illness. Some of these are directly related to the poor environmental conditions of North American Chinatowns rather than to an inherited predisposition.

Because of the stress of adjusting to American culture and the lack of family support, mental health problems among aged male Chinese have increased. Emotional

problems are also related to the bicultural conflict between the individual values of freedom, egalitarianism, and individualism and the Chinese values of filial piety, loyalty, and authoritarianism (Orque et al. 1983, p. 196).

Nursing implications   Implications relative to the care of Chinese clients include the following:

1. Nurses should always convey respect by addressing the client and family members by their given names.

2. Nurses should try to provide Chinese clients with the food to which they are accustomed. Some communities have hospitals that provide special food for their Chinese clients.

3. Chinese clients are often reluctant to be admitted to hospitals. They believe hospitals are unclean places where people go to die. They may require supportive nursing intervention for reassurance.

Japanese Americans   Japanese Americans often maintain a number of their cultural values while at the same time acculturating to the larger society. Four values of the Japanese are gaman, haji, enryo, and koko. *Gaman* means self-control. A Japanese person who is stoic when experiencing pain is probably practicing gaman. The client will not verbalize the pain and may try to deal with it. Japanese who carry on in spite of adversity are considered strong (Orque et al. 1986, p. 223).

Haji, or shame, is an important cultural concept. Japanese children are taught not to bring shame on themselves or their families by unacceptable behavior. *Enryo* is a type of behavior that encompasses politeness, respect, deference, reserve, and humility. The opposite of enryo is aggressive, boisterous, loud, rude behavior (Orque et al. 1983, p. 224). For example, a Japanese man might not turn on his signal light because he does not want to bother the nurses. *Koko* is filial piety. The Japanese perceive dependence as natural for the elderly and young children. An elderly person who is dependent and has reduced authority still maintains self-esteem. This attitude contrasts to the North American view of dependence as a sign of weakness (Kalish 1967, pp. 65–69).

Japanese Americans consider time valuable and like to use it well. They will usually follow medication schedules precisely.

Vietnamese Americans   Thousands of Vietnamese came to the United States following the Vietnamese conflict. Another, smaller, group came later. South Vietnamese have a family-centered culture in which the children are taught to value the family's interests over their own (Orque et al. 1983, p. 250). Vietnamese value propriety over time and indirectness over confrontation in a disagreement in order to preserve harmony. A Vietnamese client who is embarrassed at a nurse's question may say yes or laugh to lessen the embarrassment.

Filipino Americans

The Filipino culture is diverse. However, its central cultural values are shaped by a fatalistic view that God's will and supernatural forces determine what happens. Filipino culture is family centered, stressing interdependence among members of the family. Filipinos also emphasize achievement and social acceptance. A Filipino client is likely to avoid a disagreement with a nurse and speak evasively. By contrast, the white middle-class American may value an open expression of feelings and honest expression of thoughts. Because of their fatalistic view, Filipinos often show great patience and endurance when faced with illness.

Hispanic Americans

Hispanic Americans have their origins in a number of Spanish-speaking countries. The greatest numbers of Hispanic Americans in the United States come from Mexico, Puerto Rico, and Cuba, in that order. In recent years, increasing numbers of immigrants have come to the United States from Nicaragua, El Salvador, and other strife-torn countries of Central and South America. While the primary language of the Hispanic American is Spanish, it is important for the caregiver to know that there are differences in dialect and word usage among the different countries of origin.

There are many similarities and some differences among Hispanic Americans. Because a full discussion of each Hispanic American culture and its health care implications is beyond the scope of this book, the following pages focus on identified Mexican-American and Cuban-American beliefs and practices, many of which are common to other Hispanic cultures.

Traditional Mexican-American foods are beans and tortillas. Traditional foods for the Cuban American are beans and rice. For clients requiring a special diet, traditional foods can present problems. This situation requires special planning in consultation with dietitians. For example, Hispanics generally prefer rice to potatoes. The manner of preparing the rice is important; it differs from the Asian method, and even among Hispanic cultures there are differences in preparation. The diet of many low-income Hispanic Americans often contains a high proportion of starches: tortillas, rice, beans, corn, plantains, and so on. It is usually possible to plan diets to meet clients' preferences and thus increase the chances that the food will be eaten.

Family

Hispanic Americans have extended families that play an important part in their lives. The family is usually large, and life revolves around the home. Often the family's needs take precedence over the individual's needs. At a time of illness, the family will give a great deal of support.

In the Hispanic-American family, the woman is the primary caregiver, and often she decides when medical assistance should be sought.

Health Beliefs

Many Mexican Americans entered the United States during the early 1900s and brought with them the values, beliefs, and practices of rural Mexico; others are more recent immigrants. Cuban Americans started entering the United States in large numbers in the 1960s, escaping political and economic oppression in their homeland. Folk concepts of health and illness continue to affect the thinking of some second- and third-generation Mexican Americans and Cuban Americans today. See also Table 24–2, earlier.

Mexican Americans may hold the following health-related beliefs to varying degrees:

- Certain foods promote good health, while others can produce poor health. An example of the former is tea made from fresh orange leaves; examples of the latter are rice and coffee, which should not be taken during an evening meal.

- A person must be in tune with God to maintain good health. Thus, a person who is chronically ill is believed to have offended God and is being punished.

- Health means being free of pain and being robust, even obese, rather than thin.

In addition, health is perceived as the ability to maintain a high level of normal physical activity and illness as a state of discomfort. Some Mexican Americans also believe that certain people can use magical powers to make others ill (Abril 1977, pp. 169–70). Some Mexican Americans believe that illness is due to life-style. They often have precise ideas about the types of rest, activity, recreation, and nutrition that lead to poor and good health (Gonzalez-Swafford and Gutierrez 1983, p. 29). Illness is seen as an imbalance in the individual's body or as a punishment for wrongdoing. The causes of illness can be grouped into four categories (Spector 1985, pp. 161–63):

1. *Imbalance between "hot" and "cold" or "wet" and "dry."* The four humors, or body fluids, that must be in balance are: blood (hot and wet), phlegm (cold and wet), yellow bile (hot and dry), and black bile (cold and dry). When these fluids are not in balance, illness results. Treatment in hospitals can be based on the principles of hot and cold. For example, illnesses that are classified as hot are treated with food, drugs, and drinks that are classified as cold.

2. *Magic or supernatural forces. Mal de ojo* (evil eye) is disease caused by forces outside the body, such as a person's admiration of part of another person's body, e.g., the hair. The victim can lose the admired part or fall ill. In some places, mal de ojo is thought to be prevented by having the admirer touch the admired person while complimenting him or her, and it is believed to be cured with eggs in a ritual. The symptoms of mal de ojo include headaches, fever, fatigue, and prostration.

3. *"Dislocation" of body parts.* One example of a disease of "dislocation" is *empacho,* a disease primarily seen in children that produces swelling of the abdomen as a result of intestinal blockage. It is thought to be caused by overeating foods such as soft bread and bananas.

4. *Strong emotional states. Susto,* a disease of emotional origin, is fright caused by natural phenomena such as lightning or loud noises. The symptoms have been described as insomnia, restlessness, and nervousness. It is a common folk disease that is difficult to cure but can be treated with herbal tea. *Espanto* is a disease with symptoms similar to susto. Its origin is fright caused by seeing supernatural spirits or events and can be likened to being "spooked" in American slang. *Caraje* is a rage, a response to a particular situation. The victim may continually scream, cry, or yell and display hyperactivity.

Many Mexican and Cuban Americans, when they are ill, may believe a folk medicine diagnosis rather than a Western diagnosis, even though they may also seek help from a Western physician. Healers within the Mexican American community can be either male (a *curandero*) or female (a *curandera*). Healers consulted by Cuban Americans are called *espíritos.* They offer a number of treatments; one of the most frequently used is herb tea. Both Cuban Americans and Mexican Americans have a personal relationship with their healers in contrast to the relations in a hospital.

Puerto Rican beliefs about health and illness are not unlike those of Mexican Americans. Their diseases are also classified as hot and cold; however, food and medications are classified as hot (*caliente*), cold (*frio*), and cool (*fresco*) (Spector 1985, p. 167).

Hispanic Americans consider the appearance of blood and the presence of pain as indicators that an illness is severe. If it is "natural" for a condition to occur, it is considered harmless. When it is unnatural and folk methods fail, most Mexican Americans seek medical assistance from Western practitioners.

Health Practices   Mexican Americans are generally proud people. Those who are socially and economically deprived may well have low self-esteem and be reluctant to accept care for which they cannot pay. Therefore, Mexican American clients in the hospital may not ask for help when they have pain; a young Mexican-American male may react with hostility rather than passivity in response to nursing intervention to uphold his self-image.

As do people of diverse ethnic backgrounds, many Mexican Americans look upon the hospital as a place to die. Thus, they may avoid hospitals when they can and enter only with great fear, feeling that death is imminent. Illness is generally regarded not as a personal affair but as a family affair. Therefore, when a person is ill, many relatives generally gather around and visit. Restricting visitors can cause mistrust; nurses need to deal with such a requirement in the context of illness and discuss the matter with the entire family.

As a cultural group, Mexican Americans are very modest. Usually they consider bathing, defecating, and urinating to be very personal matters, yet they may be shy about asking a nurse to leave at such times. The sensitive nurse will provide complete privacy when possible.

Hispanic Americans encounter a number of barriers to health care: language, poverty, and time orientation. To many Hispanic Americans, time is relative; the exact time is not a primary consideration. This attitude hinders effective use of a health care system that values promptness for appointments and mandates specific intervals between doses of medications. Language is another major barrier for many Hispanic Americans seeking help from the health care delivery system. Some do not speak English, and communication is difficult and embarrassing in a system where the English language predominates. In addition, some Hispanic Americans live below the poverty level. They may not have knowledge of available health resources in the community or the money to use them.

Health Problems Drug addiction is a major health problem among Puerto Ricans. Mexican Americans who are economically deprived may be poorly nourished, e.g., have protein and vitamin deficiencies.

Nursing Implications Not all Hispanic Americans identify with their ethnic groups; many identify with white middle-class Americans.

- The nurse should not stereotype the Hispanic-American client. There are diverse beliefs and practices among various Hispanic-American groups. For example, the majority of Hispanic Americans, though not all, are Roman Catholic (Orque et al. 1983, p. 121).
- Hispanic Americans value modesty and privacy. The nurse should provide privacy when they must undress for an examination. The male client may find it especially difficult for a young, female nurse to provide personal care.
- The man in a Hispanic-American family may find it difficult to depend on other family members or even a nurse to do things for him. He expects to decide when and how things should be done and should be involved in decisions if health permits.

Appalachians

The 24 million Appalachians in the United States, 6 million of whom live in the Southern Appalachian region, are a subculture in American society (Tripp-Reimer and Freidl 1977, p. 4). A family-oriented group, Appalachians include upper, middle, and poor working classes. The upper and middle classes tend to share many values with the rest of the United States, just as the poverty group does with other poverty groups in America. Much of Appalachia is rural, encompassing parts of the states of New York, Pennsylvania, Ohio, Maryland, West Virginia, Virginia, Kentucky, Tennessee, North Carolina, South Carolina, Georgia, and Alabama (Tripp-Reimer and Freidl 1977, p. 43).

Tripp-Reimer (1982, p. 185) found that

- Appalachians tend to have large families.
- Migrants tend to move between urban areas and "the hills."
- Migrants tend to quit school at an early age.
- Many Appalachians use welfare services.
- Appalachian migrants tend to be oriented to the present.

The religion of the Appalachians tends to be fundamentalist and fatalistic. Sometimes this fatalism prevents clients from seeking help when they are ill (Lewis et al. 1985, p. 24).

Family Appalachians value family greatly. The family provides its members with a sense of belonging and a sense of identity. Appalachians value family privacy, a situation that has created some social and cultural isolation. Often many family members accompany a client to a health appointment, and they may wish to stay with the client if he or she is hospitalized. For many Appalachians, socialization begins and ends within the family.

The family is generally large and patriarchal. There are definite divisions between the work of men and women. Family ties are strong, and antagonism against another family may be intense. Time orientation is to the present, and the pressure of finances makes it difficult to plan ahead. Education is usually not high priority.

Health Beliefs Appalachians tend to define an individual as ill only when the person feels ill. They have a general distrust of health organizations and fear surgery.

Health Practices When Appalachians feel ill, they tend to try home remedies, e.g., herb teas and tonics. If these cures are not effective, they may seek the advice of a lay practitioner, e.g., "granny midwife," a herbalist, or a faith healer. In an emergency or during childbirth, an Appalachian may seek "orthodox" medical or nursing help.

Health Problems The health problems of the Appalachians are largely related to their economic circumstances and to their occupations. Nutritional problems are frequently due to the fact that they cannot afford to buy much meat, and the diet may be deficient in protein and iron. Some Appalachians work in coal mines, and prolonged exposure to coal dust can cause sarcoidosis, a disease of the lungs.

Nursing Implications The nurse caring for an Appalachian client can be guided by the following (Hicks 1976):

- Appalachians consider direct eye contact to be staring, which is impolite. Nurses should be aware that Appalachians use direct eye contact to express anger or aggression.
- Nurses should also understand that Appalachians follow the "ethic of neutrality."

a. A person must not be assertive or aggressive.

b. People should mind their own business unless asked to do otherwise.

c. A person should not assume authority over others.

d. Appalachians avoid argument and seek agreement.

Arab Americans

There are approximately three million Arabs in the United States, including people who are in America temporarily (Meleis 1981, p. 1181). These include citizens of Egypt, Lebanon, Saudi Arabia, Kuwait, and many other Arab nations. Most Arabs have a common language and share symbols, mores, and beliefs. Arabs are traditionally future oriented and value the use of time to achieve future goals.

Family   The Arab family is traditionally patriarchal and extended. The male of the household is responsible for earning the living outside the home and for making the decisions; women usually remain at home. Arabs have a need to affiliate with others and use an extensive social network to cope with daily stress (Meleis 1981, p. 1181).

Food plays an important part in Arab family life. When family members assemble, it is often around elaborate meals. Love and care are interwoven with food (Meleis 1981, p. 1182). Christian Arabs consume pork and alcohol, whereas Muslims consume neither. Sometimes Arab Americans find hospital food too bland and prefer to have food brought from home.

Health Beliefs   Arabs believe that injury or disease affects the whole person. Often Arabs provide a vague description of their illness rather than precise symptoms because they do not have a framework for signs and symptoms. Arabs usually do not refute the germ theory, but they do believe in disease-causing entities such as the evil eye. Arabs also believe that being deprived of food can cause illness.

Health Practices   Arabs do not believe in sharing a problem or asking for advice until help is offered. The person offering assistance should be able to assess the need without verifying the problem. If a nurse offers an Arab client a choice in care, the client is likely to say "No, thank you." If the nurse accepts this refusal, the client believes the nurse is not interested.

Arabs dislike disclosing information about themselves to strangers and will provide as little information as possible. Nurses must be sensitive to an Arab's dislike of re-vealing personal information. Sometimes Arabs will defer dealing with a matter until they feel more comfortable sharing information and may rely upon others, i.e., the social network, to give advice at times of stress. Arabs generally respect Western health care. Intrusive procedures are often highly regarded and thought to offer the greatest chance of cure.

Many Arabs regard health care as their right, and some may view health care professionals as their employees. Arab Americans respect expertise, which they regard as knowing about problems, making decisions for others, and being accountable for those decisions (Meleis 1981, p. 1182). Arab Americans may not question caregivers openly because of their respect for authority. Some Arabs wear amulets for protection. Even to say the number "five" is believed to increase protection. Deaths are believed to be the result of the will of God and the inadequacy of equipment and medicine.

Health Problems   One health problem that Arabs have in common with people in the Middle East is thalassemia, a genetic condition that results in anemia. It occurs in 7% to 15% of the population in the Middle East (Overfield 1985, p. 85).

Culture of Poverty

The status of being poor is often referred to as the "culture of poverty," a phrase coined by anthropologist Oscar Lewis in the 1960s. Lewis (1966, p. 19) defined the culture of poverty as a subculture of Western society with its own values and behaviors that differ from those of the nonpoor and are passed on from generation to generation. This subculture transcends ethnic and regional boundaries. Characteristics of the poor include the following (Lewis 1966, pp. 19–25):

- Lack of participation in the larger society
- Hostility toward and mistrust of bureaucratic institutions
- Inadequate use of health services
- Long periods of unemployment
- Use of public assistance

Lewis's portrayal of the poor as a subculture is challenged by other researchers, who believe this cultural viewpoint is negative, makes no attempt to question why these features exist, and fails to recognize the role of the larger society in perpetuating poverty. Some research has shown, for example, that the poor have the same values as the rest of society and that the traits Lewis identified may not be cultural but rather responses to situational circumstances. For example, the negative work behaviors associated with the lower class are not culturally derived but situationally induced. It has been shown that the poor have a strong work ethic, want to work, and do work when given equal opportunity (Mason 1981, p. 83). Lack of societal incentives prevents the poor from obtaining and holding a job. Situational theorists believe, therefore, that if society were rid of poverty, the former poor would demonstrate middle-class attitudes and behaviors.

Still other researchers suggest that all members of a society share general, abstract values but that specific, concrete values differ among subgroups and social classes. This viewpoint combines the cultural and situational perspectives of poverty into an adaptational perspective. In other words, the poor are considered a special subgroup of society in response to social structures that make it impossible for them to actualize the values and behavior forms of the dominant society.

Health Considerations
Low-income families often define health in terms of work; if people can work they are healthy. They tend to be fatalistic and believe that illness is not preventable. Because their present problems are so great and all efforts are exerted toward survival, an orientation to the future may be lacking. Most low-income people do not have regular preventive medical checkups, because they cannot afford them. It is more important to them to work than to lose a day's pay visiting a physician. Reliance on public assistance and inability to afford health care insurance limit both the low-income person's access to health care and the type of care available.

The environmental conditions of poverty-stricken areas also have a bearing on overall health. Slum neighborhoods are overcrowded and in a state of deterioration. Neglect and disorder are common. Sanitation services tend to be inadequate. Many streets are strewn with garbage, and alleys are overrun by rats. Fires and crime are constant threats. Recreational facilities are almost nonexistent, forcing children to play in streets and alleys. Parents who can work usually work long hours and earn barely enough for subsistence. They are often too tired to spend much time with their children, even though they love them. As a result, preschool children often come and go as they please, and older siblings assume the role of parent for younger children. With all of these problems confronting the poverty-stricken, it is little wonder that frustration tolerance levels are low, physical abuse is used as the form of discipline, and

value is placed on children seeking employment rather than completing their educations.

Recently attention has been focused on a subculture within the poor, the *homeless*. No longer considered derelicts, bums, or drifters, there are an estimated 250,000 to 3 million people who are homeless in the United States, including families, children, military veterans, and persons with serious and persistent alcohol, drug abuse, and mental health disorders (ANA 1987, p. 26). Recognizing that the existing health care system is not accessible to the homeless, the 1987 ANA House of Delegates adopted an emergency resolution on housing and health care for people who are homeless. In this resolution, the delegates pledged to work to ensure that funding is available to provide needed services.

The poor have the same needs and feelings as other people. They are sensitive, concerned, and easily embarrassed. When admitted to health care agencies, they are sometimes treated in humiliating, condescending, and prejudicial ways by professional caregivers. Because prejudice is usually based on fear of the unknown, and because fear is based on insecurity, it is important for nurses to examine their own values and attitudes. Nurses need to become culturally sensitive and to accept and respect the differences in the life-styles of others.

HEALTH CARE SYSTEM AS A SUBCULTURE

Nurses should remember that the health care system is also a subculture. This system has rules, customs, and a language of its own.

When obtaining an education in health care, individuals become acculturated into the system. But clients who enter the system may experience culture shock.

For example, the health care culture values cleanliness; thus, nurses wash their hands often and expect their clients to wash daily. This value may not be shared by all clients, and the practice of washing daily may be new for some people.

The health care culture has its own definition of health; often it is defined as "an optimal level of functioning." See Chapter 13 for additional information. Diagnosis and prescription are usually carried out by physicians, often in offices, clinics, or hospitals. Healing practices are based on scientific knowledge. Treatment procedures are frequently embarrassing or uncomfortable. The emotional component of disease is often ignored (Wold 1981, p. 140).

Jargon is widely used in the system and tends to make clients and support persons feel more like outsiders. Many health care workers are from the middle class; they often expect gratitude for the care they give. Strict time orientation is adhered to and highly valued. This orientation may conflict with the client's. By keeping written records, caregivers may create conflict with clients' cultural beliefs.

Traditionally, health care workers interpreted the death of a client as failure. This belief is currently being reconsidered. Measures were often taken to preserve the lives of clients but seldom to facilitate death. Currently, clinical nurse specialists called *thanatology nurses* work with families and clients coping with a terminal illness.

By recognizing that they have been acculturated into the health care system, nurses can often identify the values of the system they have adopted. It is then easier to recognize how a client's values differ from those of the system. These differing values may be a source of anxiety or frustration to clients and their support persons.

CULTURE SHOCK

Culture shock is the reaction of many people to an unfamiliar situation where former patterns of behavior are ineffective. Culture shock can occur when members of one culture are abruptly moved to another culture or setting, for example, when people of Asian background and upbringing suddenly move to the United States, or when clients are abruptly thrust into the health care subculture. When this occurs, a number of stressors impinge on the individual.

Brink and Saunders (1976, pp. 129–30) describe four phases of culture shock:

1. *Phase one*. The initial phase is identified as one of excitement and is called the *honeymoon phase*. People are stimulated by being in a new environment. Behavior that indicates this feeling varies with the ethnic origin of the person and the individual personality. Some clients, for example, may express their excitement outwardly, while others are quiet. People try to learn the norms of behavior appropriate for the new environment and often ask questions.

2. *Phase two*. Once the individual feels somewhat comfortable in the new environment, phase two begins. Phase two is the realization of having to exist in the new environment. This awareness is often accompanied by feelings of frustration and embarrassment be-

cause of errors the individual makes. Accompanying this may be feelings of inadequacy, which can diminish the individual's self-concept and self-esteem. To these feelings is added loneliness. Although many people may be around, there may be no one who enhances the individual's feelings of self-worth. Feelings of anxiety and inadequacy may be expressed through periods of withdrawal or anger.

3. *Phase three*. During the third stage, the individual seeks new patterns of behavior appropriate to the environment. The individual makes friends and can often give newcomers advice. Current friendships take on importance and occupy much of the individual's conversation. At this time, ties to the old culture become weaker.

4. *Phase four*. In the fourth phase, the individual functions comfortably and effectively. A person who returns to the former culture during this phase may experience reverse culture shock.

Nurses can assist clients and their families who are experiencing culture shock in a number of ways:

- If there is a language barrier, an interpreter can help with explanations and provide the nurse with information to incorporate into the client's care plan. The interpreter should be a trained professional. If a professional interpreter is unavailable, the nurse should obtain the services of a neutral person. The nurse should avoid having children or other family members translate for the client because the client may not wish the family to know about the health problems and because children may not understand the problem sufficiently to provide an accurate translation.

- Nurses can support clients' customs; for example, the nurse can encourage a Sikh to wear his turban in the hospital, unless this is contraindicated for health reasons. In addition, nurses can offer explanations to other health personnel about values, beliefs, and customs important to the client.

- Nurses must convey respect for a client's values, beliefs, and customs. The client will interpret an attitude of disdain or amusement as a lack of respect.

Where there is a conflict between, for example, the client's beliefs and the health care system, nurses can try to help the client find a common ground. When the client tries new behavior patterns, nurses can support the client's efforts and provide positive reinforcement. If the client experiences inadequacy or anxiety during culture shock, nurses can help by openly accepting the client and the values, beliefs, and customs.

APPLYING THE NURSING PROCESS

To provide meaningful nursing care, nurses must be aware of a client's ethnic and cultural values, beliefs, and practices as they relate to the client's health and health care. Tripp-Reimer et al. (1984) state, "A thorough cultural assessment is not necessary;" however, basic cultural data are required.

Initially, nurses must be aware of their own ethnic and cultural values, attitudes, and practices and of the relation of these beliefs to nursing practice. As the client's culture and the nurse's culture come together in the client-nurse relationship, a unique cross-cultural environment is created (see Figure 24–2) that can either improve or impair the client's outcome. Self-awareness of personal biases can enable nurses to develop modifying behaviors or (if unable to do so) to remove themselves from situations where care may be compromised. Cultural awareness can be attained by using a values clarification approach discussed in Chapter 11.

Assessing

A structured assessment guide can help nurses gather ethnic cultural data. See Table 24–3. The purpose of an ethnic-cultural assessment is "to identify deviations in cultural parameters with the goal of modifying the client's system or modifying the health care professional's system in order to increase congruence between them" (Tripp-Reimer et al. 1984, p. 81).

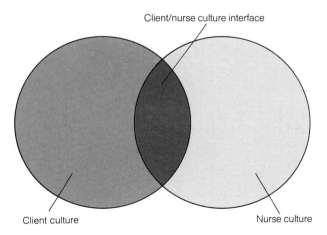

Client/nurse culture interface

Client culture

Nurse culture

Figure 24-2 When the client culture and the nurse culture come together, a new and unique cultural environment is created.

A general assessment of the client identifies significant characteristics and points out areas for in-depth assessment. At this stage, the nurse makes no conclusions but obtains information from the client. The data should be both subjective, preferably in the client's words, and objective. An example of subjective data is this client statement: "I think it is very important to be healthy." An example of objective data is "Spanish speaking, born in Cuba."

Basic cultural data that should be obtained as part of the health assessment include some information about each of the following parameters:

- *Ethnicity.* Knowledge about the client's ethnic affiliation can enable the nurse to better understand the client's needs. It is also helpful to know if the client is a recent immigrant or refugee or if the client is the child or grandchild of immigrants. The longer the client and family have lived in North America, the more acculturated they will be to their new homeland.

- *Language.* The primary language should be identified, even if the client speaks English fluently. When under the stress of illness, the client often finds it difficult to communicate in English and reverts back to the primary language. Additionally, the nurse should be sure that the client understands instructions or descriptions of procedures and treatments. Sometimes, the client exhibits behaviors of understanding, e.g., nodding the head affirmatively while instructions are given. Nurses should assess understanding by having clients repeat the instructions in their own words. If the nurse feels that the client does not understand such instructions when given in English, the nurse should obtain an appropriate interpreter.

- *Religious or spiritual requirements.* An understanding of the client's religious or spiritual beliefs is necessary for providing culture-specific care. Although the nurse is usually aware of the requirements of the religions most commonly practiced in the United States and Canada (see Chapter 26), less common religious or spiritual practices may also affect the health needs of the client. The client may wish to have a cultural healer present to conduct prayers or ritual practices. The client may be wearing protective charms or amulets. Knowing the nature of these requirements can enable the nurse to be supportive of the client's spiritual needs.

- *Family patterns.* The nurse should identify family roles and patterns and ascertain which family member is the primary decision maker. Female clients from cultures where the husband or father assumes this role
(text continues on p. 486)

TABLE 24–3   *Bloch's Ethnic/Cultural Assessment Guide*

Data Categories	Guideline Questions/Instructions
Cultural	
Ethnic origin	Does the patient identify with a particular ethnic group (e.g., Puerto Rican, African)?
Race	What is the patient's racial background (e.g., Black, Filipino, American Indian)?
Place of birth	Where was the patient born?
Relocations	Where has the patient lived (country, city)? During what years did patient live there and for how long? Has patient moved recently?
Habits, customs, values, and beliefs	Describe habits, customs, values, and beliefs patient holds or practices that affect attitudes toward birth, life, death, health and illness, time orientation, and health care system and health care providers. What is degree of belief and adherence by patients to the overall cultural system?
Behaviors valued by culture	How does patient value privacy, courtesy, respect for elders, behaviors related to family roles and sex roles, and work ethics?
Cultural sanctions and restrictions	*Sanctions*—What is accepted behavior by patient's cultural group regarding expression of emotions and feelings, religious expressions, and response to illness and death?
	Restrictions—Does patient have any restrictions related to sexual matters, exposure of body parts, certain types of surgery (e.g., hysterectomy), discussion of dead relatives, and discussion of fears related to the unknown?
Language and communication processes	What are some overall cultural characteristics of patient's language and communication process?
Language(s) and/or dialect(s) spoken	Which language(s) and/or dialect(s) does patient speak most frequently? Where? At home or at work?
Language barriers	Which language does patient predominantly use in thinking? Does patient need bilingual interpreter in nurse-patient interactions? Is patient non-English-speaking or limited-English-speaking? Is patient able to read and/or write in English?
Communication process	What are rules (linguistics) and modes (style) of communication process (e.g., "honorific" concept of showing "respect or deference" to others using words only common to specific ethnic/cultural group)?
	Is there need for variation in technique of communicating and interviewing to accommodate patient's cultural background (e.g., tempo of conversation, eye-body contact, topic restrictions, norms of confidentiality, and style of explanation)?
	Are there any conflicts in verbal and nonverbal interactions between patient and nurse?
	How does patient's nonverbal communication process compare with other ethnic/cultural groups, and how does it affect patient's response to nursing and medical care?
	Are there any variations between patient's interethnic and interracial communication process or intracultural and intraracial communication process (e.g., ethnic minority patient and white middle-class nurse, ethnic minority patient and ethnic minority nurse; beliefs, attitudes, values, role variations, stereotyping [perception and prejudice])?
Healing beliefs and practices	
Cultural healing system	What cultural healing system does the patient predominantly adhere to (e.g., Asian healing system, Raza/Latina curanderismo)? What religious healing system

▶

TABLE 24-3   (continued)

Data Categories	Guideline Questions/Instructions
Cultural, continued	
	does the patient predominantly adhere to (e.g., Seventh Day Adventist, West African voodoo, Fundamentalist sect, Pentacostal)?
Cultural health beliefs	Is illness explained by the germ theory or cause-effect relationship, presence of evil spirits, imbalance between "hot" and "cold" (yin and yang in Chinese culture), or disequilibrium between nature and man?
	Is good health related to success, ability to work or fulfill roles, reward from God, or balance with nature?
Cultural health practices	What types of cultural healing practices does person from ethnic/cultural group adhere to? Does he use healing remedies to cure *natural* illnesses caused by the external environment (e.g., massage to cure *empacho* [a ball of food clinging to stomach wall], wearing of talismans or charms for protection against illness)?
Cultural healers	Does patient rely on cultural healers (e.g., medicine men for American Indian, curandero for Raza/Latina, Chinese herbalist, hougan [voodoo priest], spiritualist, or minister for black American)?
Nutritional variables or factors	What nutritional variables or factors are influenced by the patient's ethnic/cultural background?
Characteristics of food preparation and consumption	What types of food preferences and restrictions, meaning of foods, style of food preparation and consumption, frequency of eating, time of eating, and eating utensils are culturally determined for patient? Are there any religious influences on food preparation and consumption?
Influences from external environment	What modifications if any did the ethnic group patient identifies with have to make in its food practices in white dominant American society? Are there any adaptations of food customs and beliefs from rural setting to urban setting?
Patient education needs	What are some implications of diet planning and teaching to patient who adheres to cultural practices concerning foods?
Sociologic	
Economic status	Who is principal wage earner in patient's family? What is total annual income (approximately) of family? What impact does economic status have on life-style, place of residence, living conditions, and ability to obtain health services?
Educational status	What is highest educational level obtained? Does patient's educational background influence ability to understand how to seek health services, literature on health care, patient teaching experiences, and any written material patient is exposed to in health care setting (e.g., admission forms, patient care forms, teaching literature, and lab test forms)?
	Does patient's educational background cause the patient to feel inferior or superior to health care personnel in health care setting?
Social network	What is patient's social network (kinship, peer, and cultural healing networks)? How do they influence health or illness status of patient?
Family as supportive group	Does patient's family feel the need for continuous presence in patient's clinical setting (is this an ethnic/cultural characteristic)? How is family valued during illness or death?
	How does family participate in patient's nursing care process (e.g., giving baths, feeding, using touch as support [cultural meaning], supportive presence)?
	How does ethnic/cultural family structure influence patient response to health or illness (e.g., roles, beliefs, strengths, weaknesses, and social class)?

▶

TABLE 24-3 *Bloch's Ethnic/Cultural Assessment Guide (continued)*

Data Categories	Guideline Questions/Instructions
Sociologic, continued	
	Are there any key family roles characteristic of a specific ethnic/cultural group (e.g., grandmother in black and some American Indian families), and can these key persons be a resource for health personnel?
	What role does family play in health promotion or cause of illness (e.g., would family be intermediary group in patient interactions with health personnel and making decisions regarding care)?
Supportive institutions in ethnic/cultural community	What influence do ethnic/cultural institutions have on patient receiving health services (i.e., institutions such as Organization of Migrant Workers, NAACP, Black Political Caucus, churches, school, Urban League, community clinics)?
Institutional racism	How does institutional racism in health facilities influence patient's response to receiving health care?
Psychologic	
Self-concept (identity)	Does patient show strong racial/cultural identity? How does this compare to that of other racial/cultural groups or to members of dominant society?
	What factors in patient's development helped to shape self-concept (e.g., family, peers, society labels, external environment, institutions, racism)?
	How does patient deal with stereotypic behavior from health professionals?
	What is impact of racism on patient from distinct ethnic/cultural group (e.g., social anxiety, noncompliance to health care process in clinical settings, avoidance of utilizing or participating in health care institutions)?
	Does ethnic/cultural background have impact on how patient relates to body image change resulting from illness or surgery (e.g., importance of appearance and roles in cultural group)?
	Any adherence or identification with ethnic/cultural "group identity" (e.g., solidarity, "we" concept)?
Mental and behavioral processes and characteristics of ethnic/cultural group	How does patient relate to external environment in clinical setting (e.g., fears, stress, and adaptive mechanisms characteristic of a specific ethnic/cultural group)? Any variations based on the life span?
	What is patient's ability to relate to persons outside of ethnic/cultural group (health personnel)? Is patient withdrawn, verbally or nonverbally expressive, negative or positive, feeling mentally or physically inferior or superior?
	How does patient deal with feelings of loss of dignity and respect in clinical setting?
Religious influences on psychologic effects of health/illness	Does patient's religion have a strong impact on how patient relates to health/illness influences or outcomes (e.g., death/chronic illness, cause and effect of illness, or adherence to nursing/medical practices)?
	Do religious beliefs, sacred practices, and talismans play a role in treatment of disease?
	What is role of significant religious persons during health/illness (e.g., black ministers, Catholic priests, Buddhist monks, Islamic imams)?
Psychologic/cultural response to stress and discomfort of illness	Based on ethnic/cultural background, does patient exhibit any variations in psychologic response to pain or physical disability of disease processes?

▶

TABLE 24–3 *(continued)*

Data Categories	Guideline Questions/Instructions
Biologic/Physiologic (consideration of *norms* for different ethnic/cultural groups)	
Racial-anatomic characteristics	Does patient have any distinct racial characteristics (e.g., skin color, hair texture and color, color of mucous membranes)? Does patient have any variations in anatomic characteristics (e.g., body structure [height and weight] more prevalent for ethnic/cultural group, skeletal formation [pelvic shape, especially for obstetric evaluation], facial shape and structure [nose, eye shape, facial contour], upper and lower extremities)?
	How do patient's racial and anatomic characteristics affect self-concept and the way others relate to patient?
	Does variation in racial-anatomic characteristics affect physical evaluations and physical care, skin assessment based on color, and variations in hair care and hygienic practices?
Growth and development patterns	Are there any distinct growth and development characteristics that vary with patient's ethnic/cultural background (e.g., bone density, fatfolds, motor ability)? What factors are important for nutritional assessment, neurologic and motor assessment, assessment of bone deterioration in disease process or injury, evaluation of newborns, evaluation of intellectual status, or capacity in relationship to motor/sensory development in children? How do these differ in ethnic/cultural groups?
Variations in body systems	Are there any variations in body systems for patient from distinct ethnic/cultural group (e.g., gastrointestinal disturbance with lactose intolerance in blacks, nutritional intake of cultural foods causing adverse effects on gastrointestinal tract and fluid and electrolyte system, and variations in chemical and hematologic systems [certain blood types prevalent in particular ethnic/cultural groups])?
Skin and hair physiology, mucous membranes	How does skin color variation influence assessment of skin color changes (e.g., jaundice, cyanosis, ecchymosis, erythema, and its relationship to disease processes)?
	What are methods of assessing skin color changes (comparing variations and similarities between different ethnic groups)?
	Are there conditions of hypopigmentation and hyperpigmentation (e.g., vitiligo, mongolian spots, albinism, discoloration caused by trauma)? Why would these be more striking in some ethnic groups?
	Are there any skin conditions more prevalent in a distinct ethnic group (e.g., keloids in blacks)?
	Is there any correlation between oral and skin pigmentation and their variations among distinct racial groups when doing assessment of oral cavity (e.g., leukoedema is normal occurrence in blacks)?
	What are variations in hair texture and color among racially different groups? Ask patient about preferred hair care methods or any racial/cultural restrictions (e.g., not washing "hot combed" hair while in clinical setting, not cutting very long hair of Raza/Latina patients).
	Are there any variations in skin care methods (e.g., Using Vaseline on black skin)?
Diseases more prevalent among ethnic/cultural group	Are there any specific diseases or conditions that are more prevalent for a specific ethnic/cultural group (e.g., hypertension, sickle cell anemia, lactose intolerance)?

TABLE 24-3 *Bloch's Ethnic/Cultural Assessment Guide (continued)*

Data Categories	Guideline Questions/Instructions
Biologic/Physiologic, continued	
	Does patient have any socioenvironment diseases common among ethnic/cultural groups (e.g., lead paint poisoning, poor nutrition, overcrowding [prone to tuberculosis], alcoholism resulting from psychologic despair and alienation from dominant society, rat bites, poor sanitation)?
Diseases ethnic/cultural group has increased resistance to	Are there any diseases that patient has increased resistance to because of racial/cultural background (e.g., skin cancer in blacks)?

Source From M. S. Orque, B. Bloch, and L. S. A. Monrroy, *Ethnic nursing care: A multicultural approach* (St. Louis: C. V. Mosby Co., 1983), pp. 63–69. Used by permission.

may refuse to make decisions. The nurse should recognize the significance of statements such as, "I can't make a decision until I talk to my husband," or "Ask my husband; he knows best." Another factor to determine is the client's need for the presence of family members and loved ones, especially if the client is dying.

- *Food preferences and patterns.* Beliefs about food can have great impact on the health of the client. The nurse needs to identify the foods that are forbidden in the client's culture; for example, Muslims are forbidden to eat pork products, and Orthodox Jews will not mix meat and dairy products at the same meal. At the same time, the nurses should ask the client about any food preferences that are believed to have healing qualities. Additionally, the nurse should assess the client's eating behaviors to differentiate cultural from physical manifestations; the client who does not eat, for instance, may believe that fasting will cleanse the body of impurities or atone for God's punishment.

- *Health beliefs and practices.* The nurse should assess the client's beliefs about the cause of the illness. Does the client believe that illness is caused by germs or life-style risks, or does the client believe that illness is a punishment, a curse, or an imbalance with nature? What remedies has the client already tried, and how effective have they been?

The general assessment is then followed by an assessment that is specific to the health care area of concern, e.g., preschool immunizations, diabetic teaching, home care. At this time, the nurse obtains information about the client's own reason for seeking out health care, ideas about the current problem and any previous problems, and the treatment the client anticipates. For example, the client may say, "I came to the center because I feel

ill; the world is moving around me. This happened once before. The doctor gave me some pills, and it went away."

Some questions that may elicit this information are:

- What do you think caused your problem?

- What treatment do you think you need now?

- What are the chief problems your sickness has caused you? (Kleinman et al. 1978, p. 254).

Diagnosing

The nursing diagnoses for a client who has special ethnic or cultural needs can relate to any number of factors, such as language and diet.

Impaired verbal communication is the "state in which the individual experiences, or could experience, a decreased ability to speak but can understand others" (Carpenito 1989, p. 238). Among the defining characteristics of this nursing diagnosis are the inability to speak the dominant language and difficulty in finding the correct words when speaking, both of which the person of a minority ethnic group or culture might display. In addition to the listed etiologic factor (language barrier), this diagnosis may also be related to fear, shyness, lack of privacy, or lack of a support system (all possible etiologic or contributing factors for minority group clients) as well as pathophysiologic and situational conditions.

Ineffective individual and **family coping** are discussed in Chapter 23. **Powerlessness** is the "state in which an individual perceives a lack of personal control over certain events or situations" (Carpenito 1989, p. 591). Its characteristics include expressing dissatisfaction over inability to control what is happening, refusing or being reluctant to participate in decision making, apathy, depression, or resignation to the situation. As discussed earlier in this chapter, people from some cultures are fatalistic about the meaning of illness and the purpose of hospitalization. It would be incorrect for the nurse to make this nursing diagnosis if the client values such a belief.

Social isolation is the "state in which the individual experiences a need or desire for contact with others but is unable to make that contact" (Carpenito 1989, p. 695). This is a difficult diagnosis to describe. Carpenito comments: "Since social isolation is a subjective state, all inferences made regarding a person's feelings of aloneness must be validated. Because the causes vary and people show their aloneness in different ways, there are no absolute clues to this diagnosis" (1989, p. 695). This diagnosis is most likely for the client whose family or support persons are not nearby during the hospitalization.

Planning

When planning nursing goals, the nurse needs to include appropriate cultural factors relative to the client. According to Tripp-Reimer et al. (1984, p. 81), this stage "is directed at cultural factors that may influence nursing intervention." For example, nurses can ask a client:

- What would you normally eat while you have this condition?
- What will your family do?
- Is there something I haven't mentioned that you think would be helpful?

After obtaining this information, a nurse must organize the data. According to Tripp-Reimer et al. (1984, p. 81), "the nurse is interested in the extent to which the client's beliefs, values, and customs are congruent with a trifold set of standards:

- Standards of the client's identified culture or ethnic group
- Standards of the nurse's own culture
- Standards of the health care facility that serves as the setting for the interaction"

A nurse may find that the data among the three standards are not congruent. For example, a client always eats rice as a major part of each meal. The nurse (a) learns that this practice is standard for the client's ethnic group, (b) recognizes that this practice differs from the nurse's own, and (c) realizes that the health care facility cannot provide rice for each meal. Next, the nurse re-lates this information by determining whether the treatment plan accommodates the client's eating practices. If not, then the nurse can find ways of integrating the client's practice into the nursing care plan, e.g., the client's family might bring cooked rice to the hospital. If, however, rice is contraindicated because of the client's condition, the nurse must establish ways to help the client change if the client is amenable to change or ways to understand the client if the client will not change (Tripp-Reimer et al. 1984, p. 81).

It is often important to include the client's family in the planning of nursing care, particularly if the client is a member of an extended family and if the family is a major support for the client. When planning care strategies, nurses should consider language barriers and assess the need for an interpreter. Sometimes ethnic clients require information to avoid confusion or embarrassment. For example, an ethnic client who is extremely modest may require considerable preparation and support before having an enema.

Possible client goals for the nursing diagnoses discussed earlier in this chapter are to:

- Reduce or resolve impaired communication.
- Establish effective verbal and nonverbal communication to indicate basic needs.
- Adapt to the change in environment necessitated by hospitalization.
- Maintain social contact with family, other visitors, and staff.

A goal for the family might be to establish effective coping mechanisms for dealing with the client's hospitalization.

Specific outcome criteria that make these goals measurable are as follows:

The client:

- Relates feelings, concerns, requests through interpreter.
- Uses an effective method of communication with verbal and nonverbal cues.
- Participates in the decision-making process regarding planned care.
- Uses family/friends and unit staff to assist with adaptation to changes in the environment.
- Indicates feelings of greater control over the illness and therapy.
- Interacts with staff through an interpreter or by using nonverbal cues.

The client's family:

- Uses available resources to adapt to the client's hospitalization.
- Employs effective alternative strategies for meeting those needs usually met by the extended family.

Implementing

Successful nursing interventions for clients of different cultures require supportive communication by nurses and respect for the client's values, beliefs, and practices. White (1977) stresses the importance of being culturally sensitive. Cultural sensitivity includes respecting individuals, recognizing the diversity of cultural beliefs and practices, acting on behalf of the ethnic client who is being denied safe, quality care, and modifying the care plan by incorporating those client beliefs and practices that are not life-threatening (Bello 1976, pp. 36–38, 45). Suggested guidelines for nurses are shown in the accompanying box.

RESEARCH NOTE

Are Community Health Nurses Confident in Caring for the Culturally Different Client?

Community health nurses responded to a 30-item Likert-type cultural self-efficacy scale to determine their degree of confidence in caring for three culturally distinct ethnic groups: blacks, Puerto Ricans, and Southeast Asians. The highest confidence scores were reported in the evaluation of care of the black population; the care of Southeast Asians received the lowest ratings, while scores rating the care of Puerto Ricans fell between the other two groups. Low scores were noted on items that involved knowledge of health beliefs and practices and views about respect, authority, and modesty. Higher scores were observed when an interpreter was used correctly. In no instance did ratings reach even moderate levels of confidence. Results suggest that nurses do not feel confident about caring for any of the three major ethnic groups in American communities.

Implications: Nurses need to receive adequate education and preparation in cross-cultural concepts to be able to serve ethnically diverse populations.

H. Bernal and R. Froman. The confidence of community health nurses in caring for ethnically diverse populations, *Image: Journal of Nursing Scholarship*, Winter 1987 19:201–203.

CLINICAL GUIDELINES
Interacting with Clients of Differing Culture or Ethnicity

- Convey respect for the individual and respect for the individual's values, beliefs, and cultural and ethnic practices.
- Learn about the major ethnic or cultural groups with whom you are likely to have contact.
- Analyze your own communication, e.g., facial expression and body language, and how it may be interpreted. See Chapter 18 for additional information.
- Recognize differences in ways clients communicate, and do not assume the meaning of a specific behavior, e.g., lack of eye contact, without considering the client's ethnic and cultural background.
- Understand your own biases, prejudices, and stereotypes.
- Relate clients' different cultural beliefs, e.g., the cause of swollen feet, to your own. In this way, you convey interest and respect for the clients' beliefs.
- Recognize that cultural symbols and practices can often bring a client comfort.
- Support the client's practices and incorporate them into nursing practice whenever possible and not contraindicated for health reasons; for example, provide hot tea to a client who drinks hot tea and never drinks cold water.
- Don't impose a cultural practice on a client without knowing whether it is acceptable; for example, Puerto Rican clients prefer not to be touched unnecessarily (Shubin 1980, p. 29).
- Remember that the color of a client's skin does not always determine the client's culture.
- Learn how a client views health, illness, grieving, and the health care system.
- Review your own attitudes and beliefs about health and objectively examine the logic of those attitudes and beliefs and their origins.
- Increase your knowledge about different beliefs and values and learn not to be threatened when they differ from your own.
- Remember that during illness clients may return to preferred cultural practices; for example, the client who has learned English as a second language may revert to the primary language.

Evaluating

To evaluate the effectiveness of nursing care of clients in special ethnic and cultural groups, the nurse determines the extent to which the goals have been met by comparing the client's current status with predetermined outcome or evaluation criteria.

Nurses must also evaluate their own competence in this area by asking themselves questions such as these: "How well did I communicate?" "How well did I include the client and the family in the nursing process?" "How well do I understand the client's values, beliefs, and customs?" "How well did I communicate respect for these?" "Was I able to incorporate any of the client's values, beliefs, and customs into the plan of care?" "How well did I communicate my acceptance of values, beliefs, and customs that differ from mine?" "Am I aware of my values, beliefs, and customs?"

CHAPTER HIGHLIGHTS

▶ North Americans come from a variety of ethnic and cultural backgrounds, and many North Americans retain at least some of their traditional values, beliefs, and practices.

▶ Many minority groups in North America are bicultural, i.e., they embrace two cultures: their original ethnic culture and a North American culture.

▶ An individual's ethnic and cultural background can influence beliefs, values, and customs.

▶ Through acculturation, most ethnic and cultural minority groups in North America modify some of their traditional cultural characteristics.

▶ Individual factors frequently modify an individual's cultural values, beliefs, and customs.

▶ Stereotyping individuals can lead to incorrect assumptions.

▶ When assessing a client's culture, the nurse considers values, beliefs, and customs related to health and health care.

▶ Some health problems are more prevalent in certain ethnic groups than in the general population.

▶ Nurses must understand their own cultural values, beliefs, and customs in order to provide meaningful nursing care.

▶ An ethnic and cultural assessment guide can help the nurse gather data about a client.

▶ People can experience culture shock when they enter an unfamiliar environment where previous patterns of behavior are ineffective.

LEARNING ACTIVITIES

■ Knowledge of self is important in providing culture specific nursing care. Utilizing Bloch's Ethnic/Cultural Assessment Guide, analyze your own cultural values, beliefs, and practices.

■ Select an individual of a different culture and use Bloch's Ethnic/Cultural Assessment Guide to assess their cultural values, beliefs, and practices. What factors would influence the planning of nursing care for this individual? What culture-specific nursing interventions should be planned?

■ Compare the assessment of your own cultural values, beliefs, and practices with the assessment of the individual from a different cultural background. What are the similarities (cultural universals) and differences? Are there potential areas of conflict? How would you deal with these areas of potential conflict?

READINGS AND REFERENCES

SUGGESTED READINGS

Powers, B. A. April 1982. The use of orthodox and black American folk medicine. *Advances in Nursing Science* 4:35–47.
Powers describes the function of healers in black folk culture, including their characteristics and functions. The beliefs and practices of the black folk medical system are explained. The implications for nursing practice include the possible reluctance of clients to admit using folk practices, the need for mutual respect between the nurse and client, and the use of culture brokers.

Tripp-Reimer, T., Brink, P. J., and Saunders, J. M. March/April 1984. Cultural assessment: Content and process. *Nursing Outlook* 32:78–82.
The authors present a process for assessment of a client's ethnic/cultural values, beliefs, and customs. Included is a table comparing the content of nine cultural assessment guides.

White, E. H. March 1977. Giving health care to minority clients. *Nursing Clinics of North America* 12:27–40.
White discusses black, Spanish-speaking, Native American, and Asian clients in this article. Topics covered include life-styles, health problems, health practices, and nursing implications.

RELATED RESEARCH

Aroian, K. J., Patsdaughter, C. A. Summer 1989. Multiple-method, cross-cultural assessment of psychological distress. *Image: Journal of Nursing Scholarship* 21:90–3.

Bernal, H., Froman, R. Winter 1987. The confidence of community health nurses in caring for ethnically diverse populations. *Image: Journal of Nursing Scholarship* 19:201–3.

Cameron, E., Badger, F., Evers, H. May 1989. District nursing, the disabled and the elderly: Who are the Black patients? *Journal of Advanced Nursing* 14:376–82.

SELECTED REFERENCES

Abril, I. F. May/June 1977. Mexican-American folk beliefs: How they affect health care. *The Journal of Maternal Child Nursing* 2:168–73.

American Journal of Nursing. June 1979. Black skin problems. *American Journal of Nursing* 79:1092–94.

American Nurses Association. 1987. *1987–88 Health Legislation Fact Sheets*. Kansas City, Mo.: ANA.

Anderson, A. B., and Frideres, J. S. 1981. *Ethnicity in Canada: Theoretical perspectives*. Toronto: Butterworths.

Backup, R. W. February 1980. Health care of the American Indian patient. *Critical Care Update* 7:16 + .

Bello, T. A. February 1976. The third dimension: Cultural sensitivity in nursing practice. *Imprint* 23:36–38, 45.

Bigham, G. D. September 1964. To communicate with Negro patients. *American Journal of Nursing* 64:113–5.

Bloch, B. 1976. Nursing intervention in black patient care. In

Luckraft, D., editor. *Black awareness: Implications for black patient care*. New York: American Journal of Nursing Co.

Boyle, J. 1989. Alterations in lifestyle: Transcultural concepts in chronic illness. In Boyle, J. S. , and Andrews, M. M. *Transcultural concepts in nursing care*. Glenview, Ill.: Scott, Foresman/Little-Brown.

Boyle, J. S., and Andrews, M. M. 1989. *Transcultural concepts in nursing care*. Glenview, Ill.: Scott, Foresman/Little-Brown.

Brink, P. J., editor. 1976. *Transcultural nursing. A book of readings*. Englewood Cliffs, N.J.: Prentice-Hall.

Brink, P. J., and Saunders, J. M. 1976. Culture shock: Theoretical and applied. In Brink, P. J., editor. pp. 126–38. *Transcultural nursing: A book of readings*. Englewood Cliffs, N.J.: Prentice-Hall.

Calhoun, M. A. September 1986. Providing health care to Vietnamese in America: what practitioners need to know. *Home Healthcare Nurse* 4:14–19.

Campbell, T., and Chang, T. 1981. Health care of the Chinese in America. In Henderson, G., and Primeaux, M., editors. *Transcultural health care*. Menlo Park, Calif.: Addison-Wesley Publishing Co.

Carpenito, L. J. 1989. Nursing diagnosis. *Application to clinical practice*. 3d ed. Philadelphia: J. B. Lippincott Co.

Chae, M. November 1987. Older Asians. *Journal of Gerontological Nursing* 13:10–17.

Chang, B. 1981. Asian-American patient care. In Henderson, G., and Primeaux, M., editors. *Transcultural health care*. Menlo Park, Calif.: Addison-Wesley Publishing Co.

Chapman, W. P., and Jones, C. M. 1944. Variations on cutaneous and visceral pain sensitivity in normal subjects. *Journal of Clinical Investigation* 23:81–91.

Chen-Louie, T. T. 1980. Bicultural experiences, social interactions, and health care implications. In Reinhardt, A. M., and Quinn, M. D. *Family-centered community nursing: A sociocultural framework*. St. Louis: C. V. Mosby Co.

Christian, J. L., and Greger, J. L. 1985. *Nutrition for living*. Menlo Park, Calif.: Benjamin/Cummings Publishing Co.

Chung, H. J. March 1977. Understanding the Oriental maternity patient. *Nursing Clinics of North America* 12:67–75.

Davis, M., and Yoshida, M. March 1981. A model for cultural assessment of the new immigrant. *Canadian Nurse* 77:22–23.

Drakwlic, L., and Tanaka, W. March 1981. The East Indian family in Canada. *Canadian Nurse* 77:24–26.

Flannery, R. et al. 1981. Ethnicity as a factor in the expression of pain. *Psychosomatics* 22:39–50.

Friedman, M. M. 1981. *Family nursing theory and assessment*. Norwalk, Conn.: Appleton-Century-Crofts.

Giger, J. N., Davidhizar, R. January/February 1990. Transcultural nursing assessment: A method for advancing nursing practice. *International Nursing Review*. 37(1):199–202.

Gonzalez-Swafford, M. J., and Gutierrez, M. G. November/December 1983. Ethno-medical beliefs and practices of Mexican-Americans. *Nurse Practitioner* 8:29–30, 32, 34.

Gordon, V. C.; Matousek, I. M.; and Lang, T. A. November 1980. Southeast Asian refugees: Life in America. *American Journal of Nursing* 80:2031–36.

Henderson, G., and Primeaux, M. editors. 1981. *Transcultural health care*. Menlo Park, Calif.: Addison-Wesley Publishing Co.

Hicks, G. 1976. *Appalachian valley*. New York: Holt, Rinehart and Winston.

Holleran, C. March/April 1988. Nursing beyond national boundaries: The 21st century. *Nursing Outlook* 36:72–75.

Kalish, R. A. 1967. Of children and grandfather: A speculative essay on dependency. *Gerontologist* 7:65–69.

Kleinman, A. et al. February 1978. Culture, illness, and care: Clinical lessons from anthropologic and cross-cultural research. *Annals of Internal Medicine* 88:251–58.

LaFargue, J. P. 1972. Role of prejudice in rejection of health care. *Nursing Research* 2:53–58.

———. September 1980. A survival strategy: Kinship network. *American Journal of Nursing* 80:1636–40.

Leininger, M. 1970. *Nursing and anthropology: Two worlds to blend*. New York: John Wiley and Sons.

———. 1974. Humanism, health, and cultural values. In Leininger, M., editor. *Health care dimensions*. Philadelphia: F. A. Davis Co.

———. November 1987. Transcultural eating patterns and nutrition: Transcultural nursing and anthropological perspectives. *Holistic Nursing Practice* 3:16–25.

Lewis, O. October 1966. The culture of poverty. *Scientific American* 215:19–25.

Lewis, S.; Messner, R.; and McDowel, W. August 1985. An unchanging culture: Caring for Appalachian patients and their families. *Journal of Gerontological Nursing* 11:20–24, 26.

Ludwig-Beymer, P. 1983. Transcultural aspects of pain. In Boyle, J., and Andrews, M. *Transcultural concepts in nursing care*. Boston: Little, Brown & Co.

MacDonald, J. September 1987. Preparing to work in a multicultural society. *Canadian Nurse* 83:31–32.

Martin, B. J. W. Ethnicity and health care: Afro-Americans. In *Ethnicity and health care*. 1976. New York: National League for Nursing.

Martinelli, A. M. August 1987. Pain and ethnicity: How people of different cultures experience pain. *AORN Journal* 46:273–74, 276, 278.

Mason, D. J. October 1981. Perspectives on poverty. *Image* 13:82–85.

Meleis, A. I. June 1981. The Arab American in the health care system. *American Journal of Nursing* 81:1180–83.

Murillo-Rhode, I. May 1980. Health care for the Hispanic patient. *Critical Care Update* 7:29–36.

National Center for Health Statistics. August 1985. *Charting the nation's health trends since 1960*. DHHS pub no. (PHS) 85-1251. U.S. Department of Health and Human Services, Hyattsville, Md.: Public Health Service.

Ohlson, V. M., and Franklin, M. 1985. *An international perspective on nursing practice*. Pub. No. NP-68F. Kansas City, Mo.: American Nurses' Association.

Orque, M. S.; Bloch, B.; and Monrroy, L. S. A. 1983. *Ethnic nursing care: A multicultural approach*. St. Louis: C. V. Mosby Co.

Overfield, T. 1985. *Biologic variation in health and illness*. Menlo Park, Calif.: Addison-Wesley Publishing Co.

Powers, B. A. April 1982. The use of orthodox and black American folk medicine. *Advances in Nursing Science* 4:35–47.

Primeaux, M. H. March 1977. American Indian Health care practices. *Nursing Clinics of North America* 12:55–65.

Rempusheski, V. F. September 1989. The role of ethnicity in elder care. *Nursing Clinics of North America* 24:717–24.

Richardson, E. A. W., and Milne, L. S. November/December 1983. Sickle-cell disease and the childbearing family: An update. *American Journal of Maternal/Child Nursing* 8:417–22.

Roberson, M. H. B. January 1987. Home remedies: A cultural study. *Home Healthcare Nurse*. 5:35–40.

Rothenburger, R. L. May 1987. Understanding cultural differences is the key to transcultural nursing. *AORN Journal* 45:1203, 1205–6, 1208.

———. May 1990. Transcultural nursing: Overcoming obstacles to effective communication. *AORN Journal* 51:1349–50.

Schermerhorn, R. A. 1970. *Comparative ethnic relations: A framework for theory and research*. New York: Random House.

Shubin, S. June 1980. Nursing patients from different cultures. *Nursing 80* 10:78–81. Canadian edition 10:26–29.

Smith, J. A. 1976. The role of the black clergy as allied health care professionals in working with black patients. In Luckraft, D., editor. *Black awareness: Implications for black patient care*. New York: American Journal of Nursing Co.

Spector, R. E. 1985. *Cultural diversity in health and illness*. 2d ed. New York: Appleton-Century-Crofts.

Statistics Canada. June 1989. *Census Canada* 1986. Cat. no. 93-109. Ottawa: Minister of Supplies and Services.

Tripp-Reimer, T. Spring 1982. Barriers to health care: Variations in interpretation of Appalachian client behavior by Appalachian and non-Appalachian health professionals. *Western Journal of Nursing Research* 4:179–91.

Tripp-Reimer, T. Afifi, L. A. September 1989. Cross-cultural perspectives on patient teaching. *Nursing Clinics of North America* 24:613–9.

Tripp-Reimer, T., and Freidl, M. March 1977. Appalachians: A neglected minority. *Nursing Clinics of North America* 12:41–54.

Tripp-Reimer, T.; Brink, P. J.; and Saunders, J. M. March/April 1984. Cultural assessment: Content and process. *Nursing Outlook* 32:78–82.

U.S. Department of Commerce, Bureau of the Census. April 1984. *Census of Population, General Population Characteristics United States Survey*. Washington, D.C.: Government Printing Office.

———. 1989. *Statistical abstract of the United States*. 109th ed. pp. 4–11, 15–57. Washington, D.C.: Government Printing Office.

Wang, R. M. 1976. Chinese Americans and health care. In *Ethnicity and health care*. New York: National League for Nursing.

Wauneka, A. D. 1976. Helping a people to understand. In Brink, P. R., editor. *Transcultural nursing: A book of readings*. Englewood Cliffs, N.J.: Prentice-Hall.

Weisenberg, M. 1975. Cultural influences on pain perception. In *Pain: Clinical and experimental perspectives*. pp. 141–143. St. Louis: C. V. Mosby Co.

White, E. H. March 1977. Giving health care to minority patients. *Nursing Clinics of North America* 12:27–40.

Wilson, U. M. 1983. Nursing care of American Indian patients. In Orque, M. S.; Bloch, B.; and Monrroy, L. S. A. *Ethnic nursing care: A multicultural approach*. St. Louis: C. V. Mosby Co.

Winn, M. C. 1976. A proposed tuberculosis program for Papago Indians. In Brink, P. J., editor. *Transcultural nursing: A book of readings*. Englewood Cliffs, N.J.: Prentice-Hall.

Wirth, L. 1945. The problem of minority groups. In Linton, R. *The science of man in the world crisis:* New York: Columbia University Press.

Wold, S. J. 1981. *School nursing: A framework for practice*. St. Louis: C. V. Mosby Co.

Wood, R. 1976. The American Indian and health. In *Ethnicity and health care*. New York: National League for Nursing.

Zborowski, M. 1952. Cultural components in responses to pain. *Journal of Social Issues* 8:16–30.

———. 1969. *People in pain*. San Francisco: Jossey-Bass.

CHAPTER

25

Sexuality

CONTENTS

Sex and Sexuality

The Context of Sexuality
Historical Perspectives
Ethnocultural Perspectives
Religious-Ethical Perspectives
Contemporary Perspectives

Development of Sexuality
Prenatal Period and Infancy
Early and Late Childhood
Puberty and Adolescence

Adulthood and Middle Years
Late Adulthood

Patterns of Sexual Functioning
Gender-Role Behavior
Sexual Stimulation
Sexual Response Patterns
Sexual Assault

Assessing Sexual Health
Characteristics of Sexual Health
Integrating Sexuality into the
   Nursing History
Factors Influencing Alterations in
   Sexual Functioning

Common Medical and Surgical
   Conditions Affecting Sexuality
Changes in Sexual Motivation
Problems with Genital Functioning

Diagnosing Sexuality Problems

Planning

Implementing
Developing Self-Awareness
Selecting Appropriate Interventions
Sexual Health Teaching

Evaluating

SEX AND SEXUALITY

Sexuality is an integral characteristic of every human being. We are all born with the capacity to function as sexual beings. Clients do not leave their sexuality behind when they enter the health care system—their sexuality comes along as part of the whole person. Professional nurses, as health care providers focusing on the

holistic nature of care, have a responsibility to provide effective sexual health care for their clients.

A holistic approach to client health care needs indicates that all aspects of being interact. Thus, sexuality influences and is influenced by the biologic, psychologic, sociologic, and spiritual aspects of being. The need to acknowledge and deal with issues of sexuality in health care practice cannot be overemphasized. Until

493

fairly recently, health care has treated sexuality with be-
nign neglect or has actively discouraged it as a focus of
interest.

For nurses practicing in North America today, sexuality is a much more complex issue than it was for nurses
in the past. Changes in beliefs, attitudes, and behaviors
(and the resulting conflicts) have produced uncertainty
and a need to assess nurses' understanding of and attitudes toward the many variations of sexuality. The multicultural nature of North American society has also been
a major influence on sexuality, as has the vast increase
in mass communication. The impact of such influence
groups and movements as the women's movement, gay
liberation, handicapped groups, and the "moral majority" has been powerful and is still creating change. To
help clients deal with issues of sexual health, nurses
must be aware of these multiple factors and must integrate them into effective sexual health care plans.

The words *sex* and *sexuality* are used interchangeably, and often incorrectly, to define different aspects of
sexual being. Sex is the term most commonly used to
denote biologic male or female status, but it is also used
to describe specific sexual behavior, such as sexual intercourse. Examples of such usage include the labeled
boxes on questionnaire forms to indicate male or female
(M☐, F☐) and the question "How many partners have
you had sex with since your last visit?" asked in a sexually transmitted disease clinic.

The more appropriate and descriptive term when
dealing with sexual issues is sexuality, which "includes
all of those aspects of the human being that relate specifically to being boy or girl, woman or man, and is an
entity subject to life-long dynamic change. Sexuality reflects our human character, not solely our genital nature.
As a function of the total personality, it is concerned with
the biological, psychological, sociological, spiritual, and
cultural variables of life, which, by their effect on personality development and interpersonal relations, can in
turn offer social structure" (Sex Information and Education Council of the United States 1980, p. 8). Although
sexuality is an integral part of the whole human being, it
can also be categorized and studied according to three
separate aspects: (a) biologic sex, (b) gender identity,
and (c) gender role.

Biologic sex includes all of the human being's genetically determined anatomy and physiology, which is also
influenced by intrauterine conditions. The result of genetic plus other prenatal factors usually is clearly developed primary sex characteristics or variations of these
characteristics, called ambiguous sex.

Gender identity is the individual's persisting inner
sense of being male or female, masculine or feminine.
Its development is based on biologic sex and sociocultural reinforcement, which begins at birth with identification of the baby as male or female. Ultimate congruence between biologic sex and learned sense of sexual
self is the most common outcome of this developmental
process. Variations of this congruence are common,
principally at periods of significant change in the life
span (e.g., adolescence, menopause, climacteric, old
age). The term sexual identity is sometimes equivalent
to gender identity but is more commonly used to indicate sexual orientation (e.g., heterosexual, bisexual,
homosexual).

Gender role includes all behaviors reflecting the individual's learned sense of masculinity and femininity, sex
behavior, sexual relationships, and sexual dimorphism.
The discerning of a person's gender role is based on observation of the person's behavior. The conceptual distinction between gender identity and gender is for descriptive purposes only; in reality, the two are "opposite
sides of the same coin."

THE CONTEXT OF SEXUALITY

Sexuality and the way we respond to it are influenced by
a variety of factors. A review of historical, ethnocultural,
religious-ethical, and contemporary perspectives on
sexuality will help us see sexuality in the context of the
broader human experience.

Historical Perspectives

Sexuality, as a part of the human condition, has been
with us since the beginning of time. Humankind's understanding of sexuality has evolved over time, changing to adapt to changes in knowledge, beliefs, and values. The earliest clear knowledge of sexuality comes
from writings, statues, and paintings as old as 10,000
years. Though some of the earlier paintings and sculptures indicate an awareness of sexuality, they give us no
clues as to sexual beliefs or practices. The writings,
paintings, and sculptures from 5000 B.C. onward, however, do provide clear information about sexual beliefs,
values, laws, and practices; they demonstrate the existence of circumcision, heterosexual genital intercourse,
fellatio, anal intercourse, homosexuality, prostitution
(male and female), and many other sexual practices.

Historical records from the period after the birth of
Christ are even clearer and reveal a great deal about the
development of attitudes, beliefs, and laws relating to
sexuality. The historical records from Europe (influ-

enced by the Judeo-Christian tradition), the Middle East (predominantly Muslim), India (Hindu), and China (Buddhist and Confucian) show a wide variation in approaches to sexuality. The important message of history is that contemporary approaches to sexuality are part of an ever-evolving process.

Ethnocultural Perspectives

North America is a multicultural, ethnically mixed society. Although the majority of the population traces its roots to Europe, increasingly larger proportions of the population in both the United States and Canada come from non-European roots. Citizenship ceremonies in both countries commonly have participants from up to 50 or more different countries. Native American Indians, African-Americans, Latin Americans, Chinese, East Indians (including Muslim, Hindu, and Sikh), Japanese, and Southeast Asians exemplify the ethnic groups that make up significant portions of our society.

All of these groups have their own ethnic and cultural traditions that influence the ways they view the world and interact with society. Included in these traditions are rules, practices, and values relating to sexuality. Much anthropologic and ethnocultural research indicates that the predominant North American societal approaches to sexuality based on Judeo-Christian traditions are not universal: Many North Americans have strong negative attitudes about homosexuality; in a number of subcultures, however, homosexual behavior is tolerated, and in some instances it has become an integral part of rituals such as coming of age.

Different groups hold diverse attitudes about appropriate sexual behavior, husband/wife roles, childhood sexuality, and nudity. Because clients (and, often, colleagues) may differ in their approaches to sexuality, nurses must be aware of and consider ethnocultural factors when approaching sexual issues in health care. As simple a practice as giving a bed bath can have sexual implications, depending on the cultural traditions of the client and/or nurse.

Religious-Ethical Perspectives

Probably the most obvious influences on the approach to sexuality are religion and ethics. People's dealings with sexuality are affected by beliefs and values derived from either religious traditions or some other value system. One function of religion is to provide guidelines for the conduct of human affairs. These guidelines always include sexuality. The most common approach is for a particular religious group or organization to outline ac-

ceptable sexual behavior and acceptable circumstances for the behavior, as well as prohibited sexual behavior and the consequences of breaking the sexual rules. The guidelines or rules may be detailed and rigid or broad and flexible. Within the predominant Judeo-Christian value system in North America, there are variations that, along with beliefs and values from other religious traditions, produce the potential for ongoing societal strain as people attempt to integrate all the differing rules and values.

Although ethics is integral to religion, ethical thought and ethical approaches to sexuality can be viewed separately. Many people and groups have developed written or unwritten codes of conduct based on ethical principles. These principles draw from ethical theories that often cut across religious designations while incorporating important principles from different religious traditions. Again, the crucial issue in religious-ethical matters is understanding, respecting, and working with the person's own religious-ethical value system.

Contemporary Perspectives

The ever-evolving knowledge, beliefs, values, and attitudes about sexuality cause continuing societal stress. Currently, a major influence on sexual issues is exerted by certain Christian sects. There is increasing pressure to reinforce strict guidelines for sexual behavior based on their particular view of Christian values. These efforts have been aimed not only at the members of those religious sects but also at the law, the media, health care agencies, and groups viewed unfavorably. This has created great controversy, since others in the society are comfortable with and eager to maintain the more flexible values developed over the last few decades (often labeled the "sexual revolution"). Conflict has arisen because many people accept premarital sex, unwed motherhood, homosexuality, and abortion. These conflicts appear destined to continue in the future.

Another major influence on contemporary sexuality is the information explosion. The media (TV, print, movies, video, computer networks) provide continuous output that has major impact on our views of sexuality. Media stars become the role models for acceptable male or female behavior, at the same time creating potential conflicts. The media also reflect changes in society's attitudes toward sexuality. For instance, at one time (the 1950s and 1960s), television shows always portrayed heterosexual couples as married and sleeping in twin beds. Currently they show same-sex, unmarried, and married couples, often in bed together, and—in soap operas—in varying stages of undress.

People respond emotionally to certain issues related to sexuality (e.g., teenage sexuality, contraception, homosexuality, AIDS and other sexually transmitted diseases, abortion, pornography, and sexual abuse). These issues do not have simple solutions, and nurses will certainly confront these issues in their practice. Nurses have a responsibility to be aware of the factors that contribute to possible emotional conflicts and to use this awareness in helping clients develop sexual health on their own terms.

DEVELOPMENT OF SEXUALITY

The development of sexuality in the human begins with conception and is influenced continuously by many factors throughout the life span. A variety of theories try to explain the development of sexuality, including the interaction of biologic and psychosocial factors. The one currently accepted common understanding is that sexuality as a human experience is complex and multiply influenced. Thus, the psychosocial components described here are to be understood as commonly accepted ways of looking at the interactions that influence the development of sexuality. Every society develops expectations about acceptable ways to be sexual. The components outlined in this section also reflect those societal influences and are organized according to previously identified developmental stages, including Erikson's widely accepted model of human development.

Prenatal Period and Infancy

Biologic Components   In the developing human fetus the sex chromosome pair determines whether the gonads will develop as testes or ovaries. The most common outcome of the sex-chromosome influence is an infant with a clearly defined male or female anatomy and physiology. The neurologic, vascular, and other tissues are developed well enough at birth to allow the sexual organs to respond to stimulation. This can produce penile erection in infant boys and vaginal lubrication in infant girls. The infant's behavior in response to stimulation of the genitals (either by the infant or during washing, etc.) indicates pleasure on the part of the infant. It is important to be aware that these small responses are reflexogenic and are not to be confused with postpubertal sexual responses. For the infant, this is just another pleasurable feeling.

Psychosocial Components   Much of our understanding of infant development is based on assumptions about the behavior we see. Infants behave in ways that indicate a focus on such basic needs as safety, security, comfort, nutrition, and pleasure. This is the period for development of trust, according to Erikson's model. It is during this period, in response to interactions with parenting figures and others, that infants begin to learn about gender role. From the moment of birth, the approaches and reactions to infants are based, in general terms, on society's guidelines for male and female gender roles. Little boys are talked to differently, handled differently, and expected to react differently than little girls. These adult behaviors are based on what our society believes about male or female gender roles.

There is also evidence, based on observations of behavior, that male and female infants demonstrate sexual differentiation in a variety of areas. These include motor activity, musculature, attention span, preference for stimuli, and interactions with parent figures. The origins of these differences are not clearly understood, but their existence demonstrates the complex interaction between biologic and psychosocial components of sexual development.

Early and Late Childhood

Biologic Components   In contrast to the rapid physical growth in other body systems, the anatomic and physiologic components of the sexual self change very little prior to puberty. Structurally, male and female children appear very similar in early childhood, with the genitals being the only obvious difference. Some changes become evident as late childhood progresses, with physical growth occurring fairly rapidly. Boys begin to develop a more solid musculature, and girls generally develop a slighter structure. It also becomes easier to distinguish boys' faces from girls' faces.

Psychosocial Components   The establishment of gender identity is one of the major issues in early childhood. By the age of 4 or 5 years, the combination of biologic and psychosocial factors has usually produced in the child a clear sense of being male or female. At age 3, children are usually able to identify themselves as either boy or girl. This understanding stems from the frequent use of the terms *boy, he, girl,* and *she* in describing the child. At the same time, the child is learning a sense of self through interaction with parent figures. This sense of self usually solidifies at about the same age as the sense of being a boy or a girl, 3 years. Other factors influencing the establishment of gender identity include interaction with parent figures, which provides feedback about gender-appropriate behavior, and imitation, which allows the child to mimic and receive reinforcement for same-sex parent behaviors. As with infants, parents and other adults interact differently with boys and girls. Physical as well as interpersonal interactions differ, adding to the development of gender identity.

The development of gender role, another major focus during early and late childhood, is accomplished through some of the same mechanisms by which gender identity develops. The developmental task of this period is the acquisition of sex-typed (gender-appropriate) behaviors that also are reinforced by positive responses from parents and later from others in the wider interpersonal world. These behaviors can include what clothes are worn, games played, playmates chosen, toys played with, and manner of speech, among many others. The nurse needs to be aware that there is in present-day North America a wide variation in sex-typed or gender-appropriate behaviors. Many children will develop a repertoire of behaviors as part of their gender role, including both gender-appropriate and gender-inappropriate behaviors. It is important *not* to label children on the basis of these variations. Only when there is evidence of problems in gender role or gender identity is there a potential for intervention. Such extremes are termed as *gender dysphoria*.

As development progresses, children continue to be curious about their own and others' bodies. Preschool children express this curiosity during bathing, toileting, swimming, and playing. Such curiosity is an important part of learning and should be responded to with factual information in a matter-of-fact manner. As the child learns more socially acceptable ways of expressing curiosity, usually during the early school years, the need for information is expressed as questions. School-age children ask many questions about sex, which again are best responded to with factual answers. Their questions arise from observing adults interacting, from reading, from sharing stories with peers, and from fantasies. Children develop the capacity for fantasy after the age of 4 or 5.

School-age children also express curiosity about their own and others' bodies. This takes place in individual exploration, in mutual exploration (playing "doctor" or "house"), and by watching adults whenever possible. Mutual exploration involves members of the opposite sex and, because of the sexual separation that occurs in the prepubertal period, members of the same sex. Matter-of-fact, nonjudgmental responses to such behaviors are important in order to avoid children's adopting negative feelings about their own bodies or sexual interaction.

Puberty and Adolescence

Biologic Components   Changes in sexual anatomy and physiology are more profound during puberty than at any other comparable developmental period. Puberty refers to the period of physiologic maturation, and adolescence refers to the period of psychosocial maturation.

Psychosocial Components   Changes in the psychosocial component of sexuality during adolescence are also profound. They include dealing with altered body image, dealing with changes in the body's functioning, consolidating gender identity, adjusting gender-role behavior, and learning new social-role behaviors.

Physiologic changes during puberty are relatively rapid and dramatic. The adolescent must deal with a body that is larger and proportioned differently and that requires new skills of coordination. In addition, the growth of secondary sexual characteristics and the development of physiologic functioning associated with these changes produce intense psychologic response. Conflicting emotions related to pride, embarrassment, shame, and discomfort require much adult understanding and explanation. Boys react to the comparison of their own changing body to the idealized male bodies in our culture. Height, weight, muscular development, body hair, and size of penis and testicles are all sources of anxiety as the boy compares himself to the ideal. Analogously for girls, height, weight, body shape, breast size, and menstrual cycles are all influenced by idealized norms. Adolescents need to know that there is a wide variation in healthy anatomy and physiology. This reassurance is particularly needed in response to media depictions of idealized male and female bodies. (Media stars never seem to have pimples, body odor, menstrual cramps, or spontaneous erections.)

The activation of sexual response potential during puberty puts a tremendous strain on the adolescent. Because of the hormonal triggers at work, the male body and female body become susceptible to a wide variety of sexually exciting stimuli. Adolescents respond to this new source of pleasurable sensations by engaging in erotic play, either alone through fantasy and masturbation or with others. Erotic play with a partner may include embracing, kissing, petting, and various methods of genital sexual activity.

Such sexual activity may involve partners of the same sex or the opposite sex. For the majority of adolescents, same-sex erotic play is experimental or exploratory. However, adolescents with a homosexual orientation require acknowledgment of and support for their sexual identity, to avoid anxiety, guilt, and negative self-image. Heterosexual and homosexual adolescents alike need both factual information about their bodies and support and reassurance about emotional and other psychosocial responses to their changing bodies and body functions. All adolescents are engaged in developing a clear sense of when and how to respond to intense sexual impulses.

As well as adapting to a changing body, the adolescent has opportunities to consolidate gender identity through psychosocial interactions. It is important during

---

RESEARCH NOTE

How Can Nurses Assist Gay Clients?

Nurses must meet the challenge of attending to whatever special health care needs their homosexual clients may have; indeed, the alarming rise in the incidence of AIDS brings nurses into increasing contact with the sensitivities, as well as some unusual medical needs, of gay clients.

This study asks and partially answers two questions: (1) How do gay men and lesbians learn they are gay and come to accept their gayness as a positive aspect of self? (2) What health care concerns arise in relation to "coming out" as a homosexual? The study found distinct differences between gay men and gay women in terms of their childhood upbringing and behavior patterns; the genesis of the homosexual orientation for either sex remained obscure, however. The study also found that coming out has four distinct stages: (1) identification of self as gay, (2) cognitive changes in previously held negative notions, (3) acceptance of self, and (4) action.

Implications: Kus asserts that nurses cannot provide adequate care to gay clients unless they understand this process. Nurses who do understand this process can perhaps help gay people to accept their homosexuality as a positive aspect of self.

R. Kus, Stages of coming out: An ethnographic approach. *Western Journal of Nursing Research,* May 1985, 7:177–98.

---

this period for the adolescent to understand that gender identity allows for wide variation in what constitutes male or female. The distinction between gender identity (maleness/femaleness) and sexual orientation (heterosexual/bisexual/homosexual) must be clarified for the adolescent, particularly in view of the complex signals being received. Gender-role-behavior development also is a source of stress, with frequently conflicting signals about what is gender-appropriate and what is not. There is, as well, an increased expectation for different social-role interactions on the part of the adolescent. The complexity of the influences related to psychosocial development of sexuality makes adolescence a very stressful period of growth and development. All adolescents require a factual, comprehensive knowledge base about biologic and psychosocial factors involved in the development of healthy adult sexuality.

Adulthood and Middle Years

Adulthood is the period when most developmental changes have reached maturity. The adult is both biologically and psychosocially prepared to engage in intimate psychosocial and sexual relationships. Typically, adulthood is seen as a time for developing intimacy with one partner, marrying, and parenting. Currently, a variety of alternatives to this traditional pattern is gaining wider acceptance. Regardless of the pattern of adult interpersonal relationships, sexuality is frequently a crucial component. Society continues to approve the capacity to become involved in a stable, heterosexual relationship as the ideal for adulthood.

Biologic Components   Between the ages of approximately 18 and 30 years, the young adult reaches full anatomic and physiologic maturity. Height, weight, body condition, and secondary sexual characteristics are all at their peak. These years are, for the majority of adults, the prime childbearing and child-rearing years. The earlier, unpredictable intensity of sexual feelings experienced during adolescence evens out and becomes more predictable.

Development leading to the middle years includes changes in hormone levels in both men and women. For women, development culminates in the cessation of the menstrual cycle and a decrease in estrogens, leading to such changes as the beginning atrophy of breast and vaginal tissue, delay and decrease in vaginal lubrication during sexual arousal, and loss of elasticity of skin and other tissue. For men the changes involve delay in attaining erection, decrease in size and firmness of erection, decrease in expulsive force of ejaculation, and decrease in volume of semen.

Psychosocial Components   Society's expectations for sexual development in adulthood include establishing a permanent intimate relationship with a partner of the opposite sex and bearing and raising children. This expectation may produce stress for many people as individual expectations increasingly differ from this societal "norm." The number of unmarried couples, both heterosexual and homosexual, has increased, as has the number of childless couples. Single parents are becoming more numerous, both as a result of relationship breakups and by choice. These changes in adult role relationships are not universally accepted but must be assessed by the nurse in terms of the overall health of the individual and the relationship.

The establishment of intimate adult relationships produces change in gender-role expectations. Adding to already existing role components are such expectations as partner (husband, wife, spouse), parent, and lover. These new role components require adjusting to patterns of behavior that are still developing. In addition, individual needs and preferences may encourage individuals to develop roles and role behaviors that are not congruent with broader societal expectations, for example, the househusband, woman as primary breadwinner, and commuting spouses.

Sexual interaction in adulthood is a major component of being, whether as part of a stable, intimate relationship or as part of a single life-style. The capacity to interact in sexually satisfying ways is influenced by a number of factors. A good knowledge of one's own body and its capabilities, as well as knowledge of the partner, is an essential prerequisite. Open communication about sexuality between partners is also an important factor. Knowledge and communication are frequently described as the most crucial factors determining the health of any sexual relationship. Other factors, such as parenting, role changes, and differences in sexual responsiveness, have less influence when knowledge and communication are effective. Sexuality, like any other part of interpersonal relationships, consists of learned beliefs, attitudes, and behaviors. This learning is best accomplished when it is shared by the partners in a relationship.

Late Adulthood

Biologic Components   The major biologic changes in the older female include a continued atrophy of vaginal and breast tissue (including loss of elasticity), decrease and slowing of vaginal lubrication during arousal, decreased vaginal expansion, diminished or-

gasmic intensity, and a more rapid resolution. (See the discussions of sexual stimulation and response patterns, later in the chapter.) Older women do retain the capacity for multiple orgasms.

Sexual changes in the older male include lowered sperm production, reduction in the size and firmness of the testicles, delay in achieving erection, greater ejaculatory control, less myotonia, reduced orgasmic intensity, more rapid resolution, and longer refractory period.

Psychosocial Components   Major issues influencing sexual development in late adulthood include adjusting to changing body image, adjusting to changes in family or marital status, retirement, change in body function, and decrease in mobility. Despite all these adjustments, the older adult has the capacity to continue with satisfying interpersonal and sexual relationships indefinitely.

Our society places a high value on youth and youthful beauty. The aging person is unable to match such standards and may respond to changes in body image with lowered self-esteem. Widowhood or widowerhood, loss of contact with grown children, and loss of friends have the potential for creating loneliness and depression.

Lowered self-esteem and loneliness, combined with reduced body function and loss of mobility, can lead to social isolation and loss of interaction opportunities. Society has also made it difficult for older adults to interact sexually because of negative attitudes about sexual activity among the aging. The majority of older adults retain the interest and capacity to engage in satisfying sexual relationships, whose nature is frequently more nurturing and caring and less sexually intense than in earlier years. The greatest predictor of sexual interest and activity in the later years is the pattern of sexual activity and interest throughout life, true for married adults, widowed adults, and single adults—whether heterosexual or homosexual.

PATTERNS OF SEXUAL FUNCTIONING

The interaction of contextual and developmental factors results in people's capacity to function in reciprocal ways as sexual beings. As noted earlier, biologic sex, gender identity, and gender role are the major components of individual sexuality. With a basic understanding of these components, nurses are better able to comprehend sexual functioning.

Gender-Role Behavior

Gender-role behavior is the outward expression of a person's sense of maleness or femaleness as well as the expression of what is perceived as gender-appropriate behavior. Even newborns are influenced by expectations regarding gender-appropriate role behavior, and this influence continues throughout life. Each society or culture establishes boundaries for acceptable gender-role behavior. Congruence between an individual's gender identity and expression of role behavior is the ideal, but this ideal is not always easy to achieve.

Physical structure, variations in the internal sense of what is male or female, family values, and cultural values all influence gender-role behavior. As a result, the limits of appropriate gender-role behavior are fairly flexible in North America. Expected adult male roles include breadwinner, heterosexual lover, father, and athlete. Expected male behaviors include wearing trousers, demonstrating physical strength, and expressing feelings in a controlled fashion. Women are expected to express their emotions more freely and to be more gentle in their physical responses; they also have a broader choice of clothing than men.

These descriptions represent the kinds of gender-role behaviors that are reinforced in our society. However, many individuals today express themselves with gender-role behaviors that do not conform to these stereotypes. This stretching of the boundaries can create stress for the individual and for society. Though there has been more variation in gender roles and gender-role behavior in recent years, these variations frequently are still portrayed as aberrant, humorous, or wrong.

In actuality, however, many people are challenging these stereotypes. Men sport long hair, earrings, and cosmetics. Women wear construction boots, jeans, and men's suits. Men make loving and sensitive single fathers. Women are capably functioning as competitive and assertive executives. Openly gay male and lesbian relationships are on the increase. Sexual activity in older adults is common. Such gender-role behaviors are legitimate expressions of the self as a sexual being. All individuals need sanction of and support for those gender-role behaviors that validate their sense of self. Labeling these behaviors as aberrant and intervening for change should rightly occur only when the behaviors create significant problems for individuals and their relationship with the world.

Sexual Stimulation

The sexually functional human is capable of responding to a wide variety of physical and psychologic stimuli. These erotic stimuli may be real or symbolic. In the right circumstances, imagination, sight, hearing, smell, and touch can all invoke sexual arousal.

Physical Stimulation

Physical stimulation involves touch and/or pressure to parts of the body and may be applied by one's self, by another's body contact or by inanimate objects. Examples include kissing, stroking, hugging, squeezing, breast stimulation, manual stimulation of the genitals, oral-genital stimulation, and anal stimulation. Any of these may be engaged in for sexual pleasure on their own or—as is most common in North America—as prelude to genital intercourse.

Psychologic Stimulation

Although the excitatory process involves physiology, erotic stimulation through smell, taste, hearing, sight, or fantasy is considered psychologic because the responses relate to thought processes and feelings. The stimuli evoke pleasant past experiences or hopes and desires. Certain odors (e.g., body odors, perfumes, leather, flowers) can produce erotic responses in sexual situations. Because of their specific associations, certain sights can also produce erotic responses. The more obvious sights include naked bodies and pictures of naked bodies and sexual acts. Other less obvious sights include romantic photographs, decor, lighting, and colors.

Sexual excitement is often enhanced by sound. The spoken word and music are frequent adjuncts to sexual activity. "Whispering sweet nothings" and "talking dirty" are examples. Music is frequently associated with specific sexual situations.

Most people engage in sexual fantasy. The fantasizing usually involves idealized sexual situations but may also include so-called forbidden fantasies: mental imagery of unusual or risqué activities that are out of bounds in real life. People engage in fantasy both during masturbation and when with a partner.

Sexual Response Patterns

Physiologic responses to sexual stimulation are basically the same for all individuals, male or female (see Table 25–1). However, such responses are highly variable,

TABLE 25-1 *Physiologic Changes Associated with the Sexual Response Cycle*

Phase of the Sexual Response Cycle	Signs Present in Both Sexes	Signs Present in Males Only	Signs Present in Females Only
Excitement	Increased muscle tension Moderate increase in heart rate, respirations, and blood pressure Sex flush (less prevalent in men than in women; present in 75% of women) Nipple erection (60% of men and most women)	Penile erection Tensing, thickening, and elevation of the scrotum Partial elevation and increase in size of testicles	Enlargement of the clitoral glans Vaginal lubrication Widening and lengthening of vaginal barrel Separation and flattening of the labia majora Reddening of the labia minora and vaginal wall Breast tumescence and enlarged areolae
Plateau	Increased voluntary and involuntary myotonia Abdominal, intercostal, anal, and facial muscle contraction Accelerated heart rate and respiratory rate, and increased blood pressure Sex flush (appearance in some men late in the phase; spread over the entire body in women)	Increase in penile circumference, at the coronal ridge, and deepening of color 50% increase in testicular size, and elevation close to the perineum Appearance of a few drops of mucoid secretions from the bulbourethral glands	Retraction of the clitoris under the hood Appearance of the orgasmic platform, increase in the size of the outer one-third of the vagina and the labia minora Slight increase in the width and depth of the inner two-thirds of the vagina Further reddening of the labia minora Appearance of a few drops of mucoid secretion from the Bartholin's glands Further increase in breast size and areolar enlargement
Orgasmic	Involuntary spasms of muscle groups throughout the body Diminished sensory awareness Involuntary contractions of the anal sphincter Peak heart rate, respiratory rate, and blood pressure	Rhythmic, expulsive contractions of the penis at 0.8-second intervals Emission of seminal fluid into the prostatic urethra from contraction of the vas deferens and accessory organs (stage 1 of the expulsive process) Ejaculation of semen through the penile urethra and expulsion from the urethral meatus. The force of ejaculation varies from man to man and at different times but diminishes after the first two to three contractions (stage 2 of the expulsive process)	Approximately 5 to 12 contractions in the orgasmic platform at 0.8-second intervals Contraction of the muscles of the pelvic floor and the uterine muscles Varied pattern of orgasms, including minor surges and contractions, multiple orgasms, or a simple intense orgasm similar to that of the male

▶

Phase of the Sexual Response Cycle	Signs Present in Both Sexes	Signs Present in Males Only	Signs Present in Females Only
Resolution	Reversal of vasocongestion; disappearance of all signs of myotonia within 5 minutes	A **refractory period** during which the body will not respond to sexual stimulation; varies, depending on age and other factors, from a few moments to hours or days	
	Genitals and breasts return to their preexcitement states		
	Sex flush disappears in reverse order of appearance		
	Heart rate, respiratory rate, and blood pressure return to normal		
	Other reactions include sleepiness, relaxation, and emotional outbursts such as crying or laughing		

with differences occurring between males and females, among members of the same sex, and in the same person at different times. The most common form of sexual activity with a partner is heterosexual genital intercourse, also known as coitus or copulation. Penile-vaginal intercourse can be both physically and emotionally satisfying. The choice of intercourse positions and activities depends on physical comfort and beliefs, values, and attitudes about different practices.

The other form of genital intercourse is anal intercourse, during which the penis is inserted into the anus and rectum of the partner. Anal intercourse is most commonly practiced by gay men, but some heterosexual couples engage in it as well.

Current practice dictates the use of a condom in both forms of intercourse to prevent the transmission of disease. Because anorectal tissue is not self-lubricating, a lubricant must be used on the condom. Also, since normal bacterial flora from the bowel can produce infection in other parts of the body, the used condom should be removed and another applied before inserting the penis into other body orifices. (Condoms are used for contraception as well as for preventing sexually transmitted diseases. See the discussion of sexual health teaching, later in this chapter.)

Lesbians and gay men engage in a variety of sexual activities that collectively can be labeled intercourse. Oral sex, manual sex, frottage (body rubbing), and the use of sex aids are among these. There is no evidence that this type of sexual interaction is less satisfying than heterosexual penile-vaginal intercourse.

Sexual Assault

Sexual assault, or rape, is defined as the imposition of heterosexual or homosexual intercourse against the will of the victim. By definition, both men and women can be victims of sexual assault. Complete penetration of the vagina or other body orifice by the penis or the emission of seminal fluid is not necessary for an act to be considered sexual assault. Most sexual assaults include force or violence. The assaulter may or may not be known to the victim. *Date rape* describes intercourse forced on a victim by her date. Spouses who are forced to submit to unwanted intercourse are not only victims of spouse abuse, but also victims of sexual assault. Sexual assault of children is a form of child abuse.

The victim's reaction to sexual assault, called *rape trauma syndrome,* is an acute stress reaction to a real or perceived life-threatening event. Care of the victim of sexual assault includes:

■ *Medical attention to physical trauma* Careful assessment for physical injuries or reactions directly or indirectly related to the assault is performed. Physical injuries might include bruises, lacerations, or fractures.

Other medical problems arising from the assault might include asthma, dyspnea, hyperventilation, and so on.

- *Prevention of sexually transmitted disease and pregnancy* Diagnostic studies for sexually transmitted diseases and preventive treatment such as antibiotics will be ordered. Postcoital contraceptive drugs may be given following a pregnancy test.

- *Psychological support* During the immediate assessment and treatment period, the nursing staff should provide a continuous presence of empathy, sensitivity, and support. In many communities sexual assault treatment programs are available to meet the ongoing counseling needs of the victim and her or his family. In communities where such programs are not available, referral should be made to appropriate counseling services.

- *Collection and preservation of legal evidence* Clothing, laboratory data, secretions, pubic hair, foreign material (grass, leaves, dirt), and photographs may be collected as legal evidence. It is important to label these items in accordance with requirements for evidence collection in your community. Handling and exchange of materials must also follow the rules of evidence collection and preservation. Because a nurse may be called as witness to the collection of evidence, labeling should include your signature and be accurately noted in the medical record.

ASSESSING SEXUAL HEALTH

Information about a client's sexual health status should always be an integral part of a nursing assessment. The amount and kind of data collected depend on the context of the assessment, that is, the client's reason for seeking health care and how the client's sexuality interacts with other problems. The nurse's professional preparation is another factor that influences the level of sexual health assessment.

Characteristics of Sexual Health

Lion (1982, pp. 9–10) has described the following characteristics of sexually healthy people:

- Expression of a positive body image
- Cognitive knowledge about human sexuality
- Congruence between biologic sex, gender identity, and gender-role behavior

- Behavior consistent with self-concept
- Awareness of own sexual feelings and attributes
- Capacity for physical and psychosexual responsiveness, which is enhancing to self and others
- Comfort with a range of sexual behavior and life-styles
- Acceptance of responsibility for pleasure and reproduction
- Ability to create effective interpersonal relationships with both sexes
- Value system that is developing and usable

These characteristics reflect the integral, holistic nature of sexuality as part of the human experience, and they provide a useful guide for measuring sexual health.

Integrating Sexuality into the Nursing History

Physiologic assessment should be included in any review of systems, including information on the functioning of the neurologic, cardiovascular, endocrine, and genitourinary systems. Data collected should include not only information about direct sexual functioning but also physiologic information that may relate to sexuality. For example, it is certainly important to collect data about erectile functioning in a diabetic male (cardiovascular, neurologic, and genitourinary systems), but it may also be important to note baldness (integumentary system) as a physiologic influence on sexual self-image.

Collecting such physiologic data for the nursing history does not require extensive or detailed questioning. The screening process of the systems review allows the nurse and client to identify problem areas. For example, answers to the question "Do you have any concerns about the amount or regularity of your menstrual flow?" can give clues to the presence of problems not otherwise identified. Also, questions asked about the functioning of systems directly related to sexuality often provide clients with an opportunity to give clues to sexual concerns or problems. Informing the client of the need for and use of the data reduces the reluctance of the client to talk about sexual issues. The thoroughness of the sexual assessment is directly related to the potential impact of sexuality on the health problem, or vice versa.

Psychosexual assessment should also be a part of the nursing history. Important influences include development, culture, religion, attitudes, and values. Again, specific, detailed questions about psychosexual issues are not necessary in the usual nursing history unless there are clues that potential or actual problems exist. A useful approach to psychosexual assessment is a review of sexual self-concept (see Table 25–2). Manner of dress, tone of voice, and comments about self and relationships with others can all give the nurse opportunities to explore issues of sexual self-concept more fully. Because illnesses and other health concerns can have a strong influence on sexual concept, assessment of these areas often provides the first clues to client concerns.

TABLE 25-2 *Assessment of Sexual Self-Concept*

Aspect of Self	Assessment Criteria
Sense of being (identity)	Demonstrates a clear sense of self as male or female.
	Demonstrates comfort with own identity.
Physical self (body image)	Demonstrates a realistic perception of own body.
	Demonstrates comfort with own body image.
Social self (role behavior)	Demonstrates congruence between identity and behavior.
	Demonstrates comfort with own role behavior.
Knowledge (self-awareness)	Demonstrates accurate cognitive sexual knowledge.
	Demonstrates realistic sense of self-congruence with others' view.
	Demonstrates comfort with self in relation to others.
Expectations (ideal self)	Demonstrates realistic expectations of sexual being congruent with what is possible.
	Demonstrates comfort with ideal self.
Evaluation (self-esteem)	Demonstrates realistic appraisal of sexual self.
	Demonstrates growth based on realistic evaluation.
	Demonstrates overall positive sense of self.

Watts (1979, p. 1570) outlines four levels of sexual assessment, each of which requires varying degrees of professional competence:

Level 1 focuses on screening for sexual function and dysfunction. It is conducted by the professional nurse during a health history.

Level 2 is a sexual history conducted by a professional nurse who has postgraduate education in sex education and counseling.

Level 3 is a sexual problem history conducted by qualified sex therapists.

Level 4 is a psychiatric and psychosexual history conducted by professionals who are specialized in sex therapy.

Factors Influencing Alterations in Sexual Functioning

To ensure that the assessment data base is complete, the nurse needs to gather information about factors known to alter sexual functioning. The following are some of the factors contributing to sexual dysfunction (Hurley 1986, p. 540):

- Ineffectual or absent role models
- Altered body structure or function due to disease or trauma, drugs, pregnancy or recent childbirth, or anatomic abnormalities of the genitals
- Lack of knowledge or misinformation about sexuality
- Physical abuse (e.g., sexual assault)
- Psychosocial abuse
- Value conflict
- Loss or lack of partner
- Vulnerability

When gathering a data base, the nurse also needs to be aware of common illnesses affecting sexual functioning, changes in sexual motivation, and genital sexual problems.

Common Medical and Surgical Conditions Affecting Sexuality

Heart disease and diabetes mellitus are two common illnesses that frequently influence sexual functioning. Clients with heart disease, particularly those experiencing or at risk for myocardial infarction, are often anxious about or afraid of sexual activity. Concerns about the effect of sexual activity on the heart cause people to restrict or avoid sexual activity. Many men with long-term diabetes mellitus develop erectile dysfunction related to neurologic changes secondary to the disease process.

Spinal cord injury also creates special problems. Because the level of the injury to the spinal cord determines the extent of effects on sexual functioning, individuals may be capable of erection and ejaculation and be fertile, may have psychogenic or reflexogenic genital arousal, or may have no physiologic genital responses.

Any surgical procedure has the potential to alter a person's body image, especially when the surgery involves mutilating, removing, or altering parts of the body. Examples include amputation of a leg, radical neck surgery, excision of large portions of the lower jaw, and ostomies. Impact is even greater when the surgery alters or removes body parts linked directly with sexual functioning, for instance, mastectomy, hysterectomy, and vaginal excision in women; orchiectomy (removal of the testicles), and penectomy in men. Feelings of ugliness and loss of masculinity or femininity are common after these surgeries.

Changes in Sexual Motivation

The urge or desire for sexuality activity, libido, fluctuates within each person and varies from person to person. The broad range of fluctuation is considered a problem only when the client (or those interacting with the client) identifies it as interfering with the ability to have satisfying sexual interactions.

Factors that may contribute to *decreased* sexual motivation include the following:

- *Drugs*. The following decrease sexual drive: all central nervous system depressants (e.g., alcohol, barbiturates, sedatives, morphine, heroin, and methadone), estrogens and adrenal steroids in large doses, certain psychotropic drugs, and some antihypertensive agents, e.g., reserpine (Serpasil) and methyldopa (Aldomet).

- *Depression*. This condition slows all body functions and lowers libido. It can affect both the depressed and nondepressed partner.

- *Disease*. Libido diminishes with general ill health and chronic diseases that cause debility or pain. Any disorder that causes dyspareunia (e.g., vaginitis, genital herpes, and imperforate hymen) also lowers libido.

- *Pregnancy*. Pregnancy affects sexuality if it is associated with physical discomfort, fear of injury to the fetus, or perceived loss of attractiveness. For about 4

weeks following delivery, libido is often reduced due to decreased vaginal lubrication, thinner vaginal walls, and a slower response to stimulation.

- *Stress*. The impact of emotional states on sexuality is relative to the individual. One person, for example, who is experiencing generalized anxiety may respond by becoming exceptionally sexually active. Another person may withdraw from sexual encounters to reduce anxiety or in response to his or her emotional state.

- *Aging*. Older people vary greatly in their sexual motivation. Psychosocial factors such as beliefs and attitudes about sexual functioning play an important role in this variation. Physical factors such as energy levels, pain, and immobility also have an effect.

Sexual motivation may also be enhanced by a number of various conditions and circumstances. This may or may not be a problem for the individual. Factors contributing to *increased* sexual motivation include the following:

- *Puberty and adolescence*. Both males and females experience increased sexual motivation during puberty and adolescence as a result of hormonal and body changes. This population is at risk for pregnancy and sexually transmitted disease if they do not receive appropriate sex education.

- *Drugs*. Amphetamines and cocaine enhance sexual motivation for some people for short periods. Lysergic acid diethylamide (LSD) and marijuana increase libido in some but inhibit it in others.

Problems with Genital Functioning

The ability to engage in genital intercourse is of great importance to most people. Many people experience transient problems with their ability to respond to sexual stimulation or to maintain the response. Common concerns for the male are being able to achieve and maintain an erection and to develop orgasmic timing with the partner. For women, common concerns relate to their ability to become and stay aroused and their ability to achieve orgasm.

All men have transient interferences with the ability to attain and maintain erection. *Erectile dysfunction* becomes a problem when it interferes significantly with the client's ability to satisfy himself or his partner. Such interference may occur consistently in all sexual situations, with or without a partner, or it may occur only in certain situations, such as with one partner but not with others, or with masturbation.

Erectile dysfunction is classified as primary or secondary. A man with primary erectile dysfunction has never been able to achieve an erection sufficient for intercourse. A man with secondary erectile dysfunction has functioned adequately for some time before developing erectile dysfunction. Both types of erectile dysfunction can be caused by physiologic or psychologic factors, but primary erectile dysfunction is more often associated with psychologic factors. Physiologic factors include the following:

- Neurologic disorders created by spinal cord injuries, injury to the genitals or perineal nerves, extensive surgery such as abdominal-perineal bowel resections, radical perineal prostatectomy, and diabetes mellitus
- Prolonged use of drugs such as sedatives, heroin, antidepressants, and antipsychotics (phenothiazines)
- Vascular diseases such as sickle-cell anemia and leukemia
- Endocrine disorders such as hypothyroidism and Addison's disease

Psychologic factors may include the following:

- Doubts about one's ability to perform or about one's masculinity
- Fatigue, anger, or stress caused by problems at work, in the family, or in interpersonal relationships
- Traumatic early sexual experiences (e.g., rejection)
- Pain, fear, or guilt associated with erection
- Boredom associated with a specific partner

The treatment for erectile dysfunction depends largely on the cause. Penile implants have been used to treat physiologic erectile dysfunction. Erectile dysfunction of psychologic origin often requires a change in both partners' views of sexuality. Awareness of the cause of the condition and exercises designed to increase sensations are also used.

Premature ejaculation often occurs either during penetration (of the vagina, mouth, or anus) or immediately following. The condition may relate to conditioning regarding the need for rapid orgasm or performance demands.

Treatment advocated for couples by many sex therapists includes increased sexual communication and responsiveness as well as decreased performance demands. The couple together practice sensate exercises (learning to enjoy the sensation of touch) and then work together to establish satisfying coitus.

Orgasmic dysfunction is of two types: primary and situational. A woman with primary orgasmic dysfunction has never been able to achieve orgasm. A woman with situational dysfunction has experienced at least one orgasm but is at that time nonorgasmic. Orgasmic dysfunction can be caused by drugs, alcohol, aging, and anatomic abnormalities of the genitals. However, most cases have psychologic causes, including hostility between partners, fear or guilt about enjoying the sexual act, and concern about performance.

Therapy usually involves helping both partners to establish new attitudes about sex. Pelvic muscle exercises (Kegel's exercises) can also increase the capacity of women to achieve orgasm by increasing the strength of the pubococcygeal muscle.

Vaginismus is the irregular and involuntary contraction of the muscles around the outer third of the vagina when coitus is attempted—that is, the vagina closes before penetration. Its causes can be severe sexual inhibition, often associated with early learning. Other causes can be rape, incest, and painful intercourse.

Treatment often involves sensate focus exercises and therapy to bring about psychologic changes. In some instances graduated vaginal dilators are used.

Dyspareunia describes the pain experienced by a woman during intercourse, a result of inadequate lubrication, scarring, vaginal infection, or hormonal imbalance. Treatment—such as supplying additional lubrication before intercourse—corrects the underlying cause.

DIAGNOSING SEXUALITY PROBLEMS

Nursing diagnoses for clients with problems related to sexuality are categorized as **Altered sexuality patterns.** This is a broad category that includes sexual identity, sexuality, and sexual function (Carpenito 1989, p. 666). It is defined as the state in which one expresses concern regarding one's sexuality or experiences or is at risk of experiencing a change in sexual health (Kim, McFarland, and McLane 1989, p. 57; Carpenito 1989, p. 666). **Sexual dysfunction,** the other NANDA diagnosis pertaining to sexuality, is defined as a perceived problem in achieving desired sexual satisfaction.

Examples of these nursing diagnoses and their contributing factors follow.

Altered sexuality patterns related to:

- Fear of pregnancy
- Fear of acquiring sexually transmitted disease

- Fear of effects of coitus following heart attack
- Impaired relationship with partner
- Body image disturbance secondary to trauma or radical surgery
- Current stressor (e.g., job problems, financial worries)
- Altered body function secondary to pregnancy, drugs, medications, surgery, disease process, trauma, radiation, or age (e.g., dyspareunia)
- Sexual trauma (e.g., rape or sexual exploitation)
- Unrealistic expectations of self and others

Sexual dysfunction related to:

- Excessive use of alcohol
- Painful intercourse from inadequate vaginal lubrication
- Misinformation or lack of knowledge
- Neurologic changes secondary to diabetes mellitus or spinal cord injury

Knowledge deficit (e.g., about conception or sexually transmitted diseases, contraception, or normal age-related sexual changes)

PLANNING

The overall client goals for persons with sexual problems is to maintain, restore, or improve sexual health. Outcome criteria to evaluate the achievement of client goals and the effectiveness of nursing interventions depend on the nursing diagnoses. Some suggested criteria follow.

The client:

- Verbalizes understanding of sexual anatomy and function.
- Verbalizes understanding of ways to avoid sexually transmitted disease.
- Identifies personal stressors that contribute to the dysfunction.
- Identifies attitudes restrictive to sexual behavior and sense of pleasure.
- Identifies alternative ways of dealing with sexual expression.
- Implements adaptive behaviors to accommodate altered body function, illness, or medical therapy.

- Expresses positive statements about alternative modes of sexual behavior.
- Verbalizes concerns about body image, sex role, or desirability as sexual partner.
- Expresses positive statements about gender, sex role, and/or sexual orientation.
- Reports diminished concern over sexual functioning.
- Verbalizes satisfactory/acceptable sexual practices to partner.
- States that desired sexual satisfaction has been achieved.
- Reports sense of pleasure (e.g., increased sense of erotic sensations) and gratification in sexual response.

IMPLEMENTING

Nursing responsibilities for clients with sexual problems include the following:

- Developing awareness of one's own sexual attitudes, beliefs, and knowledge
- Selecting appropriate interventions
- Providing accurate sexual information and education to clients
- Enhancing the client's body image and self-esteem (see Chapter 22).

Developing Self-Awareness

To be effective in helping clients with sexual problems, nurses must first have accurate information about sexuality, identify and accept their own sexual values and behaviors and those of others, and be comfortable acquiring and disseminating information about sexuality. Results of a study conducted at the School of Nursing, University of Wisconsin at Madison, revealed considerable misinformation and lack of information about sexual matters among graduate and undergraduate nursing students (Mims and Swenson 1978, p. 122). The following *misconceptions,* and their incidence, were reported:

- Impotence in men over 70 is nearly universal (35%).
- Certain mental and emotional instabilities are caused by masturbation (10%).
- Women are not able to respond to further stimulation for a period of time following orgasm (24%).

- A woman's chances to conceive are greatly enhanced if she has experienced orgasm (16%).
- Most homosexuals have a distinguishing body build (27%).
- Exhibitionists are latent homosexuals (32%).

Nurses who hold such misconceptions may be unable to give clients appropriate advice and assistance. Nurses need to become informed about psychosocial behaviors, sexual variations among people, and diseases and therapies that can alter sexual behavior.

Awareness of one's own attitudes (feelings, values, and beliefs) about sexuality is also essential. Before nurses can understand clients' sexuality, they must develop an awareness and tolerance of their own sexuality. This kind of self-awareness can be acquired via values clarification exercises and discussions. Nurses need to consider their feelings about matters such as masturbation, unwanted pregnancy and abortion, contraception, homosexuality and other sexual variations, nudity, and sterilization. When nurses clarify their own attitudes, they gain a greater understanding and tolerance of sexuality in others.

Selecting Appropriate Interventions

Interventions for sexual health problems are many and varied. Major components of any intervention strategy include counseling, education, and referral. Two models of intervention are presented as examples to guide nurses in selecting appropriate interventions.

Frank (1981, p. 64) suggests a three-part program for each sexual counseling session: (a) assessment, (b) information-sharing, and (c) discussion. The *assessment phase* involves asking the client questions and evaluating the answers. Frank suggests that before asking the questions of the client, the nurse should answer this question: "If I were in this client's place, what questions would I ask?" This exercise helps the nurse devise a list of questions and ways to ask them. For example, the nurse might ask a client recuperating from a heart attack the following questions:

"Now that you're recuperating and you've had some time to sort out your feelings, have you thought about how your heart attack might alter your sex life?"

"Have you and your partner discussed how you both feel about it?"

Information-sharing and discussion should follow each question. In this example, *sharing information*

means the nurse informs the client about how his heart attack might affect his sex life, including the following:

"Your heart attack will not alter your capacity for sexual response. Most people can resume intercourse in 4 to 6 weeks, but this should be confirmed by your doctor."

"Many postcoronary clients fear sexual intercourse because of increased heart and respiratory rates associated with it. However, your prescribed program of progressive physical activity will also increase your tolerance for sexual activity."

After sharing information, the nurse should encourage discussion. If the nurse cannot answer the client's questions, the nurse refers the client to someone who can. The nurse may offer helpful suggestions during *discussion,* for example:

"Many people express concern about the stress of certain positions for intercourse, but you may use whatever position is comfortable for you and your partner."

Another model to help nurses deliver sexual health care, developed by Mims and Swenson (1978, p. 123), outlines three levels of nursing intervention, all of which require use of the nursing process and communication skills. At the *basic level,* the nurse helps the client develop awareness of sexuality, which involves knowledge, attitudes, and perceptions. Mims and Swenson believe that all nurses, regardless of educational preparation, should function at this level.

The *intermediate level* includes giving permission and giving information. This level presupposes teaching skills by the nurse. *Giving permission* means that the nurse by attitude or word lets the client know that sexual thoughts, fantasies, and behaviors between informed, consenting adults are sanctioned. Giving permission begins when the nurse acknowledges the client's verbal and nonverbal sexual concerns. For example, an older male with a reduced libido may feel that he cannot discuss sex with the nurse unless the nurse broaches the subject. Other clients may need acknowledgment to feel comfortable about their virginity, homosexual activities, oral-genital sex, or masturbation. Often, many sexual concerns are alleviated when the client receives permission from the nurse to engage or not engage in certain sexual behaviors. Permission giving can be detrimental unless at the same time the nurse provides accurate information. *Giving information* should include

1. General information about sexuality, including:
   a. Anatomy and physiology of sexual organs
   b. Stages of sexual development

c. Sexual response cycles

d. Coital positions

2. Information specific to the client's needs, which may include:
   a. Alterations in sexuality made necessary by certain disease processes, medication, surgery, or therapies
   b. Alternative modes of sexual expression
   c. Contraception
   d. Sexually transmitted diseases
   e. Pregnancy
   f. Abortion
   g. Infertility

The *advanced level* of nursing intervention includes *giving suggestions,* which involves sexual therapy, educational programs, and research projects. For this level of functioning, the nurse requires specialized knowledge and skill.

For the client with **Sexual dysfunction** related to neurologic changes secondary to diabetes mellitus, implementation might involve teaching about etiology, supportive counseling related to self-image, teaching about continued ability to ejaculate, and providing information about options such as penile prostheses. Clients with **Sexual dysfunction** related to neurologic deficits secondary to spinal cord injury may need special rehabilitation programs, a good example of a third level of implementation.

Sexual Health Teaching

Providing education for sexual health is an important component of nursing implementation. Many sexual problems exist as a result of sexual ignorance; many others can be prevented with effective sexual health teaching. Examples of important areas of teaching include breast and testicular self-examination, prevention of sexually transmitted diseases, and contraception.

Sexually Transmitted Diseases   Human immunodeficiency virus (HIV) infection, or acquired immune deficiency syndrome (AIDS), is a health problem of increasing severity. According to the CDC, 186,170 cases of AIDS had been diagnosed in the United States, Canada, and Mexico by early 1991. This growing health problem has implications for nurses in health teaching as well as in providing direct care to individuals with AIDS and related conditions. Important issues noted earlier in this chapter, such as nonjudgmental attitudes and the need for accurate information, are vital to the proper understanding and care of individuals with HIV infection. AIDS is an extremely complex and sensitive issue. Information about the specifics of AIDS is available in and best sought from specialty publications, many of which are written specifically for nurses.

Common signs of sexually transmitted diseases for which people should seek medical care are shown in Table 25–3. The use of condoms is strongly advocated as a protective device against sexually transmitted diseases for homosexual and heterosexual couples. Specific strategies to prevent AIDS are shown in the accompanying box.

Strategies to Prevent AIDS

- Avoid sexual contact with persons *known* to or *suspected* to have AIDS.
- Practice "safe sex" (no exchanges of body fluids, including semen, urine, saliva, feces, or blood; no contact of body fluids with mucous membranes).
- Wear a condom during intercourse unless you have a monogamous partner who you know is not infected.
- Avoid unnecessary transfusions of blood or blood products.
- Encourage autologous transfusions for elective surgery whenever possible.
- Administer only heat-treated coagulation factor to hemophiliacs.
- Screen all potential blood donors carefully.
- Encourage AIDS clients and persons at high risk not to donate blood, plasma, organs for transplantation, or semen for artificial insemination.
- Advise parenteral drug users to use only clean, disposable needles and syringes and not to share drug equipment.
- Recommend that seropositive women delay pregnancy.
- Provide educational programs on AIDS for the public and school children.
- Use appropriate blood/body fluid precautions with known or suspected AIDS clients.

Source: Adapted from S. W. Ames and C. R. Kneisl, *Essentials of adult health nursing* (Menlo Park, Calif: Addison-Wesley Publishing Co., 1988).

TABLE 25-3 *Clinical Signs of Sexually Transmitted Diseases*

Disease	Male	Female
Gonorrhea	Painful urination; urethritis with watery white discharge, which may become purulent.	May be asymptomatic; or vaginal discharge, pain, and urinary frequency.
Syphilis	Chancre, usually on glans penis, which is painless and heals in 4 to 6 weeks; secondary symptoms—skin eruptions, low-grade fever, inflammation of lymph glands—in 6 weeks to 6 months after chancre heals.	Chancre on cervix or other genital areas, which heals in 4 to 6 weeks; symptoms same as for male.
Genital warts (condyloma acuminatum)	Single lesions or clusters of lesions growing beneath or on the foreskin, at external meatus, or on the glans penis. On dry skin areas, lesions are hard and yellow-gray. On moist areas, lesions are pink or red and soft with a cauliflowerlike appearance.	Lesions appear at the bottom part of the vaginal opening, on the perineum, the vaginal lips, inner walls of the vagina, and the cervix.
Herpes genitalis (*Herpes simplex* of the genitals)	Primary herpes involves the presence of painful sores or large, discrete vesicles that last for weeks; vesicles rupture. Recurrent herpes is itchy rather than painful; it lasts for a few hours to 10 days.	Same as for males.
Chlamydial urethritis	Urinary frequency; watery, mucoid urethral discharge.	Commonly a carrier; vaginal discharge, dysuria, urinary frequency.
Trichomonas vaginalis	Slight itching; moisture on tip of penis; slight, early morning urethral discharge. Many males are asymptomatic.	Itching and redness of vulva and skin inside thighs; copious watery, frothy vaginal discharge.
Candida albicans	Itching, irritation, discharge, plaque of cheesy material under foreskin.	Red and excoriated vulva; intense itching of vaginal and vulvar tissues; thick, white, cheesy or curdlike discharge.
Acquired Immune Deficiency Syndrome (AIDS)	Symptoms can appear anytime from several months to several years after acquiring the virus. The person has reduced immunity to other diseases. Symptoms include any of the following for which there is no other explanation: persistent heavy night sweats; extreme fatigue; severe weight loss; enlarged lymph glands in neck, axillae, or groin; persistent diarrhea; skin rashes; blurred vision or chronic headache; harsh, dry cough; thick gray-white coating on tongue or throat.	

Contraception Contraceptive methods include fertility awareness, mechanical and chemical contraception, and surgical procedures. Most people use several methods during their lives, so they need to be familiar with the various methods available. Increasingly, people are choosing methods that do not employ the use of artificial substances within the body. So-called natural methods have long been preferred by people whose religious beliefs conflict with artificial birth-control methods. Table 25–4 lists various contraceptive methods.

EVALUATING

Evaluation of goal achievement generally includes similar data collection activities implemented in the assessment phase; however, the focus is now on the expected outcomes developed in the planning phase. Evaluative activities may include (a) questioning the clients about their understanding of conception, sexual development, safer sex practices, signs of sexually transmitted diseases, and contraception; (b) asking the client about altered sexual practices; (c) observing the client demonstrate use of a condom or other contraceptive device on a model; (d) listening during an interview to the client's comments about level of sexual satisfaction and gratification of self and partner or about perception of self as being sexually acceptable.

Nurses need to appreciate that there are virtually no universals in sexual attitudes, experiences, or preferences. Attitudes toward sexuality range from the very liberal to the highly conservative. Peoples' experiences range from sexual encounters with one or more partners, long-term partnerships in marriage or other ongoing frameworks, to celibacy. Sexual preferences also vary. Many people prefer to relate exclusively to members of the opposite sex; others to the same sex; and still others to either sex. An understanding of the nurse's own perspective on human sexuality is an essential prerequisite for dealing with clients' sexual issues.

TABLE 25-4 *Contraceptive Methods*

Type	Definition/Action	Type	Definition/Action
Fertility awareness	Identification of fertile days during the month by watching for signs of ovulation.	Vaginal sponge	A spermicide-saturated sponge placed over the cervix; spermicide kills sperm and sponge prevents live sperm from entering the uterus.
Coitus interruptus	Penile withdrawal prior to ejaculation.		
Intrauterine device (IUD)	A device implanted in the cervix; prevents fertilized egg from implanting in uterus.	Oral contraceptives	Low-dosage hormones that suppress ovulation by increasing estrogen level; increased progestin level interferes with passage of sperm through the cervix.
Condom	A sheath placed over the penis; prevents sperm from entering the vagina.		
Vaginal diaphragm	A round rubber cup inserted into the vagina and placed over the cervix; prevents sperm from entering uterus. When used with spermicidal jelly or cream, destroys sperm.	Hormonal implants	Devices implanted under the woman's skin for a number of years; they release low-dosage hormones that suppress ovulation.
		Tubal ligation	Surgery that ties off the Fallopian tubes to interrupt tubal continuity.
		Vasectomy	Surgery that ligates and cuts the vas deferens to prevent the passage of sperm.

CHAPTER HIGHLIGHTS

▶ Sexuality is important in developing self-identity, interpersonal relationships, intimacy, and love.

▶ In its broad sense, sexuality involves physical, emotional, social, and ethical aspects of being and behaving. It has learned and inherited components.

▶ An understanding of the structure and function of the male and female genitals is essential for nurses.

▶ The components that contribute to the development of sexuality are numerous; both biologic and psychologic components exist at all ages.

▶ Biologic differences in the sexes are apparent at birth, but many behavioral differences are also notable throughout infancy and childhood.

▶ The establishment of sexual self-identity and gender role are critical between the ages of 18 months and 4 years.

▶ The learning of sex-typed behaviors depends on communication from parents and on imitation of parental behavior. Learning appropriate sex-typed behaviors takes several years.

▶ Adolescents may have problems establishing sexual self-identity.

▶ Adults also often experience sexual problems. A major task of the adult is to develop an intimate relationship with a partner.

▶ During the middle and later years, there are physical changes in the genitals. However, the desire and ability to maintain satisfying sexual relationships can remain.

▶ Assessing actual or potential sexual problems is conducted at four levels. The professional nurse assesses at only the first level. Assessment should be carried out when clients or support persons present cues that problems exist or when an illness could cause sexual problems.

▶ Nurses assess attitudes toward sexuality, including factors that affect attitudes and behaviors.

▶ An understanding of sexual stimuli and response patterns can help individuals have satisfying sexual relationships. This understanding is also vital for nurses wishing to help clients with psychologic problems, such as feelings of inadequacy, or medical problems, such as spinal cord injuries or myocardial infarctions.

▶ Common sexual problems of healthy adults are changes in libido, erectile dysfunction, premature ejaculation, orgasmic dysfunction, vaginismus, and dyspareunia.

▶ Illnesses that commonly affect sexuality include myocardial infarction and diabetes mellitus. Many surgical procedures also affect sexual abilities and sexual self-image, including mastectomy, hysterectomy, orchiectomy, and enterostomy.

▶ Nursing diagnoses for clients with sexual problems are related to many contributing factors, including altered body structure or function, lack of knowledge or misinformation about sexual matters, physical or psychologic abuse, value conflicts, and loss or lack of a partner.

▶ Before assisting clients with sexual problems, nurses must acquire accurate information about sexuality, identify and accept their own sexual values and behaviors as well as those of others, and be comfortable acquiring and disseminating information about sexuality.

▶ Nursing interventions include helping clients develop awareness of sexuality, giving permission, giving information, and, at an advanced level, giving suggestions.

LEARNING ACTIVITIES

■ Self-awareness about sexuality attitudes is essential. Consider each of the following sexuality issues. Write your thoughts down so that you can review them afterward. Abortion, teenage pregnancy, homosexuality, pornography, premarital sex, masturbation, heterosexuality, contraception, nudity, child pornography, prostitution, extramarital sex, bisexuality, incest.

Review your attitudes. Are they consistent? Do your attitudes about one issue impact on your beliefs about another issue? Do you have conflicting attitudes about the issues? Do your attitudes about any issue place you in potential conflict with a client or client group? How would you resolve such a conflict?

- As a nurse, how do you react to the following statements:
  - Nurses are women.
  - Astronauts are men.
  - Teachers are women.
  - Doctors are men.
  - Women are not usually athletic.
- Men are not usually tender.

What are your attitudes about male and female gender roles? What are appropriate male roles or behaviors? What are inappropriate male roles or behaviors? What are appropriate female roles or behaviors? What are inappropriate female roles or behaviors? Are there conflicts in your attitudes and beliefs about appropriate male and female gender roles?

READINGS AND REFERENCES

SUGGESTED READINGS

Chekryn, J. September 1989. Families of people with AIDS. *Canadian Nurse* 65:30–32.

In a report on a research project to identify and understand the needs of families of clients with AIDS, Chekryn identifies factors that influence nursing care decisions.

Divasto, P. February 1985. Measuring the aftermath of rape. *Journal of Psychosocial Nursing and Mental Health Services* 23:33–35.

Divasto describes an interview scale for measuring the severity of postrape symptoms and outlines symptoms and use of the data to guide client care.

Lutz, R. March 1986. Stopping the spread of sexually transmitted diseases. *Nursing* 16:47–50.

Lutz provides an overview of the most common STDs and outlines nursing activities in dealing with clients who have an STD and techniques to decrease the spread.

RELATED RESEARCH

Bullough, B.; Bullough, V.; and Smith, R. W. August 1985. Masculinity and femininity in transvestite, transsexual and gay males. *Western Journal of Nursing Research* 7:317–27.

Kus, R. May 1985. Stages of coming out: An ethnographic approach. *Western Journal of Nursing Research* 7:177–98.

Sachs, B. 1985. Contraceptive decision-making in urban, black, female adolescents: Its relationship to cognitive development. *International Journal of Nursing Studies* 22(2):116–17.

Sheehan, M. K.; Ostwald, S. K.; and Rothenberger, J. January/February 1986. Perceptions of sexual responsibility: Do young men and women agree? *Pediatric Nursing.* 12:17–21.

Webb, C. October 1987. Nurses' knowledge and attitudes about sexuality: Report of a study. *Nursing Education Today* 7:209–14.

SELECTED REFERENCES

Andrist, L. C. December 1988. Taking a sex history and educating clients about safe sex. *Nursing Clinics of North America* 23:959–73.

Benson, C. H. January/March 1988. Arthritis and sexuality. *Journal of Urological Nursing* 7:370–72.

Brunner, L. S., and Suddarth, D. S. 1988. *Textbook of medical surgical nursing.* 6th ed. Philadelphia: J. B. Lippincott Co.

Burke, P. J. 1987. Adolescents' motivation for sexual activity and pregnancy prevention. *Issues in Comprehensive Pediatric Nursing.* 10(3):161–71.

Carpenito, L. J. 1989. *Nursing diagnosis: Application to clinical practice.* 3d ed. Philadelphia: J. B. Lippincott Co.

Crooks, R., and Baur, K. 1987. *Our sexuality.* 3d ed. Menlo Park, Calif.: Benjamin/Cummings.

Douglas, C. J.; Kalman, C. M.; and Kalman, T. P. December 1985. Homophobia among physicians and nurses. *Hospital and Community Psychiatry* 36:1309–11.

Flaskerud, J. H. 1989. *AIDS/HIV infection: A resource guide for nursing professionals.* Philadelphia: W. B. Saunders Co.

Frank, D. I. January 1981. You don't have to be an expert to give sexual counseling to a mastectomy patient. *Nursing 81* 11:64–67.

Glover, J. January 16, 1985. Family planning and sexual counseling . . . The nurse's role. *Nursing Mirror* 160:28–29.

Howe, C. L. February 1986. Developmental theory and adolescent sexual behavior. *Nurse Practitioner* 11:65,68,71.

Hurley, M. E. (ed.) 1986. *Classification of Nursing Diagnoses: Proceedings of the Sixth National Conferences.* St. Louis: C. V. Mosby Co.

Kim, M. J.; McFarland, G. K.; and McLane, A. M. 1989. *Pocket guide to nursing diagnoses.* 3d ed. St. Louis: C. V. Mosby Co.

Kus, R. May 1985. Stages of coming out: An ethnographic approach. *Western Journal of Nursing Research* 7:177–98.

Lion, E. M., editor. 1982. *Human sexuality in nursing process.* New York: John Wiley and Sons.

McAndrew, T. January 1990. Elderly sexuality examined. *Pennsylvania Nurse* 45:16.

McCracken, A. L. October 1988. Sexuality practice by elders: The forgotten aspect of functional health. *Journal of Gerontological Nursing* 14:13–18.

Masters, W. H., and Johnson, V. E. 1966. *Human sexual response.* Boston: Little, Brown and Co.

———. 1970. *Human sexual inadequacy.* New York: Bantam Books.

———. 1979. *Homosexuality in perspective.* Boston: Little, Brown and Co.

Mims, F. H. September 1982. Sexual stress: Coping and adaptation. *Nursing Clinics of North America.* 17:395–405.

Mims, F. H., and Swenson, M. February 1978. A model to promote sexual health care. *Nursing Outlook* 26:121–25.

Murray, R. B., and Huelskoetter, M. M. W. 1983. *Psychiatric/mental health nursing:* Giving emotional care. Englewood Cliffs, N.J.: Prentice-Hall.

Osis, M. January/February 1986. Sexuality: An interactional perspective . . . Drugs and healthy aging. *Gerontion.* 1:6–8.

Penninger, J. A. April 1985. After the ostomy: Helping the patient reclaim his sexuality . . . a male ostomy patient. *RN* 48:46–50.

Pervin-Dixon, L. April 1988. Sexuality and the spinal cord injured. *Journal of Psychosocial Nursing and Mental Health Services* 26:31–35, 37.

Rosenberg, M. J. March 1990. Sexually transmitted diseases and the primary care provider. *Primary Care* 17:1–27.

Rothman, B. and Sebastian, H. May 1990. Intimacy and cognitively impaired elders. *Canadian Nurse* 86:32, 34.

Sex Information and Education Council of the United States. 1980. The Siecus/New York University/Uppsala principles basic to education for sexuality. *Seicus Report* 8:8–9.

Slevin, A. P., and Marvin, C. L. 1987. Safe sex and pregnancy prevention: A guide for health practitioners working with adolescents. *Journal of Community Health Nursing* 4:234–35.

Telashek, M. L., Tichy, A. M., Epping, H. April 1990. Sexually transmitted diseases in the elderly: Issues and recommendations. *Journal of Gerontological Nursing* 16:33–42.

Watts, R. September 1979. Dimensions of sexual health. *American Journal of Nursing* 79:1568–72.

Wright, D. July 31, 1985. Sex and the elderly. *Nursing Mirror* 161:18–19.

Young, E. 1984. Patient's plea: Tell us about our sexuality. *Journal of Sex Education and Therapy.* 10:53–56.

Spirituality and Religion

SPIRITUALITY, FAITH, AND RELIGION

Spirituality, faith, and religion are separate entities, yet some people use the words interchangeably. *Spirituality* or spiritual belief is a belief in or relationship with some higher power, creative force, divine being, or infinite source of energy. For example, a person may believe in "God," in "Allah," or in a "higher power." "The spiritual dimension tries to be in harmony with the universe, strives for answers about the infinite and especially comes into focus or sustaining power when the person faces emotional stress, physical illness, or death. It goes outside a person's own power" (Murray and Zentner 1989, p. 78).

Stoll (1989, p. 7) describes spirituality as a two-dimensional concept: the vertical dimension is the relationship with the transcendent/God or whatever supreme values guide the person's life; the horizontal dimension is the person's relationship with self, others, and the environment. There is a continuous interrelationship between and among the two dimensions. A *spiritual need* is a person's need to maintain, increase, or restore beliefs and faith and to fulfill religious obligations. It is often the nurse who identifies a need for spiritual assistance and obtains the desired help. According to Shelly and Fish, certain spiritual needs underlie all religions: (a) the need for meaning and purpose, (b) the need for love and relatedness, and (c) the need for forgiveness (1988, pp. 40–53). Some people believe that these needs are common to all humanity.

Faith, according to Fowler and Keen (1985, p. 18), is a universal—a feature of living, acting, and self-understanding. To have faith is to believe in or be committed to something or someone. In a general sense, religion or spiritual beliefs are an individual's attempt to understand one's place in the universe, i.e., how that person sees the self in relation to the total environment.

Religion is an organized system of worship. Religions have central beliefs, rituals, and practices usually related to death, marriage, and salvation. They also often have rules of conduct applicable to daily life. Many people satisfy their spiritual needs through a specific religion or religious framework.

Religious development of an individual refers to the acceptance of specific beliefs, values, rules of conduct, and rituals. Religious development may or may not parallel spiritual development. For example, a person may follow certain religious practices and yet not internalize the symbolic meaning behind the practices.

RELIGION AND ILLNESS

Spiritual and religious beliefs are important in many people's lives. They can influence life-style, attitudes, and feelings about illness and death. Some organized religions specify practices about diet, birth control, and appropriate medical therapy. Some religious groups condemn modern science because of "false teachings," such as evolution. Other groups support medical therapy in general but object to specific practices; e.g., the Seventh Day Adventist Church urges its members to avoid all drugs unless they are exceedingly ill.

Spiritual beliefs may assume greater importance at a time of illness than at any other time in a person's life, helping some people accept illness and explaining illness for others. Some clients may look upon illness as a test of faith; i.e., "If I have enough faith I will get well." Viewed from this perspective, illness is usually accepted by the client and the client's support persons and does not shake their religious beliefs.

Other people may look upon illness as punishment and think, "What have I done to deserve this?" These people associate disease with immoral behavior and believe their illness is punishment for past sins. They may believe that through prayer, promises, and perhaps penance, the cause of the disease will disappear. Such people may believe that health professionals treat only the symptoms of disease and that they will become well if they are forgiven. If such an individual does not get well, then the support persons either accept the "punishment" or view the "punishment" as unfair.

Usually, spiritual beliefs help people to accept illness and to plan for the future. Religion can help people prepare for death and strengthen them during life. It can provide a meaning to life and to death; a haven of strength, serenity, and faith at a time of crisis; a sense of security; and a tangible network of social support.

Certain spiritual beliefs are in conflict with accepted medical practice. When a person's faith leads the person to reject certain medical treatment, life may be threatened. For example, many practicing Jehovah's Witnesses will not accept blood transfusions because of religious doctrine.

SPIRITUAL DEVELOPMENT

James Fowler describes the development of faith in people. Fowler believes that faith, or the spiritual dimension, is a force that gives meaning to a person's life. Fowler uses the term _faith_ as a form of knowing, a way of being in relation to "an ultimate environment" (Fowler and Keen 1985, p.21). To Fowler, faith is a relational phenomenon; it is "an active 'mode-of-being-in-relation' to another or others in which we invest commitment, belief, love, risk and hope" (Fowler and Keen 1985, pp. 21–23).

RELIGIOUS BELIEFS RELATED TO HEALTH CARE

Meeting the spiritual needs of clients and their support persons is part of the function of nurses as well as designated chaplains and other clergy. Some religious groups, such as the Church of Latter-Day Saints and the Christian Scientists, do not have ordained clergy; they usually do have people whose role it is to minister to the ill, and these people must be recognized by nurses as having appropriate functions. In Christian Science, the role of ministering to the sick is carried out by a practitioner (reader).

Although nurses cannot expect to be well versed about the practices of all the religious groups in North America, it is important to be familiar with the major religious groups of the community. Representatives of a religion will usually give nurses information required in the care of clients. Some of the larger religious groups are discussed briefly here. Other reference texts can supply greater detail and information not included in this summary.

The major religions of North America are Protestantism, Catholicism, and Judaism. There are many Protestant denominations, e.g., Episcopalians, Methodists, and Baptists. The denominations share some doctrines, but each denomination has its own interpretation of scripture and its own religious practices. Catholicism also encompasses several groups, e.g., the Roman Catholic Church, the Greek Orthodox Church, and the Russian Orthodox Church. See the accompanying box for a summary of the major beliefs of Protestantism, Catholicism and Judaism.

Major religions, denominations, and some spiritual groups are listed alphabetically below. Selected facts about each group are included, but no attempt has been made to discuss broad philosophical beliefs or issues.

Agnosticism and Atheism
An *agnostic* is a person who doubts the existence of God or a supreme being or believes the existence of God has not been proved. An *atheist* denies the existence of God. *Theism* is the belief in the existence of a god or gods. *Monotheism* is the belief in the existence of one God. The moral and ethical codes of agnostics and atheists are not derived from theistic beliefs.

American Muslim Mission (Black Muslim)
The American Muslim Mission is not the same as Islam, although their beliefs are similar. Members emphasize black independence and are encouraged to obtain health care provided by the black community.

Black Muslims have a special procedure for washing and shrouding the dead and special funeral rites. Dietary considerations include prohibitions against alcoholic beverages and pork. Because the use of tobacco is forbidden, clients who are sharing a room require nonsmoking roommates.

Baptist
Baptists believe in the possibility of cure of illness by the "laying on of hands." Although some believe in faith healing to the exclusion of medical therapy, most seek competent medical help. Some Baptists do not drink coffee or tea, and many Baptists do not take alcohol. Birth control, sterilization, and abortion (therapeutic or demand) are left to individual choice. When clients are clearly terminally ill, artificial prolongation of life is discouraged. Full-term stillborn babies are buried; less than full-term fetuses are not. Infant baptism is not practiced.

Buddhism
The doctrine of avoidance of extremes is practiced by Buddhists and applied to the use of drugs, blood, or vaccines. Buddhism does not condone the taking of lives in any form, but, if a client is beyond

---

Basic Beliefs of Protestantism, Catholicism, and Judaism

Protestantism

- The Bible is the Holy Scripture.
- Sins are forgiven through faith and communication with God.
- The sacraments are baptism and Holy Communion.
- There is life after death.
- Sunday is the Sabbath.

Catholicism

- The teachings of the Lord are found in Scripture.
- Sins are confessed to a priest, who renders absolution.
- The sacraments are baptism, confirmation (acceptance of the Holy Spirit), Eucharist (Holy Communion), marriage, sacrament of the sick, penance (confession), and ordination.
- There is life eternal. For those who accept God and live faithfully, heaven is eternal home. For those who have rejected God, hell is the destination.
- Sunday is the Sabbath.

Judaism

- The laws of the Torah represent God's teachings of mercy, compassion, tolerance, and love.
- God created individuals inherently good, possessing a holy soul.
- Sabbath is observed from sunset Friday until sunset Saturday or just on Friday evening, depending on beliefs of the group.

---

recovery and can no longer strive toward "enlightenment," euthanasia *may* be permitted. Likewise, certain circumstances may warrant abortion. Buddhists approve of either burial or cremation. Last rite chanting is frequently practiced at the bedside of the deceased. Cleanliness is very important.

Buddhists generally do not practice any dietary restrictions, although members of some sects are strict vegetarians. Many Buddhists do not use tobacco, alcohol, or drugs. Buddhists have special holy days: January 1, February 15, March 21, April 8, May 21, July 15, September 1 and 23, and December 8 and 31. Buddhist clients may need to be asked how they feel about tests and treatments on those days.

Church of Christ, Scientist (Christian Science)

Members of the Church of Christ, Scientist, oppose human intervention to cure illness, seeing it as God's will. Sickness and sin are errors of the human mind and can be changed by altering thoughts rather than by medicine. People who strictly follow this religion will not accept a physician's consultation or medical treatment and rarely, if ever, enter a hospital. Christian Scientists do not permit psychotherapy, because in this process the mind is altered by others. A Christian Science "practitioner" can be called to minister to the sick, and spiritual healing is practiced. Physicians and midwives may be used during childbirth, however.

Drugs and blood transfusions are not used, and biopsies and physical examinations are not sought. Tobacco and alcohol are considered drugs and not used. Tea and coffee are often refused. Vaccines are accepted only as required by law. Christian Scientists do not have strictly defined policies about birth control, sterilization, or abortion. Autopsy is discouraged but accepted in sudden deaths, and Christian Scientists are unlikely to seek or donate organs for transplant. Whether a person wishes to rely completely upon Christian Science is up to the individual. In some areas, the church operates nursing homes in which there is complete reliance on church doctrine.

Eastern Orthodoxy

There are a number of Eastern Orthodox denominations, including Greek, Armenian, Ukrainian, Bulgarian, and Syrian. Most believe in infant baptism by immersion 8 to 40 days after birth. The last rites may be obligatory if death is impending. Dietary restrictions depend on the particular sect. During Lent, abstinence from meat and dairy products is carried out unless this is harmful to health. Eastern Orthodox beliefs and practices generally do not restrict medical science; however, the Russian Orthodox church discourages autopsy as well as donation of body parts.

The Greek Orthodox church opposes abortion. The church advocates confession at least yearly. The last rites include administration of *Holy Communion* (also referred to as the *Eucharist* or the *Lord's Supper*), a memorial sacrament in which the worshipper receives consecrated bread (or a thin wafer) representing the body of Jesus Christ, and wine or grape juice representing the blood of Jesus. The church encourages prolonging life, even for terminally ill clients.

Episcopalian (Anglican)

The Episcopal or Anglican religion places no restrictions on the use of drugs, blood, or vaccines; biopsies; or amputations or transplants for saving life. It permits birth control and sterilization, autopsy, therapeutic abortion as a life-saving measure, burial or cremation, and genetic counseling. Abortion on demand, however, is regarded as unacceptable. Episcopalians celebrate Holy Communion. Some members of this church fast before receiving Communion and abstain from meat on Fridays. The church advocates confession. The rite for anointing of the sick may be performed but is not mandatory.

Hinduism

Hindus have many dietary variations, and these vary according to the particular sect. Some do not eat veal and beef and their derivatives. Some are strict vegetarians. Alcohol may be consumed at Western social functions. Most Hindus accept modern medical practices; artificial insemination is rejected, however, because sterility reflects divine will. When giving a Hindu medications, the nurse avoids touching the client's lips, if possible.

Hindus practice special rites at death. Death is considered rebirth. The priest pours water into the mouth of the corpse and ties a thread around the wrist or neck to indicate blessing. This thread must not be removed. The body undergoes cremation, and the ashes are disposed of in holy rivers. Some injuries, such as loss of a limb, are considered signs of wrongdoing in a previous life, although the afflicted person is not an outcast from society. Hindus do believe there is a natural division among people, so that little mixing occurs among castes (hereditary social classes).

Jehovah's Witness

Jehovah's Witnesses are opposed to blood transfusions and organ transplants, although some individuals do agree to them in a crisis. Nonblood plasma expanders and autologous transfusions may be accepted. When parents refuse to have an infant transfused, a court order may be sought transferring custody to the courts or to an official of the hospital.

Members of the church eat meat that has been drained of blood. The use of alcohol and tobacco is discouraged. Some oppose modern medicine. Infant baptism is not practiced.

Jehovah's Witnesses generally have a neutral attitude toward birth control, believing it is a matter of individual conscience. Both therapeutic and demand abortions are forbidden. Burial and cremation are approved. Autopsy is approved only as required by law, and no parts of the body are to be removed. This restriction has implications for donor transplants.

Judaism

There are the three main Jewish groups: the Orthodox is the most strict; the Conservative and Reform groups are less so. Jewish law demands that Jews seek competent medical care. Jews allow the use of drugs, blood, and vaccines; biopsies and amputations are also permitted. Some Orthodox Jews believe that the entire God-given body must be returned to the earth, and they require any body tissue to be buried. Donor transplants may therefore not be acceptable to Orthodox Jews. The nurse must ensure that amputated limbs or organs are made available to such Orthodox families for burial. Cremation is discouraged. Autopsy may be permitted in less strict groups, provided that parts of the body are not removed. Bodies, even those of fetuses, are washed by the ritual burial society and buried as soon as possible after death.

Therapeutic abortion is permissible if the woman's physical or psychologic health is threatened. Demand abortion is prohibited. Vasectomy is not permitted.

Orthodox and Conservative Jews observe kosher dietary laws, which prohibit pork, shellfish, and other foods, and the eating of milk products and meat products at the same meal. Reform Jews usually do not observe kosher dietary regulations.

Circumcision is performed by Orthodox and Conservative Jews on the eighth day of a male baby's life, although it may be delayed if medically contraindicated. The rabbi and male synagogue members may be present, and a Jewish physician or *mohel* (ritual circumciser acquainted with Jewish law and hygienic medical technique) performs the circumcision. Special arrangements generally need to be made for the ceremony and the physician's approval obtained.

Orthodox and some Conservative Jews observe the Sabbath from sunset Friday to sunset Saturday and may resist hospital admission or medical procedures during that period or during major Jewish festivals, unless the treatment is necessary to preserve life. Rosh Hashanah is the first day of the Jewish new year, which occurs in September. Ten days later, Yom Kippur marks the end of the time devoted to reflecting upon life.

Lutheran

The Lutheran church imposes no restrictions on medical procedures, including autopsies and therapeutic abortions, and no dietary restrictions. Abortion on demand is not approved, however. Marriage and procreation are discouraged when offspring are likely to inherit severe physical or mental deficits. Birth control and sterilization are left to the individual's conscience. Members are baptized 6 to 8 weeks after birth, and those who wish may be anointed and blessed before death. Burial rites are generally performed on infants who die after 6 to 7 months' gestation.

Mennonite

Members of the Mennonite church are baptized in their middle teens. The church advocates no special dietary restrictions, although some congregations require abstinence from alcohol. No restrictions are placed on medical procedures, although demand abortion is not approved in some sects of the church; in others, it is left to individual conscience. Some Mennonites oppose the laying on of hands.

Mormon (Church of Jesus Christ of Latter-Day Saints)

Some Mormons believe in healing by the power of God through authorized priesthood holders. However, there is no prohibition on medical therapy—in fact, the church operates health facilities. Alcohol, tobacco, tea, coffee, and other drinks with caffeine (e.g., cola) are prohibited, and meat is eaten sparingly. Some members of the church wear a special undergarment. Mormon clients in the hospital may request the Sacrament of the Lord's Supper by a church priesthood holder. Abortion is opposed unless the life of the woman is in danger.

Muslim/Moslem (Islam)

Islam is a major religion of North Africa and the Near East. There are over 70 sects of the Islamic faith. It emphasizes strict rituals and prayers.

All pork products are prohibited, and some oppose alcoholic beverages. There is a fasting period in the ninth month of the Mohammedan year (Ramadan), but people who are ill are exempt from it. Circumcision is practiced, and cleanliness is very important.

If a fetus is aborted 130 days or more after conception, it is treated as a fully developed human being. Before that time, it is looked upon as discarded tissue. Abortion is forbidden.

The dying person must confess sins and beg forgiveness. Only relatives and family can touch the body after death. They wash and prepare it and turn it toward Mecca. Islam encourages prolonging life, even for the terminally ill.

Pentecostal (Assemblies of God)

The Pentecostal church has no doctrine against modern medical science, including blood transfusions. Members are encouraged to abstain from use of alcohol, tobacco, and illegal drugs. Some members do not eat pork. Members may pray for divine healing, and in some congregations anointing with oil is practiced.

Roman Catholicism

It is a Catholic belief that an infant has a soul from the moment of conception; therefore, a fetus must be baptized unless it is obviously dead, as must all babies whose health or life is endangered. Baptism may be performed by any person (e.g., a physician or nurse in the absence of a priest) who does what the church requires. A valid baptism requires pouring water on the baby's head while repeating the prescribed Trinitarian invocation: "I baptize thee in the name of the Father, of the Son, and of the Holy Spirit." When performed by a nurse or physician, the baptism should be recorded on the infant's chart and the family and priest informed.

The Roman Catholic church encourages anointing of the sick. The *sacrament of the sick* is now considered both a source of strength or healing and a preparation for death. The priest anoints several areas of the body with oil. Catholics can now be anointed more than once. Many older Catholics, however, may respond to this sacrament with fear or dread, considering it a sign of imminent death. Thus, before a reluctant client is anointed, the nurse or priest should interpret its current meaning to the client, to minimize apprehension. Anointing of the sick may be preceded by confession and Holy Communion. These sacraments are also performed by a priest or other commissioned person.

The Roman Catholic belief in the "principle of totality" underlies a general acceptance of medical procedures. A donor transplant is accepted as long as loss of the organ does not deprive the donor of life or functional integrity of the body. Biopsies and amputations are accepted in the same light. Autopsy is also accepted; again, all major parts of the body (those retaining human quality) must be given an appropriate burial or cremation.

Strict laws govern birth control, sterilization, and abortion. The only approved method of birth control is abstinence; artificial means are illicit. Sterilization is forbidden unless there is a sound medical indication for it. Both demand and therapeutic abortions are prohibited, even to save the mother's life.

Some Catholics observe certain dietary and fasting practices but are excused from otherwise obligatory fasting or abstaining from meat on Ash Wednesday and Good Friday when they are ill. Sunday is the day of worship, although church services are held in some churches other days of the week as well.

Salvation Army

The Salvation Army places no restrictions on medical procedures, including transplants and autopsies. Birth control and sterilization are acceptable within marriage. Demand abortions are opposed, but therapeutic ones are approved. The Army has many hospitals and social centers for people, e.g., hostels for the indigent.

Seventh-Day Adventist (Church of God, Advent Christian Church)

The Adventist church does not practice infant baptism but conducts baptism of adults by immersion. In dietary matters, it prohibits alcohol, tobacco, tea, coffee, and the use of illegal drugs, and some members advocate ovolactovegetarian diets. Some sects practice divine healing and anointing with oil. Saturday is considered the Sabbath by some.

Adventists are encouraged to avoid drugs, but they recognize that blood transfusions, vaccines, and drugs are sometimes necessary. Birth control and sterilization are left to individual conscience. Abortion is approved if the mother's life is endangered or if pregnancy is due to rape or incest. The use of hypnotism is opposed.

Unitarian Universalist Association

Unitarian Universalists emphasize reason, knowledge, individual responsibility, and personally established values. There are no dietary restrictions or official sacraments in the church, and no medical practices are prohibited. The Unitarian Universalist church encourages its members to donate parts of their bodies to research and to medical banks. Cremation is often preferred to burial.

United Church of Canada

The United Church of Canada is the largest Protestant denomination in Canada. It was formed in 1925 by the amalgamation of the Methodist, Presbyterian, and Congregationalist Churches. It operates some hospitals in underserviced areas of Canada. There are no restrictions about the use of blood or vaccines. Burial and cremation are approved.

SPIRITUAL HEALTH AND THE NURSING PROCESS

Assessing

Spiritual health, or spiritual well-being, is a feeling of being "generally alive, purposeful, and fulfilled" (Ellison 1983, p. 332). According to Pilch (1988, p. 31), spiritual wellness is "a way of living, a lifestyle that views

TABLE 26-1 *Spiritual Well-Being*

Religious component

I believe that God loves me and cares about me.

I have a personal and meaningful relationship with God.

I believe God is concerned about my problem.

My relationship with God helps me not to feel lonely.

I feel most fulfilled when I am in close communion with God.

My relationship with God contributes to my sense of well being.

Meaning and purpose in life

I feel that life is a positive experience.

I feel very fulfilled and satisfied with life.

I feel a sense of well-being about the direction my life is headed in.

I feel good about my future.

I believe there is some real purpose in life.

Source: Sample statements from a scale on religious meaning and purpose of life. © Spiritual Well-Being Scale. 1982 by Craig W. Ellison and Raymond F. Paloutzian. All rights reserved.

ASSESSMENT INTERVIEW
Spirituality

- Are any particular religious practices important to you? If so, could you please tell me about them?

- Will being here interfere with your religious practices?

- Do you feel your faith is helpful to you? In what ways is it important to you right now?

- In what ways can I help you to carry out your faith? For example, would you like me to read your prayer book to you?

- Would you like a visit from your spiritual counselor or the hospital chaplain?

- What are your hopes and your sources of strength right now?

and lives life as purposeful and pleasurable, that seeks out life-sustaining and life-enriching options to be chosen freely at every opportunity, and that sinks its roots deeply into spiritual values and/or specific religious beliefs."

Ellison and Paloutzian (1982) designed a spiritual well-being scale that includes specific questions for a client (see Table 26-1 for sample statements). They found that people who scored high on the scale tended to be less lonely, more socially skilled, and higher in self-esteem; furthermore, their religious commitment was more intrinsic to their personalities.

Nursing History

Nurses may elicit data about a client's spiritual beliefs as part of the general history. Often the information elicited is limited to the client's religious affiliation. Nurses should never assume, however, that a client follows all the practices of the client's stated religion.

Stoll (1979, p. 1574) suggests a spiritual history guide to elicit information in four areas: (a) the person's concept of God or deity, (b) the person's source of hope and strength, (c) the significance of religious practices and rituals to the person, and (d) the relationship the person perceives between the individual's spiritual beliefs and state of health. Stoll further cautions that all people have a right to their own values and beliefs and that they have a right not to discuss or reveal these beliefs to others. The spiritual assessment is best taken at the end of the assessment process or following the psychosocial assessment, once the nurse has developed a relationship with the client and/or support person and feels that it is appropriate to discuss spiritual matters. The questions provided in the box above may be suitable.

Clinical Assessment

Spiritual distress may be revealed by one or more of the following:

1. *Affect and attitude.* Does the client appear lonely, depressed, angry, anxious, agitated, apathetic, or preoccupied?

2. *Behavior.* Does the client appear to pray before meals or at other times? Does the client read religious literature? Does the client complain frequently, need unusually high doses of sedation, pace the halls at night, joke inappropriately, have nightmares and sleep disturbances, or express anger at religious representatives or a deity?

3. *Verbalization.* Does the client mention God, prayer, faith, the church, or religious topics (even briefly)? Does the client ask about a visit from the clergy? Does the client express fear of death, concern with the meaning of life, inner conflict about religious beliefs, concern about a relationship with the deity, questions about the meaning of existence, the meaning of suffering, or the moral/ethical implications of therapy?

TABLE 26-2 *Signs of Spiritual Health*

Need	Behavior or Condition
Need for meaning and purpose in life	Expresses that he has lived in accordance with his value system in the past
	Expresses desire to participate in religious rituals
	Lives in accordance with value system at present
	Expresses contentment with life
	Expresses hope in the future
Need to receive love	Expresses hope in life after death
	Expresses confidence in the health care team
	Expresses feelings of being loved by others/ God
	Expresses feelings of forgiveness by others/God
	Expresses desire to perform religious rituals leading to salvation
	Trusts others/God with the outcome of a situation in which he feels he has no control
Need to give love	Expresses love for others through actions
	Seeks the good of others
Need for hope and creativity	Asks for information about his condition realistically
	Talks about his condition realistically
	Sets realistic personal health goals
	Uses time during illness/ hospitalization constructively
	Values his inner self more than his physical self

Source: From M. F. Highfield and C. Carson, Spiritual needs of patients: Are they recognized? *Cancer Nursing,* June 1983, 6:187–192. Reprinted with permission.

4. *Interpersonal relationships.* Who visits? How does the client respond to visitors? Does a minister come? How does the client relate to other clients and nursing personnel?

5. *Environment.* Does the client have a Bible, prayer book, devotional literature, religious medals, a rosary, or religious get-well cards in the room? Does a church send altar flowers or Sunday bulletins? (Shelley and Fish 1988, pp. 61–62).

Signs of spiritual health are given in Table 26–2.

Diagnosing

The nursing diagnosis that relates to problems with spirituality is **Spiritual distress,** defined as "a disruption in the life principle that pervades a person's entire being and that integrates and transcends one's biologic and psychological nature" (Kim, McFarland, and McLane 1989, p. 62) or "the state in which the individual experiences or is at risk of experiencing a disturbance in the belief or value system which provides strength, hope, and meaning to life" (Carpenito 1989, p. 710).

O'Brien (1982, p. 81) subcategorizes spiritual distress as follows:

- Spiritual *pain,* i.e, difficulty accepting the loss of a loved one or intense suffering (physical or emotional)
- Spiritual *alienation,* i.e., separation from religious or faith community
- Spiritual *anxiety,* i.e., challenge to beliefs and value systems (e.g., by moral/ethical nature of therapy such as abortion, blood transfusion, surgery, etc.)
- Spiritual *guilt,* i.e., failure to abide by religious rules
- Spiritual *anger,* i.e., difficulty accepting illness, loss, or suffering.
- Spiritual *loss,* i.e., difficulty finding comfort in religion
- Spiritual *despair,* i.e., feeling that no one cares

Planning

Nursing interventions are identified to help the client achieve the overall goals of spiritual strength, serenity, and satisfaction.

Planning in relation to spiritual distress should be designed to meet one or more of the following needs:

- To help the client fulfill religious obligations
- To help the client draw on and use inner resources more effectively to meet the present situation

- To help the client maintain or establish a dynamic, personal relationship with a supreme being in the face of unpleasant circumstances
- To help the client find meaning in existence and the present situation
- To promote a sense of hope
- To provide spiritual resources otherwise unavailable

Sometimes clients ask directly for a visit from the hospital chaplain or their own clergyman. Others may discuss their concerns with the nurse and ask about the nurse's beliefs as a way of seeking an empathic listener. Some people are embarrassed to ask for spiritual counsel but may hint at their concern in such statements as, "I've been wondering what will happen to me when I die," or "Do you go to a church?"

Any client or support person may desire spiritual assistance. The client facing death may have accepted it, but the family and support persons may not. Often relatives are grateful for spiritual support by a nurse or pastor. Assisting them may indirectly assist the client. Among those who may desire spiritual assistance are:

- Clients who appear lonely and have few visitors
- Clients who express fear and anxiety
- Clients about to have surgery
- Clients whose illness is related to the emotions or whose illness has religious or social implications
- Clients who must change their life-style as a result of illness or injury
- Clients preoccupied about the relationship of their religion and health
- Clients whose pastor is unable to visit

It is important to ask the individual before obtaining assistance. Some people profess no religious beliefs and may be angered if the nurse makes arrangements for a chaplain to visit. The nurse needs to respect the client's wishes and not make a judgment of right or wrong, good or bad. Planning also involves establishing outcome criteria. Examples of relevant outcome criteria are listed below.

The client:

- Expresses comfort with spiritual beliefs
- Continues spiritual practices appropriate to health status
- Expresses decreased feelings of guilt
- States acceptance of moral decision

- Displays positive affect
- Expresses finding positive meaning in the present situation and in own existence
- Verbalizes relief from or acceptance of suffering
- Verbalizes relief of anger toward transcendent being, self, and others
- Verbalizes a closeness with God
- Experiences a sense of forgiveness

Implementing

Once spiritual distress has been identified as a relevant nursing diagnosis and specific strategies have been planned, the nurse is ready to implement the plan. To be effective when intervening, nurses should have already examined and clarified their own spiritual beliefs and values (see Chapter 11). A nurse who feels uncomforta-

---

RESEARCH NOTE

What Are Nurses' Attitudes About Providing Spiritual Care?

The research focused on one major explanation for the lack of spiritual care given to patients: Many nurses lack the spiritual resources and spiritual well-being to meet clients' needs effectively in this regard. Graduate students and undergraduate students in their senior year were surveyed using tools; one measured their religious and existential welfare, and the other measured attitudes regarding the role of care providers in patients' spiritual care. The study confirmed that a strong relationship existed between a nurse's spiritual well-being and the nurse's views about the provision of spiritual care by health professionals. The authors believe that an individual with a high degree of spiritual well-being has a motivating sense of direction and order that can be used to assist another. Such harmony with the self is necessary before the nurse can assist the client spiritually.

Implications: Nurses who have a high degree of spiritual well-being are most effective in helping clients spiritually.

K. L. Soeken and V. J. Carson, Study measures nurses' attitudes about providing spiritual care, *Health Progress,* April 1986, 67:52–55.

ble assisting the client spiritually (e.g., reading devotional material or praying with the client on request) should verbalize this discomfort and offer to obtain assistance for the client. It is important to respect the client's beliefs and maintain a supportive relationship. It is equally important for the nurse not to feel guilty about her or his discomfort.

To decrease spiritual distress, nurses should focus attention on the client's perception of his or her spiritual needs rather than on the practices or beliefs of the client's religious affiliation. Individual spiritual beliefs may vary greatly among members of a given religion. People join religious groups for many reasons (e.g., to have a place of worship, to find an avenue for social action such as helping the poor or homeless, to gain friends for recreational purposes, or to have a place for important life events such as weddings and funerals). Similarly, nurses should not assume that a client has no spiritual needs because the record states no religious affiliation or specifies atheist or agnostic.

To further individualize care, the nurse determines the meaning the client attaches to the situation. Such meanings can influence the client's response to an illness or condition and may either hinder nursing intervention or provide hope, courage, and strength. For example, a person who believes that illness is God's punishment may feel powerless and demonstrate little interest in therapy designed to prevent illness.

When orienting clients to the nursing unit, the nurse can provide information about hospital services to help clients meet spiritual needs and arrange for clients to participate in these as they are able. Many large hospitals have full-time chaplains who assist clients, support persons, and staff with spiritual needs. For smaller hospitals that do not have chaplains, clergy in the community usually provide this service. Many nursing units have a list of clergy who are on call when needed.

Some agencies have a chapel where religious services are regularly held for clients, support persons, and staff. Most hospitals also have quiet rooms that can be used for meditation, counsel, and even worship services. Sometimes a client prefers to meet the chaplain in a quiet, private room, particularly when the client shares his or her hospital room. A hospital may hold nondenominational religious services or several services for different denominations. If a client expresses a desire to attend services, the nurse needs to help organize the client's care so that attendance is possible if health permits.

The nurse sometimes determines that there is a true conflict between spiritual beliefs and medical therapy. In this case, the nurse encourages the client and physician to discuss the conflict and consider alternative methods of therapy. The nurse always supports the client's right to make an informed decision. If the beliefs of the nurse and client conflict, the nurse should discuss this conflict with the nurse in charge and her or his own spiritual leader. It may be preferable for the client to receive care from a nurse with compatible views. The nurse may also wish to discuss her or his feelings with other health professionals, e.g., other nurses on the team.

Evaluating

To evaluate whether or not the client achieved the goals established during the planning phase, the nurse collects data pertaining to the outcome criteria established. Skill in observation, helping relationships, and communication are required. The nurse needs to observe the client when alone and when interacting with others and listen to what the client says and does not say. See Table 26–1, earlier.

CHAPTER HIGHLIGHTS

▸ The spiritual needs of clients and support persons often come into focus at a time of illness.

▸ Nurses must respect the rights of people to hold their own spiritual beliefs and to communicate or not communicate these to others.

▸ Spiritual beliefs and practices are highly personal.

▸ Spiritual and religious beliefs can influence life-style, attitudes, and feelings about illness and death.

▸ Spiritual beliefs often help people accept illness and plan for the future.

▸ A spiritual assessment is best obtained after the nurse has developed a relationship with the client. Information about a client's concept of God or deity, the client's source of hope and strength, the significance of religious practices and rituals, and the relationship the client perceives between health and spiritual beliefs should be obtained.

▶ Spiritual distress may be reflected in a number of behaviors, including depression, anxiety, and verbalizations of fear of death.

▶ Nurses should be aware of their own spiritual beliefs in order to be comfortable assisting others.

▶ Nurses and clergy may intervene directly to help clients and support persons meet spiritual needs.

LEARNING ACTIVITIES

■ Describe the interrelationship between culture, as presented in Chapter 24, and spirituality.

■ Assess your own spiritual and religious beliefs. How might they enhance your professional ability as a nurse? How might they cause personal conflict with your role as a nurse? Are there specific areas of nursing practice where your beliefs might place you in conflict with the client? What would be the best approach to such a situation?

■ If there is a chaplain for your institution, interview him or her to identify what services are provided to clients. If there is no institutional chaplain, is there a ministerial referral list available? If not, create one, including a protestant minister, a priest, a rabbi, and other spiritual/religious support people as appropriate for your community.

READINGS AND REFERENCES

SUGGESTED READINGS

Granstrom, S. L. April 1985. Spiritual care for oncology patients. *Topics in Clinical Nursing* 7:39–45.
   Granstrom discusses how oncology nurses can help their clients clarify their experiences of suffering, doubt, and fear within a framework of faith, hope and love that brings meaning and purpose (i.e., self-actualizing), not in spite of the illness and crisis but because of it.
Henderson, K. J. May 1989. Dying, God, and anger. *Journal of Psychosocial Nursing* 27:17–21.
   Henderson describes how reading psalms from the Bible permits the release of emotional and spiritual pain for the chronically ill and dying. The train of thought in psalms of lament parallels the stages of dying as Kübler-Ross has described them.

RELATED RESEARCH

Sodestrom, K. E., and Martinson, I. M. February 1987. Patient's spiritual coping strategies: A study of nurse and patient perspectives. *Cancer Nursing* 14:41–45.
Soeken, K. L., and Carson, V. J. April 1986. Study measures nurses' attitudes about providing spiritual care. *Health Progress* 67:52–55.

SELECTED REFERENCES

Brooke, V. July/August 1987. The spiritual well-being of the elderly. *Geriatric Nursing* 8:194–95.
Burkhardt, M. A., and Nagai-Jacobson, M. G. April 1985. Dealing with spiritual concerns of clients in the community. *Journal of Community Health Nursing* 2:191–98.
Burnard, P. May 1987. Spiritual distress and the nursing response: Theoretical considerations and counselling skills. *Journal of Advanced Nursing* 12:377–82.
Carpenito, L. J. 1989. Nursing diagnosis. *Application to Clinical Practice*. 3d ed. Philadelphia: J. B. Lippincott Co.
Carson, V. B. 1989. *Spiritual dimensions of nursing practice*. Philadelphia: W. B. Saunders Co.
Ellison, C. W. April 1983. Spiritual well-being: Conceptualization and measurement. *Journal of Psychology and Theology* 11:330–40.
Fehring, R. J., and McLane, A. M. 1989. Value belief: Spiritual distress (distress of the human spirit). In Thompson, J. M.; McFarland, G. K.; Hirsch, J. E.; Tucker, S. M.; and Bowers, A. C., editors. pp. 1821–25. *Mosby's manual of clinical nursing* 2d ed. St. Louis: C. V. Mosby.
Forbis, P. A. May/June 1988. Meeting patients' spiritual needs: Helping patients to fulfill their spiritual needs is part of the nursing process. *Geriatric Nursing* 9:158–59.

Fowler, J. W., and Keen, S. 1985. *Life maps: Conversation on the journey of faith,* Waco, Texas: Word Books.

Highfield, M. F., and Cason, C. June 1983. Spiritual needs of patients: Are they recognized? *Cancer Nursing* 6:187–92.

Kim, M. J.; McFarland, G. K.; and McLane, A. M., editors. 1984. *Classification of nursing diagnoses* St. Louis: C. V. Mosby Co.

———. 1989. *Pocket guide to nursing diagnoses.* 3d ed. St. Louis: C. V. Mosby Co.

Labun, E. May 1988. Spiritual care: An element in nursing care planning. *Journal of Advanced Nursing* 13:314–20.

Lyon, J. L., and Nelson, S. May/June 1988. Mormon health. *Health Values* 12:37–44.

Murray, R. B., and Zentner, J. B. 1989. *Nursing assessment and health promotion strategies through the life span.* 4th ed. Norwalk, Conn.: Appleton & Lange.

Nagai-Jacobson, M. G., and Burkhardt, M. A. May 1989. Spirituality: Cornerstone of holistic nursing practice. *Holistic Nursing Practice* 3:18–26.

O'Brien, M. E. 1982. The need for spiritual integrity. In Yura, H., and Walsh, M., editors. pp. 81–115. *Human needs 2 and the nursing process.* Norwalk, Conn.: Appleton-Century-Crofts.

Pilch, J. J. May/June 1988. Wellness spirituality. *Health Values* 12:28–31.

Piles, C. L. January/February 1990. Providing spiritual care. *Nurse Education Today* 15:36–41.

Saylor, D. February 1990. Pastoral care: The chaplain's perspective. *Journal of Nursing Administration* 20:15–19.

Shelly, J. A., and Fish, S. 1988. *Spiritual care: The nurse's role.* 3d ed. Downers Grove, Ill.: Inter Varsity Press.

Stoll, R. T. September 1979. Guidelines for spiritual assessment. *American Journal of Nursing* 79:1574–77.

———. 1989. The essence of spirituality. In Carson, V. B., editor. *Spiritual dimensions of nursing practice.* Philadelphia: W. B. Saunders Co.

Coping with Loss, Grieving, and Death

LOSS

Loss is an actual or potential situation in which a valued object, person, or the like is inaccessible or changed so that it is missing from the person's life. People can experience the loss of body image, a significant other, a sense of well-being, a job, personal possessions, beliefs, a sense of self, and so on. Illness and hospitalization often produce losses.

Death is a fundamental loss, both for the dying person and for those who survive. Although death is inevitable for everyone, it is a lonely experience that each person ultimately faces alone. Yet even death, like loss, can stimulate people to grow in perception of both themselves and others. Death can be viewed not simply as loss of life, but as the dying person's final opportunity to experience life in ways that bring meaning and fulfillment.

Types and Sources of Loss

There are two general types of loss, actual and perceived. Both actual losses and perceived losses can be anticipatory. An actual loss can be identified by others and can arise either in response to or in anticipation of a situation. For example, a woman whose husband is dying may experience actual loss in anticipation of his death. A perceived loss is experienced by one person but cannot be verified by others. Psychologic losses are often perceived losses, in that they are not directly verifiable. For example, a woman who leaves her employment to care for her children at home may perceive a loss of independence and freedom. An *anticipatory loss* is experienced before the loss really occurs.

There are many sources of loss: (a) loss of an aspect of oneself—a body part, a physiologic function, or a psychologic attribute, (b) loss of an object external to oneself, (c) separation from an accustomed environment, and (d) loss of a loved or valued person.

Aspect of Self The loss of an aspect of self changes a person's body image, even though the loss may not be obvious to others. A face scarred from a burn is generally obvious to people; loss of part of the stomach or loss of ability to feel emotion may not be as obvious. The degree to which these losses affect a person largely depends on the integrity of the person's body image (part of self-concept). Sometimes changes in self-image affect a person's social roles, such as employee, father, and husband. Any change that the person perceives as negative in the way the person relates to the environment can be considered a loss of self.

Losses such as divorce can have considerable impact. A divorce may mean loss of financial security, a home, and daily routines. Therefore, even when the divorce was desired, the sense of loss can last for some time afterward.

During old age, dramatic changes occur in physical and mental capabilities. Again the self-image is vulnerable, and support and reassurance are important. Old age is when people usually experience many losses: of employment, of usual activities, of independence, of health, of friends, and of family.

External Objects Loss of external objects includes (a) loss of inanimate objects that have importance to the person, such as the loss of money for a person without financial means, or the burning down of a family's house, and (b) loss of animate objects such as pets that provide love and companionship.

Accustomed Environment Separation from an environment and people who provide security can result in a sense of loss. The 6-year-old sheltered by home and family is likely to feel loss when first attending school and relating to more people. The university student who moves away from home for the first time also experiences a sense of loss.

Loved Ones The loss of a loved one or valued person through illness, separation, or death can be very disturbing. In illness such as brain damage from viral infec-

tion or stroke, a person may undergo personality changes that make friends and family feel they have lost that person.

The death of a loved one is a permanent and complete loss. In primitive societies, death was considered a normal, natural event, and life was seldom long. The death of a young man brought greater grief than the deaths of women, children, or elderly people. In contemporary North American society, death is considered unacceptable and usually occurs in private, unless there is an accident. Death often happens in a hospital or in a home in the presence of immediate family. There is a tendency to prolong and preserve life. The culture reveres youthfulness; although people expect to live to old age, this is not considered as attractive as youth.

Loss as Crisis

Loss, especially loss of life or a loved one, can be viewed as either a situational or developmental crisis. The loss of a job or the loss of a young child, for example, is usually an unexpected situational crisis. On the other hand, losses incurred in the process of normal development—such as the departure of grown children from the home, retirement from a career, and the death of aged parents—are developmental crises that can be anticipated and, to some extent, prepared for.

How individuals deal with loss is closely related to their stage of development, personal resources, and social support systems. In dealing with loss of life, the nurse needs to consider the influence of these factors on the dying person and the surviving loved ones. As with all people in crisis, the experience of a dying person cannot be properly understood apart from the social context (Hoff 1984). In crisis situations, including the crisis of death, it is important for the nurse to consider the entire family as the client of care.

Bereavement and Grief

Bereavement is the subjective response to a loss through the death of a person with whom there has been a significant relationship. *Grief* is the total response to the emotional experience of the loss and is manifested in thoughts, feelings, and behaviors (Martocchio 1985, p. 327). *Mourning* is the behavioral process through which grief is eventually resolved or altered; it is often influenced by culture and custom.

Bereavement and grief cannot be viewed as a single crisis but rather are a series of crises that constitute a "life transition period" (Demi and Miles 1986). To view death as a single crisis can mislead caregivers into believing that short-term crisis intervention will bring positive resolution of the grief experience. In fact, normal bereavement can last as long as a year or more. Dealing with death loss is complex and intensely emotional and should not be oversimplified.

Age and the Impact of Loss

Age affects a person's understanding of and reaction to loss. With experience, people usually increase their understanding and acceptance of life, loss, and death. As in other aspects of human development, children show more rapid and dramatic variation and changes in their understanding of death. Their understanding is susceptible to influence by outside events, such as life-threatening illness, which usually deepens the child's understanding of death and makes it more like that of an adult

(Fetsch 1984). Table 27–1 outlines the development of the concept of death through the life span.

People do not usually experience the loss of life or loved ones at regular intervals. As a result, preparation for these experiences is difficult. Coping with other losses of life, such as the loss of a pet, the loss of a friend, and the loss of youth or a job, can help people anticipate the more severe loss of death by teaching them successful coping strategies.

Childhood   Children differ from adults not only in their understanding of loss and death, but also in how they are affected by the loss of others. The child's patterns progress rapidly; adult patterns of growth and development are generally stable. The loss of a parent or other significant person can threaten the child's ability to develop, and regression sometimes results. Assisting the child with the grief experience includes helping the

TABLE 27-1   *Development of the Concept of Death*

Age	Beliefs/Attitudes	Age	Beliefs/Attitudes
Infancy to 5 years	Does not understand concept of death	12 to 18 years	Fears a lingering death
	Infant's sense of separation forms basis for later understanding of loss and death		May fantasize that death can be defied, acting out defiance through reckless behaviors, e.g., dangerous driving, substance abuse
	Believes death is reversible, a temporary departure, or sleep		Seldom thinks about death, but views it in religious and philosophic terms
	Emphasizes immobility and inactivity as attributes of death		May seem to reach "adult" perception of death but be emotionally unable to accept it
5 to 9 years	Understands that death is final		
	Believes own death can be avoided		May still hold concepts from previous developmental stages
	Associates death with aggression or violence	18 to 45 years	Has attitude toward death influenced by religious and cultural beliefs
	Believes wishes or unrelated actions can be responsible for death	45 to 65 years	Accepts own mortality
9 to 12 years	Understands death as the inevitable end of life		Encounters death of parents and some peers
	Begins to understand own mortality, expressed as interest in afterlife or as fear of death		Experiences peaks of death anxiety
			Death anxiety diminishes with emotional well-being
	Expresses ideas about death gathered from parents and other adults	65 years +	Fears prolonged illness
			Encounters death of family members and peers
			Sees death as having multiple meanings, e.g., freedom from pain, reunion with already deceased family members

child regain the normal continuity and pace of emotional development.

Adults often assume that children do not have the same need as an adult to grieve the loss of others. In situations of crisis and loss, children are sometimes pushed aside or protected from the pain. They can feel afraid, abandoned, and lonely. Careful work with bereaved children is especially necessary, because experiencing a loss in childhood can have serious effects later in life. Research suggests a connection between early loss of a parent through death or divorce and increased risk of depression or suicide in adulthood (Taylor 1983–84).

Early and Middle Adulthood   As people grow, loss comes to be experienced as part of normal development. By middle age, for example, the loss of a parent through death seems a normal occurrence compared to the death of a younger person. Coping with the death of an aged parent has even been viewed as a necessary developmental task of the middle-aged adult. Society does not support intense or prolonged mourning for such a normal event (Moss and Moss 1983–84).

For the middle-aged adult, the loss of a parent can signal the disintegration of the family of origin. It is also a forceful reminder that the adult child is part of the older generation and therefore closer to death. The challenge of this developmental crisis for adult children is to assess the psychologic legacy of the parent, integrating what is valuable into their own identity. If the relationship with the parent was full of conflict, the parent's death can help release the child's energy for more productive use.

Late Adulthood   For older adults, the loss through death of a long-time mate is profound. Though individuals differ in their ability to deal with such a loss, research suggests an increase in health problems for widows and widowers during the first year following the death of spouse (Richter 1984). Because the majority of deaths occur among the elderly, and because the number of elderly is increasing in North America, nurses will need to be especially alert to the potential problems of older grieving adults.

Educating the Nurse About Loss

People in North America are socialized to think of death as the worst occurrence in life. They therefore do their best to avoid thinking or talking about death—especially their own. Death is thought about rarely, and almost exclusively in negative terms. Nurses are not immune to such attitudes. They need to take time to analyze their own feelings about death before they can effectively help others with a terminal illness. Nurses who are unconsciously uncomfortable with dying clients tend to impede the clients' attempts to discuss dying and death in these ways:

- Changing the subject, e.g., "Let's think of something more cheerful," or "You shouldn't say things like that."

- Offering reassurance, e.g., "You are doing very well."

- Denying what is happening, e.g., "You don't really mean that," or "You're going to live until you are a hundred."

- Being fatalistic, e.g., "Everyone dies sooner or later," or "God will take you when He wants you."

- Blocking discussion, e.g., "I don't think things are really that bad," conveying an attitude that stops further discussion of the subject

- Being aloof and distant or avoiding the client

- "Managing" the client's care and making the client feel increasingly dependent and powerless

The curricula of many nursing schools include education about death. Agencies and associations sponsor continuing education programs aimed at reducing death anxiety among nursing staff. Other programs help nurses explore the specific problems of direct contact with terminally ill clients and around-the-clock responsibility for their care. In all such programs nurses learn not only their own attitudes and concerns but also ways to support and comfort each other when they experience anger and frustration in the grief that follows the death of clients whom they not only cared for but also cared about.

Caring for the dying and the bereaved is one of the nurse's most complex and challenging responsibilities, bringing into play all the skills needed for holistic physiologic and psychosocial care. To be effective, nurses must come to grips with their own attitudes toward loss, death, and dying, because these attitudes will directly affect their ability to provide care. Each nurse is personally responsible for actively engaging in a career-long process of education through reading, listening, and self-examination.

GRIEF

Grieving, the normal subjective emotional response to loss, is essential for good mental and physical health. It permits the individual to cope with the loss gradually and to accept it as part of reality. Grief is a social process; it is best shared and carried out with the assistance of others.

Grief work is important, because bereavement has been shown to have potentially devastating effects on health. Among the symptoms that can accompany grief are anxiety, depression, weight loss, difficulties in swallowing, vomiting, fatigue, headaches, dizziness, fainting, blurred vision, skin rashes, excessive sweating, menstrual disturbances, palpitations, chest pain, dyspnea, and infection (Gonda and Ruark 1984). The bereaved may also experience alterations in libido, concentration, and patterns of eating, sleeping, activity, and communication.

Although bereavement can threaten health, a positive resolution of the grieving process can enrich the individual with new insights, values, challenges, openness, and sensitivity. This applies to both the dying person and surviving loved ones, for the dying person is also living. If the quality of life permits, the dying person also should have the opportunity to grow emotionally and spiritually in the time that remains.

Stages of Grieving

Many authors have described stages or phases of grieving, perhaps the most famous of them being Kübler-Ross, who has described five stages: denial, anger, bargaining, depression, and acceptance (Kübler-Ross 1969, pp. 38–137). See Table 27–2. Engel (1964, pp. 94–96)

TABLE 27-2 *Kübler-Ross's Stages of Grieving*

Stage	Behavioral Responses	Nursing Implications
Denial	Refuses to believe that loss is happening Is unready to deal with practical problems, such as prosthesis after loss of leg May assume artificial cheerfulness to prolong denial	Verbally support client's denial for its protective function. Examine your own behavior to ensure that you do not share in client's denial.
Anger	Client or family may direct anger at nurse or hospital staff about matters that normally would not bother them	Help client understand that anger is a normal response to feelings of loss and powerlessness. Avoid withdrawal or retaliation with anger; do not take anger personally. Deal with needs underlying any angry reaction. Provide structure and continuity to promote feelings of security. Allow clients as much control as possible over their lives.
Bargaining	Seeks to bargain to avoid loss May express feelings of guilt or fear of punishment for past sins, real or imagined	Listen attentively, and encourage client to talk to relieve guilt and irrational fears. If appropriate, offer spiritual support.
Depression	Grieves over what has happened and what cannot be May talk freely (e.g., reviewing past losses such as money or job), or may withdraw	Allow client to express sadness. Communicate nonverbally by sitting quietly without expecting conversation. Convey caring by touch. Help support persons understand importance of being with the client in silence.
Acceptance	Comes to terms with loss May have decreased interest in surroundings and support persons May wish to begin making plans, e.g., will, prosthesis, altered living arrangements	Help family and friends understand client's decreased need to socialize and need for short, quiet visits. Encourage client to participate as much as possible in the treatment program.

TABLE 27-3 Engel's Stages of Grieving

Stage	Behavioral Responses
Shock and disbelief	Refusal to accept loss
	Stunned feelings
	Intellectual acceptance but emotional denial
Developing awareness	Reality of loss begins to penetrate consciousness
	Anger may be directed at hospital, nurses, etc.
	Crying and self-blame
Restitution	Rituals of mourning, e.g., funeral
Resolving the loss	Attempts to deal with painful void
	Still unable to accept new love object to replace lost person
	May accept more dependent relationship with support person
	Thinks over and talks about memories of the dead person
Idealization	Produces image of dead person that is almost devoid of undesirable features
	Represses all negative and hostile feelings toward deceased
	May feel guilty and remorseful about past inconsiderate or unkind acts to deceased
	Unconsciously internalizes admired qualities of deceased
	Reminders of deceased evoke fewer feelings of sadness
	Reinvests feelings in others
Outcome	Behavior influenced by several factors: importance of lost object as source of support, degree of dependence on relationship, degree of ambivalence toward deceased, number and nature of other relationships, and number and nature of previous grief experiences (which tend to be cumulative)

Source: G. L. Engel, Grief and grieving. *American Journal of Nursing,* September 1964, 64:93–98. Used by permission.

has identified six stages of grieving: shock and disbelief, developing awareness, restitution, resolving the loss, idealization, and outcome. See Table 27–3.

Nurses also have begun to write about the components of grief. Clark (1984) describes a three-phase course through which the bereaved progresses, lasting 6 months to 2 years. Martocchio (1985) discusses five clusters of grief and maintains that there is no single correct way, nor a correct timetable, by which a person progresses through the grief process. Whether a person can succeed in integrating the loss, and how this is accomplished, is related to that person's individual development and personal makeup. Individuals responding to the very same loss cannot be expected to follow the same pattern or schedule in resolving their grief, even while they support each other. Martocchio's five clusters of grief include the following:

1. *Shock and disbelief.* A feeling of numbness is a common response immediately following the death of a loved one. The bereaved may feel depressed, angry, guilty, and sad. Disbelief or denial may persist even though the loss has been accepted intellectually.

2. *Yearning and protest.* The anger that the bereaved feel may be directed at the deceased for having died, at God, at others whose loved ones are still alive, or at the caregivers. The bereaved may begin to fear their own mental deterioration and withdraw from sharing their thoughts and feelings with others.

3. *Anguish, disorganization, and despair.* When the reality of the loss is genuinely admitted, depression can set in. Weeping is common at this time. The bereaved lose interest and motivation in pursuing the future, are unable to make decisions, and lack confidence and purpose. Activities that were once enjoyed with the deceased are now without attraction. Coping strategies such as excessive drinking may compromise health.

4. *Identification in bereavement.* The bereaved may take on the behavior, personal traits, habits, and ambitions of the deceased. Sometimes they may also experience the same symptoms of physical illness.

5. *Reorganization and restitution.* Achieving stability and a sense of reintegration can take a period of time that ranges widely, from less than a year to several years. Although the bereaved are able to experience a sense of well-being and can resume most normal patterns of functioning, the feelings of grief do not simply cease. For many the pain of loss, though diminished, recurs for the rest of their lives.

A normal grief reaction may be abbreviated or anticipatory. _Abbreviated grief is brief but genuinely felt._ The lost object may not have been sufficiently important to the grieving person or may have been replaced immediately by another, equally esteemed object. _Anticipatory grief is experienced in advance of the event._ The wife who grieves before her ailing husband dies is anticipating the loss. A beauty queen may grieve in advance of an operation that will leave a scar on her body. Because many of the normal symptoms of grief will have already been expressed in anticipation, the reaction when the loss actually occurs may be quite abbreviated.

Unhealthy grief—that is, _pathologic_ or _dysfunctional grief_—may be unresolved or inhibited. Both normal and unhealthy grief may be delayed. Many factors can contribute to dysfunctional grief, including a prior traumatic loss in childhood and the circumstances of the present loss. For instance, the sudden, untimely death of an adolescent or young adult can complicate the expression and resolution of grief. Other influences include family or cultural barriers to the emotional expression of grief.

Unresolved grief is extended in length and severity. The same signs are expressed as with normal grief, but the bereaved may also have difficulty expressing the grief, may deny the loss, or may grieve beyond the expected time. With _inhibited grief,_ many of the normal symptoms of grief are suppressed, and other effects, including somatic, are experienced instead.

Burgess and Lazare (1976, p. 100) state that dysfunctional grief may be inferred from the following data or observations:

- The client fails to grieve following the death of a loved one; e.g., a husband does not cry at, or absents himself from, his wife's funeral.

- The client becomes recurrently symptomatic on the anniversary of a loss or during holidays (especially Thanksgiving and Christmas).

- The client avoids visiting the grave and refuses to participate in religious memorial services of a loved one, even though these practices are a part of the client's culture.

- The client develops persistent guilt and lowered self-esteem.

- Even after a prolonged period, the client continues to search for the lost person. Some make the search while in fugue states. Others may wander from town to town or act as if they were expecting the deceased to return. Some may consider suicide to effect reunion.

- A relatively minor event triggers symptoms of grief.

- Even after a period of time, the client is unable to discuss the deceased with equanimity, e.g., the client's voice cracks and quivers, eyes become moist.

- An interview of the client is characterized by themes of loss.

- After the normal period of grief, the client experiences physical symptoms similar to those of the person who died.

- The client's relationships with friends and relatives worsen following the death.

Many factors contribute to _unresolved grief_ (Burgess and Lazare 1976, pp. 97–100):

- Ambivalence (intense feelings of both love and hate) toward the lost person. The bereaved is often afraid to grieve for fear of discovering unacceptable negative feelings.

- A perceived need to be brave and in control; fear of losing control in front of others.

- Endurance of multiple losses, such as the loss of an entire family, which the bereaved finds too overwhelming to contemplate.

- Extremely high emotional value (overcathexis) invested in the dead person. Failure to grieve in this instance helps the bereaved avoid the reality of the loss.

- Uncertainty about the loss—for example, when a loved one is "missing in action."

- Lack of support persons.

- Subjection to socially unacceptable loss that cannot be spoken about, e.g., suicide, abortion, or giving a child up for adoption.

Assessing Loss and Grieving

To gather a complete database that allows accurate analysis and identification of appropriate nursing diagnoses for clients experiencing losses and grieving, the nurse first needs to recognize the state of awareness the client and family manifest, the symptoms of grief, and the factors influencing a loss reaction.

States of Awareness   In cases of terminal illness, the state of awareness shared by the dying person and the family affects the nurse's ability to communicate freely with clients and other health care team members and to assist in the grieving process. Three types of awareness that have been described are closed awareness, mutual pretense, and open awareness (Strauss and Glaser 1970, p. 300).

In *closed awareness,* the client and family are unaware of impending death. They may not completely understand why the client is ill, and they believe the client will recover. The physician may believe it is best not to communicate a diagnosis or prognosis to the client or family. Nursing personnel are confronted with an ethical problem in this situation, and they have several choices. One course is to answer questions evasively or falsely. But ultimately the client and family will know the truth, and when they do they may recognize that information given them earlier was false. See Chapter 11 for further information on ethical dilemmas.

With *mutual pretense,* the client, family, and health personnel know that the prognosis is terminal but do not talk about it and make an effort not to raise the subject. Sometimes the client refrains from discussing death to protect the family from distress. The client may also sense discomfort on the part of health personnel and therefore not bring up the subject. Mutual pretense permits the client a degree of privacy and dignity, but it places a heavy burden on the dying person, who then has no one in whom to confide fears.

With *open awareness,* the client and people around know about the impending death and feel comfortable about discussing it, even though it is difficult. This awareness provides the client an opportunity to finalize affairs and even participate in planning funeral arrangements. One study indicates that nurses prefer the state of open awareness and prefer to become emotionally involved with their clients, since it "allows them to fully implement their ideal of nursing care" (Field 1984, p. 67).

Not all people can handle open awareness. For example, a 45-year-old man who knows he is dying may be unable to discuss his forthcoming death without becoming angry at people around him. Whether to inform dying clients that their condition is terminal is a difficult issue for physicians. Some authorities believe that terminal clients acquire knowledge of their condition even if they are not directly informed. Others believe that many clients remain unaware of their condition until the end. It is difficult, however, to distinguish what clients know from what they are willing to accept. A study by Cappon (1970) asked groups of healthy persons, physically ill clients, psychiatric clients, and dying clients whether they would like to know if a serious illness was terminal. The majority responded yes; however, of the four groups, the dying least desired this information (33% did not want to be told). Cappon concluded that

physicians should be cautious and not give more information than the client wants.

Symptoms of Grief   The nurse assesses the grieving client and/or family members following a loss to determine the phase or stage of grieving. The following clinical symptoms of grief are described by Schulz (1978, pp. 142–43):

- Repeated somatic distress
- Tightness in the chest
- Choking or shortness of breath
- Sighing
- Empty feeling in the abdomen
- Loss of muscular power
- Intense subjective distress

Physiologically, the body responds to a current or anticipated loss with a stress reaction. The nurse can assess the clinical signs of this response (see Chapter 23). See also coping mechanisms and responses in Chapter 23.

Factors Influencing a Loss Reaction   The influence of age and developmental level on a person's reaction to loss has already been discussed. Other factors include the personal significance of the loss, culture, spiritual beliefs, sex role, and socioeconomic status.

Significance of the loss   The significance of a loss depends on the perceptions of the individual experiencing the loss. One person may experience a great sense of loss over a divorce; another may find it only mildly disrupting. A number of factors affect the significance of the loss:

- Age of the person
- Value placed on the lost person, body part, and so on
- Degree of change required because of the loss
- The person's beliefs and values

Expectations can also greatly affect significance. For elderly people who have already encountered many losses (e.g., family, health, independence), an anticipated loss such as their own death may not be important; they may be apathetic about it instead of reactive. More than fearing death, some may fear loss of control or becoming a burden (Charmaz 1980, p. 77).

Culture   Culture influences an individual's reaction to loss. How grief is expressed is often determined by the customs of the culture. It has been suggested that the Protestant ethic—individualism, self-reliance, independence, and hard work—leads to the practice of handling grief only with significant others, not a larger community (Charmaz 1980, p. 284). In the United States and Canada, unless an extended family structure exists, grief is handled by the nuclear family, which, because of its small size, emphasizes self-reliance and independence.

Many Americans appear to have internalized the belief that grief is a private matter to be endured internally. Therefore, feelings tend to be repressed and may remain unidentified. People who have been socialized to "be strong" and "make the best of the situation" may not express deep feelings or personal concerns when they experience a serious loss.

Some cultural groups value social support and the expression of loss. In certain black churches, the expression of emotion plays a prominent part. In Hispanic American groups where strong kinship ties are maintained, support and assistance are provided by family members, and the free expression of grief is encouraged.

Spiritual beliefs　Spiritual beliefs and practices greatly influence both a person's reaction to loss and subsequent behavior. Most religious groups have practices related to dying, which are often important to the client and support persons. For additional information, see Chapter 26. To provide support at a time of death, nurses need to understand the client's particular beliefs and practices.

Sex role　The sex roles into which many people are socialized in the United States and Canada affect their reactions at times of loss. Men are frequently expected to "be strong" and show very little emotion during grief, whereas it is acceptable for women to show grief by crying. Often when a wife dies, the husband, who is the chief mourner, is expected to repress his own emotions and to comfort sons and daughters in their grieving.

Sex roles also affect the significance of body image changes to clients. A man might consider a facial scar to be "macho," but a woman might consider it ugly. Thus, the woman, but not the man, would see it as a loss.

Socioeconomic status　The socioeconomic status of an individual often affects the support system available at the time of a loss. A pension plan or insurance, for example, can offer a widowed or disabled person choices of ways to deal with a loss: A woman who loses a hand and can no longer do her previous work may be able to pursue vocational reeducation; a man whose wife has died may be able to afford to take a cruise or visit relatives in Europe. Conversely, a person who is confronted with both severe loss and economic hardship may not be able to cope with either.

Diagnosing

Many of the NANDA nursing diagnoses apply to grieving clients, depending on the information obtained from individual assessment. Some diagnoses that may be applicable are **Anticipatory grieving, Dysfunctional grieving, Impaired adjustment,** and **Social isolation. Anticipatory grieving** is often a healthy response. It is used as a diagnosis when the client expresses sorrow, anger, or guilt about the potential loss and experiences changes in eating habits, sleep patterns, activity levels, and communication.

Dysfunctional grieving is the state in which an individual or group experiences prolonged unresolved grief and engages in detrimental activities (Carpenito 1989, p. 364). This diagnosis is not appropriate until several months or a year after the loss. It is appropriate when the nurse assesses that the client is not performing usual expected roles, denies the loss, has continued difficulty in expressing the loss, has continued alterations in sleep patterns, and fails to develop new relationships or interests. See also the manifestations described earlier.

Impaired adjustment may be the diagnosis for clients with loss of a body part or physiologic function. It is the "state in which the individual is unable to modify his/her behavior or lifestyle in a manner consistent with a change in health status" (Kim et al. 1989, p. 2). Such clients may verbalize nonacceptance of the change in health status, lack movement toward independence, or be unable to limit expectations of self. This diagnosis can be applied either to the person suffering the loss or to a significant other. For instance, the husband of a woman hospitalized with a life-threatening illness may feel unable to assume unaccustomed domestic duties, such as child care, and he may feel resentment because the disease has removed the person who maintained the stability of family life. The athlete who suffers a sudden heart attack might also be diagnosed with **Impaired adjustment.** The reduced capacity for physical exertion that the condition imposes may threaten self-image and self-esteem.

Social isolation occurs when the painful nature of grief causes those experiencing it to withdraw from their normal social support systems. These clients may have a

RESEARCH NOTE

What Responses Can Nurses Expect of the Bereaved?

The purpose of this study was to identify themes associated with bereavement. An analysis of 30 narrative accounts revealed nine themes: five core themes, three meta-themes, and one contextual theme. The *core themes* are *being stopped* (the interruption of life's usual flow following the death of a loved one, characterized by varying degrees of inability, frequently stated in terms of "I can't"); *hurting* (cluster of intensely painful emotions); *missing* (acute awareness of all that has been lost); *holding* (desire to maintain all, particularly that which was good, from the loved one's lost existence); and *seeking* (a search for help).

The *meta-themes* are *change* (the dynamic, change-inducing character, or wavelike quality, of bereavement); *expectations* (a sense of "rightness" or "ought-ness" that hovers over bereavement); and *inexpressibility* (inadequacy of words to describe the experience).

The one *contextual theme, personal history,* is the theme in which the five core themes are embedded and is the one essential to understanding the quality of bereavement. These themes were compared with three theoretical perspectives on bereavement by Freud, Kübler-Ross, and one existential-phenomenological perspective. Features of bereavement that are dissimilar or unaddressed by the theoretical perspectives are (a) the quality of grief's changing character, (b) holding, (c) expectations of how the bereaved should overlay the experience, and (d) how the personal history affects the quality and meaning of the loss.

Implications: Using these themes as a guide, nurses can expect a broad range of unique responses from the bereaved. In particular, nurses need to understand the changing character of grief that may be triggered years after the death. Obtaining a personal history is critically important in determining the quality and meaning of the person's bereavement.

S. L. Carter, Themes of grief, *Nursing Research,* November/December 1989, 38:354–58.

sad, dull affect, be uncommunicative and withdrawn, express feelings of loneliness, and lack supportive others. Some people feel the need to display mastery of the situation or wish not to burden friends. They may be afraid to test the strength of friendships. A new widow, for example, might feel awkward maintaining a social relationship in the circle of married couples she had participated in with her husband.

Social support is a major positive influence on the successful resolution of grief (Richter 1984). **Social isolation,** as a nursing diagnosis, can therefore be useful in directing nursing interventions that help the client to build the necessary support network.

Altered family processes occur when a family that normally functions effectively experiences a dysfunction. Discussion about this diagnosis is in Chapter 16.

Examples of these diagnoses and contributing factors follow.

Anticipatory grieving related to:

- Perceived potential loss of loved one
- Perceived potential loss of body part or function
- Perceived potential loss of physiopsychosocial well-being
- Perceived potential loss of personal possessions
- Perceived potential loss of social role
- Perceived impending death of self

Dysfunctional grieving related to:

- Multiple past or current losses
- Lack of resolution of previous grieving response
- Unresolved guilt related to the deceased
- Lack of adequate social supports
- Unconscious gain from others to maintain grieving
- Difficulty or inability to express feelings freely

Impaired adjustment related to:

- Disability requiring change in life-style
- Inadequate or unavailable support systems
- Impaired cognition
- Ineffective denial

Social isolation related to:

- Inability to engage in satisfying personal relationships
- Inadequate personal resources

- Alterations in physical appearance
- Altered state of wellness

Planning

The goals of grieving are to be able to remember the lost object or person without intense pain and to be able to redirect emotional energy into one's own life and regain the capacity to love. More specifically, the client needs to (a) feel free from emotional bondage to the deceased person, (b) be able to adjust to the changed environment, (c) be capable of developing new relationships and renewing old ones, and (d) feel comfortable with both positive and negative memories of the deceased (Martocchio 1985).

Examples of outcome criteria for grieving clients follow.

The client:

- Verbalizes feelings of sorrow (or anger or loss).
- Shares thoughts and feelings with significant others.
- Uses appropriate resources (e.g., friends, clergy, support groups).
- Resumes usual activities (e.g., activities of daily living, work, recreation).
- Maintains constructive interpersonal relationships.
- Establishes new relationships.
- Verbalizes sense of progress toward resolution of the grief.
- Identifies alternative plans for meeting goals that were important before the loss.

Implementing

The skills most relevant to situations of loss and grief are attentive listening, silence, open and closed questioning, paraphrasing, clarifying and reflecting feelings, and summarizing. Less helpful to clients are responses that give advice and evaluation, those that interpret and analyze, and those that give unwarranted reassurance (Martocchio 1985). To ensure effective communication, the nurse must make an accurate assessment of what is appropriate for the client.

Communication with grieving clients needs to be relevant to their stage of grief. Whether the client is angry or depressed affects how the client hears messages and how the nurse interprets the client's statements. Implications for nurse-client communication are related to Kübler-Ross's five stages in Table 27–2, earlier.

Assisting Clients with Their Grief

- Provide opportunity for the persons involved to "tell their story."
- Recognize and accept the varied emotions that people express in relation to a significant loss.
- Provide support for the expression of difficult feelings, such as anger and sadness, recognizing that people must do this in their own way and at their own pace.
- Include children in the grieving process.
- Encourage the bereaved to maintain established relationships.
- Acknowledge the usefulness of mutual-help groups.
- Encourage self-care by family members—in particular, the primary caregiver.
- Acknowledge the usefulness of counseling for especially difficult problems.

Source: J. Q. Benoliel, Loss and terminal illness, *Nursing Clinics of North America,* June 1985, 20:445.

The guidelines in the box above can assist nurses in helping the bereaved.

Evaluating

Evaluating the effectiveness of nursing care of the grieving client is difficult because of the long-term nature of the life transition. Criteria for evaluation must be based on goals set by the client and family, and not on an arbitrary standard of success (Benoliel 1985). A follow-up visit to the surviving family members may be an appropriate nursing measure not only to obtain information for evaluation but also to assist nurses in working through their own grief by expressing their continuing concern for the family.

CARE OF THE DYING CLIENT

Assessing

Nursing care and support for the dying client and family include making an accurate assessment of the physiologic signs of approaching death. In addition to signs related to the client's specific disease, certain other physical signs are indicative of impending death. The four main characteristic changes are loss of muscle tone, slowing of the circulation, changes in vital signs, and sensory impairment.

Various consciousness levels occur just before death. Some clients are alert, whereas others are drowsy, stuporous, or comatose. Hearing is thought to be the last sense lost.

The traditional *clinical signs of death* were cessation of the apical pulse, respirations, and blood pressure. However, since the advent of artificial means to maintain respirations and blood circulation, identifying death is more difficult. In 1968, the World Medical Assembly adopted the following guidelines for physicians as indications of death (Benton 1978, p. 18):

- Total lack of response to external stimuli
- No muscular movement, especially breathing
- No reflexes
- Flat electroencephalogram

In instances of artificial support, absence of electric currents from the brain (measured by an electroencephalogram) for at least 24 hours is an indication of death. Only a physician can pronounce death, and only after this pronouncement can life-support systems be shut off.

Another definition of death is cerebral death, which occurs when the higher brain center, the cerebral cortex, is irreversibly destroyed. The client may still be able to breathe but is irreversibly unconscious. Brain death can be determined only when the client is not under the influence of CNS depressant drugs.

A special concern for the nurse is the family of the client who has been determined "brain dead" and is a candidate for donor organs. In this situation, the family and loved ones may feel guilty or confused as they view their loved one's normal heart function on a cardiac monitor. Careful explanations will ensure that the family understands the finality of the client's injury despite the appearances of normal function.

Diagnosing

The full range of nursing diagnoses, addressing both physiologic and psychosocial needs, can be applied to the dying client, depending on the assessment data. Three diagnoses that may be particularly appropriate are **Fear, Hopelessness,** and **Powerlessness.**

Fear   The diagnosis of **Fear** was discussed in detail in Chapter 23. Many fears are associated with death, and the nurse needs to determine a client's specific fears. Gonda and Ruark (1984, pp. 31–32) discuss three objects of the dying person's fear: the process of dying, nonexistence, and what comes after death. The nurse is usually better able to assist a client with the complex process of dying than with the spiritual fears of nonexistence and the hereafter.

Schulz (1978, p. 27) outlines the following fears related to a person's own death: pain, body misfunction, humiliation, rejection or abandonment, nonbeing, punishment, interruption of goals, and negative impact on survivors (e.g., psychologic suffering, economic hardship).

Sheehy (1981, pp. 27–62), in his discussion about common fears of dying, includes fear of pain, loneliness, dependence, the moment of death, and annihilation. Although there is no pain at the moment of death and the transition from life to death seems easy, many people fear this moment. Sheehy believes that fear of the moment of death is the result of the emotional sting and pain experienced during the death of a parent. People remember this previous pain and, therefore, believe that dying is painful. Fear of annihilation, or being reduced to nothingness after death, and questions about immortality need to be faced. Does immortality rest in what the individual achieved in this life, or does the soul survive after death? Whatever a person believes about life after death, both body and mind may be viewed as reentering the universe and becoming part of it as some form of energy.

Hopelessness   The very nature of a terminal illness or any other dying process can lead to a client's loss of hope. The nurse can identify this subjective state by noting some of the following behaviors: (a) passivity, (b) decreased verbalization, (c) decreased affect, (d) verbal cues (sighing, "I can't," or "Why bother?"), (e) lack of initiative, and (f) decreased response to stimuli. Feelings of hopelessness often follow an awareness of the reality of the loss and may be expressed in the despair phase of mourning (Gonda and Ruark 1984, p. 38). Real or perceived abandonment can also mean a diagnosis of **Hopelessness.** A loss of belief in religious and spiritual values or powers may be related to the development of hopelessness. The return of realistic hope can be facilitated by the nurse through assisting the client and/or family to focus on the outcomes of specific, short-term goals (Gonda and Ruark 1984, pp. 89–90).

Powerlessness   The dying client or the family may express a lack of control over the situation. **Powerlessness** is a likely diagnosis when the impending death is sudden and unexpected or when the dying client is a child. However, this diagnosis is not limited to such situations. Dying clients who have confronted chronic debilitating diseases may perceive that they can no longer control their conditions. The nurse can identify powerlessness by observing the following behaviors: (a) verbal expression of having no control or influence over the situation or outcome, (b) frustration about inability to perform previously mastered activities, (c) aggressive behavior when goals are not achieved, (d) lack of participation in decision making, and (e) feelings of depression or resentment.

Examples of these nursing diagnoses and possible contributing factors follow.

Fear related to:

- Knowledge deficit (concern about pain and inability to cope)
- Lack of social support in threatening situation
- Negative impact on survivors

Hopelessness related to:

- Prolonged restriction of activity resulting in isolation
- Deteriorating physiologic condition
- Terminal illness
- Long-term stress (e.g., chronic pain)
- Perceived significant loss of loved one, youth, influence, opportunity

Powerlessness related to:

- Chronic debilitating disease
- Terminal illness
- Institutional environment
- Interpersonal behavior of others

Planning

Major goals of dying clients are (a) maintaining physiologic and psychologic comfort and (b) achieving a dignified and peaceful death. Outcome criteria for clients with diagnoses of **Fear, Hopelessness,** and **Powerlessness** follow.

The client:

- Is free of pain.
- Participates in self-care activities in accordance with health status.
- Makes choices related to care and treatment.

- Verbalizes feelings of anger, sorrow, or loss.
- Maintains open relationship with support persons and staff.
- Identifies areas of personal control.
- Expresses sense of control over the present situation.
- Expresses feelings of optimism about the present and future.
- Expresses positive feelings about relationships with significant others.
- Shares values and personal meaning of life.
- Reminisces and reviews personal life positively.
- Accepts limitations and seeks help as needed.

Implementing

The major nursing responsibility for clients who are dying is to assist the client to a peaceful death. More specific responsibilities are:

1. To provide relief from loneliness, fear, and depression
2. To maintain the client's sense of security, self-confidence, dignity, and self-worth
3. To maintain hope
4. To help the client accept his or her losses
5. To provide physical comfort

People facing death need help facing the fact that they will have to depend on others. Some dying clients require only minimal care and can be cared for at home; others need continuous attention and the services of a hospital and its staff. People need help, well in advance of death, in planning for the period of dependence. They need to consider what will happen and how and where they would like to die.

Helping Clients Die with Dignity   Dignity may be defined as the ability to function as a significant and integrated person (Sheehy 1981, p. 56). True dignity comes from within. Generally, dependence on others and loss of control over oneself and interactions with the environment are associated with loss of dignity. Dying clients often feel they have lost control over their lives and over life itself. By introducing options available to the client and significant others, nurses can restore and support feelings of control. Some choices that clients can make are the location of care, e.g., hospital, home, or hospice; times of appointments with health professionals; activity schedule; use of health resources; and times of visits from relatives and friends.

Most clients interviewed about dying indicate that they want to be able to manage the events preceding death so they can die peacefully. Nurses can help clients to find meaning and completeness and to determine their own physical, psychologic, and social priorities. Dying people often strive for self-fulfillment more than self-preservation, and they need to find meaning in continuing to live while suffering. Part of the nurse's challenge, then, is to help maintain, day to day, the client's will and hope.

Salter (1982, p. 21) believes it is important for nurses and clients to focus not on the end, but on three stages of living fully until death:

1. *Developing and growing.* In this stage, the client can be assisted to paint, sculpt, go to a library, visit an art gallery, etc. An occupational therapist can help clients do what they still can do and what is pleasurable.

2. *Lying fallow.* In this stage, physiotherapy measures, such as breathing exercises and passive exercises, help the client to relax and enhance self-esteem.

3. *Letting go and becoming dependent.* In this stage, nursing intervention is usually required to meet both physical and psychologic needs.

Hospice and Home Care

Hospice care, palliative care, and home care focus on support and care of the dying person and family, with the goal of facilitating a peaceful and dignified death. Hospice care is based on holistic concepts that emphasize care rather than cure. Its goals are

- Control and relief of pain and symptoms of the illness
- Provision of physical comfort for the terminally ill
- Provision of social, emotional, and spiritual comfort for the client, family, and friends throughout the final stage of illness, at the time of death, and during the bereavement period of the survivors

The principles of hospice care can be carried out in a variety of settings, the most common being the autonomous hospice and the hospital-based palliative-care unit. Palliative care is challenging and requires skillful interpersonal relationships and compassion (see Suggested Readings at the end of this chapter). Services range from fully comprehensive to a focus on selected areas, such as symptom control and pain management, in some palliative care units. Home care services for the dying client maintain the client in the natural home environment until that is no longer possible or until death. Hospice care is always provided by a team of both health professionals and nonprofessionals to ensure a full range of care services. In the United States these services have been delivered primarily through autonomous, community-based hospices. In Canada most hospice programs are hospital-based. This difference may be a function of different methods for funding health care (Corless 1983, pp. 336–39). Both countries have established standards and guidelines for the development and operation of hospice programs (Health and Welfare Canada 1981; National Hospice Organization 1981).

Meeting Physiologic Needs of the Dying Client

The physiologic needs of the dying are related to a slowing of body processes and to homeostatic imbalances. Interventions include personal hygiene measures; pain control; relief of respiratory difficulties; assistance with movement, nutrition, hydration, and elimination; and measures related to sensory changes.

Pain control is essential to enable clients to maintain quality life activities, including eating, moving, and sleeping. Many drugs have been used to control the pain associated with terminal illness: morphine, heroin, methadone, alcohol, marijuana, and LSD. In hospitals the most frequently used agents are morphine, methadone, and alcohol. Usually the physician determines the dosage, but the client's opinion should be considered; the client is the one ultimately aware of personal pain tolerance and fluctuations of internal states. Because of decreased blood circulation, analgesics may be administered by intravenous infusion rather than subcutaneously or intramuscularly.

Spiritual Support

Spiritual support is of great importance in dealing with death. Although not all clients identify with a specific religious faith or belief, the majority have a need for meaning in their lives, particularly as they experience a terminal illness. Conrad (1985, pp. 417–19) has categorized the spiritual needs of the dying as follows:

1. Search for meaning
2. Sense of forgiveness
3. Need for love
4. Need for hope

The nurse has a responsibility to ensure that the client's spiritual needs are attended to, either through direct intervention or by arranging access to individuals who can provide spiritual care. Death-related beliefs and practices of selected religious groups are shown in Table 27–4. Nurses need to be aware of their own comfort

text continues on p. 543

TABLE 27–4 Death-Related Beliefs and Practices of Selected Religious Groups

Group	Afterlife	Rituals/ Funerals	Autopsy	Organ Donation	Cremation	Prolonging Life
American Indian	Beliefs vary	Practices vary; most want family present	Prohibited		Practices vary	
Black Muslim		Special procedures for washing and shrouding the dead; special funeral rites				
Buddhist in America	Reincarnation; after reaching state of enlightenment, may attain nirvana	Last rite; chanting at bedside	No restriction		No restriction	Permit euthanasia in hopeless illness
Church of Christ Scientist	Yes	No last rites	Only in sudden death	No	Individual decision	
Church of Jesus Christ of Latter Day Saints (Mormon)	Yes	Baptism of dead essential; may preach gospel to the dead	No restriction	No restriction	Discouraged	
Eastern Orthodox (Greek and Russian Orthodox)	Yes	Last rites (administration of Holy Communion obligatory for some)	Discouraged		Discouraged	Encouraged
Episcopal (Anglican)	Yes	Last rites not mandatory	No restriction	No restriction	No restriction	
Hindu	Reincarnation; after leading a perfect life, may join Brahma	Priest pours water into mouth of corpse and ties string around wrist or neck as sign of blessing; string must not be removed; family washes body	No restriction	No restriction	Preferred; ashes cast in holy river	
Islam (Moslem, Muslim)	May join Allah by being a good Moslem and observing rituals daily	Dying person must confess sins and ask forgiveness in presence of family; family washes and prepares body (female body cannot be washed by male) and turns body toward Mecca	May oppose	Prohibited	Prohibited	Encouraged

TABLE 27–4 *(continued)*

Group	Afterlife	Rituals/Funerals	Autopsy	Organ Donation	Cremation	Prolonging Life
Jehovah's Witness			Prohibited unless required by law. No body parts may be removed	Prohibited	No restriction	
Judaism	Dead will be resurrected with coming of Messiah; man lives on through survival of memory	Body ritually washed by members of Ritual Burial Society; burial as soon as possible after death; dead not left unattended; five stages of mourning extending over a year; no embalming; no flowers at funeral because flowers are a symbol of life	Orthodox prohibit; some liberals permit; no body parts removed	Beliefs vary	Largely prohibited; beliefs vary	Generally oppose after irreversible brain damage
Lutheran	Yes	Last rites optional	No restriction	No restriction	No restriction	
Roman Catholicism	Yes; resurrection with second coming of Christ	Rites for anointing the sick not mandatory; receiving Holy Communion mandatory	Permitted, but all body parts must be given appropriate burial	No restriction	No restriction	Discouraged
Seventh Day Adventist	Dead are asleep until return of Christ, when final rewards and punishments will be given					
Unitarian	Beliefs vary		No	No	Encouraged	Preferred

Sources: H. M. Ross, Societal/cultural views regarding death and dying, *Topics in Clinical Nursing*, 1981, 3(3):1–16; H. M. Ross and J. B. Pumphrey (consultant), Recognizing your patient's spiritual needs, *Nursing 77*, December 1977, 7:64–70; and L. J. Carpenito, *Nursing diagnosis: Application to clinical practice*. 3d ed. (Philadelphia: J. B. Lippincott Co., 1989), pp. 713–19.

with spiritual issues and be clear about their own ability to interact supportively with the client. Nurses have a responsibility to not impose their own religious/spiritual beliefs on a client, but to respond to the client in relation to the client's own background and needs. Communication skills are most important in helping the client articulate needs and in developing a sense of caring and trust.

Specific interventions may include facilitating expressions of feeling, prayer, meditation, reading, and discussion with appropriate clergy/spiritual advisor. It is important for nurses to establish an effective interdisciplinary relationship with spiritual support specialists. For a further discussion of spiritual issues, see Chapter 26.

Evaluating

Examples of outcome criteria are listed on page 539.

Caring for the dying client and the family is a nursing challenge that, when performed in a caring and humane manner, will not only afford dignity to the dying client and comfort for the family, but will also enable the nurse to enhance his or her knowledge and explore feelings about death.

CHAPTER HIGHLIGHTS

▸ Nurses help clients deal with all kinds of losses, including loss of body image, loss of a loved one, loss of a sense of well-being, and loss of a job.

▸ Loss, especially loss of a loved one or a valued body part, can be viewed as a crisis event, either situational or developmental, and either actual or perceived (both of which can be anticipatory).

▸ How an individual deals with loss is closely related to the individual's stage of development, personal resources, and social support systems.

▸ Caring for the dying and the bereaved is one of the nurse's most complex and challenging responsibilities.

▸ Nurses' attitudes about death and dying directly affect their ability to provide care.

▸ Nurses must consider the entire family as the client of care in situations involving loss, especially the crisis of death.

▸ Grieving is a normal, subjective emotional response to loss; it is essential for mental and physical health. Grieving allows the bereaved person to cope with loss gradually and to accept it as part of reality.

▸ Knowledge of different stages or phases of grieving and factors that influence the loss reaction can help the nurse understand the responses and needs of clients.

▸ Nurses caring for clients who are suffering loss or dying need effective communication skills.

▸ Dying clients require physical help and emotional support to ensure a peaceful and dignified death.

LEARNING ACTIVITIES

■ Review your own personal experiences of death—of a family member, a loved one, or a client. What were your feelings about the death experiences? What behaviors did you manifest? How did you resolve your feelings of loss?

■ What are your beliefs about death? What happens to the individual after death? How do your beliefs affect your care of the dying client and the family?

■ Visit a hospice in your community. What services does the hospice provide for the client and for the family? Where do they provide service? How do you obtain hospice support for a client? What criteria are required for a client to receive hospice support? How is the hospice funded?

■ What specific cultural or religious groups are indigenous to your community? Analyze beliefs and practices related to dying and death for these groups. Prepare a plan of care for a dying client from one of these groups and share it with nursing colleagues.

READINGS AND REFERENCES

SUGGESTED READINGS

Bennett, J. December 1988. Helping people with AIDS live well at home. *Nursing Clinics of North America* 23:731–48.
Over two-thirds of those living with AIDS are not in a hospital or hospice situation, i.e., they are neither acutely ill nor dying. Bennett discusses nursing care goals for the person with AIDS, the challenge of living with AIDS, assessment, recurrent problems, and needs. Individual decision making is encouraged; physical comfort and symptom relief is emphasized.

Benoliel, J. Q. June 1985. Loss and terminal illness. *Nursing Clinics of North America* 20:439–48.
This leading nurse-scholar writing on loss and grief presents a succinct overview of loss and the implications for the individual, the family, and nursing care.

Campbell, A. June 21–27, 1989. Hospices are for living . . . from patient profiles. *Nursing Times* 85:39–41.
With four patient profiles, Campbell illustrates how patients are allowed to be home as much as possible and how families treat the hospice as an extension of their own homes. Campbell emphasizes the importance of liaison between the hospice home care team, the general practitioner, and the community nurse.

RELATED RESEARCH

Carter, S. L. November/December 1989. Themes of grief. *Nursing Research* 38:354–58.

Kirschling, J. M., and McBride, A. B. April 1989. Effects of age and sex on the experience of widowhood. *Western Journal of Nursing Research* 11:207–18.

Masters, M., and Shontz, F. C. August 1989. Implications of problems and strengths of the hospice client by clients, caregivers, and nurses: Implications for nursing. *Cancer Nursing* 12:226–35.

Pfost, K. S.; Stevens, M. J., and Wessels, A. B. 1989. Relationship of purpose in life to grief experiences in response to the death of a significant other. *Death Studies* 13(4):371–78.

SELECTED REFERENCES

Alexander, J., and Kiely, J. March/April 1986. Working with the bereaved. *Geriatric Nursing* 7:85–86.

Benoliel, J. Q. June 1985. Loss and terminal illness. *Nursing Clinics of North America* 20:439–48.

Benton, R. E. 1978. *Death and dying: Principles and practices in patient care.* New York: D. Van Nostrand Co.

Burgess, A. W., and Lazare, A. 1976. *Community mental health: Target populations.* Englewood Cliffs, N.J.: Prentice-Hall.

Cappon, D. February 1970. Attitudes towards death. *Coast Graduate Medicine* 47:257.

Carpenito, L. J. 1989. *Nursing diagnosis: Application to clinical practice.* 3d ed. Philadelphia: J. B. Lippincott Co.

Charmaz, K. 1980. *The social reality of death.* Reading, Mass.: Addison-Wesley Publishing Co.

Clark, C.; Curley, A.; and Hughes, A. December 1988. Hospice care: A model for caring for the person with AIDS. *Nursing Clinics of North America* 23:851–62.

Clark, M. D. December 1984. Healthy and unhealthy grief behaviors. *Occupational Health Nursing* 32:633–35.

Conrad, N. L. June 1985. Spiritual support for the dying. *Nursing Clinics of North America* 20:415–26.

Corless, I. B. 1983. The hospice movement in North America. In Corr, C. A., and Corr, D. M. (editors). *Hospice care: Principles and practice.* New York: Springer Publishing Co.

Demi, A. S., and Miles, M. S. 1986. Bereavement. *Annual Review of Nursing Research* 4:105–23.

Dobratz, M. C. April 1990. Hospice nursing: Present perspectives and future directives. *Cancer Nursing* 13:116–22.

Engel, G. L. September 1964. Grief and grieving. *American Journal of Nursing* 64:93–98.

Fetsch, S. H. November/December 1984. The 7- to 10-year-old child's conceptualization of death. *Oncology Nurses' Forum* 11:52–56.

Field, D. January 1984. "We didn't want him to die on his own"—Nurses' accounts of nursing dying patients. *Journal of Advanced Nursing* 1:59–70.

Gabriel, R. M., and Kirschling, J. M. 1989. Assessing grief among the bereaved elderly: A review of existing measures. *Hospice Journal* 5:29–54.

Gifford, B. J., and Cleary, B. B. February 1990. Supporting the bereaved. *American Journal of Nursing* 90:48–55.

Gonda, T. A., and Ruark, J. E. 1984. *Dying dignified: The health professional's guide to care.* Menlo Park, Calif.: Addison-Wesley.

Hoff, L. A. 1984. *People in crisis.* Menlo Park, Calif.: Addison-Wesley.

Kim, M. J.; McFarland, G. K., and McLane, A. M. 1989. *Pocket guide to nursing diagnoses,* 3d ed. St. Louis: C. V. Mosby.

Kübler-Ross, E. 1969. *On death and dying.* New York: Macmillan Publishing Co.

———. 1975. *Death: The final stage of growth.* Englewood Cliffs, N.J.: Prentice-Hall.

———. 1978. *To live until we say good-bye.* Englewood Cliffs, N.J.: Prentice-Hall.

Martocchio, B. C. June 1985. Grief and bereavement: Healing through hurt. *Nursing Clinics of North America* 20:327–41.

Morris, E. October 19–25, 1988. A pain of separation . . . How can nurses best assist the dying and the bereaved? *Nursing Times* 84:54–56.

Moss, M. S., and Moss, S. Z. 1983–84. The impact of parental death on middle-aged children. *Omega* 14(1):65–75.

National Hospice Organization. 1981. Standards of a hospice

program of care. Arlington, Va: National Hospice Organization.

Richter, J. M. July 1984. Crisis of mate loss in the elderly. *American Nursing Society* 6(4):45–54.

Salter, R. March 1982. The art of dying. *Canadian Nurse* 78:20–21.

Schulz, R. 1978. *The psychology of death, dying and bereavement.* Reading, Mass.: Addison-Wesley Publishing Co.

Sheehy, P. F. 1981. *On dying with dignity.* New York: Pinnacle Books.

Strauss, A. L., and Glaser, B. G. 1970. Awareness of dying. In Schoenberg, B., Carr, A. C., Peretz, D., and Kutcher, A. H., editors. *Loss and grief.* New York: Columbia University Press.

Taylor, D. A. 1983–84. View of death from sufferers of early loss. *Omega* 14(1):77–82.

Tschudin, V. March 21–27, 1990. Essentials of management: Support yourself. *Nursing Times* 86:40–2.

A

Significant Events in Nursing History

1–500 (circa)   Care (mostly hygienic and comfort measures) for the destitute, homeless, and sick provided mainly by early Christians, working as committed individuals or in association with an organized church.

500–1500 (circa)   Male and female religious, military, and secular orders with the primary purpose of caring for the sick came into being. Conspicuous among them were the Knights Hospitalers of St. John; the Alexian Brotherhood, organized in 1431; and the Augustinian sisters, the first purely nursing order.

1633   Sisters of Charity founded by St. Vincent de Paul in France. It was the first of many such orders with the same name (sometimes Daughters of Charity) organized under various Roman Catholic church auspices and largely devoted to caring for the sick.

1639   Augustinian sisters came to Canada, eventually establishing the Hotel Dieu in Quebec City.

1644   Jeanne Mance, known as the Florence Nightingale of Canada, founded the Hotel Dieu in Montreal.

——Mother Elizabeth Seton established the first American order of Sisters of Charity of St. Joseph, in Maryland.

1738   Mother d'Youville organized a noncloistered group of women to care for the sick in both hospitals and homes. These women became the Soeurs Grises or Grey Nuns.

1836   Theodor Fliedner reinstituted the Order of Deaconesses from earlier days, opening a small hospital and training school in Kaiserswerth, Germany. This was where Florence Nightingale received her "training" in nursing. The deaconess movement spread to four continents, the first motherhouse being established in Pittsburgh, Pennsylvania, in 1849.

1854–56   Florence Nightingale, long concerned with care of the sick, was named Superintendent of the Female Nursing Establishment of the English General Hospitals in Turkey, in charge of the nursing care of the soldiers during the Crimean War.

1859   Publication of *Notes on nursing: What it is and what it is not,* by Nightingale, in London. It was intended for the ordinary woman, not as a text for nurses.

1860   With a fund of 45,000 pounds (over $220,000 at that time) contributed by the grateful British public and soldiers, Nightingale established the first "modern" school of nursing

at St. Thomas's Hospital in London. This date is considered the beginning of nursing as an organized profession. Nightingale believed not only in nursing the sick but also in promoting health.

1861–65   Dorothea Lynde Dix, better known for her earlier work in improving conditions of care for the mentally ill, was appointed superintendent of the first nurse corps of the United States Army during the Civil War.

1864   Jean Henri Dunant of Switzerland established the international conference that founded the Red Cross, for the relief of the suffering in war, in the Geneva Convention signed by 14 nations (the United States not among them).

1872   Woman's Hospital, Philadelphia, opened a training school for nurses.

——New England Hospital for Women and Children, Boston, opened a training school for nurses. Linda Richards, who graduated from the school in 1873, became known as America's first trained nurse.

——American Public Health Association established. Its primary concern at that time was with sanitary and environmental conditions. Later nurses became a significant part of its membership.

1873   First three schools of nursing patterned after (but not strictly according to) Nightingale principles were established at Bellevue Hospital, New York; Massachusetts General Hospital, Boston; and New Haven Hospital, Connecticut.

1874   First hospital training school (Mack Training School) for nurses formed in Canada at St. Catharines, Ontario.

1879   Mary Eliza Mahoney, first trained black nurse, graduated from the nursing school of New England Hospital for Women and Children.

1882   American National Red Cross organized by Clara Barton and linked with the international organization when the United States Congress ratified the Geneva Convention.

1885   Publication of *Textbook of nursing for the use of training schools, families and private students,* the first textbook written by an American Nurse (Clara Weeks Shaw) for nurses.

1893   Henry Street Settlement, New York, established by Lilian D. Wald and Mary Brewster to care for the sick and poor in their homes.

——American Society of Superintendents of Training Schools for Nurses (renamed the National League of Nursing Education [NLNE] in 1912) became the first organized nursing group in the United States and Canada.

1897 Nurses' Associated Alumnae of United States and Canada organized. Renamed the American Nurses' Association (ANA) in 1911.

——Victorian Order of Nurses established in Canada by Lady Aberdeen. It conducted practically all public health nursing.

1899 International Council of Nurses (ICN) established by Mrs. Bedford Fenwick of Great Britain, United States and Canadian nurses were among its founders, and their national associations were among the first admitted to membership.

1900 *American Journal of Nursing,* first nursing journal in the United States to be owned, operated, and published by nurses, launched. Its publisher, incorporated in 1902, now also publishes *Nursing Research,* established in 1952; *Nursing Outlook,* 1953; *International Nursing Index,* 1966; *MCN: American Journal of Maternal–Child Nursing,* 1976; and *Geriatric Nursing: American Journal of Care for the Aging,* 1980.

1901 United States Army Nurse Corps formally established by act of Congress.

1903 First nurse practice acts passed in North Carolina, New Jersey, Virginia, and New York.

1905 *Canadian Nurse* journal inaugurated. By 1959 it was published in both English and French.

1908 Canadian National Association of Trained Nurses (CNATN) established. It later became the Canadian Nurses' Association (CNA).

——National Association of Colored Graduate Nurses (NACGN) established.

——United States Navy Nurse Corps formed.

1912 National Organization for Public Health Nursing (NOPHN) established.

——United States Children's Bureau created by Congress as part of the Department of Commerce and Labor.

1916 Criteria for a profession, set forth by Abraham Flexner in "Is social work a profession?" (published in *School and society,* volume 1), became yardsticks for nursing and continue to serve this function.

1917 NLNE published its first *Standard curriculum for schools of nursing;* revised editions, under slightly different titles, appeared in 1927 and 1937.

1919 Ethyl Johns established the first baccalaureate degree program in nursing in the British Empire at the University of British Columbia, Vancouver.

1922 Sigma Theta Tau, national honor society of nursing in the United States, founded by six nursing students at Indiana Training School for Nurses.

1923 Publication of *Nursing and nursing education in the United States,* better known as the Goldmark (or Winslow-Goldmark) Report. Originally intended to study education for public health nursing, the study committee extended its work to include all of nursing education, criticizing the low standards, inadequate financing, and lack of separation of education from service.

——Yale University (New Haven, Connecticut) and Western Reserve University (Cleveland, Ohio), each with the aid of endowments, established independent schools of nursing. In 1934, both started requiring a baccalaureate degree for admission to the schools and granted masters of nursing degrees.

1928 Publication of *Nurses, patients, and pocketbooks,* first report of the Committee on Grading of Nursing Schools appointed two years earlier. The report indicated that there was an oversupply of nurses in general but an undersupply of adequately prepared ones.

1929 American Association of Nurse-Midwives formed. It merged in 1969 with the American College of Nurse-Midwifery to become the American College of Nurse-Midwives.

1931 Weir Report in Canada recommended integration of nursing education into the provincial education system.

1932 Association of Collegiate Schools of Nursing (ACSN) established to promote nursing education on a professional and collegiate level and to encourage research.

1933 ANA launched campaign for hospitals to employ graduate nurses instead of relying heavily on nursing students for patient care.

1934 Publication of *Nursing schools today and tomorrow,* final report of the Grading Committee (which never did grade schools publicly). It confirmed the weaknesses in nursing education pointed out in the Goldmark Report, recommended graduate instead of student nursing staffs, and called for public support of nursing education.

1939 Graduate School of Midwifery created by the Frontier Nursing Service, Hyden, Kentucky.

1940 Formation of the Nursing Council on National Defense (retitled the National Nursing Council for War Service [NNCWS] in 1941), with representation from major nursing organizations and nursing service agencies, to unify all nursing activities directly or indirectly related to war.

1942 Committee appointed to develop what became the State Board Test Pool Examination (SBTPE). By 1950 all states were using the SBTPE.

——American Association of Industrial Nurses (now the American Association of Occupational Health Nurses) formed.

1943 United States Cadet Nurse Corps established. Through this corps, the federal government subsidized the cost of nursing education, in accelerated programs, for all students agreeing to serve after graduation in civilian or military nursing services for the duration of the war. It was discontinued in 1945.

1946 ANA adopted its economic security (now economic and general welfare) program legitimizing collective bargaining for nurses through their state nurses' associations.

1947 Passage of the Taft-Hartley Act, exempting nonprofit hospitals and other charitable institutions from the obligation to bargain collectively with their employees.

1948 Publication of *Nursing for the future,* report of a far-reaching study of "who would organize, administer, and finance *professional* schools of nursing." Commissioned by the National Nursing Council for War Services and carried out by anthropologist Esther Lucile Brown, the report recommended, among other things, that education for nursing belonged in colleges and universities, not in hospitals.

——NLNE formally established the National Nursing Accrediting Service for nursing educational programs.

——Nationwide movement toward "team nursing" started at Hartford Hospital, Connecticut.

——Metropolitan Demonstration School of Nursing in Windsor, Ontario, operated a 2-year nursing education program (from 1948 to 1952). The Lord Report in 1952 concluded that nurses could be trained at least as satisfactorily in 2 years as in 3 years.

1949 United States Air Force Nurse Corps created.

1950–53 United States nurses served in the Korean war, in Mobile Army Surgical Hospitals (M.A.S.H.).

1951 National Association of Colored Graduate Nurses dissolved itself, to be absorbed into the ANA.

1952 After years of study, the nursing profession in the United States was restructured into two national organizations: the ANA, which remained the membership organization, and the newly formed National League for Nursing (NLN), merging the former NLNE, NOPHN, and ACSN.

——Associate degree education for nursing begun in an experimental project at Teachers College, Columbia University, New York.

——*Nursing Research* launched due to the efforts of the ACSN.

1953 National Student Nurses' Association (NSNA) founded.

——United States Department of Health, Education, and Welfare (HEW) created. It became the Department of Health and Human Services (HHS) in 1980.

1954 Association of Operating Room Nurses formed.

1955 American Nurses' Foundation established by the ANA for research purposes.

1956 Federal nurse traineeship program established to aid registered nurses in advanced study.

1960 Publication of *Spotlight on nursing education* by Helen K. Mussallem, report of a pilot project for the evaluation of schools of nursing in Canada.

1963 Publication of *Toward quality in nursing,* report of the Surgeon General's Consultant Group in Nursing, another study of nursing and nursing education that projected the need for more and better prepared nurses.

1964 Ryerson Polytechnical Institute, Toronto, started the first diploma nursing program in Canada within a college institution.

——First Nurse Training Act allocated federal aid for nursing education in the United States.

1965 ANA issued its first (and famous) "Position paper on nursing education," calling for all nursing education to take place in institutions of higher education and stipulating the baccalaureate as minimum preparation for professional nursing practice, the associate degree for technical nursing practice.

1967 Pediatric nurse practitioner program initiated at University of Colorado, Boulder; a program at the University of California, San Francisco, gave nurses increased responsibility in ambulatory care. These marked the beginning of the "nurse practitioner" or "expanded role of the nurse" movement.

1969 Nurses' Association of the American College of Obstetricians and Gynecologists formed.

——American Association of Cardiovascular Nurses formed. It was broadened in 1972 to become the Association of Critical-Care Nurses.

——American Association of Colleges of Nursing (AACN) formed after two years of informal meetings.

1970 Canadian Nurses' Association established a national Testing Service (CNATS) to prepare examinations for graduate nurses seeking provincial registration.

——Publication of *An abstract for action,* report of the national Commission on Nursing and Nursing Education, and often referred to as the Lysaught report, after the study director. The report categorized nursing into episodic (illness) and distributive (preventive and health maintenance) care.

——Publication of *Extending the scope of nursing practice,* by HEW, endorsing extension of the nurse's traditional functions and responsibilities.

——Introduction of primary nursing as an alternative to team nursing.

——National Association of School Nurses formed.

1971 National Black Nurses' Association created.

——Lucille Kinlein became the first nurse to hang out her shingle as an independent practitioner. Today many nurses are in independent practice singly or in groups.

——Emergency Department Nurses' Association established.

1972 New York State amended its Nurse Practice Act to define professional nursing practice as diagnosing and treating human responses to actual or potential health problems.

——Nurses for Political Action, now Nurses' Coalition for Action in Politics (N-CAP), established to promote legislation in behalf of nursing; associated with the ANA.

1973 Federation of nursing specialty organizations and the ANA was created, after 2 years of preliminary meetings.

——ANA started certification program for nurses in specialty practice.

——American Academy of Nursing established, with appointment of 36 charter fellows. It was associated with the ANA.

——"External" associate degree program in nursing launched in New York. It permitted a degree to be awarded on the basis of independent study validated by examination. This was extended to the bachelor's degree in nursing in 1976.

——National Association of Pediatric Nurses formed.

——First national conference on nursing diagnoses held in St. Louis, Missouri.

1974 Amendments to the Taft-Hartley Act removed exemption of nonprofit institutions from the obligation to engage in collective bargaining.

——Association of Rehabilitation Nurses formed.

1975 Oncology Nursing Society started.

1976 Robert Wood Johnson Foundation launched a program of faculty fellowships in primary care.

1978 ANA House of Delegates resolved that "by 1985" minimum preparation for "entry into professional practice" would be the baccalaureate in nursing.

——Council of State Boards of Nursing separated from the ANA to form an autonomous body, the National Council of State Boards of Nursing.

1979 Committee on Credentialing in Nursing called for establishment of a free-standing national credentialing center, not endorsed by the ANA.

——Case Western Reserve University, Cleveland, initiated the first professional education program in nursing awarding the ND (Doctor of Nursing) degree.

1982 NLN endorsed the baccalaureate in nursing as minimum preparation for professional practice.

——ANA converted to a federation of constituent nurses' associations rather than an association of individual nurse members.

——National Association of Orthopedic Nurses established.

——North American Nursing Diagnosis Association (NANDA) established.

1983 Congress passed legislation changing Medicare reimbursement to hospitals to a system of prospective payment based on Diagnosis Related Groups (DRGs).

——Institute of Medicine report called for federally funded entity to place nursing research in the mainstream of scientific investigation.

——Center for Research for Nursing created by the American Nurses' Association.

1985 ANA House of Delegates voted to recommend titles for two levels of professional nursing practice: "registered nurse" for the baccalaureate-prepared nurse, and "associate nurse" for the associate degree (technical) nurse.

——National Institute of Nursing established.

1986 N-CAP (Nurses' Coalition for Action in Politics) renamed ANA-PAC.

——National Center for Nursing Research (within the National Institutes of Health in Bethesda, Maryland) established.

1988 The Secretary's Commission on Nursing, DHHS, issued its final report, which included 16 recommendations to improve recruitment and retention of an adequate supply of registered nurses.

1990 NCNIP (National Commission on Nursing Implementation Project) and the Advertising Council of America launched a multimillion dollar national advertising campaign to provide a more accurate image of nurses and nursing that would attract new recruits to the profession.

B

Nursing's Agenda for Health Care Reform

EXECUTIVE SUMMARY

America's Nurses have long supported our nation's efforts to create a health care system that assures access, quality, and services at affordable costs. This document presents nursing's agenda for immediate health care reform. We call for a basic "core" of essential health care services to be available to everyone. We call for a restructured health care system that will focus on the consumers and their health, with services to be delivered in familiar, convenient sites, such as schools, workplaces, and homes. We call for a shift from the predominant focus on illness and cure to an orientation toward wellness and care.

The basic components of nursing's "core of care" include:

1. A restructured health care system which:

- Enhances consumer access to services by delivering primary health care in community-based settings.
- Fosters consumer responsibility for personal health, self care, and informed decision making in selecting health care services.
- Facilitates utilization of the most cost-effective providers and therapeutic options in the most appropriate settings.

2. A federally-defined standard package of essential health care services available to all citizens and residents of the United States, provided and financed through an integration of public and private plans and sources:

- A public plan, based on federal guidelines and eligibility requirements, will provide coverage for the poor and create the opportunity for small businesses and individuals, particularly those at risk because of preexisting conditions and those potentially medically indigent, to buy into the plan.
- A private plan will offer, at a minimum, the nationally standardized package of essential services. This standard package could be enriched as a benefit of employment or individuals could purchase additional services if they so choose. If employers do not offer private coverage, they must pay into the public plan for their employees.

3. A phase-in of essential services, in order to be fiscally responsible:

- Coverage of pregnant women and children is critical. The first step represents a cost-effective investment in the future health and prosperity of the nation.
- One early step will be to design services specifically to assist vulnerable populations who have had limited access to our nation's health care system. A "Healthstart Plan" is proposed to improve the health status of these individuals.

4. Planned change to anticipate health service needs that correlate with changing national demographics.

5. Steps to reduce health care costs include:

- Required usage of managed care in the public plan and encouraged in private plans.
- Incentives for consumers and providers to utilize managed care arrangements.

551

- Controlled growth of the health care system through planning and prudent resource allocation.

- Incentives for consumers and providers to be more cost efficient in exercising health care options.

- Development of health care policies based on effectiveness and outcomes research.

- Assurance of direct access to a full range of qualified providers.

- Elimination of unnecessary bureaucratic controls and administrative procedures.

6. Case management will be required for those with continuing health care needs. Case management will reduce the fragmentation of the present system, promote consumers' active participation in decisions about their health, and create an advocate on their behalf.

7. Provisions for long-term care, which include:

- Public and private funding for services of short duration to prevent personal impoverishment.

- Public funding for extended care if consumer resources are exhausted.

- Emphasis on the consumers' responsibility to financially plan for their long-term care needs, including new personal financial alternatives and strengthened private insurance arrangements.

8. Insurance reforms to assure improved access to coverage, including affordable premiums, reinsurance pools for catastrophic coverage, and other steps to protect both insurers and individuals against excessive costs.

9. Access to services assured by no payment at the point of service and elimination of balance billing in both public and private plans.

10. Establishment of public/private sector review—operating under federal guidelines and including payers, providers, and consumers—to determine resource allocation, cost reduction approaches, allowable insurance premiums, and fair and consistent reimbursement levels for providers. This review would progress in a climate sensitive to ethical issues.

Additional resources will be required to accomplish this plan. While significant dollars can be obtained through restructuring and other strategies, responsibility for any new funds must be shared by individuals, employers, and government, phased in over several years to minimize the impact.

NURSING'S AGENDA FOR HEALTH CARE REFORM

Nurses provide a unique perspective on the health care system. Our constant presence in a variety of settings places us in contact with individuals who reap the benefits of the system's most sophisticated services, as well as those individuals seriously compromised by the system's inefficiencies.

More and more, nurses observe the effects of inadequate services and of the declining quality of care on the nation's health. Firsthand experience tells us that the time has come for change. Patchwork approaches to health care reform have not worked. While preserving the best elements of the existing system, we must build a new foundation for health care in America. It is this realization that drives *Nursing's Agenda For Health Care Reform*.

Nursing's plan for reform converts a system that focuses on the costly treatment of illness to a system that emphasizes primary health care services and the promotion, restoration, and maintenance of health. It increases the consumer's responsibility and role in health care decision making and focuses on partnerships between consumers and providers. It sets forth new delivery arrangements that make health care a more vital part of individual and community life. And it ensures that health services are appropriate, effective, cost efficient, and focused on consumer needs.

A HEALTH CARE SYSTEM IN CRISIS

The strengths and weaknesses of our nation's health care system are well documented. Every day, many Americans profit from the system's technological excellence, extensive medical research, well-educated health professionals, diverse range of providers, and myriad of facilities. Millions of people live longer lives because of the care they receive.

But America's health care system in also very costly, its quality inconsistent, and its benefits unequally distributed. Although the system provides highly sophisticated care to many, millions of Americans must overcome enormous obstacles to get even the most elementary services. In short, health care is neither fairly nor equitably delivered to all segments of the population.

As caregivers in a diversity of settings, responsible for providing care and coordinating health care services 24 hours-a-day, nurses clearly understand the implications of the system's failings. The more than two million nurses in America are at the front lines—in hospitals, nursing homes, schools, home health agencies, workplaces, community clinics, and managed care programs. And what nurses see are the alarming effects of a system that has lost touch with the communities it is supposed to serve:

1. More and more people must overcome major barriers to gain access to even the most elementary services.

2. Too many Americans receive treatment too late because they live in inner cities or in urban or rural areas where service levels are inadequate.

3. People enter hospitals daily in advanced stages of illness, suffering from problems that could have been treated in less costly settings or avoided altogether with adequate disease prevention and health promotion services.

4. The lack of access to prenatal care contributes to an alarming number of infant deaths and low birth weights each year.

5. Obstacles to obtaining fundamental services, such as childhood immunizations, are largely responsible for a resurgence in preventable diseases.

6. Disproportionate amounts of resources are used for expensive medical interventions, which all too often provide neither comfort nor cure.

7. Every year, expensive nursing home care impoverishes an alarming number of residents and their families.

Major changes in the health care system can no longer be put on hold. Further analysis and investigation will neither change the facts nor diminish the problems.

Today, more than 60 million Americans are either uninsured or underinsured. This fact alone cries out for health care reform. Now, the system's inability to contain costs is placing more and more Americans with "adequate" insurance coverage at risk of hardship when major illnesses do occur. Employers and employees alike are desperately seeking solutions to the dual problems of rising health care costs and increased premium rates that threaten basic coverage for most American workers and their dependents.

Americans cannot afford to sit idly and do nothing. Health care costs are approaching 12 percent of the gross national product (GNP). Health care is expected to cost over $756 billion in 1991.[1] If nothing is done to control expenditures, health care spending is expected to reach $1.2 to $1.3 trillion by 1995 – an increase of some $500 billion in less than five years. At this rate, if the system remains unchanged, spending will reach between $2.1 and $2.7 trillion by the year 2000.[2]

THE FRAMEWORK FOR CHANGE

Nurses strongly believe that the health care system must be restructured, reoriented, and decentralized in order to guarantee access to services, contain costs, and ensure quality care. Our plan—the product of consensus building within organized nursing—is designed to achieve this goal. It provides central control in the form of federal minimum standards for essential services and federally defined eligibility requirements. At the same time, it makes allowances for decentralized decision making which will permit local areas to develop specific programs and arrangements best suited to consumer needs.

Nursing's plan is built around several basic premises, including the following:

- All citizens and residents of the United States must have equitable access to essential health care services (a core of care).

- Primary health care services must play a very basic and prominent role in service delivery.

- Consumers must be the central focus of the health care system. Assessment of health care needs must be the determining factor in the ultimate structuring and delivery of programs and services.

- Consumers must be guaranteed direct access to a full range of qualified health care providers who offer their services in a variety of delivery arrangements at sites which are accessible, convenient, and familiar to the consumer.

- Consumers must assume more responsibility for their own care and become better informed about the range of providers and the potential options for services. Working in partnership with providers, consumers must actively participate in choices that best meet their needs.

- Health care services must be restructured to create a better balance between the prevailing orientation toward illness and cure and a new commitment to wellness and care.

- The health care system must assure that appropriate, effective care is delivered through the efficient use of resources.

- A standardized package of essential health care services must be provided and financed through an integration of public and private plans and sources.

- Mechanisms must be implemented to protect against catastrophic costs and impoverishment.

The cornerstone of nursing's plan for reform is the delivery of primary health care services to households and individuals in convenient, familiar places. If health is to be a true national priority, it is logical to provide services in the places where people work and live. Maximizing the use of these sites can help eliminate the fragmentation and lack of coordination which have come to characterize the existing health care system. It can also promote a more "consumer friendly" system where services such as health education, screening, immunizations, well-child care, and prenatal care would be readily accessible.

At the same time, consumers must be the focus of the health care system. Individuals must be given incentives to assume more responsibility for their health. They must develop both the motivation and capability to be more prudent buyers of health services. Promotion of healthy lifestyles and better informed consumer decisions can contribute to effective and economical health care delivery.

Finally, in implementing reforms, attention must be directed to the unique needs of special population groups whose health care needs have been neglected. These individuals include children, pregnant women, and vulnerable groups such as the poor, minorities, AIDS victims, and those who have difficulty securing insurance because of preexisting conditions. Lack of preventive and primary care for this sector has cost the nation enormously—both in terms of lives lost or impaired and dollars spent to treat problems that could have been avoided or treated less expensively through appropriate intervention.

Access to care alone may not be sufficient to resolve the problems of these vulnerable groups. For those individuals whose health has been seriously compromised, a "catch up" program characterized by enriched services is justified. Coverage of pregnant women and children is critical. This first step represents a cost effective investment in the future health and prosperity of the nation.

It is this set of values that distinguishes nursing's plan from other proposals and offers a realistic approach to health care reform.

A PLAN FOR REFORM

Nursing's plan for health care reform builds a new foundation for health care in America. It shifts the emphasis of the health care system from illness and cure to wellness and care. While preserving key components of the existing system, it sets forth new strategies for guaranteeing universal coverage; making health care a more vital part of community life; and ensuring that the health care services provided are appropriate, effective, and cost efficient.

The following pages provide a general overview of nursing's vision for a better health care system.

Universal Access to a Standard Package of Essential Services

Nursing's plan envisions a new and bold approach to universal access to a standard package of essential health care services and the manner in which these services are delivered.

The federal government will delineate the essential services (core of care) which must be provided to all U.S. citizens and residents. This standard package will include defined levels of:

- Primary health care services, hospital care, emergency treatment, inpatient and outpatient professional services, and home care services.

- Prevention services, including prenatal and perinatal care; infant and well-child care; school-based disease prevention programs; speech therapy, hearing, dental, and eye care for children up to age 18; screening procedures; and other preventive services with proven effectiveness.

- Prescription drugs, medical supplies and equipment, and laboratory and radiology services.

- Mental health services and substance abuse treatment and rehabilitation.

- Hospice care.

- Long-term care services of relatively short duration.

- Restorative services determined to be essential to the prevention of long-term institutionalization.

By taking this approach, traditional illness services are balanced with provisions for health maintenance services which prevent illness, reduce cost, and avoid institutionalization. Thus, hospital coverage and emergency care are covered, as are such services as immunizations, physical examinations, and prenatal and perinatal care.

The creation of federal minimum standards for essential services will necessitate modifications in existing public programs. The ultimate goal will be, over time, to merge all government-sponsored health programs into a single public program.

Coverage Options

Universal coverage for the federally defined package of essential services will be accessed through an integration of public and private plans and resources.

- A public plan, administered by the states, will provide coverage for the poor (those below 200% of the federal poverty level), high-risk populations, and the potentially medially indigent. Any employer or individual will also have the option of buying into this plan as their source of coverage.

- Private plans (employment-based health benefit programs and commercial health insurance) will be required to offer, at a minimum, the nationally standardized package of essential services. This package could be enriched as a benefit of employment or individuals could purchase additional services from commercial insurers if they so choose.

All citizens and residents will be required to be covered by one of these options. Under both the public plan and private plans, no one will be denied insurance because of preexisting conditions. If employers do not offer private coverage, they will be required to pay into the public plan for their employees. Employer payments will be actuarially equivalent to the costs of employee and dependent coverage. Financial relief will be made available to small businesses (25 employees or less) for whom this provision would not be feasible. Individuals with no source of private coverage could also buy into the public plan. To assure universal access to essential services, systems will be developed to identify the insurance option through which each individual's needs are met.

Premiums and Payment Rates

Access to health care services will be enhanced by offering insurance premiums that the public can afford and payment rates to providers that are equitable and inclusive.

Both the public and private plans will utilize deductibles and copayments to ensure that beneficiaries continue to pay for a portion of their own care and, therefore, have financial incentives to be economical in their use of services. Deductible amounts and copayment rates, however, will never serve as barriers to care. Provisions will be made to waive or subsidize deduc-tions and copayments for households with incomes below 200% of the federal poverty level. Deductibles for certain types of programs and services (e.g., health promotion, such as well-child care, immunizations, and mammograms; and managed care plans) will be held to a minimum to encourage wider use of cost-efficient, wellness-oriented options.

Public and private payers will be required to offer fair and consistent rates of payment to providers. To protect access to care, providers will not seek payment at the point of service; nor will they be permitted to engage in balance billing. Because providers will be reimbursed fairly through insurance and the problems of uncompensated care will be largely eliminated, there will be no need for providers to charge consumers amounts above the established rate. Consequently, the consumer's financial responsibility for health care services will be more predictable.

To make insurance more affordable to individuals and to reduce costs to insurers and employers, nursing's plan calls for reforms in the private insurance market. These reforms may encompass a variety of strategies, including:

- Community rating for all insurers.

- A cap on the out-of-pocket expenses individuals must pay for catastrophic care, including nursing home and other long-term care.

- State reinsurance pools to protect insurers and consumers against the high costs of insuring a broader range of patients.

Special Programs for Vulnerable Groups

Countless individuals suffer from long-term health problems associated with inadequate access to basic health services over time. Often, the poor and many members of minority groups are in this category. Special programs will provide services and outreach to vulnerable populations in order to compensate for formerly inadequate care and its consequences.

For infants and children (e.g., low birthweight babies, battered and neglected children, pregnant teenagers, children who abuse drugs, and young victims of violence and homelessness), such programming could be viewed as a health service ("Healthstart") equivalent to the Headstart Program for those who are educationally disadvantaged. An expanded version of the Women's, Infants and Children (WIC) Program may be needed to produce quality outcomes in maternal-child health for poor and minority populations. Other special population groups also may warrant compensatory health programs beyond the scope of essential health benefits and services.

It is important to note that the ultimate goal of improved health is not achievable exclusively within the confines of the health sector. Social failures also have serious health consequences. Improvements in the broader environment have a major impact on health status and health care costs. While the focus of this plan is on the health care system, nursing's long-term policy agenda for the nation is much broader. National health reform must also consider the interrelationships between health and such factors and education, behavior, income, housing and sanitation, social support networks, and attitudes about health. Better health cannot be the nation's only goal when hunger, crime, drugs, and other social problems remain. Consequently, nursing is committed to pursuing reform in other areas affecting health. Discussion of such reform, however, is beyond the scope of this paper.

Long-Term Care

The high costs of long-term care often threaten to impoverish patients and their families. Nursing's plan seeks to prevent impoverishment and the potential loss of dignity by recognizing both public responsibility for long-term care and continued personal commitment to planning for such care. Financing arrangements will provide "front-end" coverage for chronic care and long-term care services of short duration through a variety of public and private options.

Beyond addressing short-term needs, individuals will be expected to assume personal responsibility for long-term care through strengthened private insurance programs and a variety of innovative financing arrangements. Such strategies will include privately purchased long-term care insurance, new savings and tax incentives, and home equity conversion opportunities, Such steps are essential to prevent individuals and their families from becoming impoverished by necessary care that can be anticipated and planned for. Emphasis on personal responsibility, however, does not ignore the fact that there will always be some individuals who will be left without resources and who must reach out for public assistance.

Catastrophic Expenses

Length and/or intensity of illness may generate catastrophic costs. Given this fact, limits will be placed on individuals' out-of-pocket payments for catastrophic health care expenses. Costs to insurers or individuals that exceed preset limits will be covered through a state reinsurance pool, to which all insurers must contribute. Under nursing's plan, insurers will tap into the pool when their total costs or costs per patient exceed preset limits. When costs decline, they will resume normal financing.

Decentralized Delivery System

Although standards for essential health services and eligibility requirements are to be mandated at the federal level, delivery mechanisms for health services will be decentralized in terms of planning and administration to foster greater consumer orientation. Because local needs differ, states will have the authority to modify implementation in order to reflect geographical diversity.

To promote greater use of disease prevention and primary health care, services will be delivered, whenever possible, in convenient, familiar sites readily accessible to households and individuals. Maximizing the use of local settings, including schools, homes, places of work, and other community facilities, will help reduce the fragmentation of primary health care delivery and promote a more consumer-friendly system.

Cost Effective, Quality Care

By properly balancing individual health needs and self-care responsibilities with provider capabilities, care can be provided in a more efficient and coordinated manner. It can be more effectively directed at health promotion activities that will ultimately improve outcomes and reduce costs. Nursing's plan for reform is designed to achieve such a balance.

Provider Availability

Financial and regulatory obstacles, as well as institutional barriers, that deny consumer access to all qualified health professionals will be removed. The wider use of a range of qualified health professionals will increase access to care, particularly in understaffed specialties, such as primary health care, and in underserved urban and rural geographical areas. It will also facilitate selection of the most cost-effective option for care.

Under this arrangement, health providers must be reasonably and fairly compensated for their services. Where fee-for-service payment arrangements continue, payments for patient services must be made directly to providers.

Consumer Involvement

Consumers will be encouraged to assume more responsibility for their own health. Health professionals will work in partnership with consumers to evaluate the full range of their needs and available services. Together, the consumer and the health professional will determine a course of action that is based on an understanding of the effectiveness of treatment.

Outcome and Effectiveness Measures

Development of multidisciplinary clinical practice guidelines is essential to the proper functioning of the health care system. These guidelines will be used to sensitize providers and others to the proven effectiveness of practices and technologies. With clear-cut information on the value of various procedures, payers, providers, and consumers can work together to eliminate wasteful and unnecessary services. Moreover, increased dissemination of research findings regarding health care outcomes will enhance provider and consumer involvement in making the most effective choices about care and treatment. By taking this approach, the likelihood of serious disputes or litigation over appropriateness of care will be minimized. Likewise, the need for defensive practices designed to protect providers against malpractice suits will be greatly reduced.

Practice guidelines and directives derived from research, while providing an element of control, will be supportive of innovation. Coverage will be extended to procedures shown to be significantly more effective and less costly than existing approaches, and/or useful in improving patient outcomes and quality of life. At the same time, an effort will be made to carefully weigh new therapeutic approaches with high start-up costs that may ultimately be less expensive than present methods.

Use of advancements in clinical practice and technology will be conditioned on satisfying criteria related to cost efficiency and therapeutic effectiveness. Such an approach will not deny people essential services. It will, however, carefully assess the appropriateness of providing high-tech curative medical care to those who simply require comfort, relief from pain, supportive care, or a peaceful death.

Review Mechanisms

State and local review bodies — representative of the public and private sectors and composed of payers, providers, and consumers —will be established. These groups, operating under federal guidelines, will determine resource allocation, cost reduction approaches, allowable insurance premiums, and fair and consistent reimbursement levels for providers. Such review will be sensitive to ethical issues.

Managed Care

Managed care will be instituted both to reduce costs and to assure consumer access to the most effective treatments. Nursing's plan envisions managed care as organized delivery systems which link the financing of health care to the delivery of services — serving to maximize the quality of care while minimizing costs. To promote the use of managed care, enrollment in approved provider networks will be a requirement for those covered by the public plan. Managed care will also be encouraged for recipients of private coverage through reductions in deductibles and copayments.

In the past, managed care has been used, in many instances, to protect the pocketbooks of insurers rather than the rights of consumers. Managed care must be restructured to retain the maximum possible consumer choice and to place a premium on services that address the health of consumers.

Case Management

In contrast to managed care systems, case management is rooted in the client-provider relationship. Case management services will be used to integrate, coordinate, and advocate for people requiring extensive services. The aim of case management is to make health care less fragmented and more holistic for those individuals with complex health care needs. A variety of health care professionals are qualified to provide this service. The first allegiance of these providers will be to their clients. Acting as advocates, they will provide both direct care and negotiate with systems on behalf of their clients. They will be authorized to access services for a given client. Both case management (provider) and managed care (delivery systems) models are important to the smooth functioning of the health care system.

A Realistic Plan of Action

Under nursing's plan, universal coverage will be achieved through implementation of both the public and private plan options. Employers will be motivated to collaborate with employees in shaping private plans which best satisfy their needs. At the same time, as larger numbers of more diverse groups participate in the public plan, the attractiveness of this option in terms of cost, quality, and image will be enhanced.

While the public and private sector plans can move forward simultaneously, it may be necessary to expand coverage to segments of the population in sequential steps. These steps would be introduced at an acceptable and financially reasonable rate until the ultimate goal of universal coverage is achieved. This approach would avoid excessive shocks to the health care system and allow the public to adjust to changing patterns of service.

Given this perspective, the first targeted population would include all pregnant women, children under age six, and those individuals who demonstrate a health status seriously compromised by a history of inadequate care. Improvements in coverage and benefits for these groups will have the greatest impact on the nation's future health and productivity.

As expeditiously as possible, other segments of the population would be covered. These groups might be targeted as outlined below; this sequence, however, is not necessarily intended as a rigid order:

- All children and young people, ages 6-18.
- All those above age 18 with incomes below 100% of the federal poverty level.
- All employees and dependents.
- All those with incomes below 200% of the federal poverty level.

The process will culminate with the merger of all entitlement plans into a single public program to provide coverage to all citizens and residents who do not have or cannot obtain coverage through a private plan.

The Fiscal Implications of Reform

It is impossible to predict the dollar amount which will be associated with the expansion of services or the efficiencies in nursing's plan. It is predictable that additional funding will be necessary to support start-up costs and transition. It is also possible that such expenditures will be recaptured over time.

A number of proposals for reform have been introduced. Among those proposals with cost estimates, additional health care costs range from $60-$90 billion.[3, 4] While nursing's plan for expanded coverage is similar in a number of ways to some of these proposals, offsetting proposed efficiencies integral to the plan will create significant dollars for reallocation. These resources will be directed to areas currently underfunded or excluded, including long-term care and primary care services.

While precise financial estimates are not possible at this time, several general observations can be made:

Cost Impact

Extension of coverage for essential services to the uninsured and underinsured will result in the dedication of more dollars. One source estimated that such coverage, if provided in 1990, would have added approximately $12 billion to health spending.[5]

It will also be necessary to dedicate more dollars to the expansion of long-term care services. Cost estimates for improved long-term care coverage vary. One 1990 study suggests that provision of comprehensive long-term care services, if implemented in 1990, would have cost $45 billion — $34 billion of which would have been new costs.[6] Nursing's plan, however, calls for more limited coverage supported through a combination of public dollars and enhanced personal responsibility.

In the initial phases of nursing's health care reform, the emphasis on preventive services will require dollars. Over time, however, improved health resulting from the availability of comprehensive primary health care services will produce a cost-reducing "health dividend." By placing greater emphasis on health promotion and disease prevention in community-based settings, the system will reach out aggressively to individuals and households to foster an increased commitment to healthy lifestyles, prevention of disease, periodic screening for early detection of illness and earlier treatment, and promote informed decision making by the consumer. All of this will contribute to cost-effective, early interventions which, over time, will reduce the need for more costly care.

Cost Savings

New costs associated with nursing's plan will be offset to a considerable degree by the following cost-saving initiatives:

- Required usage of managed care in the public plan and encouraged use in private plans.
- Incentives for consumers and providers to utilize managed care arrangements.
- Controlled growth of the health care system through planning and prudent resource allocation.
- Assurance of direct access to a full range of qualified providers.
- Development of health care policies based on effectiveness and outcomes research.
- Incentives for consumers and providers to be more cost efficient in selecting health care options.
- Elimination of unnecessary bureaucratic controls and administrative procedures, through such mea-

sures as standardized billing, simplified utilization review, stream-lined administrative procedures, regulatory reforms, and consolidation of plans.

Sources of Revenue

To the extent that any additional dollars are needed, sources can be found. Responsibility for financing health care reform must be distributed equitably among individuals, employers, and government.

Individuals will continue to pay a portion of health costs through copayments by households and individuals with incomes above 200% of the poverty level, and through reduced copayments for those whose incomes are 100-200% of the poverty level.

Employers will provide private health insurance that meets or exceeds minimum federal standards for their employees and dependents, or will provide coverage through the public plan. Accommodations will be made to provide small businesses with the necessary financial relief to meet this obligation.

State governments currently pay a portion of health care expenses for the poor and fund certain other health programs. Nursing's health care reform plan calls for consolidation of existing government health plans into a single public program. When this occurs, all states will contribute revenues to the program through maintenance-of-effort arrangements.

Revenues to pay for any increased costs could be derived from some combination of higher tobacco and alcohol taxes, additional payroll taxes, higher marginal income tax rates, and the increase of elimination of the income ceiling for FICA tax collection. A value-added tax (similar to a national sales tax) could also be considered.

A LOOK TOWARD THE FUTURE

The existing health care system stands as evidence of the futility of patchwork approaches to health care reform. America's nurses say it is time to frame a new vision for reform — time for a bold departure from the present. Reform of any single component of the system will not do the job. Insurance reform alone will not guarantee access to care if the health care delivery system is not restructured. Conversely, many people will remain unserved or underserved if health care services are so costly that millions of Americans cannot afford to purchase care.

To be most effective, a health care system must do more than provide equipment, supplies, facilities, and manpower. It must guarantee universal access to an assured standard of care. It must use health resources effectively and efficiently — balancing efforts to promote health with the capacity to cure disease. It must provide care in convenient, familiar locations. And it must make full use of the range of qualified health professionals and diverse settings for care. It is this insight that underlies nursing's plan for reform — making it the most viable solution to the nation's health care crisis.

SOURCES

1. U.S. Department of Commerce, 1991, *U.S. Industrial Outlook 1991*, Chapter 44, "Health and Medical Services," pp. 1-6.

2. National Leadership Coalition for Health Care Reform, 1991, "A Comprehensive Reform Plan for the Health Care System," p. 2.

3. *The Pepper Commission, A Call For Action: Final Report*, September 1990, p. 137.

4. Mark G. Battle, January 8, 1991, National Association of Social Workers, remarks during NASW's National Health Care Press Conference.

5. Lewin/ICF estimates, November 1990, *To The Rescue: Toward Solving America's Health Care Crisis*, Families USA Foundation, p. 13.

6. Pepper Commission, p. 151.

This information is provided courtesy of the American Nurses Association: A Supplement to The American Nurse, June 1991.

INDEX

NOTE: A *t* following a page number indicates a tabular material and an *f* following a page number indicates an illustration. Page numbers listed in boldface indicate definitions of terms.

Food and fluid, withdrawing or withholding, 198
Formal groups, **347–348**
Formally designated change agent, **209**
Framework, **44**
Fraud, **169**
Frequently used rates, 312–313, 314*t*
Freud, Sigmund, 182–184, 184*t*
Friendship groups, 348
Full disclosure, **78–80**
Functional method of management, 379
Functional self-esteem, **412**

Gait, 333
Gaman, 474
Gaps, data, **113**
GAS. *See* General adaptation syndrome
Gay clients, 498
Gay family, **299–300**
Gender dysphoria, **497**
Gender identity, **494**, 496, 498
Gender role, **494**, 497
Gender-role behavior, **500**
General adaptation syndrome (GAS), **430–431**
General inhibition syndrome, **433**
General leads, 342
General systems theory, 62–63
Genetics, 233, 236, 303–304
Genital functioning, 505–506
Genuineness, **328**
Geographic Information Systems (GISs), **313**
Geography, 237
Gerontology, **389–390**
  See also Aging
Gestures, 333–334
Gilligan, Carol, 187–188
Girth measurements, 278, 278*t*
GISs. *See* Geographic Information Systems
Global self, **410**
Global self-esteem, **412**
Goals
  of client, 128–131, 132*t*, 146
  community health, 320
  definition of, **365**
  health care, 287
  learning, 365–366, 365*t*
  self-concept, 420
  stress, 444

Goodrich, Annie, 22
Good Samaritan acts, 175
Goods and services, production, distribution, and consumption of, 310
Gordon's typology of 11 functional health patterns, 100, 101
Governance, **11**
Government, 215, 218, 274
  See also Politics
Graphs, 84
Greece, 19
Greek Orthodox church, 518
Grief
  abbreviated, 533
  anticipatory, 533
  bereavement and, 528–529
  client and, 537
  definition of, **527**, **528**
  importance of, 530–531
  inhibited, 533
  loss and, 528–529
  pathologic, 533
  symptoms of, 534
  types of, 527–528, 533
  unresolved, 533
  See also Grieving
Grievances, **168**, 168*t*
Grieving
  assessing, 533–535
  diagnosing, 535–537
  elderly clients and, 395–396
  Engel's stages of, 531–532, 532*t*
  evaluating, 537
  implementing, 537
  Kübler-Ross's stages of, 531, 531*t*
  planning, 537
  stages of, 531–533, 531*t*, 532*t*
  See also Grief
Group dynamics
  cohesiveness, 353–354
  commitment, 350, 352
  decision-making, 352–353
  definition of, **350**
  group process and, 350
  interaction patterns, 353, 354*f*
  leadership style, 352
  managing and, 384
  power, 354–355
Group process, **350**
  See also Group dynamics
Groups
  bicultural, 458
  classification of, 344, 347–348
  convenience, 348
  definition of, **344**

dominant, 458
dynamics, assessing
  cohesiveness, 353–354
  commitment, 350, 352
  decision-making, 352–353
  group process and, 350
  interaction patterns, 353, 354*f*
  leadership style, 352
  power, 354–355
  effective, 350, 351*t*
  formal, 347–348
  friendship, 348
  growth, 350
  health care, 348–350
  hobby, 348
  ineffective, 351*t*
  informal, 348
  life-style changes and, 290
  minority, 458
  primary, 344, 347
  secondary, 347
  self-awareness, 350
  self-evaluation, 355
  self-help, 252, 348–350
  self-protective, 348
  semiformal, 348
  task, 384
  teaching, 348, 369
  therapy, 350
  verbal communication within, 354*f*
  work, 348
  work-related social support, 384
Growth groups, 350
Guided imagery, 449–450, 449*t*

Haji, 474
Hall, Lydia E., 227, 227*t*
Hand movements, 333–334
Havelock, Ronald, 212
HBM. *See* Health belief model
Healing power, **61**
Health
  continuum of, with illness, 234–235, 235*f*
  definition of
    adaptive model, 226, 230
    adult, 230
    changing concept of, 225
    clinical model, 226
    ecological model, 226
    eudaemonistic model, 229–230
    nurse theorists' views of, 227–229*t*
    personal, 230–231
    role performance model, 226
      (continued)

Health risk appraisal (HRA), **279**
Health Self-Determination Index (HSDI), 284–285
Health status, **107**, **235**, 236–237
Health subsystem, **315**
Hearing loss, 391
Heart disease, 504–505
Helping relationship
  definition of, **325–326**
  developing, 328
  persons involved in, 325
  phases of, 326, 328
  skills for, 327t
  tasks for, 327t
Henderson, Virginia, 3, 227t
Hereditary factors. *See* Genetics
Heterosexual orientation, 498
HHA. *See* Health hazard appraisal
Hierarchy of needs, 55–56, 55f
Hierarchy of virtues, 186–187
High-empathy nurses, 326
Hinduism, 518
Hinshaw, Ada Sue, 33
Hispanic Americans, 466–467t, 475–477
Hitting, 436, 436–437
HIV. *See* Human immunodeficiency virus
HMO. *See* Health maintenance organization
Hobby groups, 348
Holding, 437
Holism, **54–55**
Holistic approach, **54**, 493
Holistic health, 54–55
Holy Communion, **518**, 519, 520
Home health care agencies, **258**, 540
Homeless, 264–265, 479
Homeodynamics, **63**
Homeostasis, **63**, **440–441**
Homicide, 470
Homosexual orientation, 498
Honeymoon phase of culture shock, **480**
Hopelessness, 538
Hospice services, **259–260**, 540
Hospitalization, effects of, 243
Hospitals., **258**, 276–277
Hostility, **434**
Hotel Dieu, 21
HPLP. *See* Health Promoting Lifestyle Profile
HRA. *See* Health risk appraisal
HSDI. *See* Health Self-Determination Index

Human beings
  needs of, 55–58
  as research subjects, 78–81, 79t
  response patterns of, 119, 120
  theory of
    holism, 54–55
    influence of, 53
    needs, 55–58
    person as adoptive system, 54
    person as system, 53–54
  See also Client
Human immunodeficiency virus (HIV), 509
Humanism, **360**
Humanistic theory, **59**
Human Tissue Act, 175
Humor, 448
Hypertension, 245, 462, 471
Hypothermia, 399
Hypotheses, **75**
Hypothesizing, **132**

ICD. *See International Classification of Diseases*
ICN. *See* International Council of Nurses
Id, 183
Ideal self, **412**
Identifying, **436**
Identity, 423, 494
Identity stressors, 417
Illness
  of Appalachians, 477
  of Arab Americans, 478
  behaviors, 240–242
  of black Americans, 471
  of Chinese Americans, 474
  continuum of, with health, 234–235, 235f
  definition of, **232**
  disease and, 234f
  in family, 243–245, 306–307
    intervening in, 306–307
  of Hispanic Americans, 477
  of Native Americans, 470
  needs and, 57
  religion and, 516
  See also Disease
Imagery, 449–450, 449t
Immoral act, **187**
Immunization, 398
Impaired nurses, **171–172**
Impaired verbal communication, 338
Implementing
  accountability in, 95

communication
  nontherapeutic techniques, 342–344
  therapeutic techniques, 339–342
community health, 320–321
culture and, 488
definition of, **138**
dying client care, 539–540, 543
grieving, 537
health promotion, 288–292
loss, 537
models and, 47
nursing actions, 138–140, 139t
nursing strategies, 141
process of, 140–141
self-concept goals, 420–424
sexual health, 507–508, 511
spiritual health, 523–524
stress strategies, 445–447
teaching plan, 367–370
Implied contract, **165**
Incidence rate, **312**
Incident report, 173, 174
Inconsistencies, data, **113**
Incontinence, 392
Incorrect perceptions, 213
Independent nursing action, 139
Independent variable (IV), **83**
Indirect services, **258–259**, 311
Individual decisions, **352**
Individual practice associations (IPA), **257**
Inductive reasoning, **64–65**
Inductive theory, **76**
Industrial clinic, **257**
Ineffective coping, 433
Infants, 369, 496
Influence, **216**
  See also Power
Informally designated change agent, **209**
Information dissemination programs, **276**
Information power, **216**
Informative statements, 341–342
Informed consent, **172–173**
Inhibited grief, **533**
Innovation-decision process, **212**
Input, **63**
Inquest, **175**
Insurance, 175–176, 255–256
Integrative power, **61**
Intellectual dimension of wellness, 232, 232f
Intentional torts, 170t
Interactions, 325–326, 353, 354f

(continued)

Person as adaptive system, 54
Personal distance, **336**
Personal identity, 411
Personality types, 437, 440, 450
Personal power. *See* Referent power
Personal self, 416
Personal space, **335, 461**
Personal standards, 187
Personal systems, **54**
Personal values, 189–190, 192–193
Person-role conflict, **411**
Person as system, 53–54
PES format, **115**
Peters, R. S., 185–187
Petrissage, **448**
PET. *See* Positron emission tomography
Pew Memorial Trust, 265
PhD. *See* Doctor of philosophy
PHO. *See* Preventive health orientation
PHS. *See* Public Health Service
Physical appearance, 390
Physical assessment, 100, 278
Physical dimension of wellness, 231, 232*f*
Physical-fitness assessment, 278
Physical self, 416
Physician's office, 256–257
Physiologic adaptation, **441**
Physiologic factors
    of adaptation, 441
    of aging, 390–393
    disease and, 233
    of dying client, 540
    elderly clients and, 390–393
    of homeostasis, 440–441
    learning and, 361
    of sexuality
        adolescents, 497
        adults, 498, 499
        children, 496
        infants, 496
    of sexual stimulation, 500, 501–502*t*
    of stress, 432*f*, 434
Pilot study, 76
Plaintiff, **162**
Planned change, **209, 211**
Planning
    accountability in, 95
    communication, 334
    community health, 319
    components of
        client goals, 128–131

consulting, 137–138
nursing care plan, 135, 137
nursing orders, 134–135, 136*t*
nursing strategies, 131–134, 133*t*
priority setting, 126–128
computers and, 381–382, 381*f*
culture and, 487–488
definition of, **125**
discharge, 138
dying client care, 539
family health, 304–305
grieving, 537
health beliefs and, 126
health promotion, 287–288
loss, 537
models and, 47
nursing strategies, 131–134
process of, 125–126
self-concept, 419–420
sexual health, 507
spiritual health, 522–523
stress strategies, 444–445
of teaching, 365
Politeness, 474
Political action
    American Nurses' Association and, 25
    for care policy-making, 25
    change and, 218–220
    in community, 218
    in government, 218
    in professional organizations, 218
    in workplace, 218
Politics
    change and, 217–218
    health care services and, 254–255
    subsystem, **315**
    See also Government
Population
    aging, 253
    epidemiology and, 312
    health care services and, 253
    in North America, 253*f*
    research process and, 76
    in research terminology, 84
    study of, 25
Positional power. *See* Legitimate power
Positive affect, **269**
Positive feedback, 422
Positive health, **275**
Positive health promotion, **275**
Positive reinforcement, **364**
Positive self-evaluation, 422
Positivism, **332**

Positron emission tomography (PET), 397
Possum response. *See* General inhibition syndrome
Postconventional level, **184**, 186*t*
Postmortem examination. *See* Autopsy
Posture, 333, 450
Poverty
    culture and, 478–479
    family health and, 304
    health care services and, 254
    Native Americans and, 470
Power
    advocacy, 61
    of caring, 61–62
    change and, 216–217
    coercive, 216
    connection, 216
    definition of, **216**
    expert, 216–217
    group dynamics and, 354–355
    healing, 61
    information, 216
    integrative, 61
    legitimate, 216
    participative/affirming, 61
    referent, 216
    reward, 216
    transformative, 61
Power-coercive strategies, **213**
Powerlessness, 216, 538–539
PPO. *See* Preferred provider organization
PPS. *See* Prospective payment system
Praise, 420
Prayer, **436**, 465
Preceptor, **383**
Preconventional level. *See* Premoral level
Preferred provider organization (PPO), **257**
Pregnancy, 473
Prehelping phase. *See* Introductory phase
Preinteraction phase of helping relationship, 326, 327*t*
Premature closure, **96**
Premature ejaculation, **506**
Premoral level, **184**, 186*t*
Presbycusis, **391**
Presbyopia, **391**
Preschoolers, 369, 437, 497
    See also Children

(continued)

Theory *(continued)*
    Erikson, 184, 185*t*
    Freud, 182–184, 184*t*
    Gilligan, 187–188
    Kohlberg, 184–185, 186*t*
    Peters, 185–187
    Schulman and Mekler, 187
    terms in, 182
  nursing
    conceptual framework of,
      43–45
    development of, 43–45
    nursing research and, 52–53
  nursing research, 83
  perception, 65–66
  problem-solving, 63–65
  stress, 430–431, 433
  structural-functional, 297
  systems, 296–297
  See also Models
Therapeutic communication, **330**,
  339–342
Therapeutic model of
  communication, **334**
Therapeutic relationship. *See*
  Helping relationship
Therapeutic touch (TT), 451
Therapist, **350**
Therapy groups, 350
Threatened self-interest, 213
*Timeline for Transition into the
  Future System for Two
  Categories of Nurses*
  (NCNIP), 9, 9*f*
Time orientation, 461
Timing in verbal communication,
  331–332
Toddlers, teaching, 369
Tolerance, low, 213
Tort, **169–170**, 170*t*, 171
Tort law, **161**
Tort liability, **169**
Total body relaxation technique, 449
Total care. *See* Case method of
  management
Touch
  elderly clients and, 391
  forms of, 342
  stress and, 437
  therapeutic, 451
Traditional family, **297**
Traditional Western medicine,
  463–464, 464*t*
Trainees, **350**
Trainer, **350**
Transactional stress theory, 431, **433**

Transaction, stress as, 431, 433
Transferring energy, **451**
Transformative power, **61**
Trial, **162**
Trial-and-error problem-solving, 63
Tri-Council for Nursing, 23
Trust, 422
Truth, Sojourner, 21, 26
TT. *See* Therapeutic touch
Tuberculosis, 474
Tubman, Harriet, 21, 26
Two-career family, **297–298**
Two-parent family, 24
Type A personalities, 437, 440, 450
Type B personalities, 437, 440

Unanimous decisions, **352**
Unconscious clients, 172
Uncontrolled variables, **83**
Undernutrition, **399**
Unemployment, 254
Unfreezing stage, **211–212**, 290–291
Uniform Anatomical Gift Act, 175
Unintentional torts, 170*t*
Unitarian Universalist Association,
  520
United Church of Canada, 520
United States Army Nurse Corps, 21
United States Cadet Nurse Corps, 22
United States Constitution, 160
United States Navy Nurse Corps, 21
United States Sanitary Commission,
  21
United States. *See* North America
Unplanned change, **211**
Unresolved grief, **533**
Unruffling, **451**
Unwarranted reassurance, 342–343
Urinary elimination, 392, 401
Urinary tract infection (UTI), 401
Utilitarianism, **201**
UTI. *See* Urinary tract infection

Vaccines, 518, 519, 520
Vaginismus, **506**
Validation, **120**
Validity, **84**
Value conflicts, **194**
Values
  acquisition of, 188–189
  of Asian Americans, 472–473
  attitudes and, 191
  being, 56
  beliefs and, 191

  clarification, 191–192
  of client, 193–194
  conflicts, 194, 202
  definition of, **181**, 182
  ethical dimensions and, 181–182
  feelings and, 191
  health, 126
  nursing, 31–32
  personal, 189–190, 192–193
  professional, 188, 189–191
  transmission of, 189
Values clarification, **191–192**
Value set, **188**
Value system, **45**, **181**
Variables, **83**
VA. *See* Veterans administration
  hospitals
"Vassar Training Camp", 22
Vegetative client, 25
Verbal abuse, 436
Verbal communication, **330–332**,
  338, 354*f*
Verbal and motor factors, of stress,
  436–437
Verdict, **162**
Verifying, 341
Veterans Administration (VA)
  hospitals, 256
Vietnam Conflict, 22
Vietnamese Americans, 474–475
  See also Asian Americans
Violence, **434**
Virtues, hierarchy of, 186–187
Vision changes, 391
Vision problems, 474
Visualization, 422
Vocation, **6**
Voluntary insurance, 255
Vulnerable subjects, **80**

Wald, Lillian, 22
Walking, 402
War, 22–23
Warmth, **337**
Well-being, 232, 521, 521*t*
  See also Health
Well-intentioned act, **187**
Wellness, **231–232**, 232*f*, 275*t*, 286
Wellness assessment programs, **276**
Wellness Index, 283, 284*f*
Western Interstate Commission on
  Higher Education (WICHE),
  89–90
WHO. *See* World Health
  Organization

WICHE. *See* Western Interstate Commission on Higher Education
Wide Range Achievement Test (WRAT), 363
Wills, **173–174**, 199, 199*t*
Women's Central Association for Relief, 21
Woolsey, Jane Stuart, 21
Work groups, 348
Working capacity of heart, 392

Working phase of helping relationship, 326, 327*t*, 328
Workmen's compensation, 255
Workplace, 34, 215, 218
Work-related social support groups, 384
Worksite wellness programs, **276**, 277
World Health Organization (WHO), 225–226, 266, 275
World War I, 21–22

World War II, 22
WRAT. *See* Wide Range Achievement Test

Yama, **450**
Yang, 448, 473
Yin, 448, 473
Yoga, **450–451**